Engineering Materials

This series provides topical information on innovative, structural and functional materials and composites with applications in optical, electrical, mechanical, civil, aeronautical, medical, bio- and nano-engineering. The individual volumes are complete, comprehensive monographs covering the structure, properties, manufacturing process and applications of these materials. This multidisciplinary series is devoted to professionals, students and all those interested in the latest developments in the Materials Science field, that look for a carefully selected collection of high quality review articles on their respective field of expertise.

Indexed at Compendex (2021)

Stevo Najman · Vojislav Mitić · Thomas Groth ·
Mike Barbeck · Po-Yu Chen · Ziqi Sun ·
Branislav Randjelović
Editors

Bioceramics, Biomimetic and Other Compatible Materials Features for Medical Applications

Springer

Editors
Stevo Najman
Faculty of Medicine
University of Niš
Niš, Serbia

Thomas Groth
Department of Biomedical Materials
Institute of Pharmacy
Martin Luther University Halle-Wittenberg
Halle (Saale), Germany

Po-Yu Chen
Department of Materials Science
and Engineering
National Tsing Hua University
Hsinchu, Taiwan

Branislav Randjelović
Department of Mathematics
Faculty of Electronic Engineering
University of Niš
Niš, Serbia

Vojislav Mitić (Deceased)
Niš, Serbia

Mike Barbeck
BerlinAnalytix GmbH
Berlin, Germany

Ziqi Sun
School of Chemistry and Physics
Queensland University of Technology
Brisbane, QLD, Australia

ISSN 1612-1317 ISSN 1868-1212 (electronic)
Engineering Materials
ISBN 978-3-031-17268-7 ISBN 978-3-031-17269-4 (eBook)
https://doi.org/10.1007/978-3-031-17269-4

This Springer imprint is published by the registered company Springer Nature Switzerland AG
The registered company address is: Gewerbestrasse 11, 6330 Cham, Switzerland

Preface I

In honor of Prof. Mitić, the late editor

The Book and the Serbian Ceramic Society

The work on this book started already at the end of 2020 under the leadership and guidance of our late colleague Prof. Dr. Vojislav V. Mitić (1955–2021), who made great efforts, expended enormous energy, and exerted great influence. He initiated this book together with Prof. Dr. Stevo Najman. They invited and connected colleagues, co-editors, authors, and researchers from different scientific fields from all over the world to strengthen the research toward biomimetic and other biocompatible materials for medical purposes and applications. The result is now available in the form of this amazing collection of multidisciplinary research that provides a current cross section of the research in the field of biomimetic applications in medicine. While working on this book, Prof. Dr. Vojislav V. Mitić lost his battle with COVID-19 (on September 27, 2021, in Belgrade).

The publication of the book entitled *Bioceramics, Biomimetic and Other Compatible Materials Features for Medical Applications* by Springer Nature was initiated by the Serbian Ceramic Society (SeCerS) when Prof. Mitić was President of the Society. Prof. Mitić was a member of the Yugoslav Ceramic Society since 1997 and was one of the founders of the Serbian Ceramic Society in 2011. In the same year, he was elected as the first president of SeCerS. In 2018, he founded the Serbian section of the American Ceramic Society. He was also the organizer of ten international conferences on "Advanced Ceramics and Applications."

An Overview of the Scientific and Academic Contributions and Achievements of Prof. Dr. Vojislav V. Mitić

Prof. Dr. Vojislav V. Mitić was born in Niš in 1955 and finished his basic academic studies at the Faculty of Electronics, University of Niš.

His career was very fruitful. He left as a full professor at the Faculty of Electrical Engineering, University of Niš, and as a principal research fellow at the Institute of Technical Sciences, Serbian Academy of Sciences and Arts, Belgrade. The main research areas he was engaged in and in which he asserted himself in worldwide dimensions were electroceramics, BaTiO3-based ceramics, and fractal theory. As part of his pedagogical teaching activities at the University of Niš, he taught about ten subjects in the field of materials, especially electronic materials. He is the author of the monograph *Structure and Electrical Properties of BaTiO3-Ceramics* and co-author of textbooks for students.

Prof. Dr. V. Mitić has published more than 550 scientific papers and participated in more than 110 conferences and symposia, and he was a member of the organizing and scientific committees of several scientific conferences. He has given numerous invited lectures at many European and international universities and institutes. He was a reviewer for numerous journals, reviewed scientific projects, and was a member of the editorial board of several journals and collaborated in many scientific projects.

Prof. Dr. V. Mitić was elected a member/fellow of several high-ranking organizations, including the prestigious World Academy of Ceramics, International Institute for Sintering (IS), Fellow American Ceramic Society (Electronic Ceramics Division), National Institute of Ceramic Engineering (NICE), Order of Ceramic Engineers USA, International Society for Stereology, European Microstructure Analysis Society (EMAS), Royal Microscopic Society (GB), Material Research Society of Japan, Australian Ceramic Society, International Ceramic Federation (IFC), American Ceramics Society (Chapter for Serbia, Chairman), Association for electronics, telecommunication, computer science, automatics and nuclear technique—ETRAN, IEEE, and he was President of Serbian Ceramic Society.

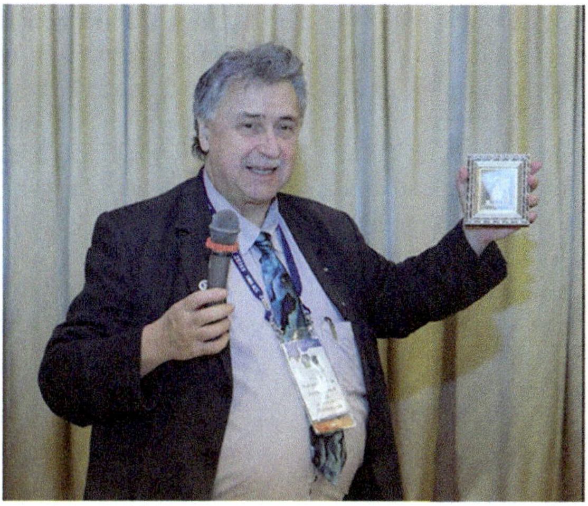

Prof. Dr. Vojislav V. Mitić (Photo taken at the 18th Asian Chemistry Congress, Taipei, Taiwan on December 9, 2019).

Scientific Contribution and Achievements Prof. Vojislav V. Mitić pioneered various applications of fractal geometry and analysis in the fields of ceramic materials, energy issues, and Brownian motion. He developed unprecedented mathematical-physical methods for controlling chaotic motion (Mitić et al., 2020). The results explain certain processes in the nature of materials science, especially for ceramic structures. He also contributed greatly to the development of methods related to fractal nature analysis in the reconstruction of material structures. Nowadays, it is considered a novel and reliable method used to characterize the microstructure of materials in the form of grains or pores (Mitić et al., 2010, 2011, 2013 and 2015). Constructive fractal theory can be applied to identify microcapacitors with fractal electrodes. The results of applied fractal mathematics provide a completely new perspective for evaluating intergranular capacitance and understanding the spatial distribution of microimpedance. This is beneficial for the development of electronic circuit integration and miniaturization.

In addition, Prof. Mitić's research results are significant for the aspect of energy storage (Mitić et al., 2015). They include the development of various approaches and solutions for advanced miniaturization, integration of electronic parameters at multiple levels, packaging of electronic circuits, and properties of circuits and components. These achievements demonstrate Prof. Mitić's scientific contribution over a long period of his academic career (Mitić et al., 2012, 2015 and 2020). The unique approach with the combination of the Voronoi model and fractals provides a much more natural approach to physical structures of advanced technology than Euclidean geometry. The method parameters have fractal nature with energy variation and Brownian walk (Mitić et al., 2020 and 2021; Randjelović et al. 2021; Hwu et al., 2021; Aleksić et al., 2021).

Many methods for modeling the microstructure, grain geometry, and grain boundary surface have been developed by Prof. Mitić. The research results are crucial for the optimization of a wide range of electrical properties. He also worked on artificial neural networks to solve problems such as pattern recognition, clustering, and functional optimization (Mitić et al., 2020). His research team analyzed thermophysical parameters of samples based on Murata powders consolidated by sintering processes (Mitić et al., 2020 and 2021). In order to avoid lengthy and even erroneous experiments that waste time, material, and energy, he introduced an artificial neural network method (Mitić et al., 2020). The solution he provided was original and practical for real microstructure projection, especially for phenomena in thin films surrounding grains.

Professor Mitić and his collaborators explored Brownian motion of particles and presented a breakthrough idea about the morphology of microstructure in relation to material properties (Mitić et al., 2012). One of their pioneering works is that they have developed a new protocol for understanding and predicting Brownian motion of coronaviruses (Mitić et al., 2021). It is the first time in biophysics that results on coronavirus case are revealed by mathematical-physical interval fractal analysis. Under his leadership and together with his colleagues from Taiwan, Ukraine, and the USA, the research teams investigated the relationship between the movement of microparticles and microorganisms in nature (Mitić et al., 2020). Moreover, the results of their 3D trajectories confirmed the real images of the movement of sub-microorganisms in space. The approach is truly original and leads to understanding and recognizing the various biological phenomena.

Professor Mitić was an outstanding scientist with a profound vision and great leadership. In this era, Prof. Mitić has illuminated a new direction and opened the frontiers for future research.

Social and Other Activities and Achievements

In addition to his remarkable and significant achievements in science and education, Prof. Mitić made impressive contributions in social life, politics, national economy, international relations, and his community.

From 1997 to 2006, Dr. V. Mitić was Chairman of the Board of Directors of EI (Electronic Industry) Corporation. He was also a member of the Board of Directors of the Chamber of Commerce of Yugoslavia, the American Chamber of Commerce in Belgrade, and the Serbian American Chamber in Chicago. He led the project of consolidation, restructuring, and privatization of EI Corporation with the World Bank (IFC), as well as the project of integration of industrial and development capacities in the countries of Southeastern Europe after war and crisis.

He had important socio-political functions—from 1989 to 1992, he was the president of the Executive Council of the City of Niš and a member of the Honorary Senate of Europe, the European Movement in Serbia, and the Pan-European Union Serbia.

He was also an active sports official as President of the Tennis Club in his hometown Niš and in the Tennis Federation of Yugoslavia and Serbia.

Professor Mitić was a very active Rotarian. He participated in the establishment of Rotary clubs in Serbia and the spread of the Rotary idea in Southeastern Europe and held several important positions, including District Governor of the Balkans in 2006/2007.

He visited or established contacts with scientific, educational, economic, political, and sports institutions and organizations in over 30 countries around the world.

Our Voja

Professor Vojislav—Voja Mitić possessed an exceptional character and was deeply committed to the flourishing of our societies and the welfare of the humanity.

He was also a husband and the father of the two sons.

Finally, he was a respected colleague and a good person.

Niš, Serbia — Branislav Randjelović
Taipei, Taiwan — Jih Ru Hwu
Niš, Serbia — Stevo Najman
Belgrade, Serbia — Nina Obradović
May 2022

Preface II

Biomaterials represent an important category of materials which have been engineered to interact with biological systems for a large variety of medical purposes to support, enhance, or replace the biological functions of tissues and organs. Biomaterials could be either natural or artificial materials which should be highly compatible with living tissues and cells and biofunctional for appropriate use. To support health and quality of life of human beings, biomaterials have been widely employed in medicine and dentistry, such as bone and soft tissue replacement, dental applications, cardiovascular, and other organ support, as well as other fields of reconstructive and regenerative medicine. Most of implanted biomaterials made from either natural or artificial materials, unfortunately, have different composition, microstructures, and surface chemistry, which creates a microenvironment different from the natural tissues and organs as a reflection of their physico-chemical properties. In most cases, the organism will recognize such biomaterials as "foreign bodies", which will induce positive or negative impacts to the implant and surrounding biological systems. In some cases, the so-called foreign body reactions resulting from the implanted biomaterials may trigger undesired blood clotting, inflammation, tissue degradation, and can even result in treatment failure. Furthermore, the interfacial reactions between implant and tissue can also lead to desired or undesired corrosion, and degradation of the implant, which will challenge the integrity and functionality of the biomaterial and hence the biological systems, too. While the nano-/micro-scale structures and the biomaterial/tissue or cell interfaces have been well understood to play vital roles in wound healing, engrafting of implants and further biological responses, the detailed interfacial reactions and interactions are yet to be fully clarified to achieve further progress in this field.

Besides the direct use of conventional biomaterials in medical applications, the terms "biomimicry" and "bioinspiration" convey an idea of designing artificial materials with better performance by learning from natural structures. The fabrication of bioinspired or biomimicking materials integrates the unique physical and chemical properties of artificial materials with the well-evolved biological structures and functions. This represents a novel direction for mining the potential of existing materials in combination with biomimicking approaches to realize unique properties that cannot be obtained from their original forms. Inspired by these interesting properties present in nature, researchers have endeavored to develop novel artificial biomimicking/bioinspired materials for adjust the biocompatibility and interfacial interactions of biomaterials. This can be achieved by coatings of biomaterials that mimic the composition of the surrounding tissue matrix components in terms of microstructure, mechanical properties, and chemical composition.

To address the critical challenges in the design, fabrication, and application of biomaterials in this book, we put special attention on the fabrication and testing of biomaterials for their applications in bone substitutions, orthopedic surgery, bioresorbable vascular stents, and others. The key issues in the biomaterials/cells or tissues interactions are typically noted and discussed, with the new concept of biomimicry in some cases. This book includes six well-defined parts based on the major challenges in biomaterials development and application, in which 19 chapters facing the cutting-edge problems of the field are assembled.

The first part is about the topic of "Bone Substitutes and Osteogenic Biomaterials". In this part, the first chapter discusses the effect of the microenvironment mimicking tissue composition on controlling human adipose-derived stem cells' behavior, which provides a fundamental understanding how to tailor implants and scaffolds for regeneration of bone and other tissues. The next two chapters show that composition of ceramic materials with presence of specific metal ions and design of bioceramics can promote the healing response of bone. The second chapter describes the physiological phenomenon of bone tissue remodeling and the different ceramic bone substitute materials (BSMs), which sheds a light on tissue responses to biomaterials, as well as inflammation in physiological bone tissue healing and inflammation induced by implanted BSMs. Thus, this chapter provides insight into the topic of interaction between bioceramics and the immune system. Chapter "Bioceramics in Orthopedic Surgery" introduces the progress and main features of few generations of bioceramics employed in orthopedic surgery as joint implants, bioactive coatings, or bearing coatings, and provides an outlook on designing next generation bioceramics.

The second part gives an introduction to "Materials in Biomedical Applications," in which one chapter introduces Copper(II)-loaded polyphosphazenes as a novel detoxicant for efficient hydrolysis of chemical warfare agents for nerve, such as sarin. The synthesis protocol of the bifunctional copolymers was provided in this chapter and the half-life time of the hydrolysis was examined.

The third part provides detailed understanding on the critical "Biomaterials-Cells/Tissues Interactions". In this part, four chapters ("Stimuli-responsive Multilayers Based on Thiol Chemistry Controlling Adhesion and Growth of Fibroblasts"–"Biomimetics in Orthopedic Surgery and Traumatology") are included. Chapter "Stimuli-responsive Multilayers Based on Thiol Chemistry Controlling Adhesion and Growth of Fibroblasts" studies stimuli-responsive multilayers based on chondroitin sulfate and chitosan by modifying polysaccharides with free thiol groups to control the adhesion and growth of fibronectin or human fibroblasts onto the surface.

Such surface coating can be made responsive to environmental stimuli such as redox or pH sensitive which provides also further opportunities for controlled release of bioactive drugs that promote healing responses. Chapter "Properties of Hydroxyapatite-Based Biomaterials Important for Interactions with Cells and Tissues" concentrates on the interaction between the hydroxyapatite (HAp)-based biomaterials and the cells and tissues. Research data on various multifunctional and hybrid materials with calcium phosphates and HAp for potential application in diagnostic, preventive, oncological, reconstructive, and regenerative medicine are described. The effect of some major properties of HAp and HAp-based biomaterials, such as composition, particle size, material shape, porosity, surface charge, topography, on the cell adhesion and proliferation was systematically discussed. Authors also present the results of their research with different hydroxyapatite-based biomaterials in different in vitro and in vivo experimental models in the field of bone tissue engineering and regenerative medicine. Chapter "Comparative in Vitro Study on Anti-inflammatory Activity of Covalent Versus Layer-by-Layer-Bound Heparin and Hyaluronan Including Signal Transduction Through Transcription Factor NF-κB" develops novel anti-inflammatory coatings through chemical bonding of a glycosaminoglycan monolayer or physical adsorption of a glycosaminoglycan-chitosan multilayer to enhance the biocompatibility of the biomaterials to resist chronic inflammation and subsequent fibrotic encapsulation after implantation. Chapter "Biomimetics in Orthopedic Surgery and Traumatology" introduces the way of biomimicry in producing biomaterials with imitating compositions and properties with the natural tissues in orthopedic surgery and traumatology, which provide new approaches to design advanced biomaterials with improved interfacial affinity and enhanced cell/tissue interactions.

The fourth part gives ideas on "Production Methods and Testing of Materials for Medical Applications" (chapters "Multifunctional Bio-ceramic Scaffolds and Composites Fabricated by the Freeze Casting Techniques"–"The Nanomaterials Fractal Characterization and Bioforensic Science"). Freeze casting technique has become one of novel approaches to fabricate ceramic-based scaffolds with anisotropically aligned and micrometer-sized channels. It is a relatively facile, low-cost, andeco-friendly method with wide material selectivity, scalability, and controllability of microstructures and properties. In the chapter "Multifunctional Bio-ceramic Scaffolds and Composites Fabricated by the Freeze Casting Techniques", the authors utilized natural ceramic-based sources, namely the diatomaceous earth and Tilapia fish scale powder, as raw materials to fabricate silica- and hydroxyapatite-based scaffolds for a variety of applications, for example, wastewater treatment, oil–water separation, water absorption and retention, thermal insulation, and potentially biomedical materials. The chapter "Preparation and Analysis Methods of Bone Ceramic Substitutes" provides an overview of the different classes of bone substitute materials in combination with the most common fabrication techniques for ceramic bone substitute materials in consideration of certain material properties that are matching with the process of bone regeneration. In this context, a focus in the further development of ceramic bone substitutes is to create biomimicking materials. Therefore, characterization is an essential step in the development of a novel bone substitute.

This chapter also sheds a light on structural, physical, and chemical characterization methods. Chapter "Comparison of Numerical Model with Experimental Measurements for the Purpose of Testing Partially and Fully Biodegradable Stents" presents interesting results regarding a numerical approach in the investigation of partially and fully bioresorbable vascular stents for applications against coronary artery disease. The author concludes that *in silico* mechanical tests can partially or fully replace in vitro stent tests, which can open a new avenue for regulatory submission and change regulatory ISO standard procedures. Chapter "Structural and Morphological Characterization of Strontium Ferrite-Ethylcellulose Nanocomposite for Application in Membrane Technology" presents the fabrication and characterization of magnetic ethyl-cellulose-strontium ferrite (EC-SrFe12O19) nanocomposite membranes which have potential application in membrane technology. Chapter "Unusual Chemical Reactivity at Low Temperatures of Buckminsterfullerene C_{60}" explores some unusual properties of buckminsterfullerene C_{60} with the formation of a charge-transfer complex at low temperatures in different solvents, which provides a solution to modify the materials for enhance the biological and medicinal applicability. Chapter "The Nanomaterials Fractal Characterization and Bioforensic Science" presents the synthesis and characterization of photoluminescent Bi, Y, and Ag-doped zeolite LTA topology nanopowders, potential nanomaterials for taking fingerprints in bioforensics, by applying the X-ray powder diffraction, crystallographic analysis, and scanning electron microscopy. Also, it was shown that fractal nature analysis, based on self-similarity, is an outstanding scientific approach for determination and prediction of material's properties.

The fifth part of this book pays attention on "Natural Patterns, Theoretical Models and New Insights in Material Characterization," which includes four chapters ("Medical Devices Based on Mimicry in Light-Matter Interaction: "Structured Matter Meets Structured Light""–"Neural Networks from Biophysical Applications in Microelectronics Parameters Measurements"). Within the chapters of this part, the authors expand the boundaries of the field of materials science with their specific approach. In the chapter "Medical Devices Based on Mimicry in Light-Matter Interaction: "Structured Matter Meets Structured Light"," methods and designs of mimicry taken from nature and biology and implemented in photonic science and engineering are presented as well as order of geometrical features and process based on the symmetry and harmony. Chapter provides some good examples of mimicry in the application of the principles of light-matter interactions (mirror effect and absorption effect) in either matter characterization and diagnostics in medicine (without damage) or phototherapy (absorption). Chapter "Brownian Motion Fractal Nature Frontiers Within the Matter" presents Brownian motion fractal nature frontiers within in the matter that explains a connection between the Brownian motion of microorganisms within fractal nature, with the idea of developing an appropriate procedure and method to control the microorganism's motion direction and predict the position of the microorganism in time. Authors defined the diagrams in two and three dimensions in order to establish the control of Brownian chaotic motion as a bridge between chaotic disorders to control disorder which can be applied on particle physical systems and matter, generally. In the last two chapters of this part, authors present a good way of modeling problems from material science, especially regarding biomimetic materials and synthetized diamonds, using a new, effective, but also very simple mathematical disciplines: graph theory and neural networks. Graph applications and artificial neural networks can replace theoretical models that are hard to be presented analytically with data obtained using these models. All these extended applications are the quite new tool and methods for obtaining parameters values at the real microstructure level what is opening a new perspectives in microelectronics miniaturization designing, especially in biomimetic materials. In the chapter "Graph Theory Approach in Synthetized Diamonds Electrophysical Parameters Defining," a graph theory approach is applied for defining the electrophysical parameters on micro and nano level of grains and pores of ultra-nanocrystalline synthetized diamonds, which provides an overview of complex relationship between graph theory and electrophysical parameters for further designing microelectronic structures and advance miniaturization. The authors of chapter "Neural Networks from Biophysical Applications in Microelectronics Parameters Measurements" performed a neural network study on the biophysical parameters, such as electric, dielectric, and ferroelectric characteristics, to predict the grain sizes in the function of temperature and time as distribution function between them which could be a new approach in microelectronics miniaturization designing.

The sixth part, which is also the last part, discusses "Ceramics in Socio-political Fields." The final chapter ("Bioceramics and Politics: (Un)likely Encounters") provides an opinion on possible interactions and intersections between bioceramics research and applications and politics in its widest sense and explores possible approaches to social study of bioceramics with focus on political science paradigms, such as biopolitics.

This book is contributed by a group of outstanding researchers and scientists from different countries and disciplines oriented in research toward biomimetic and other related compatible materials for medical purpose and applications. This remarkable collection of multidisciplinary articles gives research overview covering a survey covering diverse aspects of biomaterials from the synthesis and fabrication, their characterization and testing, the understanding of interfacial phenomena, to their biomedical application and the socio-political discussion of their use. The broad discussion on biomaterials presented in this book will be hopefully interesting to a wide range of readers from different fields of biomedical, materials, and health science, biochemistry and chemistry, nanotechnology, and engineering. We hope this book will be a good reference for not only undergraduate and graduate students but also researchers and engineers by providing inspiring insights into materials design, structure characterizations, property evaluations, mechanism investigations, and biomedical applications.

Niš, Serbia — Stevo Najman
Halle (Saale), Germany — Thomas Groth
Brisbane, Australia — Ziqi Sun
Berlin, Germany — Mike Barbeck
Hsinchu, Taiwan — Po-Yu Chen
Niš, Serbia — Branislav Randjelović
July 2022

Contents

Bone Substitutes and Osteogenic Biomaterials

Tailoring the Microenvironment of Cells Towards Osteogenic Differentiation Using Multilayers of Glycosaminoglycans and Growth Factor Immobilization

Reema Anouz, Mingyan Zhao, Fan Gong, and Thomas Groth

Abstract The extracellular matrix (ECM) provides the structural support and signals important for cell fate, tissue homeostasis and regeneration. Layer-by-Layer technique can apply ECM components like glycosaminoglycans (GAGs) and proteins due to their intrinsic charge to make ECM-like multilayers. Here, the effect of microenvironment on controlling human adipose-derived stem cells' (hADSCs) behavior was studied using multilayers composed of native GAGs (nGAGs) such as, hyaluronic acid (HA) and chondroitin sulfate (CS) or their oxidized forms "oGAGs" (oHA & oCS) in combination with collagen I; based primarily on ion pairing and on additional intrinsic covalent cross-linking by imine bond formation. Osteogenic differentiation of hADSCs was found to be stronger, when collagen I was combined with CS and in case of intrinsic cross-linking using oCS. While these studies still required osteogenic media to achieve differentiation, the second part of this study was conducted using heparin (H) and CS that were combined with chitosan as polycation. oH and oCS permitted not only intrinsic cross-linking to enhance the multilayer stability, but also controlled the release of the osteogenic growth factor BMP-2. There, the oGAGs systems were superior to nGAGs in controlling osteogenic differentiation of C2C12 muscle cells. Overall, multilayers made of oxidized CS with either collagen I or

---

Reema Anouz and Mingyan Zhao are contributed equally.

R. Anouz · T. Groth (✉)
Biomedical Materials Department, Institute of Pharmacy, Martin Luther University Halle-Wittenberg, 06120 Halle, Saale, Germany
e-mail: thomas.groth@pharmazie.uni-halle.de

M. Zhao · F. Gong
Stem Cell Research and Cellular Therapy Center, Affiliated Hospital of Guangdong Medical University, Zhanjiang, China

F. Gong
Department of Spinal Surgery, Affiliated Hospital of Guangdong Medical University, Zhanjiang, China

T. Groth
Interdisciplinary Center of Materials Science, Martin Luther University Halle-Wittenberg, Heinrich-Damerow Strasse 4, 06120 Halle, Saale, Germany

S. Najman et al. (eds.), *Bioceramics, Biomimetic and Other Compatible Materials Features for Medical Applications*, Engineering Materials,
https://doi.org/10.1007/978-3-031-17269-4_1

chitosan as polycations, seem to be useful to direct cell differentiation towards osteogenic and other lineages

Keywords Glycosaminoglycans · Cell Adhesion · Osteogenic differentiation

1 Introduction

In native tissues, cells reside in an extracellular matrix (ECM)-based microenvironment composed of proteins such as fibrillar collagens, but also adhesive proteins like fibronectin and proteoglycans with glycosaminoglycans (GAGs), as well as, soluble factors like cytokines which regulate the development of tissues, their function and their regeneration [1–3]. The ECM acts not only as a structural support for cells but also provides them with mechanical and chemical signals, which determine their cellular fate [4]. In particular, the biochemical and biophysical properties represent two main cues of ECM, which show direct and strong effects on cell behaviors and functions [5]. For instance, the ECM proteins such as collagen and fibronectin can interact with cells via integrin adhesion receptors [6], which are involved in signal transduction processes [7]. GAGs like chondroitin sulfate, which represent side chains of proteoglycans; are present in the ECM, on cells' surface, and are involved in collagen fibrillization, but also storage and presentation of cytokines, thus, tissue formation like in bone [8]. Hyaluronan is as another highly abundant GAG that represents part of ECM in cartilage and other connective tissues. In addition, it binds to hyaladherins such as, the cell surface receptor CD44 which is present in a multitude of cells (e.g. mesenchymal stem cells) and induces signal transduction processes as well [9]. Hence, the molecular composition of ECM plays a pivotal role in regulating cellular processes like adhesion, proliferation and differentiation with subsequent formation, remodeling and regeneration of tissues [10, 11]. In addition, biophysical cues such as topological and mechanical properties of ECM like topography, stiffness, elasticity and viscosity result in profound effects on cellular morphology and function [12–14], through mechano-transduction mechanisms [15, 16]. For example, it has been observed that many types of cells spread more on a stiffer substrata [17] and migrate towards regions of higher elastic modulus [18]. Moreover, spreading has been shown to be a strong modulator of cell differentiation showing that mesenchymal stem cells (MSCs) develop towards osteogenic lineage as spread phenotype and towards adipogenic if cell spreading is low [19]. Beside insoluble ECM components, diffusible components such as cytokines and hormones can interact with cells via corresponding receptors involved in signal transduction, regulating by that cell growth and differentiation. For example, binding of growth factor bone morphogenic protein (BMP) to corresponding cellular receptors promotes chondrogenesis and osteogenesis of stem and other cells [20, 21]. It should be noted that insoluble matrix components like fibronectin, and ECM proteoglycans provide also binding sites for cytokines regulating their stability and biological activity. Particularly, proteoglycans of ECM (e.g. perlecan) and of cell surface like syndecans containing chondroitin and heparan sulfate side chains that can bind cytokines specifically, like BMPs having heparin-binding domains [8, 22].

Biomaterials have a long tradition to replace lost or damaged tissues or support healing [23]. So far, various synthetic polymers [24], metals [25] and ceramics [26] have been used as implant materials to replace and regenerate damaged tissues. However, these biomaterials still have many flaws related to tissue necrosis, infection, and even rejection [27]. One reason of failure of many man-made biomaterials is the lack of a favorable surface for cell attachment missing specific cell-recognizable signals such as adhesive ligands for integrins [28–30]. Therefore, surface functionalization of implant materials has emerged to obtain a more biocompatible and bioactive interface between implants and tissues [28, 31]. An emerging technique of biomaterials' surface functionalization is the Layer-by-Layer (LbL) technique that was first discovered by Iler [32] and became more popular when it was re-established by Decher and Hong in 1991 using alternating adsorption of polyanions and polycations [33]. LbL which represents a simple method to modify material surfaces with polyelectrolyte multilayers (PEM), has shown to be applicable also in medical areas such as tissue engineering and drug delivery [34]. Selection of polyelectrolytes and complexation conditions like pH value, ionic strength and temperature can be used to control surface features such as wettability, surface charge, topography and intrinsic PEM properties like thickness and viscoelasticity [34]. ECM proteins and GAGs represent polyelectrolytes due to the presence of charged side groups such as amino, carboxylic, sulfate and other groups. Hence, they are suitable as building blocks for PEM that can mimic the ECM composition; addressing cell adhesion receptors (e.g. integrins, hyaladherins) and providing also bindings sites for cytokines permitting storage, presentation and release of growth factors to control cell fate [35, 36].

This study aims to investigate the effect of microenvironment based on biogenic PEM as a tool to control spreading and osteogenic differentiation of cells. For that purpose, multilayer systems based on GAGs as polyanions were developed here. An additional impact on the bioactivity was introduced by using oxidized GAGs (oGAGs) [37] that were able to achieve intrinsic cross-linking of multilayers by formation of imine bonds with the polycations collagen I and chitosan [38]. A first study was carried out with collagen I as polycation and either native or oxidized chondroitin sulfate and hyaluronan as polyanions showing that the composition of PEM affects osteogenic differentiation of human adipose-derived stem cells (hADSCs). Since it was found in the first part of these studies that intrinsic cross-linking particularly of sulfated GAG chondroitin sulfate promotes osteogenesis, we were curious whether uploading of osteogenic growth factor bone morphogenic protein 2 (BMP-2) to multilayer systems with sulfated oGAG heparin or chondroitin sulfate as polyanions, would trigger osteogenic differentiation of C2C12 myoblasts used as a sensitive model cell system here. A further difference from the first multilayer systems was; the use of chitosan as polycation for the bulk of multilayer and only a terminal collagen I layer, and the addition of a specific pH change from pH 4, for the initial part, to pH 9 for the terminal part of multilayers which was found to be adhesion promoting to cells, in a previous study [39]. Both studies provide an insight into the power of multilayer systems, especially when using oxidized GAGs in cooperation with growth factors to control microenvironment of cells as biogenic and bioactive surface coatings and thus are of high interest for application as coatings for implants and scaffolds for regeneration of bone and other tissues.

2 Experimental Part

2.1 Materials

Poly (ethylene imine) (PEI, M_w ~ 750 kDa, Sigma, Germany) dissolved in sodium chloride (0.15 M, Roth, Germany) solution was obtained at a concentration of 5 mg mL^{-1}. Native hyaluronan (nHA M_w ~ 1.3 MDa) was provided by Innovent (Jena, Germany) while native chondroitin sulfate (nCS, M_w ~ 25 kDa) was purchased from Sigma. From HMC Heppe Medical Chitosan GmbH (Halle, Germany), native Chitosan (Chi) was purchased. Native heparin (H) was provided by AppliChem (Darmstadt, Germany). Oxidized CS, HA and H (oCS, oHA, oH, respectively) were prepared according to a previously published method with slight modification [40, 41] Native GAGs (nCS, nHA, nH) and oxidized GAGs (oCS, oHA, oH) were used as polyanions and adjusted to a concentration of 0.5 mg mL^{-1} or in excess as 2 mg mL^{-1} in 0.15 M NaCl. Collagen I (Col I) derived from porcine skin (M_w ~ 100 kDa, Sichuan Mingrang Bio-Tech, China) was utilized as polycation and adjusted to a concentration of 0.5 mg mL^{-1} in 0.2 M acetic acid supplemented with 0.15 M sodium chloride; while chitosan was used as a further polycation at 2 mg mL^{-1} in 0.15 M NaCl. Prior to use, the pH value of all polyelectrolyte solutions was adjusted to pH 4 or pH 4 and 9 depending on the system except for PEI (pH adjusted to 7.4) (Fig. 1).

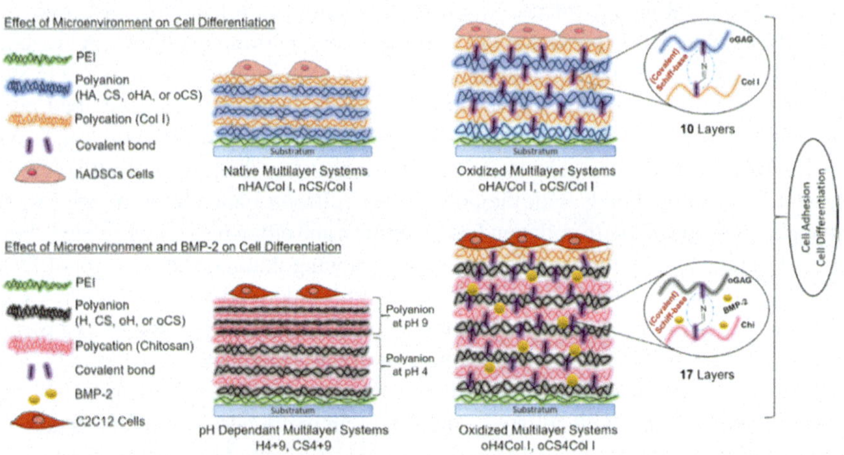

Fig. 1 An illustration scheme showing the multilayer systems used in both studies, where PEI is poly (ethylene imine), HA is hyaluronic acid, CS is chondroitin sulfate and H is heparin. The "n" before the abbreviations stands for "native". The oxidized version of the used glycosaminoglycans are abbreviated as; oHA (oxidized hyaluronic acid), oCS (oxidized chondroitin sulfate) and oH (oxidized heparin)

2.2 Preparation of Polyelectrolyte Multilayers (PEM)

Polyelectrolyte multilayers were fabricated on silicon substrates, gold sensors or on cleaned glass coverslips depending on the experimental methods. PEI was used as anchoring base layer; multilayers were formed on top of the PEI layer using nGAGs (nCS, nHA, nH) or oGAGs (oCS, oHA, oH) as polyanions and either; Col I for the 8 layers systems (Col-PEM) or Chitosan for the 17 layers systems (CHI-PEM), as polycation. The polyanions were adsorbed for 15 min at pH 4.0 for all systems except for pH dependent systems, where pH 4 was used for the first 4 layers of native GAGs and pH 9 for the subsequent 4 layers of nGAGs according to a previous publication [39]. Col I or chitosan were adsorbed for 20 and 15 min, respectively, at pH 4. Each adsorption step was followed by washing with sodium chloride solution (0.15 M, pH 4.0) for 3 × 5 min. As a result, multilayer systems with 8 and 17 layers were obtained. The Col-PEM (4 bilayers of Col I paired with either nGAG or oGAG) were denoted as: nCS/Col I; nHA/Col I; oCS/Col I and oHA/Col I. while the CHI-PEM systems with 17 layers were abbreviated as CS4 + 9 (native CS & Chitosan, depending on pH change), H4 + 9 (native Heparin & Chitosan, depending on pH change), oCS4Col (oxidized CS at pH 4 combined with chitosan and a terminal layer of Col I) and oH4Col (oxidized H at pH 4 combined with chitosan and a terminal layer of Col I).

2.3 Characterization of Polyelectrolyte Multilayers and Surface Properties

The layer growth and multilayer formation were monitored using SPR (IBIS Technologies B.V., Enschede, The Netherlands) to detect the changes in the refractive index (RI) due to the adsorption of molecules at the gold-liquid interface of the sensor. The measurements were performed in situ in the flow cell of the device using MUDA modified gold sensors [39]. Briefly, 0.15 M NaCl solution (pH 4.0) was brought into the flow cells to achieve a stable baseline. Then, the PEI solution was injected to the sensor surface for 15 min followed by washing with NaCl (0.15 M) solution for 15 min. Afterwards, polyelectrolyte solutions of nGAGs (nCS, nHA, nH) or oGAGs (oCS, oHA, oH) and Col I or Chi were alternatively adsorbed up to either 8 layers for Col-PEM or 17 layers for CHI-PEM, with the incubation of nGAGs, oGAGs and Chi for 15 min, while Col I for 20 min. After each adsorption step, samples were rinsed with NaCl solution as described above to remove the unbound molecules. The average of the 10 angle shift values (m°) at the end of each rinsing step was taken for plotting the layer growth.

The PEM thickness was determined using an M-2000 V scanning ellipsometer (J.A. Woollam Co. Inc., Lincoln, NE) that is equipped with a liquid cell (J.A. Woollam Co. Inc.) for solution injection. The measurement of multilayer thickness was conducted after 8 layers or 17 layers of PEM that were obtained. The thickness of multilayers was calculated by fitting the experimental data to an additional Cauchy layer. A refractive index of 1.36 that corresponds to native PEM values [42] was used for thickness calculation of the natural polymers. The experimental data were analyzed using the software of the device (WVase32).

Static Water Contact Angle (WCA) measurements were performed to measure the wettability of the multilayer surfaces using an OCA15 + device from DataPhysics (Filderstadt, Germany). One milliliter ultrapure water was used as test liquid and automatically dropped onto the samples; WCA values were obtained using Ellipse-fitting method. The experiments were conducted in triplicate, and each sample measured with five droplets.

The surface topography of the PEM was investigated using AFM (Nano-R, Pacific Nanotechnology, Santa Clara, CA). Cleaned and multilayers coated silicon wafers were investigated under ambient (air) laboratory conditions in close-contact mode, and scans of (3 × 3) μm^2 were recorded. The images were processed using the topography section analysis software "Gwyddion 2.30, Gwyddion 2.49.

2.4 *BMP-2 Loading and Release Study via ELISA*

In a 96-well plate, the CHI-PEM with nGAGs (pH 4 + 9) and oGAGs were fabricated and BMP-2 was adsorbed for all samples at 4 °C for over-night at 5 $\mu g\ mL^{-1}$ in 1 mM HCl (50 μL each well). Collecting samples was done over 4 days and each day replaced by fresh PBS (pH 7.4). The released amounts of BMP-2 were checked, using an ELISA kit from PeproTech (Hamburg, Germany). For cell studies, the BMP-2 at a concentration of 5 $\mu g\ mL^{-1}$ in 1 mM HCl was prepared from the stock solution (50 $\mu g\ mL^{-1}$) and loaded to the multilayers (200 μL each sample) for over-night at 4 °C. Then, the BMP-2 solution was aspirated, the multilayers were rinsed quickly with 0.15 M NaCl pH 7.4 followed by C2C12 cells seeding.

2.5 *Cell Adhesion Studies*

Adhesion of hADSCs and C2C12 cells was studied by viewing the focal adhesion (FA) complexes formation and actin organization. hADSCs (2×10^4 cells mL^{-1}) were seeded onto the Col-PEM surfaces and grown in Dulbecco's modified Eagle's medium (DMEM/F12, Gibco, Alcobendas, Spain) for 4 h, while C2C12 were seeded on CHI-PEM at a density of (5×10^4 cells mL^{-1}) in DMEM supplied with 10% FBS for 24 h. Then, for Col-PEM, cells were labeled using a primary monoclonal anti-vinculin antibody (1:400, Sigma) and subsequently incubated with a secondary antibody, namely, AlexaFluor 488 goat anti-mouse IgG (1:400, InVitrogen, USA). The actin cytoskeleton was stained by parallel incubation with AlexaFluor 555 Phalloidin (1:100, inVitrogen). For CHI-PEM, similar process was used. A mouse vinculin antibody was used as a primary antibody (7F9) (1:50, Santa Cruz Biotechnology) followed by a secondary CY2-conjugated goat anti-mouse antibody (1:100, Dianova); for actin cytoskeleton and cell nuclei using BODIPY-Phalloidin (1:50, Invitrogen) and TO-PRO-3 (1:400, Invitrogen), respectively, for 30 min each. Afterwards, for both studies, samples were mounted with Mowiol (Merck, Germany), investigated and photographed using a confocal laser scanning microscope (CLSM 710, Carl Zeiss Micro-Imaging GmbH, Germany). Images were processed with the ZEN2011 (Carl Zeiss) and later, images were analyzed by ImageJ software.

2.6 Osteogenic Differentiation of Cells

Osteogenic differentiation of hADSCs and C2C12 cell was studied by alkaline phosphatase assay and Alizarin Red S staining. Briefly, hADSCs were induced with osteogenic media (OM) consisting of basal medium containing osteogenic supplements namely, 50 mg mL^{-1} ascorbic acid (Sigma), 10 nM dexamethasone (Sigma), 50 ng mL^{-1} BMP2 (Peprotech, USA) and10 mM β-glycerophosphate (Alfa Aesar, Ward Hill, USA) while C2C12 cell were incubated in a DMEM medium with 10% FBS + 1% penicillin/streptomycin and supplied with 10 nM dexamethasone and 50 mg mL^{-1} ascorbic acid for PEM samples and positive controls. For negative controls, DMEM with 10% FBS + 1% penicillin/streptomycin was used without further supplements. At the predetermined time point, the activity of alkaline phosphatase (ALP) was determined to evaluate the osteogenic differentiation. Cell lysis was done using 0.2% Triton X-100 (Sigma), then the lysates were incubated with substrate solution, 2 mM *p*-nitrophenyl phosphate (*p*NPP, Sigma) dissolved in 1 M diethanolamine (pH 9.8), in the dark at 37 °C for 30 min, and the absorbance was measured at 405 nm using a plate reader. The total protein amount of the lysates was measured by BCA assay. ALP activity was calculated by normalization to the protein content of the lysates. Alizarin Red S staining was conducted to investigate the calcium phosphate deposition. Briefly, the samples were rinsed once with PBS and followed by fixing with 4% paraformaldehyde for 10 min. After rinsing twice with distilled water, Alizarin Red solution (2%, pH 4.2, Roth) was added and left working for 45 min in the dark. Finally, the excess dye was removed by thoroughly rinsing with distilled water. Images were captured using an Axiovert 100 equipped with a CCD camera or 10 × lens via Leica DM IL microscope (Germany).

For the development of a Col I matrix of hADSCs cultured on Col-PEM, cells were stained with a primary mouse antibody Col I (Sigma) followed by a secondary Cy2-conjugated goat anti mouse antibody (Dianova), and examined with CLSM. The expression levels of Runx2 and Col I of hADSCs were assessed by qRT-PCR using specific primers (Table 1) and *β-actin* was taken as the endogenous control. The data was calculated by 2^-ddct method based on Livak et al. [43].

Table 1 Primers used for qRT-PCR. "Adapted from [*Acta Biomaterialia*, Vol 41, Zhao et al., Molecular composition of GAG-collagen I multilayers affects remodeling of terminal layers and osteogenic differentiation of adipose-derived stem cells, Pages 86–99], Copyright 2016, with permission from Elsevier"

	Forward primer	Reverse primer	Size
β-actin	ACTCCTACGTGGGCGACGAGG	CAGGTCCAGACGCAGGATGGC	389 bp
Col IA	GCCAAGACGAAGACATCCCA	CACCATCATTTCCACGAGCA	891 bp
Runx 2	CTCACTACCACACCTACCTG	TCAATATGGTCGCCAAACAGATTC	320 bp

3 Results

3.1 Physicochemical Characterization of Polyelectrolyte Multilayers (PEM)

The multilayer growth of Col-PEM was monitored using the surface sensitive SPR technique (Fig. 2a). In general, the trend in layer growth was similar for PEM based on the same GAG, either nCS/Col I and oCS/Col I or nHA/Col I and oHA/Col I. However, slight differences were observed in the growth regimes of Col-PEM with CS when compared to Col-PEM with HA. For Col-PEM with nHA (nHA/Col I) and with oHA (oHA/Col I), a linear increase in angel shifts was observed up to three (nHA) or five deposited layers (oHA) on top of the PEI anchoring layer, after that, the adsorption of polyelectrolytes reached a plateau. It was visible that the angle shifts of Col-PEM with oHA were significantly higher probably owing to an additional intrinsic cross-linking. Conversely, the increase in angle shifts of Col-PEM with nCS and oCS were roughly linear. Again, a higher angle shift was observed for Col-PEM with oCS. Furthermore, here the SPR curves found a much higher increase in angle shifts of Col I (even numbers) when compared to nCS and oCS deposition (odd numbers), which was in contrast to HA. Further, a higher increase in angle shifts was observed for PEM based on oGAGs in comparison to their natives.

The SPR studies of CHI-PEM showed that growth of all PEMs was linear (Fig. 2b). A higher increase in angle shifts was observed in oGAGs systems compared to native depending on pH variations (H4 + 9 & CS4 + 9). The latter showed a decrease in angle shifts after switching from pH4 to pH 9. Additionally, the increase in angle shifts in CHI-PEM with pH dependence was higher in heparin than CS.

Multilayers thickness, under wet and dry conditions, determined by ellipsometry is shown in Fig. 3a, b. The overall averaged thickness of Col-PEM before PBS washing was between 3 and 6 nm per bilayer resembling the thickness of polyelectrolyte multilayer films found by another group [44]. It is interesting to note that a decrease in thickness of Col-PEM with nGAGs occurred when multilayers were challenged with PBS (pH 7.4) to simulate physiological conditions. In contrast, the decrease in layer thickness was significantly lower for Col-PEM with oGAGs. In the other study on CHI-PEM, the thickness of the various PEM is shown in both dry and wet state, as well (Fig. 3b). The type of GAG did not influence the thickness of

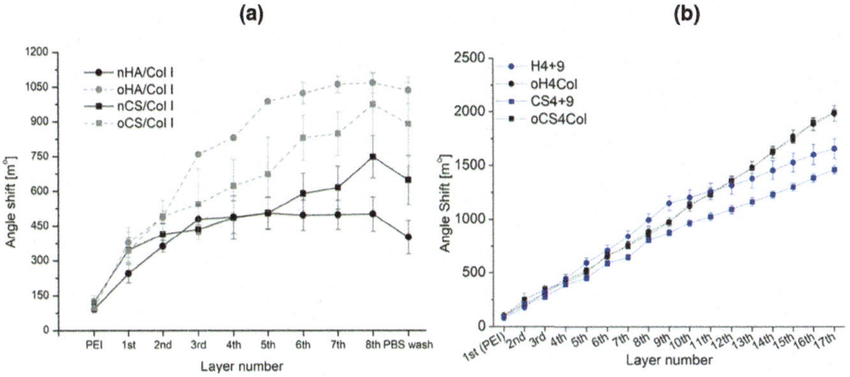

Fig. 2 Layer growth of PEM systems of native and oxidized polysaccharides determined by surface plasmon resonance angle shifts, plotted as a function of the layer number; **a** Col-PEM, odd numbers refer to native or oxidized glycosaminoglycans (nGAG or oGAG), even numbers refer to collagen I (Col I); **b** CHI-PEM, CHI-PEM with oGAGS [oCS4Col (black square), oH4Col (black circle)], CHI-PEM with nGAGs [CS4 + 9 (blue square), H4 + 9 (blue circle)]. pH 4 was kept constant for chitosan (Chi). For CS4 + 9 and H4 + 9 samples, the pH of GAGs solution was 4.0 until 8th layer and 9.0 after 10th layer. First layer was always PEI, even layers: polyanion, odd layers: polycation; the 17th layer was Chi for (CS4 + 9 and H4 + 9) or Col I for (oCS4Col and oH4Col); (mean ± SD). "Adapted from [Anouz et al. Novel Surface Coatings Using Oxidized Glycosaminoglycans as Delivery Systems of Bone Morphogenetic Protein 2 (BMP-2) for Bone Regeneration, *Macromolecular Bioscience*, 2018] with permission from [John Wiley and Sons], [https://doi.org/10.1002/mabi.201800283], [Copyright 2018, WILEY]"

PEM significantly. However, CHI-PEM with pH dependence (4 + 9) showed significantly lesser thickness than the CHI-PEM with oGAGs. After water immersion, the thickness increased; hydrated CHI-PEM made of oGAGs showed significantly higher thickness compared to CHI-PEM with nGAGs.

WCA measurements were performed to monitor the surface wetting properties after each single layer adsorption to follow the multilayer formation process regarding composition of each layer [45]. In Fig. 3c, an oscillation of WCA was observed during the adsorption of native or oxidized GAGs and Col I. Interestingly, the WCA trend of the Col-PEM with CS differed strongly from that of HA from the 5th layer onwards, while no significant difference was found between Col-PEM with nGAGs and oGAGs. There, in Col-PEM with CS, an increase in WCA with increasing layer number was observed. This is contradictory to Col-PEM with HA, where the WCA of the multilayers increased to a lesser extent after the adsorption of Col I, but decreased more after subsequent HA deposition. The WCA of the terminal HA (nHA, oHA) layer was similar to that of the previous HA (nHA, oHA) layer.

Furthermore, Fig. 3d shows WCA measurements of CHI-PEM, of which all PEMs showed alternating WCA values which were lower for GAGs and higher for Chi. Native and oxidized heparin showed lower WCA than CS with large differences between alternating layers of H and Chi. On the contrary, smaller differences of

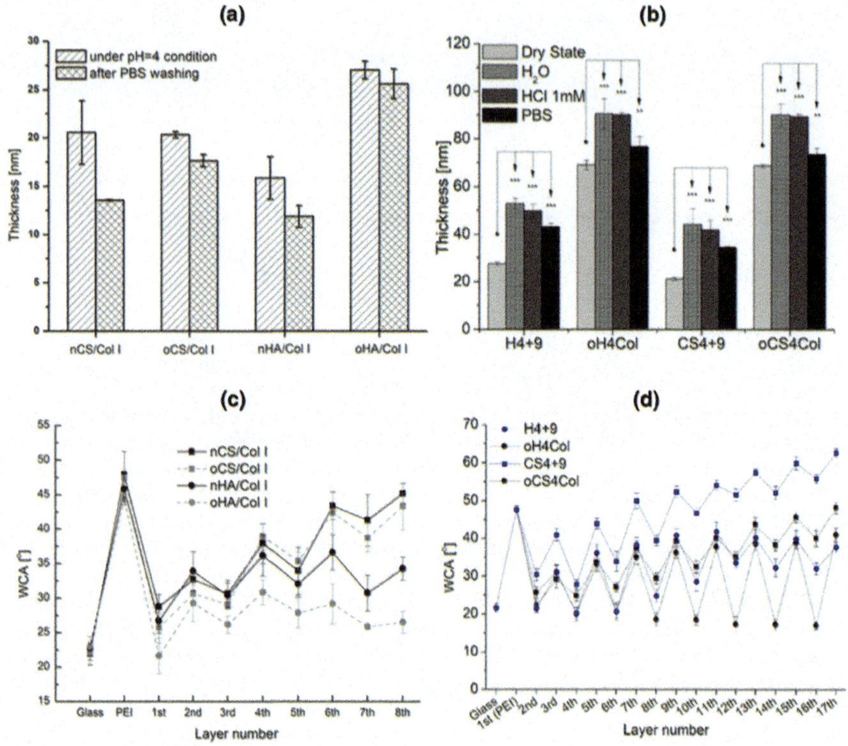

Fig. 3 **a** In situ thickness and change of thickness of the four different Col-PEM measured with ellipsometry. [Under pH = 4 condition: thickness of the PEM was measured in sodium chloride (0.15 M, pH 4); after PBS washing: PBS (pH 7.4) was brought into the measuring cell, and measurement was done thereafter; **b** Thickness of CHI-PEM measured by ellipsometry (dry condition is represented by light gray columns, H_2O immersion condition is in grey, HCl immersion condition is in dark grey, and black is for PBS immersion); $n = 9$, (mean ± SD); **($p \leq 0.01$), ***($p \leq 0.001$); **c** Static water contact angle (WCA) measurement during multilayers deposition up to eight layers of Col-PEM; odd numbers represent native or oxidized glycosaminoglycans (nGAGs or oGAGs), even numbers represent collagen I (Col I);; **d** Static WCA during multilayer formation of CHI-PEM up to 17 layers plotted as a function of the layer number; oCS4Col (black square), oH4Col (black circle), CS4 + 9 (blue square), H4 + 9 (blue circle). pH 4 was kept constant for chitosan (Chi). For CS4 + 9 and H4 + 9 samples, the pH of GAG solution was 4.0 until 8th layer and 9.0 after 10th layer. Layer 1 was always PEI, even layers: polyanion, odd layers: polycation; the 17th layer was Chi (CS4 + 9 and H4 + 9) or Col I (oCS4Col and oH4Col). Results are means ± SD of three independent experiments. "Adapted with permission from [Zhao et al. Improved Stability and Cell Response by Intrinsic Cross-Linking of Multilayers from Collagen I and Oxidized Glycosaminoglycans, *Biomacromolecules*, 2014], [https://doi.org/10.1021/bm501286f], [Copy right 2014, American Chemical Society]." "Adapted from [Anouz et al. Novel Surface Coatings Using Oxidized Glycosaminoglycans as Delivery Systems of Bone Morphogenetic Protein 2 (BMP-2) for Bone Regeneration, *Macromolecular Bioscience*, 2018] with permission from [John Wiley and Sons], [https://doi.org/10.1002/mabi.201800283], [Copyright 2018, WILEY]"

WCA values were between CS and Chi. CHI-PEM with CS had an overall higher WCA compared to CHI-PEM with heparin.

The topography of all PEM was studied by AFM in dry state. Figure 4a, shows that the topography of Col-PEM was related to the type of GAG as well as the mechanism (ion pairing or covalent binding) of the multilayer formation. It is of note that there was a well-distinguished interconnected network of Col I fibrils on both Col-PEM, with nCS and oCS. By contrast, only a small quantity of short fibrils was found in both Col-PEM, with nHA and oHA. In Col-PEM with HA, Col I molecules tended to assemble into elongated globules, which is well in line with the results reported by Jiang et al. (pH 4.5) [46]. Figure 4b, shows the surface topography of CHI-PEM. In all CHI-PEM, a granular surface morphology was noticed and the topography of the terminal layers was highly related to the pH conditions used during multilayer formation and the terminal layer used (Chitosan or Col I). It was found that when chitosan was the terminal layer in the PEM prepared at pH 4 + 9 regime (H4 + 9 & CS4 + 9) a finer granularity was seen, while collagen I as terminal molecule led to more coarse granularity.

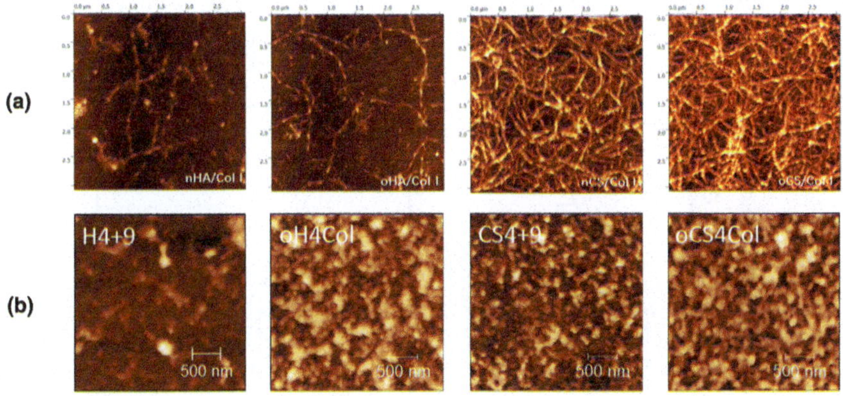

Fig. 4 **a** Atomic force microscopy (AFM) images of the outermost Col I layer of Col-PEM. Four bilayers of native and oxidized hyaluronic acid (nHA, oHA) or native and oxidized chondroitin sulfate (nCS, oCS) were prepared with collagen I (Col I) as polycation. Scan size of all images is (3 × 3) μm^2. **b** Atomic force microscopy images of CHI-PEM with collagen I (Col) terminated PEMs (oCS4Col and oH4Col) and chitosan (Chi) terminated PEMs (CS4 + 9 and H4 + 9); scale bar: 500 nm. "Adapted with permission from [Zhao et al. Improved Stability and Cell Response by Intrinsic Cross-Linking of Multilayers from Collagen I and Oxidized Glycosaminoglycans, *Biomacromolecules,* 2014], [https://doi.org/10.1021/bm501286f], [Copy right 2014, American Chemical Society]." "Adapted/Reproduced from [Anouz et al. Novel Surface Coatings Using Oxidized Glycosaminoglycans as Delivery Systems of Bone Morphogenetic Protein 2 (BMP-2) for Bone Regeneration, *Macromolecular Bioscience,* 2018] with permission from [John Wiley and Sons], [https://doi.org/10.1002/mabi.201800283], [Copyright 2018, WILEY]"

3.2 BMP-2 Release Study

All CHI-PEM were able to load and release BMP-2 over 4 days (Fig. 5). In general, CHI-PEM with heparin, released higher amounts of BMP-2 whereas CHI-PEM with oCS (oCS4Col) released the least amount of BMP-2 over time. It was interesting to see that despite the similar release profile of CHI-PEM with native and oxidized heparin, there was still different effects of the released BMP-2 regarding cell adhesion and differentiation (shown later). Moreover, heparin was expected to release less BMP-2 due to the binding of BMP-2 with heparin via heparin binding sites. However, CHI-PEM with heparin released more BMP-2 than CHI-PEM with CS. CHI-PEM with CS were able to store and control the release of BMP-2 more than heparin. Further, the least released amounts of BMP-2 in CHI-PEM with oCS system was shown to be highly effective than other higher released amounts by other systems (shown later).

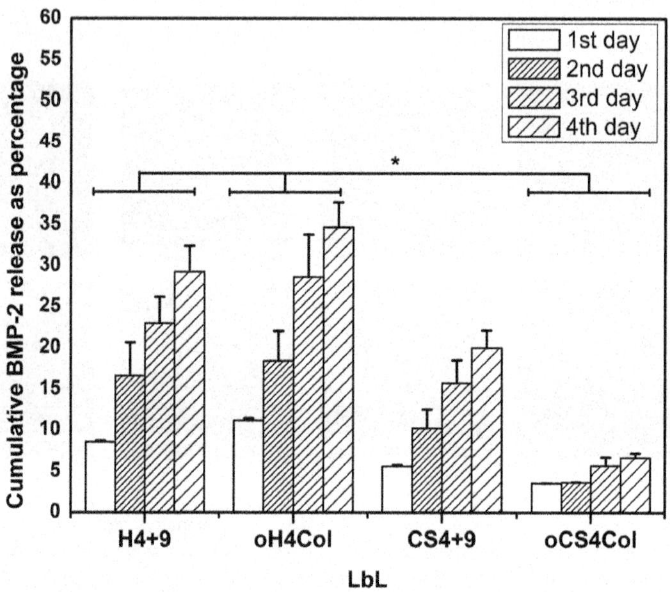

Fig. 5 Cumulative BMP-2 release over 4 days, from CHI-PEM, as percentage of the total loaded amount of BMP-2. Release study was done using ELISA. Values represent means ± standard deviations (SD), $n = 10$ replicates of each. "Adapted from [Anouz et al. Novel Surface Coatings Using Oxidized Glycosaminoglycans as Delivery Systems of Bone Morphogenetic Protein 2 (BMP-2) for Bone Regeneration, *Macromolecular Bioscience*, 2018] with permission from [John Wiley and Sons], [https://doi.org/10.1002/mabi.201800283], [Copyright 2018, WILEY]"

3.3 Adhesion and Spreading of Cells Seeded on Native and Oxidized Multilayers

To understand the organization of cell adhesive machinery, the focal adhesions (FA) formation was investigated by staining of vinculin and the organization of actin cytoskeleton after 4 h of cell culture. Figure 6a demonstrates that a significant spreading of hADSCs was visible on Col-PEM. In addition, a pronounced difference was observed in the overall appearance of FA plaques. Much larger and elongated FA plaques with longitudinal actin stress fibers (yellow color of the merged images) were found in hADSCs plated on Col-PEM with CS, while much less extended and rather dot-like FA plaques were detected when cells were plated on Col-PEM with HA. Particularly, the quantitative evaluation of vinculin-positive FA indicated higher quantities in cells placed on Col-PEM with CS compared to HA, and on Col-PEM with oCS compared to nCS (see Fig. 6b). We further investigated the expression and organization of $\alpha_2\beta_1$, since integrins are the important components of FA plaques that connected ECM proteins with the signaling complexes and cell cytoskeleton. Indeed, as shown in Fig. 6c, d, $\alpha_2\beta_1$ integrins were much more expressed and better organized in FA of hADSCs cultured on Col-PEM with CS (either nCS/Col I or oCS/Col I), forming clusters similar to small FA plaques. In contrast, on Col-PEM with HA, hADSCs exhibited a weaker expression of integrin and a rather diffuse distribution tending to accumulation of these integrins at the cell edges (see Fig. 6c, d as well).

To see whether the composition of CHI-PEM and loading of BMP-2 affected cell adhesion and spreading, two sets of BMP-2 loaded and non-loaded CHI-PEM were studied using C2C12 cells in this experiment. (Fig. 7a, upper row) shows results of all CHI-PEM without BMP-2. It was found that C2C12 cells cultured on CHI-PEM with native heparin (H4 + 9) were mostly rounded with no visible actin or vinculin organization. In control samples where cells were seeded directly on glass, no vinculin in focal adhesion sites was expressed, either. However, a general increase in cell adhesion with strong organization of focal adhesions and actin filaments was observed when C2C12 cells were seeded on BMP-2 loaded CHI-PEM. The increase in cell spreading, appearance of stress fibers and focal adhesion were visible in C2C12 cells cultured on all surfaces except when glass was used as control surfaces; despite the addition of BMP-2 to the culture medium, no big difference observed. The quantification of cell area was done using these immunofluorescence images (IF). Figure 7b demonstrates an increase in cell area on all BMP-2 loaded CHI-PEM. It was also interesting to see that such increase was absent in case of soluble BMP-2 (+Ctrl) where BMP-2 was added directly to the cell culture medium.

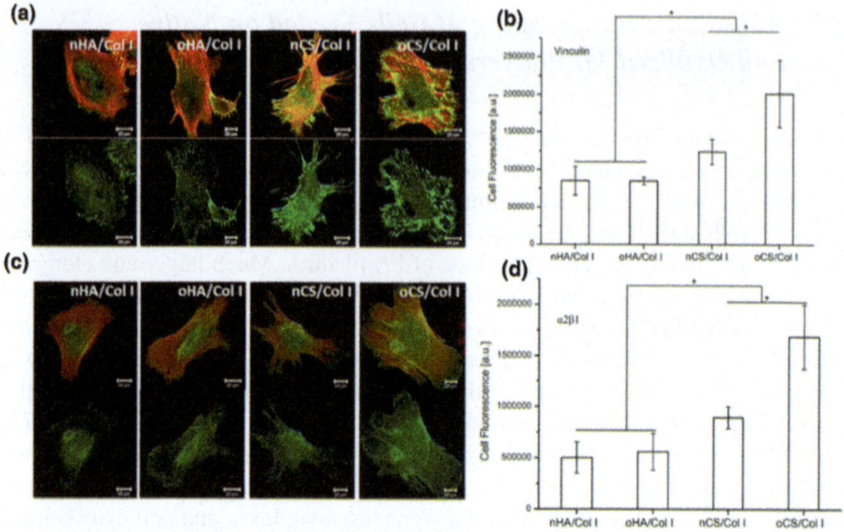

Fig. 6 **a** Confocal laser scanning microscopy (CLSM) observations showing the expression and organization of actin (red) and vinculin (green) of hADSCs plated on Col-PEM after 4 h culture; **b** Quantification of fluorescence signals of vinculin in FA by ImageJ and determination of corrected total cell fluorescence by fluorescence signal with subtraction of background signal; **c** Expression of α2β1 integrin (green) in hADSCs after 4 h incubation on Col-PEM and the respective merged images with filamentous actin (red); **d** fluorescence signals of α2β1 integrin was quantified by ImageJ and corrected total cell fluorescence was evaluated by fluorescence signal with subtraction of background signal. Cells were incubated in serum free medium for the first 1 h and then supplemented with 10% serum for the next 3 h of culture. "Adapted from [*Acta Biomaterialia*, Vol 41, Zhao et al., Molecular composition of GAG-collagen I multilayers affects remodelling of terminal layers and osteogenic differentiation of adipose-derived stem cells, Pages 86–99], Copyright 2016, with permission from Elsevier"

3.4 Osteogenic Differentiation of Cells Seeded on Multilayers Composed of Native and Oxidized GAGs

To learn about the effect of Col-PEM on the osteogenesis of hADSCs, ALP activity was determined at day 5, 11 and 15 post-differentiation (Fig. 8a). A first important finding was neither a remarkable increase nor a difference among the different PEM of ALP activity, when hADSCs were incubated in basal medium (BM). However, ALP activity of hADSCs was greatly increased after being supplied with osteogenic medium (OM) between days 5 and 15 on all the PEM. It is of note that pronounced differences were observed when comparing the ALP activity of cells cultured in OM on the different tested samples. As seen in Fig. 8a, hADSCs on Col-PEM with CS and oCS exhibited a dramatically higher ALP activity in comparison to cells on Col-PEM with nHA and oHA. On the other hand, there were also no differences of ALP activity between Col-PEM with nGAGs and oGAGs. A further observation was that Alizarin Red Staining revealed no evident staining when cells were

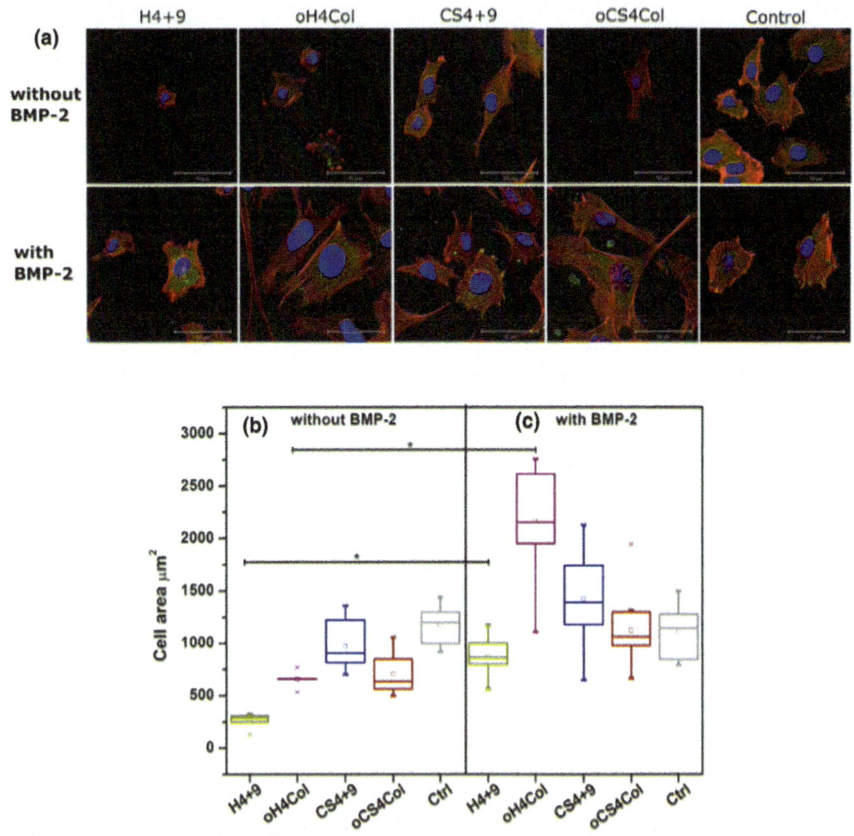

Fig. 7 Adhesion of C2C12 cells seeded on CHI-PEM, after 24 h of incubation. **a** Confocal laser scanning microscopy (CLSM) images show C2C12 cells after 24 h on CHI-PEM with native and oxidized GAGs. The cells were stained for vinculin (green) present in focal adhesions, filamentous actin (red), and nucleus (blue) on multilayers without BMP-2 (upper row) and with BMP-2 loading (lower row). As a control, cells were seeded on plain glass slides either without or with BMP-2 in the medium. Cells were suspended in DMEM 10% FBS and imaged with CLSM 63 × oil immersion objective; scale bar: 50 µm. Measurement of cell area done using image analysis software; **b** cells seeded on CHI-PEM with no BMP-2 loading; **c** with BMP-2 loaded to the multilayers. "Adapted from [Anouz et al. Novel Surface Coatings Using Oxidized Glycosaminoglycans as Delivery Systems of Bone Morphogenetic Protein 2 (BMP-2) for Bone Regeneration, *Macromolecular Bioscience*, 2018] with permission from [John Wiley and Sons], [https://doi.org/10.1002/mabi.201800283], [Copyright 2018, WILEY]"

cultured in BM (upper panel of Fig. 8b). However, a strong staining of cells was found when hADSCs were incubated in OM (lower panel of Fig. 8b). It was also seen there that staining was more intense when hADSCs were cultured on Col-PEM with CS compared to HA. It was also found that Col-PEM with oCS induced the most extensive calcium deposition in hADSCs indicated by a strong red staining of these preparations. Immunofluorescence staining (see Fig. 8c) that was applied to investigate de novo expression of osteogenic-specific ECM protein Col I (green staining) secreted by hADSCs (blue staining), showed no staining when cells were incubated in BM (upper panel in Fig. 8c). Conversely, strong staining with observation of a fibrillar structure of newly developed Col I became visible especially when hADSCs were placed on Col-PEM with CS in OM (lower panel in Fig. 8c). To further study the osteogenic differentiation of hADSCs on the different PEM, the osteogenic marker genes Runx2 and Col I were studied by qRT-PCR at day 14 post-differentiation. As displayed in Fig. 8d, Col-PEM with CS, particularly oCS, caused a much higher expression of Runx2 compared to Col-PEM with HA, when cells were incubated in OM, while no remarkable differences were seen when cells were cultured in BM. Notably, a significantly increased Col I expression was found in hADSCs adhering on Col-PEM with oCS. However, no pronounce differences were detected among the other three groups (see Fig. 8d).

To evaluate the effect of loaded BMP-2 on the osteogenic differentiation of C2C12 cells, ALP activity and Alizarin red S staining were performed as described in the previous section for hADSC. Figure 9a, shows that the highest ALP activity was seen when C2C12 cells were grown on CHI-PEM with oCS. A similar ALP activity was found with CHI-PEM with oH. On the other hand, the ALP activity, induced by CHI-PEM with nGAGs, was more comparable to the negative control where no BMP-2 was added to the medium. Similar findings were found during the investigation of

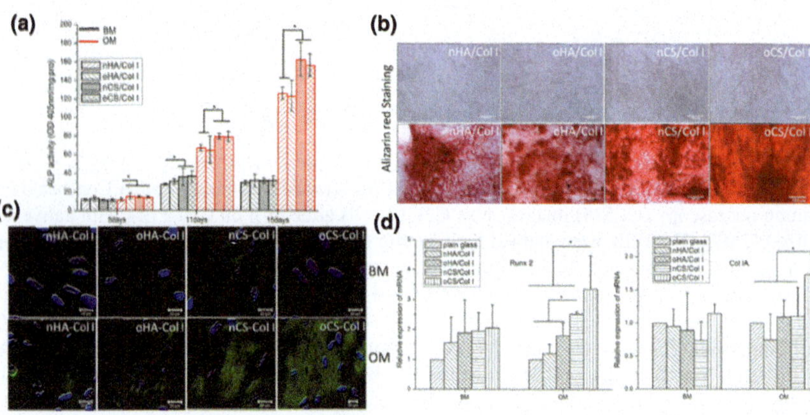

Fig. 8 Osteogenic differentiation of hADSCs seeded on Col-PEM with native and oxidized GAGs, either with basal medium (BM) or osteogenesis medium (OM). **a** Alkaline phosphates (ALP) activity of hADSCs adhering on the Col-PEM after 3 weeks culture with (BM) and (OM), respectively. **b** Alizarin Red S staining of calcium phosphate at day 21 post-differentiation. **c** Immunofluorescence staining of collagen I (Col I) in hADSCs at day 21 post-differentiation incubated with BM (upper panel) and OM (lower panel). **d** Bar charts displaying the Runx 2 and Col IA expressions in hADSCs at day 14 post-differentiation determined by qRT-PCR. Relative gene expression is shown as normalized to gene expression in hADSCs plated on plain glass. "Adapted from [*Acta Biomaterialia*, Vol 41, Zhao et al., Molecular composition of GAG-collagen I multilayers affects remodeling of terminal layers and osteogenic differentiation of adipose-derived stem cells, Pages 86–99], Copyright 2016, with permission from Elsevier"

the formation of mineralized matrix, shown in Fig. 9b. A remarkable mineralization indicated by the presence of red staining was observed when C2C12 cells were cultured on CHI-PEM with oGAGs. However, it should be also noted that staining was cluster like when cells were cultured on CHI-PEM with oCS in contrast to oH where red staining was more diffuse. On the other hand, C2C12 cells grown on CHI-PEM with nGAGs, either H or CS, did not produce a mineralized matrix since there was no remarkable staining observed. Further, the positive control having the 5 $\mu g\ mL^{-1}$ BMP-2 added to the medium and C2C12 cells seeded directly on tissue culture polystyrene, showed positive alizarin red staining indicating the obvious formation of mineralized matrix. By contrast, the negative control together with CHI-PEM with nGAGs (H4 + 9 and CS4 + 9) did not show any positive staining.

4 Discussion

4.1 *Effect of Polyanion and Polycation on Multilayer Formation*

It was shown here that the type of GAG, the pH value during polyelectrolyte deposition and the additional intrinsic cross-linking largely affected the multilayer formation, surface properties, and subsequent cellular behavior in terms of cell adhesion, spreading and differentiation. The comparison of two different systems that differed in term of polycations; with one based on collagen I throughout multilayer formation (Col-PEM) and the other with chitosan as building block for the bulk of multilayer (CHI-PEM), but using both native and oGAGs permitted to clarify effects of terminal multilayer composition and additional factors like BMP-2 on osteogenic differentiation of cells.

The comparison of multilayer formation between the two major PEM systems (Col & CHI-PEM) using SPR studies showed a linear increasing growth for CHI-PEM, while the use of Col I as polycation (Col-PEM) led to some kind of saturation with decreasing mass deposition at higher layer numbers. Studies with ellipsometry showed that the type of GAG did not affect significantly the overall thickness of PEM. However, the use of nGAGs in both Col-PEM and CHI-PEM showed a significantly lower overall thickness compared to those with oGAGs, which suggests that the covalent cross-linking caused more adsorption of polyelectrolytes in comparison to ion pairing alone. The pronounced decrease in thickness of Col-PEM with nGAGs multilayer systems after switch from NaCl of pH 4.0 to PBS with pH 7.4 corresponds obviously to a loss of material due to de-charging Col I whose isoelectric point (pI) is around 5.5 [47]. Similar observations of reduced layer thickness were made during multilayer formation with chitosan as polycation (CHI-PEM) using the specific pH regime during formation of multilayers from pH 4 to pH 9, which was applied like in a previous study because such PEM promoted cell adhesion, while those formed at pH 4 only were rather cell-repellent [39].

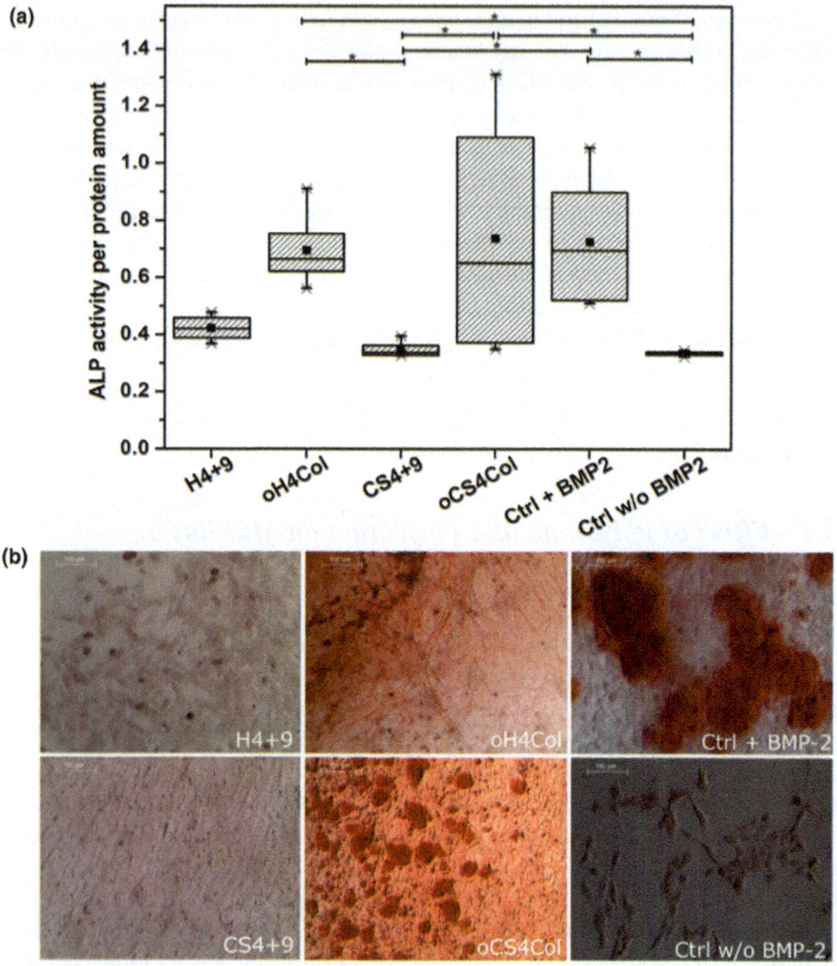

Fig. 9 Osteogenic differentiation of C2C12 cells seeded on CHI-PEM with native and oxidized GAGs. **a** ALP activity measurements in C2C12 cells seeded directly on BMP-2 loaded CHI-PEM fabricated in 24-well plate, determined after 4 days' incubation time via absorbance measurements at 405 nm, using plate reader. The total protein amount (BCA values) was used to normalize the measurements. **b** Bright-field images (10 ×) of C2C12 cells seeded on CHI-PEM for 14 days and stained with alizarin red-S solution to investigate the formation of mineralized matrix; scale bar: 100 μm. "Adapted from [Anouz et al. Novel Surface Coatings Using Oxidized Glycosaminoglycans as Delivery Systems of Bone Morphogenetic Protein 2 (BMP-2) for Bone Regeneration, *Macromolecular Bioscience*, 2018] with permission from [John Wiley and Sons], [https://doi.org/10.1002/mabi.201800283], [Copyright 2018, WILEY]

Studies of wetting properties showed that all PEM expressed alternating WCA values, lower for GAGs and higher for either Col I or Chi, indicating a change in the terminating molecule after each layer deposition. Both native and oxidized H and HA layers showed WCA lower than CS layers. While WCA of these PEM remained almost constant with increase in layer number, PEM with nCS and oCS as polyanion showed increasing WCA with increasing layer number. Since pure films from the polycations used are quite hydrophobic such as Col I (WCA$\sim$110°) [48] and CHI (WCA$\sim$100°) [49], this increase in WCA in PEM with CS as polyanion must be related to the presence of larger amounts of polycations (Col I or Chi) bound in those systems, as proven by SPR and also in previous studies [50]. Further, the use of oGAGs led to slightly lower WCA in all PEM systems. Probably, the additional cross-linking in oGAGs PEM might have stabilized the binding of GAG to surface regions of Col-PEM, which increased the wettability owing to the more hydrophilic nature of GAGs compared to the polycations [48].

Since Col I was used as the terminal layer in most studied PEM, it was interesting to look at the topography and potential fibrillogenesis of collagen that is known to be highly affected by the microenvironment [51, 52]. Here, Col I fibrillogenesis was observed in Col-PEM when nCS or oCS were used as polyanions, but not with nHA or oHA, which further demonstrates that the presence of GAG influences the assembly and organization of Col I fibrils [51]. Additionally, we could show here that the additional crosslinking in PEM with oGAGs does not hamper the Col I fibrillogenesis, significantly. The AFM studies of CHI-PEM even when Col I was used as terminal layer showed only a granular topography with no signs of fibrillogenesis, also when CS was used as polyanion, which is probably due to the low quantity of the protein that could be adsorbed as a single layer.

4.2 Biological Studies

Cell adhesion and spreading are considered as strong regulators of gene expression as well as cell differentiation [19]. The first study with Col-PEM was dedicated to check whether controlling these modulators alone is enough to induce osteogenesis of hADSCs. More adhesion, spreading and integrin clustering of hADSCs were seen on Col-PEM with CS as polyanion that were also related to more Col I deposition and fibrillization, which enhanced adhesion of various cells through an $\alpha_2\beta_1$ integrin-mediated mechanism in other studies [53]. Hence, the apparently lower spreading and lower organization of $\alpha_2\beta_1$ integrin in hADSCs on Col-PEM with HA as polyanion might be related to lower quantity and fibrilization of Col I. However, the higher wettability of Col-PEM with HA as polyanion might contributed to this reduced hADSCs adhesion and spreading because cells adhere and spread more on moderately wettable surfaces [54]. This effect of wettability was also relevant for CHI-PEM where CS4 + 9 supported more cell adhesion and spreading of C2C12 myoblasts compared to the other systems due to its moderate wettability (WCA $\approx$ 62°). Similar findings on the effect of hydrophilicity of multilayers on adhesion of C2C12 myoblast cells were made in one of our previous studies [10]. Apart from the wettability and composition of the PEM studied here, potential differences in substrate stiffness that were not studied here might contribute to different degree of spreading because it has been shown that intrinsic chemical cross-linking of PEM increase their stiffness compared to PEM made from nGAGs, which promotes cell adhesion and spreading [55, 56].

ALP is considered as an early stage marker at which osteoblasts start synthesizing their own ECM which starts to calcify at later stage of osteogenesis [57]. Therefore, osteogenesis of both hADSCs and C2C12 cells was studied by measuring ALP activity and histochemical staining. In addition, for hADSCs, we applied also immunofluorescence staining and qRT-PCR to detect gene products that are related to osteogenic differentiation. Studies with Col-PEM using CS as polyanion, particularly oCS showed an enhanced osteogenic differentiation in comparison to cells cultured on Col-PEM with HA as polyanion. The superior osteogenic activity of Col-PEM with CS *vs* HA, is most probably related the larger quantity and fibrillar organization of Col I in these PEM. It is also fitting to more spreading and stronger formation of FA and integrin clustering of hADSCs on Col-PEM with CS as polyanion. It has been demonstrated that osteogenesis is regulated by integrins, with β1 and β3 integrins each has shown to be important in mediating the osteoblastic differentiation of hMSCs [58]. For example, interaction of hMSCs with Col I through β1 integrins triggers phosphorylation of focal adhesion kinase (FAK) and downstream signaling by MAP kinase pathway which is also related to expression of osteogenic transcription factors [59, 60]. However, the more pronounced osteogenic differentiation of hADSCs on Col-PEM with CS compared to Col-PEM with HA as polyanion occurred only in the presence of osteogenic medium while no significant osteogenesis was seen in medium without osteogenic inducers. Hence, a composition of the matrix that promotes attachment and spreading of stem cells including ligation of β1 integrins to collagen may support osteogenesis. However, the presence of soluble osteogenic inducers like the higher concentration of dexamethasone and other inducers is still required. Therefore, the second study with CHI-PEM was focusing on the efficiency of similar oGAGs systems for upload and release of the growth factor BMP-2 to have an optimal system that control both the microenvironment and release of signaling molecules.

For this part of study, C2C12 cells that transdifferentiate from myoblasts to osteoblasts, provided a good model to investigate whether the PEM together with growth factor represents a versatile system to control cell differentiation. Here, heparin was used in comparison to CS due to the fact that BMP-2 binds to negatively charged sulphated GAGs via electrostatic interaction because of heparin binding domain [61]. It was somewhat surprising to see that BMP-2 had obviously a higher affinity to CHI-PEMs with CS than H as polyanion, because CHI-PEM with heparin released more BMP-2. It was also interesting to note that the binding was more significant for CHI-PEM with oCS (oCS4Col) that released the least amounts over-time, possibly because of their intrinsic cross-linking. Further, cell adhesion and spreading were studied here considering them prerequisites for cell differentiation and gene expression [19] as well as, for GFs receptor activation for further differentiation [62].

Thus, immunohistochemical staining of C2C12 cells for the nucleus, actin filaments and vinculin in FA was performed for C2C12 cells. First, on BMP-2 non-loaded CHI-PEM, cells on CHI-PEM with nCS (CS4 + 9) were characterized with actin filaments formation and expression of vinculin in FA, which indicated more cell adhesion on CS4 + 9 compared to the other non-loaded CHI-PEM where cells were almost rounded and the formation of actin filaments was poor with no vinculin-positive FA. This was related to the moderate wettability of CS4 + 9 system, as discussed previously [39]. Further, on all BMP-2 loaded CHI-PEM, an increase in cell adhesion was observed. This increase was represented by strong actin filaments alignment with more cell polarization and expression of vinculin-positive FA plaques, which demonstrates the BMP-2 synergistic effect on cell adhesion. BMP-2 binding to its receptor results in the initiation of β3 integrin adhesive phenotype through gathering and reorganization of the cytoskeleton via stress fibers and filopodia. Stimulation of β3 via BMP-2 is considered to be the first event of β3 integrin-BMPR cross-talk that is responsible for the transient phenotype of C2C12 cells before converting them from myoblasts to osteoblasts. Additionally, β3 stimulation is required for adhesion and migration, as well as, for Smad signalling initiation [63]. Moreover, osteogenic differentiation of C2C12 cells was studied by measuring the ALP activity at early stage and by the formation of mineralized matrix by staining with Alizarin Red as later sign of osteogenesis. Cells on CHI-PEM with oGAGs (oCS4Col & oH4Col), exhibited the highest ALP activity similar to the positive control where BMP-2 was added directly to the medium. Heparin is able to bind and protect BMP-2 from degradation promoting the activity of growth factor [61]. However, lower osteogenic activity of cells on CHI-PEM with H as polyanion was observed despite the higher release of BMP-2, indicates an inhibition of BMP-2 activity possibly by sequestering and mediating heparin internalization by cells [64]. This could be the reason why CHI-PEM with oH (oH4Col) promoted less formation of mineralized matrix when compared to CHI-PEM with oCS (oCS4Col). However, in general it was seen that CHI-PEM with oGAGs induced higher ALP activity and more formation of mineralized matrix than CHI-PEM with nGAGs (pH 4 + 9). Indeed, it should be also mentioned that the CHI-PEM with oGAGs possessed a terminal layer of collagen I that was applied unlike the pH4 + 9 regimes, as a cell adhesion promoter which affects cell differentiation to some extent, too. However, despite the supportive role of a Col I terminal layer on osteogenesis that was described above for hADSCs; here the presence and the impressive effect of BMP-2 on cell spreading and, hence, signal transduction plays obviously the most important role in the osteogenic differentiation of C2C12 myoblast.

5 Conclusion

It was shown in this study that LbL technique can be used to tailor the microenvironment of cells by selection of matrix molecules like CS and collagen I, and also the additional uploading of growth factors that permits controlled presentation of them.

In particular the use of oxidized GAGs like oCS showed that intrinsic cross-linking is not only promoting cell adhesion to a higher extent than the native forms, but also osteogenic differentiation in the presence of osteogenic medium supplements. Even the use of another polycation chitosan during the multilayer formation process in combination with oCS and only a terminal layer of collagen I that did not fibrillize provided a system of superior osteogenic stimulation to C2C12 muscle cells; if it was used as a reservoir for BMP-2 uploading. It was also found that not the release, but rather keeping and probably the presentation of BMP-2 is the key to superior osteogenic activity in oCS that was exceeding that of PEM with heparin. Further, triggering cell adhesion alone was not enough to induce osteogenesis, the presence of soluble osteogenic inducers was still needed. Altogether, these studies demonstrate in an impressive manner the potency of LbL technique to fabricate bioactive surface coatings on implants and scaffolds to direct differentiation of cells into the desired direction to support healing and regeneration of tissues.

Acknowledgements The financial support to R.A by the International Graduate School AGRIPOLY supported by the European Regional Development Fund (ERDF) and the Federal State Saxony-Anhalt is greatly acknowledged. We are also thankful for the financial support that was also provided by a grant form Deutsche Forschungsgemeinschaft to TG (Gr1290/11-1). The National Natural Science Foundation of China (32071326), the Natural Science Foundation of Guangdong Province, China (2019A1515011613, 2021A1515011196), the Zhanjiang competitive funding project, China (2018A01032, 2020A01018) and the Characteristic innovation projects of Guangdong Province universities (2018KTSCX076).

References

1. Frantz, C., Stewart, K.M., Weaver, V.M.: The extracellular matrix at a glance. J. Cell Sci. **123**(24), 4195 (2010). https://doi.org/10.1242/jcs.023820
2. Mecham, R.P.: Overview of extracellular matrix. Curr. Protoc. Cell Biol. **57**, 10.1.1–10.1.16 (2012). https://doi.org/10.1002/0471143030.cb1001s57
3. Schaefer, L.S.R.: Proteoglycans: from structural compounds to signaling molecules. Cell Tissue Res. **339**, 237–246 (2010)
4. Hynes, R.O.: The extracellular matrix: Not just pretty fibrils. Sci. **326**, 1216–1219 (2009). https://doi.org/10.1126/science.1176009
5. Von der Mark, K.P.J., Bauer, S., Schmuki, P.: Nanoscale engineering of biomimetic surfaces: cues from the extracellular matrix. Cell Tissue Res. **339**, 131–153 (2010)
6. Kechagia, J.Z., IJaR-CP: Integrins as biomechanical sensors of the microenvironment. Nat. Rev. Mol.Cell Biol. **20**, 457–473 (2019)
7. Sainio, A.J.H.: Extracellular matrix-cell interactions: focus on therapeutic applications. Cell. Signal. **66**, 109487 (2020)
8. Köwitsch, A., Zhou, G., Groth, T.: Medical application of glycosaminoglycans: a review. J. Tissue Eng. Regen. Med. **12**(1), e23–e41 (2018)
9. Leng, Y., Abdullah, A., Wendt, M.K., Calve, S.: Hyaluronic acid, CD44 and RHAMM regulate myoblast behavior during embryogenesis. Matrix Biol. **78–79**, 236–254 (2019). https://doi.org/10.1016/j.matbio.2018.08.008
10. Aggarwal, N., Altgärde, N., Svedhem, S., Zhang, K., Fischer, S., Groth, T.: Effect of molecular composition of heparin and cellulose sulfate on multilayer formation and cell response. Langmuir **29**(45), 13853–13864 (2013). https://doi.org/10.1021/la4028157

11. Murphy, C.M., Matsiko, A., Haugh, M.G., Gleeson, J.P., O'Brien, F.J.: Mesenchymal stem cell fate is regulated by the composition and mechanical properties of collagen–glycosaminoglycan scaffolds. J. Mech. Behav. Biomed. Mater. **11**, 53–62 (2012). https://doi.org/10.1016/j.jmbbm.2011.11.009
12. Dvir, T., Timko, B.P., Kohane, D.S., Langer, R.: Nanotechnological strategies for engineering complex tissues. Nat. Nanotechnol. **6**(1), 13–22 (2011). https://doi.org/10.1038/nnano.2010.246
13. Niepel, M.S., Fuhrmann, B., Leipner, H.S., Groth, T.: Nanoscaled surface patterns influence adhesion and growth of human dermal fibroblasts. Langmuir **29**(43), 13278–13290 (2013). https://doi.org/10.1021/la402705r
14. Rehfeldt, F., Engler, A.J., Eckhardt, A., Ahmed, F., Discher, D.E.: Cell responses to the mechanochemical microenvironment—implications for regenerative medicine and drug delivery. Adv. Drug Deliv. Rev. **59**(13), 1329–1339 (2007). https://doi.org/10.1016/j.addr.2007.08.007
15. Chu, G., Yuan, Z., Zhu, C., Zhou, P., Wang, H., Zhang, W., Cai, Y., Zhu, X., Yang, H., Li, B.: Substrate stiffness- and topography-dependent differentiation of annulus fibrosus-derived stem cells is regulated by Yes-associated protein. Acta Biomater. **92**, 254–264 (2019). https://doi.org/10.1016/j.actbio.2019.05.013
16. Aragona, M.P.T., Manfrin, A., Giulitti, S., Michielin, F., Elvassore, N., Dupont, S., Piccolo, S.: A mechanical checkpoint controls multicellular growth through YAP/TAZ regulation by actin-processing factors. Cell **154**(5), 1047–1059 (2013)
17. Ye, K., Cao, L., Li, S., Yu, L., Ding, J.: Interplay of matrix stiffness and cell-cell contact in regulating differentiation of stem cells. ACS Appl. Mater. Interfaces. **8**(34), 21903–21913 (2016). https://doi.org/10.1021/acsami.5b09746
18. Lo, C.-M., Wang, H.-B., Dembo, M., Wang, Y.-l: Cell movement is guided by the rigidity of the substrate. Biophys. J . **79**(1), 144–152 (2000). https://doi.org/10.1016/S0006-3495(00)76279-5
19. McBeath, R., Pirone, D.M., Nelson, C.M., Bhadriraju, K., Chen, C.S.: Cell shape, cytoskeletal tension, and RhoA regulate stem cell lineage commitment. Dev. Cell **6**(4), 483–495 (2004)
20. Duan, Y., Yu, S., Xu, P., Wang, X., Feng, X., Mao, Z., Gao, C.: Co-immobilization of CD133 antibodies, vascular endothelial growth factors, and REDV peptide promotes capture, proliferation, and differentiation of endothelial progenitor cells. Acta Biomater. **96**, 137–148 (2019). https://doi.org/10.1016/j.actbio.2019.07.004
21. Levinson, C., Lee, M., Applegate, L.A., Zenobi-Wong, M.: An injectable heparin-conjugated hyaluronan scaffold for local delivery of transforming growth factor β1 promotes successful chondrogenesis. Acta Biomater. **99**, 168–180 (2019). https://doi.org/10.1016/j.actbio.2019.09.017
22. Schnabelrauch, M., Scharnweber, D., Schiller, J.: Sulfated glycosaminoglycans as promising artificial extracellular matrix components to improve the regeneration of tissues. Curr. Med. Chem. **20**(20), 2501–2523 (2013)
23. Zhu, L., Luo, D., Liu, Y.: Effect of the nano/microscale structure of biomaterial scaffolds on bone regeneration. Int. J. Oral Sci. **12**(1), 6 (2020). https://doi.org/10.1038/s41368-020-0073-y
24. Hosoyama, K., Lazurko, C., Muñoz, M., McTiernan, C.D., Alarcon, E.I.: Peptide-based functional Biomaterials for soft-tissue repair. Front. Bioeng. Biotechnol. **7**(205) (2019). https://doi.org/10.3389/fbioe.2019.00205
25. Fu, J., Su, Y., Qin, Y.-X., Zheng, Y., Wang, Y., Zhu, D.: Evolution of metallic cardiovascular stent materials: a comparative study among stainless steel, magnesium and zinc. Biomaterials **230**, 119641 (2020). https://doi.org/10.1016/j.biomaterials.2019.119641
26. Montazerian, M., Zanotto, E.D.: Bioactive and inert dental glass-ceramics. J. Biomed. Mater. Res. Part A **105**(2), 619–639 (2017). https://doi.org/10.1002/jbm.a.35923
27. Helmus, M.N., Gibbons, D.F., Cebon, D.: Biocompatibility: meeting a key functional requirement of next-generation medical devices. Toxicol. Pathol. **36**(1), 70–80 (2008). https://doi.org/10.1177/0192623307310949

28. Rashidi, H., Yang, J., Shakesheff, K.M.: Surface engineering of synthetic polymer materials for tissue engineering and regenerative medicine applications. Biomater. Sci. **2**, 1318–1331 (2014)
29. Corobea, M.S., Albu, M.G., Ion, R., Cimpean, A., Miculescu, F., Antoniac, I.V., Raditoiu, V., Sirbu, I., Stoenescu, M., Voicu, S.I., Ghica, M.V.: Modification of titanium surface with collagen and doxycycline as a new approach in dental implants. J. Adhes. Sci. Technol. **29**(23), 2537–2550 (2015). https://doi.org/10.1080/01694243.2015.1073661
30. Silva, A.D.R., Pallone, E.M.J.A., Lobo, A.O.: Modification of surfaces of alumina-zirconia porous ceramics with Sr2+ after SBF. J. Aust. Ceram. Soc. **56**(2), 517–524 (2020). https://doi.org/10.1007/s41779-019-00360-4
31. Hu, C., Ashok, D., Nisbet, D.R., Gautam, V.: Bioinspired surface modification of orthopedic implants for bone tissue engineering. Biomaterials **219**, 119366 (2019). https://doi.org/10.1016/j.biomaterials.2019.119366
32. Iler, R.: Multilayers of colloidal particles. J. Colloid Interface Sci. **21**(6), 569–594 (1966)
33. Decher, G., Hong, J.D.: Buildup of ultrathin multilayer films by a self-assembly process, 1 consecutive adsorption of anionic and cationic bipolar amphiphiles on charged surfaces. In: Makromolekulare Chemie. Macromolecular Symposia, vol. 1, pp. 321–327. Wiley Online Library (1991)
34. Borges, J., Mano, J.F.: Molecular interactions driving the layer-by-layer assembly of multilayers. Chem. Rev. **114**(18), 8883–8942 (2014)
35. Capila, I., Linhardt, R.J.: Heparin–protein interactions. Angew. Chem. Int. Ed. **41**(3), 390–412 (2002)
36. Niepel, M.S., Kirchhof, K., Menzel, M., Heilmann, A., Groth, T.: Controlling cell adhesion using pH-modified polyelectrolyte multilayer films. In: Layer-by-Layer Films for Biomedical Applications, pp. 1–30 (2015)
37. Yang, Y., Köwitsch, A., Ma, N., Mäder, K., Pashkuleva, I., Reis, R.L., Groth, T.: Functionality of surface-coupled oxidised glycosaminoglycans towards fibroblast adhesion. J. Bioact. Compat. Polym. **31**(2), 191–207 (2016)
38. Martins, G.V., Mano, J.F., Alves, N.M.: Nanostructured self-assembled films containing chitosan fabricated at neutral pH. Carbohyd. Polym. **80**(2), 570–573 (2010)
39. Aggarwal, N., Altgärde, N., Svedhem, S., Michanetzis, G., Missirlis, Y., Groth, T.: Tuning cell adhesion and growth on biomimetic polyelectrolyte multilayers by variation of pH during layer-by-layer assembly. Macromol. Biosci. **13**(10), 1327–1338 (2013)
40. Dawlee, S.S.A., Balakrishnan, B., Labarre, D., Jayakrishnan, A.: Oxidized chondroitin sulfate-cross-linked gelatin matrixes: a new class of hydrogels. Biomacromol **6**(4), 2040–2048 (2005)
41. Wang, D.-A.V.S., Sharma, B., Strehin, I., Fermanian, S., Gorham, J., Fairbrother, D.H., Cascio, B., Elisseeff, J.H.: Multifunctional chondroitin sulphate for cartilage tissue-biomaterial integration. Nat. Mater. **6**(5), 385–392 (2007)
42. Johansson, J.Å., Halthur, T., Herranen, M., Söderberg, L., Elofsson, U., Hilborn, J.: Build-up of collagen and hyaluronic acid polyelectrolyte multilayers. Biomacromol **6**(3), 1353–1359 (2005). https://doi.org/10.1021/bm0493741
43. Livak, K.J., Schmittgen, T.D.: Analysis of relative gene expression data using real-time quantitative PCR and the 2鑒拾斘擟T method. Methods **25**(4), 402–408 (2001). https://doi.org/10.1006/meth.2001.1262
44. Boura, C., Menu, P., Payan, E., Picart, C., Voegel, J.C., Muller, S., Stoltz, J.F.: Endothelial cells grown on thin polyelectrolyte mutlilayered films: an evaluation of a new versatile surface modification. Biomaterials **24**(20), 3521–3530 (2003). https://doi.org/10.1016/S0142-9612(03)00214-X
45. Yoo, D., Shiratori, S.S., Rubner, M.F.: Controlling bilayer composition and surface wettability of sequentially adsorbed multilayers of weak polyelectrolytes. Macromolecules **31**(13), 4309–4318 (1998). https://doi.org/10.1021/ma9800360
46. Jiang, F., Hörber, H., Howard, J., Müller, D.J.: Assembly of collagen into microribbons: effects of pH and electrolytes. J. Struct. Biol. **148**(3), 268–278 (2004). https://doi.org/10.1016/j.jsb.2004.07.001

47. Barbani, N., Lazzeri, L., Cristallini, C., Cascone, M.G., Polacco, G., Pizzirani, G.: Bioartificial materials based on blends of collagen and poly (acrylic acid). J. Appl. Polym. Sci. **72**(7), 971–976 (1999)
48. Taraballi, F., Zanini, S., Lupo, C., Panseri, S., Cunha, C., Riccardi, C., Marcacci, M., Campione, M., Cipolla, L.: Amino and carboxyl plasma functionalization of collagen films for tissue engineering applications. J. Colloid Interface Sci. **394**, 590–597 (2013). https://doi.org/10.1016/j.jcis.2012.11.041
49. Leceta, I., Guerrero, P., De La Caba, K.: Functional properties of chitosan-based films. Carbohyd. Polym. **93**(1), 339–346 (2013)
50. Zhao, M., Li, L., Zhou, C., Heyroth, F., Fuhrmann, B., Maeder, K., Groth, T.: Improved stability and cell response by intrinsic cross-linking of multilayers from collagen I and oxidized glycosaminoglycans. Biomacromol **15**(11), 4272–4280 (2014). https://doi.org/10.1021/bm501286f
51. Wood, B.C.: The formation of fibrils from collagen solutions 3. Effect of chondroitin sulfate and some other naturally occurring polyanions on the rate of formation. Biochem. J. **75**(3), 605–612 (1960)
52. Kvist, A.J., Johnson, A.E., Mörgelin, M., Gustafsson, E., Bengtsson, E., Lindblom, K., Aszódi, A., Fässler, R., Sasaki, T., Timpl, R., Aspberg, A.: Chondroitin sulfate perlecan enhances collagen fibril formation. Implications for perlecan chondrodysplasias. J. Biol. Chem. **281**(44), 33127–33139 (2006)
53. Coelho, N.M., Gonzalez-Garcia, C., Planell, J.A., Salmeron-Sanchez, M., Altankov, G.: Different assembly of type IV collagen on hydrophilic and hydrophobic substrata alters endothelial cells interaction. Eur. Cell. Mater. **19**, 262–272 (2010)
54. Köwitsch, A., Yang, Y., Ma, N., Kuntsche, J., Mäder, K., Groth, T.: Bioactivity of immobilized hyaluronic acid derivatives regarding protein adsorption and cell adhesion. Biotechnol. Appl. Biochem. **58**(5), 376–389 (2011). https://doi.org/10.1002/bab.41
55. Zhao, M.A.R., Groth, T.: Effect of microenvironment on adhesion and differentiation of murine C3H10T1/2 cells cultured on multilayers containing collagen I and glycosaminoglycans. J. Tissue Eng. (2020). https://doi.org/10.1177/2041731420940560
56. Kirchhof, K., Andar, A., Yin, H.B., Gadegaard, N., Riehle, M.O., Groth, T.: Polyelectrolyte multilayers generated in a microfluidic device with pH gradients direct adhesion and movement of cells. Lab Chip **11**(19), 3326–3335 (2011). https://doi.org/10.1039/c1lc20408d
57. Jikko, A., Harris, S.E., Chen, D., Mendrick, D.L., Damsky, C.H.: Collagen integrin receptors regulate early osteoblast differentiation induced by BMP-2. J. Bone Miner. Res. **14**(7), 1075–1083 (1999)
58. Shekaran, A., García, A.J.: Extracellular matrix-mimetic adhesive biomaterials for bone repair. J. Biomed. Mater. Res. Part A **96A**(1), 261–272. https://doi.org/10.1002/jbm.a.32979
59. Lund, A.W., Stegemann Jp Fau-Plopper, G.E., Plopper, G.E.: Inhibition of ERK promotes collagen gel compaction and fibrillogenesis to amplify the osteogenesis of human mesenchymal stem cells in three-dimensional collagen I culture. (1557-8534 (Electronic))
60. Salasznyk, R.M., Klees Rf Fau-Hughlock, M.K., Hughlock Mk Fau-Plopper, G.E., Plopper, G.E.: ERK signaling pathways regulate the osteogenic differentiation of human mesenchymal stem cells on collagen I and vitronectin. (1541-9061 (Print))
61. Kisiel, M., Klar, A.S., Ventura, M., Buijs, J., Mafina, M.-K., Cool, S.M., Hilborn, J.: Complexation and sequestration of BMP-2 from an ECM mimetic hyaluronan gel for improved bone formation. PloS one **8**(10) (2013)
62. Salmerón-Sánchez, M., Dalby, M.J.: Synergistic growth factor microenvironments. Chem. Commun. **52**(91), 13327–13336 (2016)
63. Fourel, L., Valat, A., Faurobert, E., Guillot, R., Bourrin-Reynard, I., Ren, K., Lafanechère, L., Planus, E., Picart, C., Albiges-Rizo, C.: β3 integrin–mediated spreading induced by matrix-bound BMP-2 controls Smad signaling in a stiffness-independent manner. J. Cell Biol. **212**(6), 693–706 (2016)
64. Jiao, X., Billings, P.C., O'Connell, M.P., Kaplan, F.S., Shore, E.M., Glaser, D.L.: Heparan sulfate proteoglycans (HSPGs) modulate BMP2 osteogenic bioactivity in C2C12 cells. J. Biol. Chem. **282**(2), 1080–1086 (2007)

Biology of Ceramic Bone Substitutes

Mike Barbeck, Said Alkildani, and Ole Jung

Abstract The human skeleton has the miraculous capacity of healing itself when needed through a cascade known as bone remodeling. However, bone tissue is not able to regenerate itself in case of a broad variety of defects. In these cases, bone substitution is necessary to enable and support the process of bone remodeling. The gold standard for the regeneration of critical-sized bone defects is the transplantation of patient's own bone tissue harvested from another body region. This harvested bone tissue is called an autograft. Due to its donor site morbidity and limited availability, the use of bone tissue harvested from another individual (allografts) or from another species (xenograft) or synthetic materials that are chemically and structurally mimicking to native bone tissue (alloplastic grafts) has been established. This book chapter covers the physiological phenomenon of bone tissue remodeling and the different bone substitute materials (BSMs). The chapter also sheds a light on tissue responses to biomaterials, as well as inflammation in physiological bone tissue healing and inflammation induced by implanted BSMs. Inflammation generally has a negative connotation, but this chapter intends to elaborate on inflammation as an inherent and important process in bone tissue healing.

Keywords Bone tissue regeneration · Synthetic bone substitutes · Tissue responses · Inflammation · Immune response · Degradation · Macrophages · Multinucleated giant cells · Implant vascularization

1 Introduction

The regeneration of bone fractures and defects of different sizes due to different causes such as traumata, tumor diseases, bone infections as well as the loss of teeth

M. Barbeck (✉) · S. Alkildani
BerlinAnalytix GmbH, Ullsteinstrasse 108, 12109 Berlin, Germany
e-mail: mike.barbeck@icloud.com

M. Barbeck · S. Alkildani · O. Jung
Clinic and Policlinic for Dermatology and Venereology, Rostock University Medical Center, Strempelstraße 13, 18057 Rostock, Germany

S. Najman et al. (eds.), *Bioceramics, Biomimetic and Other Compatible Materials Features for Medical Applications*, Engineering Materials,
https://doi.org/10.1007/978-3-031-17269-4_2

with consecutive resorption processes is one of the major challenges in medicine, especially in oral and maxillofacial surgery. Autologous bone grafts (autografts), as parts of patients´ own body, are still considered the gold standard [1]. In addition to its osteoconductive properties, autologous bone also exhibits osteoinductive and osteogenic properties [2, 3]. The autologous bone tissue graft contains the inorganic bone hard substance, matrix proteins and the typical bone cells: osteoblasts, osteoclasts, osteocytes, and endothelial cells as well as their precursor cells [2, 4]. In addition, regulatory cell types such as osteal macrophages ("OsteoMacs"), which are a special macrophage subpopulation found in bone tissue, are present [2, 5]. However, their specific role in bone regeneration is still largely unknown. Overall, the transfer of an autologous bone graft is of fundamental importance for the healing process, as it transfers physiologically active and vital tissue into a defected area. Thus, an autologous graft is intended to optimally contribute to remodeling in the course of bone integration, in which the implanted bone matrix is subjected to undergo a gradual osteoclastic degradation process, while allow for a parallel formation of new bone hard substance through osteoblastic activity [2, 6, 7]. On a cellular level, the structural integrity of healthy bone is maintained through the adaptation to the change of mechanical loading on the skeletal system by continuous bone formation and degradation processes, that are ensured by the cell-mediated activities known as "physiological remodeling" [1, 4]. Thereby, it is of fundamental importance that autologous bone grafts do not lead to rejection reactions [2]. This is a major reason for the known high success rate of autologous bone grafts. However, autologous bone grafting from intra- and extraoral sites is often associated with complications [3]. In addition to the risks associated with the need for a second surgical intervention, pain, secondary bleeding, nerve injury, and even fractures at the donor site are considered as other comorbidities [8–12]. Furthermore, the availability of autologous grafts is limited [13].

Another important argument in favor of applying alternatives to support bone tissue regeneration in everyday clinical practice is the increasing aging of our society. More and more patients with age-related diseases such as postmenopausal osteoporosis and tumor diseases of different entities (e.g., multiple myeloma) will have to be treated. However, these patients show a disturbed bony remodeling, that can be described as pronounced osteoclast function with associated bone resorption [11, 14]. These patients suffer from a predominant and massive disturbance of bony integrity [15, 16]. In case of transplantation of this pathologically altered bone substance, the consequences are an altered architecture of the trabecular bone with microfractures [17, 18]. For this reason, the transplantation of bone tissue with a disturbed metabolism and reduced regenerative capacity is controversial and can be seen as counterintuitive.

Various biomaterials are considered as alternatives to autologous transplant for defect filling and bone tissue regeneration, which are referred to the large group of bone substitute materials (BSMs) and are available. This group of materials, which is very varied, includes not only replacement materials of natural origin—allografts and xenografts—but also materials of synthetic or alloplastic origin [19, 20] (Table 1).

Table 1 Definitions of the different bone tissue healing properties and their presence in the different bone grafts [21–23]

Healing Properties	Osteoinduction	Osteoconduction	Osteogenesis
Definition	The recruitment and stimulation of precursor cells to differentiate into osteogenic cell lineages	The process of host vasculature and tissue ingrowth on and within an implant	The synthesis of new bone tissue via donor cells
Bone grafts			
Autograft	*	*	*
Allograft	Sometimes	*	–
Xenograft	–	*	–
Alloplastic grafts	–	*	–

The research in recent decades has shown that material-related inflammatory tissue reactions are induced during the application of such biomaterials [24, 25]. In this context, macrophages, in particular, are involved in these inflammatory tissue reactions towards BSMs, depending on their physicochemical characteristics [26, 27]. It has been shown that macrophages represent a crucial regulatory cell type in this material-induced reaction due to their expression of pro- and anti-inflammatory molecules (e.g. CCR-7, COX-2, CD-206 and CD-163) [7, 26–28].

Thus, macrophages are involved in the process of tissue healing and bone regeneration as an important control element. It is generally assumed that a biomaterial should induce the expression of a predominantly anti-inflammatory tissue response in order to optimally support the process of (bone) tissue regeneration and promote tissue healing (Fig. 1) [29–31]. However, it is assumed that the expression of proinflammatory molecules is also of crucial importance for the successful application of a BSM, since material degradation is processed via such molecules [32, 33].

In addition, macrophages have been shown to play a crucial role in implant bed vascularization and perfusion, which is an important factor in (bone) tissue healing, through the expression of signal molecules such as the vascular endothelial growth factor (VEGF) [35, 36].

Furthermore, the biocompatibility of BSMs is often discussed in this context, especially regarding their induction of the so-called multinucleated giant cells (MNGCs) [37, 38]. These giant cells are often declared as pathological cell types in the literature even in comparison to multinuclear cell types involved in different diseases such as Langhans giant cells related to tuberculosis [39–41]. However, research in recent decades has shown that MNGCs, just like their mononuclear precursor cells, i.e., monocytes or macrophages, can express both pro- and anti-inflammatory molecules [26, 42]. Therefore, it is assumed that the biomaterial-associated MNGCs as well as macrophages are likely to be involved in the process of bone regeneration as important control elements [41, 43]. This means that this cell type seems to occupy direct regulatory functions in the process of tissue regeneration in combination with indirect roles such as the induction of the implant bed vascularization through their

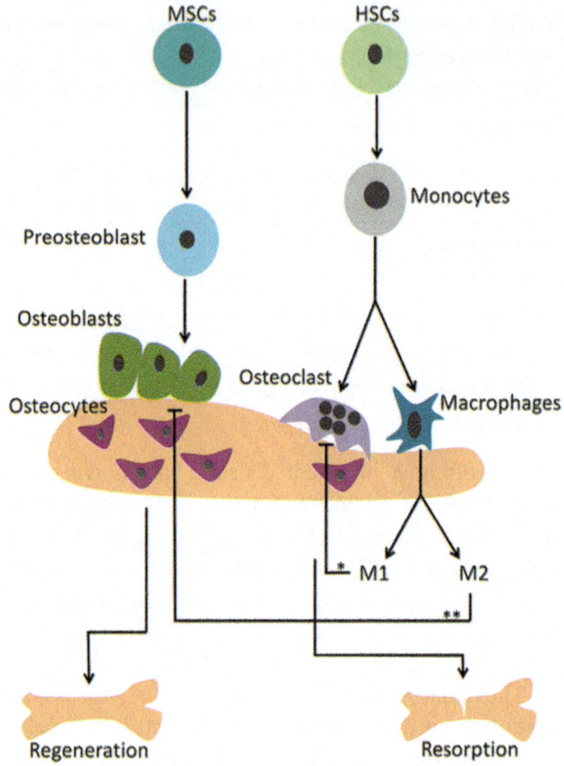

Fig. 1 Cell types involved in the physiological bine remodeling process. (*Pro-inflammatory subtype of macrophages, **Anti-inflammatory subtype of macrophages) [34]

VEGF expression (Fig. 1) [43]. Furthermore, the biomaterial-induced MNGCs are involved in the degradation of biomaterials through their ability to lyse and phagocytose, which indicates a significant function also in the context of the creeping substitution of BSMs [42, 44]. It was shown that the process of cellular degradation of biomaterials may involve various pro-inflammatory molecules such as molecules of the reactive oxygen species (ROS) group [44]. However, the exact involvement of MNGCs in the processes of bone healing and material degradation is still unknown. In summary, this means that in addition to the pure anti-inflammatory tissue response for the purpose of tissue healing, pro-inflammatory effectors are also required for their degradation, especially in the case of the application of resorbable biomaterials such as various BSMs.

Overall, it is still unknown to what extent of the (biomaterial-mediated) inflammatory tissue response is consistent with the best possible extent of (bone) tissue regeneration. It is also unclear to what extent inflammation is consistent with a simultaneous degradation process and the associated osteoconductive material functionality. Biomaterial research aims at a deeper understanding of the molecular mechanisms of these processes in order to reconcile the optimal material characteristics of different BSMs with the best possible inflammatory cell and tissue reaction for bone integration. These findings are of crucial importance to promote material-supported regeneration of bone defects.

2 Bone Substitute Materials (Bioceramics)

2.1 Natural Bioceramics

Allogeneic BSMs are derived from the bone tissue of human donors. Tissue from living donors is mostly used for this purpose, most often from femoral heads that are removed during hip replacement surgeries [45]. Since the tissue is from donors of the same species but not from the recipient, the application of allogeneic BSMs needs to perform a purification process of the donor bone tissue [46, 47]. All immunologically active components, such as the various cellular components of the donor bone tissue as well as potentially contained pathogens, must be removed before application to prevent rejection or exaggerated inflammatory responses, which may lead to clinical "failure" of the implant [48, 49]. Finally, the bone matrix composed of hydroxyapatite (HA) is the main component to be used as the allogenic biomaterial (Fig. 2) [49].

Moreover, xenogeneic BSMs have become established in clinical practice over the last decades due to recurrent discussions about the safety of allogenic materials and not least their overall improved availability [36, 50, 51]. This material group is extracted from animal bone tissue [52]. The purified HA-based bone matrix, which is mostly derived from the femoral head of cattle, is also used as a BSM Fig. 3.

In comparison to allogenic materials, the application of xenogeneic BSMs makes a decellularization of the bone tissue before its clinical application mandatory to prevent undesired immunological or inflammatory tissue reactions [53, 54]. The purification of this class of materials is also repeatedly discussed and investigated in

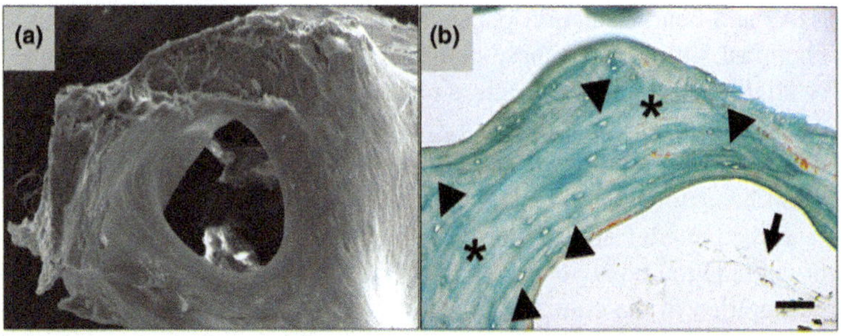

Fig. 2 Exemplary images of an allogenic BSMs. **a** Scanning electron microscopic image of the allogenic BSM, showing the trabecular porous structure of the biomaterial (100× magnification). **b** Light microscope image of the allogenic BSM. The image shows the calcified matrix (stars) with decellularized osteocyte lacunae (arrowheads) as well as small fiber portions of the intertrabecular connective tissue (arrow) (Masson Goldner stain, 400× magnification, scale bar = 50 μm)

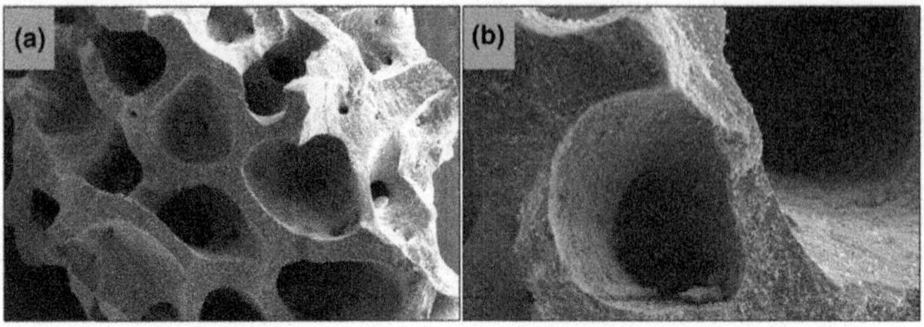

Fig. 3 Exemplary scanning electron microscopic images of a xenogeneic BSM. **a** Overview of the trabecular structure of the biomaterial (30× magnification). **b** View of a pore and the material surface (100× magnification)

terms of the potential transmission of pathogens. An example of a potential risk is prions of bovine spongiform encephalopathy (BSE), which have been described in recent decades [36, 55, 56].

As a natural alternative to allo- and xenogeneic materials, the so-called phytogenic or plant-based BSMs have been developed [36, 57–59]. In case of this material class, special processes have been developed, which make it possible to convert the calcium carbonate-based exoskeleton of corals and red algae to calcium phosphate through a hydrothermal conversion process [60]. The original structure of the exoskeleton is preserved, resulting in porous BSMs [61].

2.2 Synthetic Bioceramics

Different synthetic materials have been established in the last decades as an important alternative to the natural BSMs [58, 60]. Within the large and heterogeneous group of synthetic BSMs, materials based on calcium phosphates, i.e., mainly hydroxyapatite (HA) and beta-tricalcium phosphate (β-TCP), are still most prominent due to the chemical similarity of these compounds to the native calcified bone matrix [62, 63]. Highly porous biomaterials, similar to the morphology of the natural bony extracellular matrix, are seen in Fig. 4.

However, it has been shown that HA and β-TCP have different solubility and degradation behaviors [63, 64]. HA is degraded very slowly in the body, while β-TCP is resorbed much faster [65, 66]. In this context, it has been reported that these different degradation behaviors are usually not optimally suited for the purpose of bony regeneration in the context of creeping substitution [65]. For this reason, the two compounds were combined to the so-called biphasic calcium phosphates, which have revealed to be suitable for bone regeneration in different indications in a broad number of studies [66]. Thus, biphasic BSMs are now mainly used in everyday clinical practice [66]. In this context, mixing ratios of 60% HA and 40% β-TCP has been established since the degradation behavior of this combination seems to be best suited to support the process of bone regeneration [65].

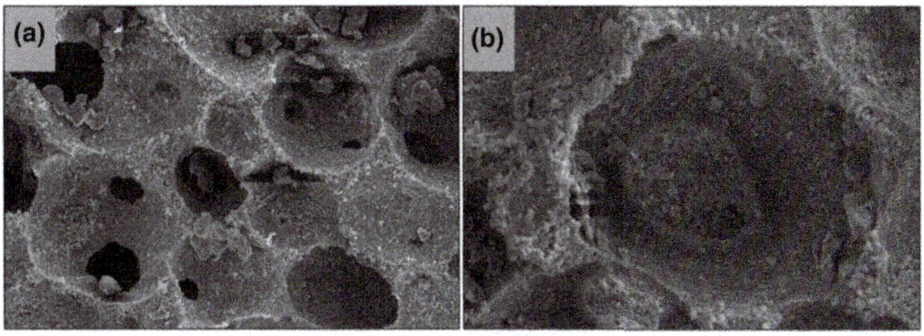

Fig. 4 Exemplary scanning electron microscopic images of a synthetic biphasic BSM. **a** Overview of the porous structure of the material (100× magnification). **b** View of a pore and the material surface (200× magnification)

Another synthetic group of BSMs is the group of the so-called bioglasses or bio-active glasses [65–67]. This class of materials is classified as bioceramics and contains silicon oxide or silicate as its main component and three other basic compounds that are sodium oxide, calcium oxide and/or phosphorus [68]. The variation of these compounds allows for the production of different bioglasses [69]. Bioglasses have been extensively investigated for several decades for their regenerative properties in the context of bone healing [69]. In particular, the release of bioactive ions plays an important role in the regenerative properties of bioglasses [69, 70]. The production processes of these material classes allow the inclusion of ions such as magnesium, which could further increase the regenerative potential of bioglasses (Fig. 5) [71–73].

2.3 3D Printing for Manufacturing of Bone Substitute Material

Over the last decades, biomaterials and BSMs, fabricated via additive manufacturing techniques, have excessively been studied; particularly through the further development of various 3D printing technologies [74]. The hopes for the application of 3D printing technologies lie not only in the improvement of many medical applications, but also in the simplified production of patient-specific implants [74, 75]. 3D printing has already proven its feasibility, particularly in the manufacturing of prosthetics, orthotics and surgical instruments [76–78]. Overall, it is expected that 3D printing techniques will also find widespread application in the field of patient-specific BSMs, which are still offered primarily on an allo- or xenogeneic material basis. However, 3D printing has not yet become established, since, among other things, no basic materials have yet been developed with similar characteristics compared to the BSMs described above. Although synthetic materials based on calcium phosphates, i.e., based on HA and β-TCP as well as on biphasic mixtures, have already been printed and tested, this class of materials has not yet been able to be established, particularly

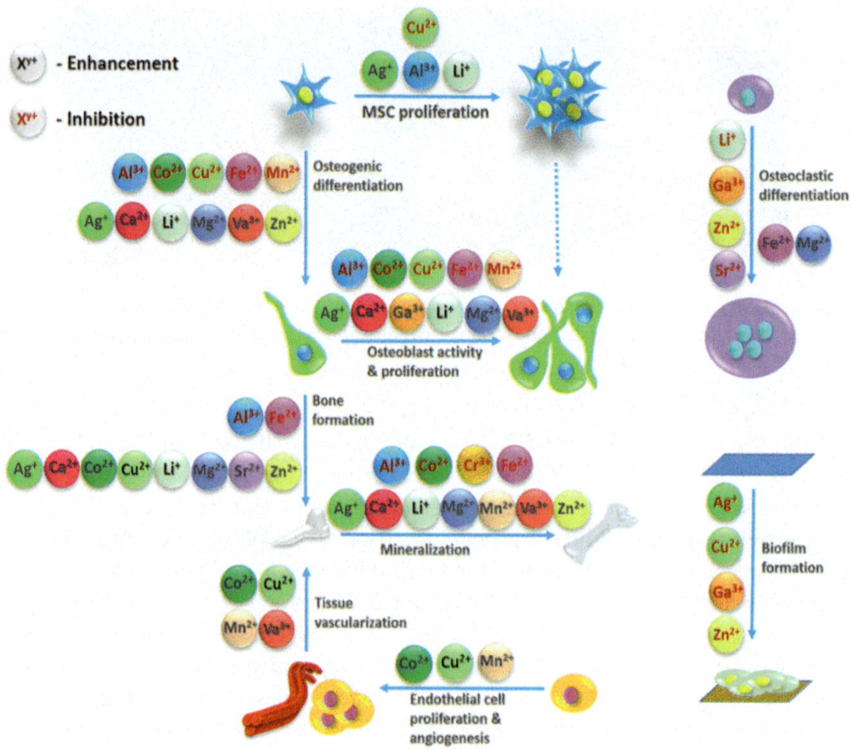

Fig. 5 Overview of the involvement of different ions in the processes of bone metabolism [73]

due to its limited mechanical properties [79, 80]. Additionally, the biocompatibility and printability of biomaterials for such application purposes are yet not completely understood.

Currently, BSMs produced by the printing process of Fused Deposition Modeling (FDM) or Fused Filament Fabrication (FFF) are favored [81, 82]. This manufacturing process involves the layer-by-layer production of a material that is based on a meltable plastic, whereby advanced technologies also enable the utilization of molten metal [82]. In the field of 3D printing for bone regeneration, the use of biodegradable polymers is again the preferred option. Synthetic polymers have been the primary focus of research due to their superior mechanical properties and printability compared to natural polymers such as collagen [82]. In this context, polymers based on polylactic acid (PLA) and polyglycolic acid (PGA), as well as the co-polymer poly(lactide-co-glycolide) (po-ly(lactic-co-glycolic acid), PLGA) and polycaprolactone (PCL) are at the center of current research in this field [82, 83]. However, the applicability of these polymers has been limited up to now. As an example, the acidic degradation products in the case of PCL and the resulting low bioactivity are considered a limiting concern [84, 85]. For this reason, mixtures of "classical BSM" such as biphasic calcium phosphates and bioglasses in combination with the above-described polymers, were and are most often investigated as scaffold materials in the field of 3D-printed bone tissue regeneration [86–88].

2.4 Natural Polymer-Based Bone Substitute Materials

Collagen is the most widely used natural polymers for biomedical applications based on its biological features and its good biocompatibility [82, 89]. Thus, collagen is a basis material for biomaterials in a variety of medical applications including especially medical devices for bone regeneration, e.g., dental composites in combination with calcium phosphates [89–91]. Especially collagen type I is mainly used as biomaterial as it is the most abundant component of the extracellular matrix (ECM) [89]. Thus, it is also used as a bone BSM as the bone ECM is very rich in collagen type I (Fig. 6) [92]. Interestingly, it has been shown that collagen can be produced in a wide variety of forms such as granules, gels or pastes, membranes, scaffolds and composites (combined with calcium phosphates) [93].

In addition to collagen-based biomaterials, other natural polymers such as silk fibroin are used for (bone) tissue regeneration because they are seem also to be very similar to the extracellular matrix of native bone [88, 94]. Further advantages of using silk fibroin-based biomaterials are their controlled degradability and mechanical stability compared to collagen-based materials Silk fibroin-based biomaterials are repeatedly tested as scaffolds for bone tissue engineering, especially in combination with cell types such as (pre-) osteoblasts [95–97].

Another category of natural polymers used in bone tissue regeneration most often combined with bone substitute granules to injectable BSMs, are polysaccharides [94, 98]. Hyaluronic acid is a polysaccharide found in every tissue of vertebrates [98]. It

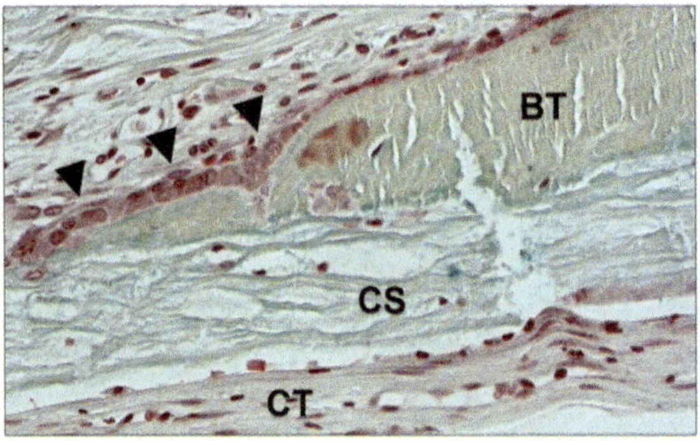

Fig. 6 Exemplary microscopic image of a collagen scaffold (CS) based on bovine pericardium promoting the formation of bone matrix (BT) within a calvaria defect area of a Wistar rat. Areas of active bone formation (black arrowheads = osteoblasts) were visible at two weeks post-implantation (Movat Pentachrome staining, 40× magnification)

is commonly extracted from bovine or avian sources [98]. Hyaluronic acid is water-soluble and can form solutions that are viscoelastic and form 3D structures. This biopolymer encourages angiogenesis and regeneration via recruiting different cells in vivo; hence, it is used in wound healing and (bone) tissue regeneration [98–100].

Plant-based polysaccharides are also of interest in the field of biomaterials and regenerative medicine [94]. For example, cellulose is a biopolymer that is biocompatible, bioactive and has shown to provide mechanical properties making it suitable for bone tissue engineering [101, 102]. Also, cellulose allows cell attachment and induces osteogenic differentiation [101]. Cellulose crystals can be used along with other biopolymers and BSMs, enhancing the regenerative properties of the biomaterial [101, 103]. Another plant-based polysaccharide, which is intensively investigated in biomedical applications, is alginate [94, 104]. Alginate is known for its gel-forming properties and biocompatibility [94]. Composites of alginate with other polymers and BSMs can be promising in bone tissue engineering [104]. Interestingly, cellulose and alginate are not biodegradable via physiological enzymes by mammals and, thus, there are still studies on their biodegradability mechanisms [101, 104].

In summary, all of the mentioned bone graft substitute classes—without the addition of cells—can contribute to bone tissue regeneration only through the process of osteoconduction (Fig. 7) [22, 23]. This means that no adequate substitute for autologous bone tissue grafts has been developed up to date as the exact composition (e.g. individual bone-tissue-associated proteins) and topography (i.e. porosity and surface morphology) of the bone matrix or the exact functionality of bone-associated proteins have not been fully clarified.

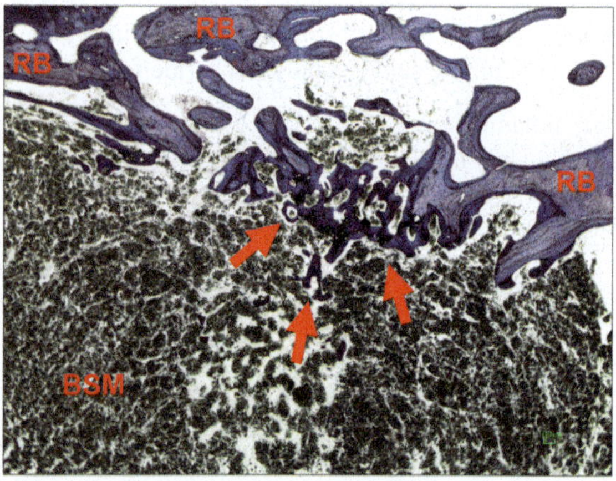

Fig. 7 Exemplary image from an implantation site of an injectable BSM (BSM) one month post implantation. Bone growth is starting from the residual bone (RB) along the material granules (red arrows) (Toluidine staining, 100× magnification, scale bar = 100 μm)

3 Inflammatory Tissue Reaction to Biomaterials and Bone Tissue Healing

Another important factor that has a decisive influence on the application and functionality of biomaterials in general, and also of BSMs, is the material-associated inflammatory tissue reaction. Research over the last decades has shown that the implantation of all biomaterials—whether of natural or synthetic origin—induces an inflammatory process in different degree [26, 105]. This process has so far been referred to as "foreign body response to biomaterials" [26]. Although the term "inflammation" is usually associated with negative connotations and complications, it should be noted that this term overall includes both pro- and anti-inflammatory processes [26, 42].

3.1 Inflammation in Physiological Bone Tissue Healing

Also, the process of bone healing is accompanied by inflammatory processes, even without the application of biomaterials [106, 107]. A precisely coordinated interaction of the cells and (inflammatory) signaling molecules takes place at the molecular level [106]. Thereby the process of bone healing can take place in two different ways: On the one hand, bone fractures can heal via the process of primary ossification, i.e. by direct ingrowth of bone tissue starting from the fracture boundaries directly into the defect, with stable and direct apposition of the fracture ends (fracture gap up to one millimeter) [108, 109]. Secondary bone healing takes place in case of fractures with a wider and/or unstable fracture gap, including various consecutive inflammatory phases [108–110]. This regeneration process is the most common form of fracture healing. The initial phase of secondary bone healing, the so-called early inflammatory phase, is characterized by the formation of a fracture hematoma, which mainly involves cell types such as monocytes and macrophages, thrombocytes, granulocytes, endothelial cells and, in addition to osteoblasts and mesenchymal stem cells [106, 111]. These cell types express or secrete a multitude of pro- and anti-inflammatory mediators, which among other things initiate the remodelling of the fracture hematoma into granulation tissue [108, 109, 111, 112]. Based on the granulation tissue, the so-called soft callus finally forms within the fracture area and leads to a stabilization of the defect site [14]. Furthermore, collagen II is degraded within the soft callus and the production of collagen I increases, which then mineralizes forming the so-called hard callus [113]. These processes are also controlled by various inflammatory signal molecules such as transforming growth factor beta (TGF-β) and members of the bone morphogenetic protein (BMP) family [108, 112]. Subsequently, the hard callus is converted into lamellar bone. This healing cascade involves different immune cells, while macrophages play a special role [114]. This means that macrophages are not only involved in wound cleansing, but according to recent findings, they are also involved in the process of bone healing [108, 114]. In this context it should be noted that several inflammatory macrophage subtypes

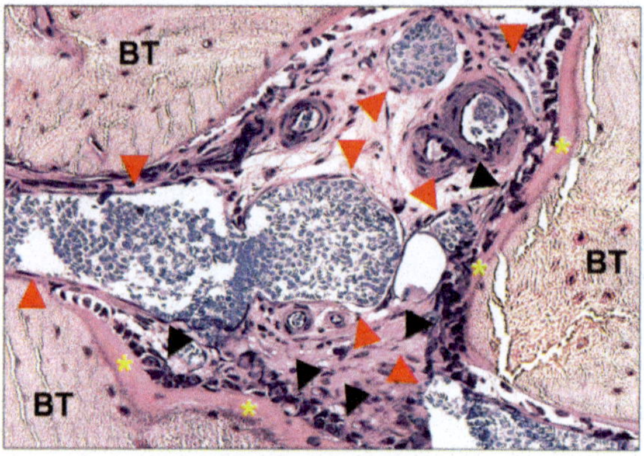

Fig. 8 Exemplary microscopic image of the bone defect area of the tibia of a rabbit. Within the intertrabecular connective tissue, various blood vessels (red arrowheads) are visible in the direct vicinity of areas of active bone formation (yellow asterisks = osteoid) with associated active osteoblasts (black arrowheads) (BT = bone tissue) (Giemsa staining, 20× magnification)

have been roughly defined [108, 115]. In particular, the so-called anti-inflammatory M2-macrophages are believed to play a decisive role in tissue or bone regeneration (Fig. 1) [114, 116].

The vasculature of the fracture site is another decisive basis for the processes of degradation and tissue regeneration, which not only allows the supply of nutrients and the removal of metabolic end products, but also the targeted migration of cells (Fig. 8) [117–119]. Therefore, the process of angiogenesis is essential for bone healing, with signal molecules such as angiopoietins and especially VEGF playing important roles [120, 121]. In addition, VEGF is not only directly involved in the induction of angiogenesis, but also indirectly in the process of ossification by promoting osteoblastic differentiation [121]. This brief introduction to the process of secondary bone healing reflects the importance of inflammatory processes in tissue healing up to the condition of a restitutio in integrum and shows their important contribution to (bone) tissue healing even without biomaterial application.

3.2 *Relationships Between BSM-Associated Tissue Reaction and Bone Tissue Healing*

As already mentioned, every biomaterial also triggers an inflammatory reaction within the implantation area [26, 105, 122]. In various studies, it was shown that the extent of tissue reactions to a biomaterial, i.e. the extent of the cells involved, the secretion of pro- and anti-inflammatory cytokines, the integration behavior and the blood supply of the implantation sites, depends on the composition of the physicochemical properties of the biomaterial [44–46, 65, 123–126]. In the case of synthetic

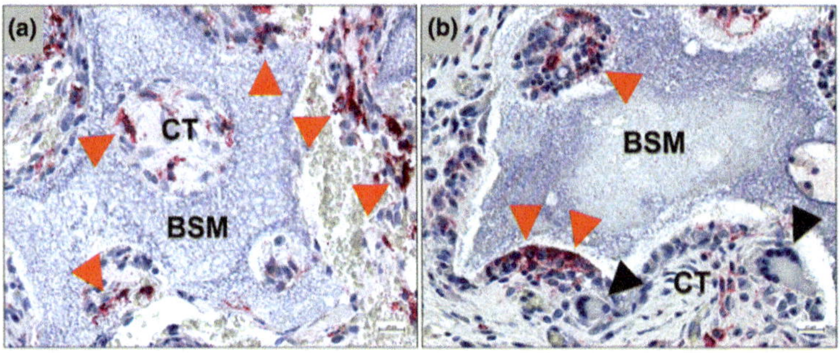

Fig. 9 Exemplary microscopic images from the implantation area of a synthetic BSM after immunohistochemical detection of **a** anti-inflammatory M2-macrophages (red arrowheads) and **b** pro-inflammatory M1-macrophages (red arrowheads) (black arrowheads = multinuclear giant cells) (CT: connective tissue, BSM: bone substitute material). (A: CD163 detection, B: NF-κB detection, 400× magnification, scale bar = 20 μm)

BSMs, for example, correlations have been discovered between the chemical composition, as well as different physical factors (such as the shape and morphology of the material and the porosity), and the extent of the inflammatory tissue reaction [44–46, 65, 123–126]. For example, the two calcium phosphate compounds HA and β-TCP induced different degrees of inflammatory tissue response, which is expressed in different numbers of MNGCs and different degrees of implantation bed vascularization. As a result, both compounds exhibit different degradation behaviors [65]. Furthermore, the influence of the addition of other material components such as collagen and other organic components on the effects regarding the modulation of the tissue reactions was also analyzed [127–129]. In this reaction cascade, macrophages as a regulatory cell type are also in the focus of research (Fig. 9) [26, 105, 129].

It is generally assumed that a biomaterial—after an early phase with a predominantly pro-inflammatory tissue response—should induce the expression of an overall anti-inflammatory tissue response in order to be optimally regenerative [43, 97, 129]. However, this very general hypothesis represents the biomaterial-associated tissue reaction process only in a very one-sided way, as it has been further shown that the degradation of a biomaterial, such as various BSMS, is processed by expression and secretion of pro-inflammatory mediators [26, 43, 97, 130, 131]. Overall, the extent to which the biomaterial-mediated inflammatory tissue reaction is consistent with the best possible degree of (bone) tissue regeneration, including a simultaneous degradation process, is still unknown.

In this context, the so-called biocompatibility of biomaterials is often discussed [36]. For example, biomaterials that induce the formation of multinucleated giant cells are still considered non-biocompatible (Fig. 10) [102, 132].

However, it has been shown that biomaterial-induced multinucleated giant cells, similar to macrophages, may be involved in the process of bone regeneration as an important control element [42, 97]. It has been shown that giant cells resulting from the fusion of macrophages also express both pro- and anti-inflammatory factors [42].

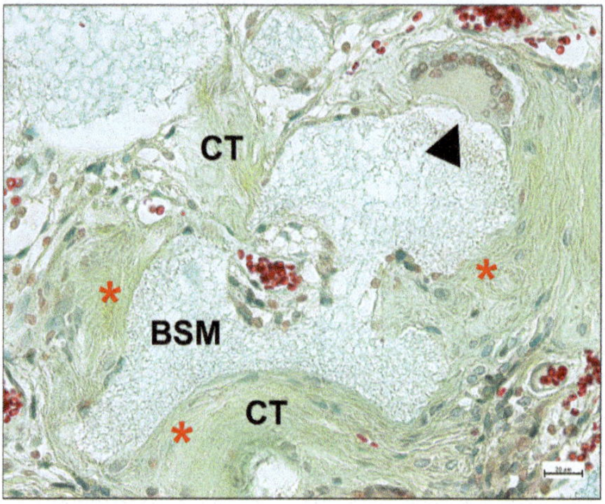

Fig. 10 Exemplary histological image of an implantation area of a synthetic BSM. On the surface of the BSM, multinucleated giant cells (black arrowhead) were frequently found, while in other areas a ring-like fibrotic tissue reaction (red stars) could be detected. (CT = connective tissue, BSM: bone substitute material) (Movat Pentachrome staining, 400-fold magnification, scale bar = 20 μm)

In addition, both cell types, besides their regulatory functions in the process of tissue regeneration, also play a crucial role in the process of vascularization of an implant site, for example through their expression of VEGF [44]. Furthermore, biomaterial-induced multinucleated giant cells are involved in the degradation of biomaterials through their ability to lyse and phagocytose, which indicates a significant function in the creeping replacement of BSMs (Fig. 11) [36].

To date, however, it has not been conclusively clarified which cellular differentiation this multinucleated cell type undergoes and what significance this cell type has for material degradation, particularly for bone tissue healing. On the one hand, the multinuclear giant cells are called "osteoclast-like cells" due to their multinucleated nature and their expression of the osteoclast marker tartrate-resistant acid phosphatase (TRAP) and last but not least due to their induction by calcium phosphate-based chemistries [42, 97]. This material-induced cell type is also found in implantation sites of various other biomaterials based on collagen or silk protein (Silk Fibroin) and expresses the enzyme TRAP (Fig. 12) [26, 30, 133–137].

Overall, it has been shown that there are various overlaps between the material-induced (inflammatory) tissue response and the process of bone tissue healing (Fig. 13) [42–44, 138, 139].

4 Conclusion

In summary, the understanding of the differentiation, the inflammatory characteristics, and the precise involvement of degradation of both macrophages and multinucleated giant cells is crucial for the understanding of biomaterial-mediated tissue

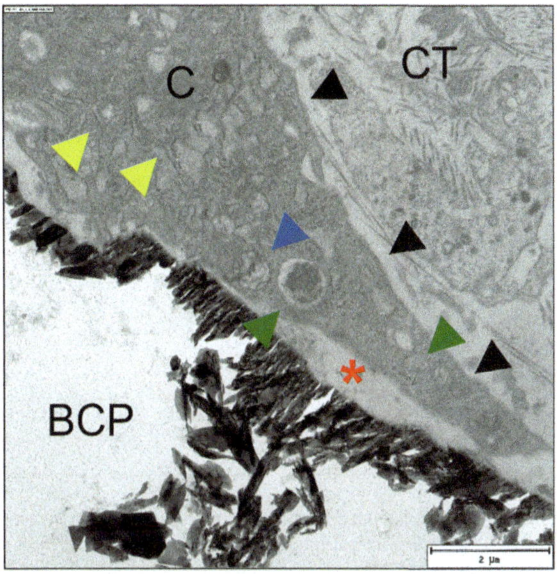

Fig. 11 Exemplary trans-electron microscopic image from the implantation site of a biphasic calcium phosphate BSM (BCP). At the surface of the BSM, multinucleated giant cells (black arrowheads) are detected, which have formed a sub-cellular compartment (red star) at the material surface. Within the cytoplasm (C) vacuoles with material fragments (green arrowheads) as signs of material phagocytosis were observed (yellow arrowheads = rough endoplasmic reticulum, blue arrowhead = mitochondrion, CT: connective tissue) (4800-fold magnification, scale bar = 2 μm) [45]

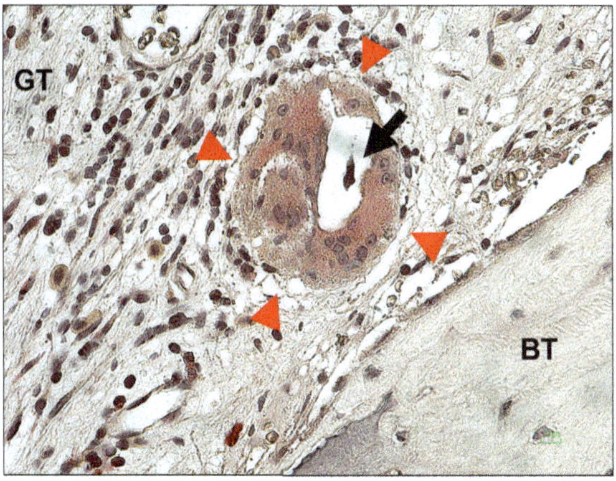

Fig. 12 Exemplary microscopic image from the implantation site of a silk fibroin (SF)-based biomaterial on day 30 post implantation with a TRAP-positive giant multinuclear cell (red arrowheads). SF fragments (arrow) were detected intracellularly (GT = granulation tissue, BT = bone tissue) (TRAP staining, 40-fold magnification, scale bar = 10 μm)

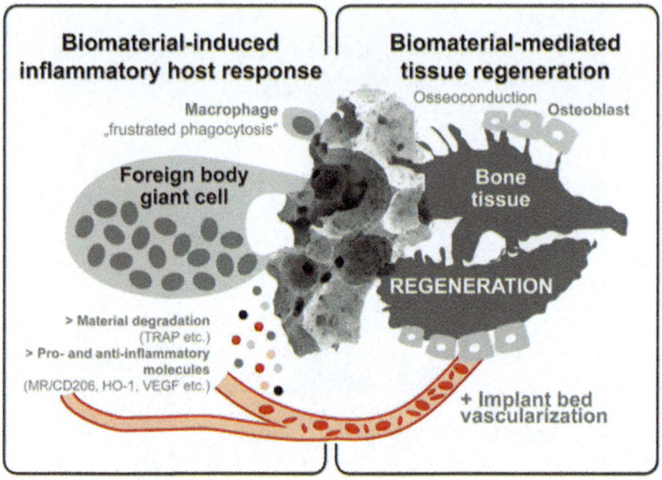

Fig. 13 Schematic relationship between the inflammatory tissue reaction in response to the implantation of a biomaterial and the processes of bone tissue regeneration in the case of BSMs. It should be noted that the physicochemical properties of a biomaterial (center) influence the reactivity of macrophages and their fusion into multinucleated giant cells through the process of frustrated phagocytosis. The multinucleated giant cells, which besides macrophages process the degradation of a biomaterial, secrete pro- and anti-inflammatory signaling molecules and other signaling factors such as the angiogenesis factor (VEGF) like their mononuclear precursors. Thus, the inflammatory tissue reaction in response to a biomaterial application can support the vascularization of the implant bed and the formation of new bone tissue. The material-induced inflammatory tissue response and bone tissue regeneration are thus linked in this way [140]

regeneration. However, very little knowledge exists about these processes and especially about the interrelation of different material factors and the orientation of material-induced inflammation.

Therefore, research in the field of biomaterials research is aimed at a deeper understanding of the mechanisms of these processes to identify the optimal material characteristics of different biomaterials with an optimal inflammatory cell and tissue reaction for tissue healing. These findings are also of crucial importance in identifying the "right biomaterial" for the "right clinical application".

References

1. Giannoudis, P.V., Dinopoulos, H., Tsiridis, E.: Bone substitutes: an update. Injury **36**(Suppl), S20–S27 (2005). https://doi.org/10.1016/j.injury.2005.07.029
2. Goldberg, V.M., Akhavan, S.: Biology of bone grafts. In: Friedlaender, J.R., G.E. (eds.) Bone Regeneration and Repair; Liebermann, SpringerLink (2005)
3. Bauer, T.W., Muschler, G.F.: Bone graft materials. An overview of the basic science. Clin. Orthop. Relat. Res. 10–27 (2000)

4. Pape, H.C., Evans, A., Kobbe, P.: Autologous bone graft: properties and techniques. J Orthop Trauma **24**(Suppl), S36-40 (2010). https://doi.org/10.1097/BOT.0b013e3181cec4a1
5. Khan, S.N., Cammisa F.P.J., Sandhu, H.S., Diwan, A.D., Girardi, F.P., Lane, J.M.: The biology of bone grafting. J. Am. Acad. Orthop. Surg. **13**, 77–86 (2005)
6. Le, B.Q., Nurcombe, V., Cool, S.M., van Blitterswijk, C.A., de Boer, J., LaPointe, V.L.S.: The components of bone and what they can teach us about regeneration. Mater. **11** (2017). https://doi.org/10.3390/ma11010014
7. Miron, R.J., Bosshardt, D.D.: OsteoMacs: key players around bone biomaterials. Biomaterials **82**, 1–19 (2016). https://doi.org/10.1016/j.biomaterials.2015.12.017
8. Arrington, E.D., Smith, W.J., Chambers, H.G., Bucknell, A.L., Davino, N.A.: Complications of iliac crest bone graft harvesting. Clin. Orthop. Relat. Res. 300–309 (1996). https://doi.org/10.1097/00003086-199608000-00037
9. Nkenke, E., Weisbach, V., Winckler, E., Kessler, P., Schultze-, S., Wiltfang, J., Neukam, F.W.: Morbidity of harvesting of bone grafts from the iliac crest for preprosthetic augmentation procedures: a prospective study. Int. J. Oral Maxillofac. Surg. **33**, 157–163 (2004). https://doi.org/10.1054/ijom.2003.0465
10. Schaaf, H., Lendeckel, S., Howaldt, H.P., Streckbein, P.: Donor site morbidity after bone harvesting from the anterior iliac crest. Oral. Surg. Oral. Med. Oral. Pathol Oral. Radiol. Endod. **109**, 52–58 (2010). https://doi.org/10.1016/j.tripleo.2009.08.023
11. Klijn, R.J., Meijer, G.J., Bronkhorst, E.M., Jansen, J.A.: Sinus floor augmentation surgery using autologous bone grafts from various donor sites: a meta-analysis of the total bone volume. Tissue Eng. Part B Rev. **16**, 295–303 (2010). https://doi.org/10.1089/ten.TEB.2009.0558
12. Raghoebar, G.M., Louwerse, C., Kalk, W.W., Vissink, A.: Morbidity of chin bone harvesting. Clin. Oral. Implant. Res. **12**, 503–507 (2001). https://doi.org/10.1034/j.1600-0501.2001.120511.x
13. Raghoebar, G.M., Meijndert, L., Kalk, W.W., Vissink, A.: Morbidity of mandibular bone harvesting: a comparative study. Int. J. Oral. Maxillofac. Implant. **22**, 359–365 (2007)
14. Dimitriou, R., Mataliotakis, G.I., Angoules, A.G., Kanakaris, N.K., Giannoudis, P.: V Complications following autologous bone graft harvesting from the iliac crest and using the RIA: a systematic review. Injury **42**(Suppl), S3-15 (2011). https://doi.org/10.1016/j.injury.2011.06.015
15. Zhang, W.B., Zheng, L.W., Chua, D., Cheung, L.K.: Bone regeneration after radiotherapy in an animal model. J. Oral. Maxillofac. Surg. **68**, 2802–2809 (2010). https://doi.org/10.1016/j.joms.2010.04.024
16. Tarantino, U., Cerocchi, I., Scialdoni, A., Saturnino, L., Feola, M., Celi, M., Liuni, F.M., Iolascon, G., Gasbarra, E.: Bone healing and osteoporosis. Aging. Clin. Exp. Res. **23**, 62–64 (2011)
17. Henriksen, K., Bollerslev, J., Everts, V., Karsdal, M.A.: Osteoclast activity and subtypes as a function of physiology and pathology–implications for future treatments of osteoporosis. Endocr. Rev. **32**, 31–63 (2011). https://doi.org/10.1210/er.2010-0006
18. Ginaldi, L., Di Benedetto, M.C., De Martinis, M.: Osteoporosis, inflammation and ageing. Immun. Ageing. **2**, 14 (2005). https://doi.org/10.1186/1742-4933-2-14
19. Al-Sayyad, M.J., Abdulmajeed, T.M.: Fracture of the anterior iliac crest following autogenous bone grafting. Saudi. Med. J. **27**, 254–258 (2006)
20. Hu, R., Hearn, T., Yang, J.: Bone graft harvest site as a determinant of iliac crest strength. Clin. Orthop. Relat. Res. 252–256 (1995)
21. Miron, R.J., Bosshardt, D.D.: Osteoinductive potential of a novel biphasic calcium phosphate bone graft in comparison with autographs. Xenografts DFDBA. 668–675 (2015). https://doi.org/10.1111/clr.12647
22. Stewart, S., Bryant, S.J., Ahn, J., Hankenson, K.D.: Bone regeneration. In: Translational Regenerative Medicine. Elsevier Inc.; pp. 313–333. ISBN: 9780124103962
23. Roberts, T.T., Rosenbaum, A.J., Roberts, T.T., Rosenbaum, A.J., Roberts, T.T., Rosenbaum, A.J.: Healing bone grafts, bone substitutes and orthobiologics the bridge between basic science and clinical advancements in fracture healing. 6278 (2012). https://doi.org/10.4161/org.23306

24. Pryor, L.S., Gage, E., Langevin, C.J., Herrera, F., Breithaupt, A.D., Gordon, C.R., Afifi, A.M., Zins, J.E., Meltzer, H., Gosman, A., et al.: Review of bone substitutes. Craniomaxillofac. Trauma. Reconstr. **2**, 151–160 (2009). https://doi.org/10.1055/s-0029-1224777
25. Kao, S.T., Scott, D.D.: A review of bone substitutes. Oral. Maxillofac. Surg. Clin. North Am. **19**(vi), 513–521 (2007). https://doi.org/10.1016/j.coms.2007.06.002
26. Anderson, J.M., Rodriguez, A., Chang, D.T.: Foreign body reaction to biomaterials. Semin. Immunol. **20**, 86–100 (2008). https://doi.org/10.1016/j.smim.2007.11.004
27. Mountziaris, P.M., Mikos, A.G.: Modulation of the inflammatory response for enhanced bone tissue regeneration. Tissue Eng. Part B Rev. **14**, 179–186 (2008). https://doi.org/10.1089/ten.teb.2008.0038
28. Muldashev, E.R., Muslimov, S.A., Musina, L.A., Nigmatullin, R.T., Lebedeva, A.I., Shangina, O.R., Khasanov, R.A.: The role of macrophages in the tissues regeneration stimulated by the biomaterials. Cell Tissue Bank **6**, 99–107 (2005). https://doi.org/10.1007/s10561-004-5805-2
29. Sheikh, Z., Brooks, P.J., Barzilay, O., Fine, N., Glogauer, M.: Macrophages, foreign body giant cells and their response to implantable biomaterials. Mater **8**, 5671–5701 (2015). https://doi.org/10.3390/ma8095269
30. Xia, Z., Triffitt, J.T.: A review on macrophage responses to biomaterials. Biomed. Mater. **1**, R1-9 (2006). https://doi.org/10.1088/1748-6041/1/1/r01
31. Mantovani, A., Biswas, S.K., Galdiero, M.R., Sica, A., Locati, M.: Macrophage plasticity and polarization in tissue repair and remodelling. J. Pathol. **229**, 176–185 (2013). https://doi.org/10.1002/path.4133
32. Forbes, S.J., Rosenthal, N.: Preparing the ground for tissue regeneration: from mechanism to therapy. Nat. Med. **20**, 857–869 (2014). https://doi.org/10.1038/nm.3653
33. Chazaud, B.: Macrophages: supportive cells for tissue repair and regeneration. Immunobiology **219**, 172–178 (2014). https://doi.org/10.1016/j.imbio.2013.09.001
34. Kačarević, Ž.P., Rider, P.M., Alkildani, S., Retnasingh, S., Smeets, R., Jung, O., Ivanišević, Z., Barbeck, M.: An introduction to 3D bioprinting: Possibilities, challenges and future aspects. Materials (Basel) **11** (2018). https://doi.org/10.3390/ma11112199
35. Barbeck, M., Najman, S., Stojanovic, S., Mitic, Z., Zivkovic, J.M., Choukroun, J., Kovacevic, P., Sader, R., Kirkpatrick, C.J., Ghanaati, S.: Addition of blood to a phycogenic bone substitute leads to increased in vivo vascularization. Biomed. Mater. **10**, 55007 (2015). https://doi.org/10.1088/1748-6041/10/5/055007
36. Peric Kacarevic, Z., Kavehei, F., Houshmand, A., Franke, J., Smeets, R., Rimashevskiy, D., Wenisch, S., Schnettler, R., Jung, O., Barbeck, M.: Purification processes of xenogeneic bone substitutes and their impact on tissue reactions and regeneration. Int. J. Artif. Organs, 391398818771530 (2018). https://doi.org/10.1177/0391398818771530
37. Hsiong, S.X., Mooney, D.J.: Regeneration of vascularized bone. Periodontol **41**, 109–122 (2000 2006). https://doi.org/10.1111/j.1600-0757.2006.00158.x
38. Bingle, L., Lewis, C.E., Corke, K.P., Reed, M.W., Brown, N.J.: Macrophages promote angiogenesis in human breast tumour spheroids in vivo. Br. J. Cancer **94**, 101–107 (2006). https://doi.org/10.1038/sj.bjc.6602901
39. Anderson, J.M.: Multinucleated giant cells 40–47
40. Brodbeck, W.G., Anderson, J.M.: Giant cell formation and function. Curr. Opin. Hematol. **16**, 53–57 (2009). https://doi.org/10.1097/MOH.0b013e32831ac52e
41. Miron, R.J., Bosshardt, D.D.: Multinucleated Giant cells: good guys or bad guys? Tissue Eng. Part B Rev. **24**, 53–65 (2018). https://doi.org/10.1089/ten.TEB.2017.0242
42. Barbeck, M., Motta, A., Migliaresi, C., Sader, R., Kirkpatrick, C.J., Ghanaati, S.: Heterogeneity of biomaterial-induced multinucleated giant cells: possible importance for the regeneration process? J. Biomed. Mater. Res. - Part A **104**, 413–418 (2016). https://doi.org/10.1002/jbm.a.35579
43. Miron, R.J., Zohdi, H., Fujioka-Kobayashi, M., Bosshardt, D.D.: Giant cells around bone biomaterials: osteoclasts or multi-nucleated giant cells? Acta Biomater **46**, 15–28 (2016). https://doi.org/10.1016/j.actbio.2016.09.029

44. Ghanaati, S., Barbeck, M., Orth, C., Willershausen, I., Thimm, B.W., Hoffmann, C., Rasic, A., Sader, R.A., Unger, R.E., Peters, F., et al.: Influence of beta-tricalcium phosphate granule size and morphology on tissue reaction in vivo. Acta Biomater **6**, 4476–4487 (2010). https://doi.org/10.1016/j.actbio.2010.07.006
45. Barbeck, M., Dard, M., Kokkinopoulou, M., Markl, J., Booms, P., Sader, R.A., Kirkpatrick, C.J., Ghanaati, S.: Small-sized granules of biphasic bone substitutes support fast implant bed vascularization. Biomatter **5**, e1056943 (2015). https://doi.org/10.1080/21592535.2015.1056943
46. Wissing, T.B., Bonito, V., van Haaften, E.E., van Doeselaar, M., Brugmans, M., Janssen, H.M., Bouten, C.V.C., Smits, A.: Macrophage-driven biomaterial degradation depends on scaffold microarchitecture. Front Bioeng. Biotechnol. **7**, 87 (2019). https://doi.org/10.3389/fbioe.2019.00087
47. Goldberg, V.M., Stevenson, S.: Bone graft options: fact and fancy. Orthopedics **17**, 809–810,821 (1994)
48. Gilbert, T.W., Sellaro, T.L., Badylak, S.F.: Decellularization of tissues and organs. Biomaterials **27**, 3675–3683 (2006). https://doi.org/10.1016/j.biomaterials.2006.02.014
49. Somuncu, O.S.: Decellularization concept in regenerative medicine. Adv. Exp. Med. Biol. (2019). https://doi.org/10.1007/5584_2019_338
50. Hofmann, G.O., Kirschner, M.H., Wangemann, T., Falk, C., Mempel, W., Hammer, C.: Infections and immunological hazards of allogeneic bone transplantation. Arch. Orthop. Trauma. Surg. **114**, 159–166 (1995). https://doi.org/10.1007/bf00443390
51. Weyts, F.A., Bos, P.K., Dinjens, W.N., van Doorn, W.J., van Biezen, F.C., Weinans, H., Verhaar, J.A.: Living cells in 1 of 2 frozen femoral heads. Acta. Orthop. Scand. **74**, 661–664 (2003). https://doi.org/10.1080/00016470310018162
52. Lorenz, J., Schlee, M., Al-, S., Chia, P., Sader, R.A., Ghanaati, S.: Variant purification of an allogeneic bone block. Acta. Stomatol. Croat. **51**, 141–147 (2017). https://doi.org/10.15644/asc51/2/7
53. Baldini, N., De Sanctis, M., Ferrari, M.: Deproteinized bovine bone in periodontal and implant surgery. Dent. Mater. **27**, 61–70 (2011). https://doi.org/10.1016/j.dental.2010.10.017
54. Wong, M.L., Griffiths, L.G.: Immunogenicity in xenogeneic scaffold generation: antigen removal vs. decellularization. Acta Biomater **10**, 1806–1816 (2014). https://doi.org/10.1016/j.actbio.2014.01.028
55. Badylak, S.F.: Xenogeneic extracellular matrix as a scaffold for tissue reconstruction. Transpl. Immunol. **12**, 367–377 (2004). https://doi.org/10.1016/j.trim.2003.12.016
56. Barbeck, M., Udeabor, S., Lorenz, J., Schlee, M., Holthaus, M.G., Raetscho, N., Choukroun, J., Sader, R., Kirkpatrick, C.J., Ghanaati, S.: High-temperature sintering of xenogeneic bone substitutes leads to increased multinucleated giant cell formation: in vivo and preliminary clinical results. J. Oral. Implant. **41**, e212–e222 (2015). https://doi.org/10.1563/aaid-joi-D-14-00168
57. Barbeck, M., Witte, F., Wenisch, S., Schnettler, R.: Xenogeneic bone grafting materials. Implants, 34–36 (2017)
58. Kolk, A., Handschel, J., Drescher, W., Rothamel, D., Kloss, F., Blessmann, M., Heiland, M., Wolff, K.D., Smeets, R.: Current trends and future perspectives of bone substitute materials—from space holders to innovative biomaterials. J. Craniomaxillofac. Surg. **40**, 706–718 (2012). https://doi.org/10.1016/j.jcms.2012.01.002
59. Hermann, J.S., Buser, D.: Guided bone regeneration for dental implants. Curr. Opin. Periodontol **3**, 168–177 (1996)
60. Felício-Fernandes, G., Laranjeira, M.C.M.: Calcium phosphate biomaterials from marine algae Hydrothermal synthesis and characterisation. Quim. Nova. **23**, 441–446 (2000)
61. Damien, E., Revell, P.A.: Coralline hydroxyapatite bone graft substitute: a review of experimental studies and biomedical applications. J. Appl. Biomater Biomech. **2**, 65–73 (2004)
62. Lu, L., Bradford, L., Yaszemski, M.J.: Synthetic bone substitutes: current opinion in orthopaedics. Curr. Opin. Orthop. **11**, 383–390 (2000)

63. Eppley, B.L., Pietrzak, W.S., Blanton, M.W.: Allograft and alloplastic bone substitutes: a review of science and technology for the craniomaxillofacial surgeon. J. Craniofac. Surg. **16**, 981–989 (2005). https://doi.org/10.1097/01.scs.0000179662.38172.dd
64. Horowitz, R.A., Mazor, Z., Foitzik, C., Prasad, H., Rohrer, M., Palti, A.: β-tricalcium phosphate as bone substitute material: properties and clinical applications. J. Osseointegration, **2** (2010). https://www.journalofosseointegration.eu/index.php/jo/article/view/65
65. Ghanaati, S., Barbeck, M., Detsch, R., Deisinger, U., Hilbig, U., Rausch, V., Sader, R., Unger, R.E., Ziegler, G., Kirkpatrick, C.J.: The chemical composition of synthetic bone substitutes influences tissue reactions in vivo: histological and histomorphometrical analysis of the cellular inflammatory response to hydroxyapatite, beta-tricalcium phosphate and biphasic calcium phosphate cer. Biomed. Mater. **7** (2012). https://doi.org/10.1088/1748-6041/7/1/015005
66. Bouler, J.M., Pilet, P., Gauthier, O., Verron, E.: Biphasic calcium phosphate ceramics for bone reconstruction: a review of biological response. Acta Biomater **53**, 1–12 (2017). https://doi.org/10.1016/j.actbio.2017.01.076
67. Hench, L.L.: The story of Bioglass. J. Mater. Sci. Mater Med. **17**, 967–978 (2006). https://doi.org/10.1007/s10856-006-0432-z
68. Jones, J.R.: Bioactive glasses, Woodhead Publishing Limited (1971)
69. Abbasi, Z., Bahrololoom, M.E., Shariat, M.H., Bagheri, R.: Bioactive glasses in dentistry: a review. J. Dent. Biomater. **2**, 1–9 (2015)
70. Gerhardt, L.C., Widdows, K.L., Erol, M.M., Burch, C.W., Sanz-Herrera, J.A., Ochoa, I., Stampfli, R., Roqan, I.S., Gabe, S., Ansari, T., et al.: The pro-angiogenic properties of multifunctional bioactive glass composite scaffolds. Biomaterials **32**, 4096–4108 (2011). https://doi.org/10.1016/j.biomaterials.2011.02.032
71. Ohura, K., Nakamura, T., Ebisawa, Y., Kokubo, T., Kotoura, Y., Oka, M.: Bioactivity of CaO·SiO_2 glasses added with various ions | SpringerLink. J. Mater. Sci. Mater. Med. **3**, 95–100 (1992). https://doi.org/10.1007/BF00705275
72. Souza, M.T., Crovace, M.C., Schröder, C., Eckert, H., Peitl, O., Zanoto, E.D.: Effect of magnesium ion incorporation on the thermal stability, dissolution behavior and bioactivity in Bioglass-derived glasses. J. Non. Cryst. Solids **382**, 57–65 (2013)
73. Glenske, K., Donkiewicz, P., Kowitsch, A., Milosevic-Oljaca, N., Rider, P., Rofall, S., Franke, J., Jung, O., Smeets, R., Schnettler, R., et al.: Applications of metals for bone regeneration. Int. J. Mol. Sci. **19** (2018). https://doi.org/10.3390/ijms19030826
74. Asa'ad, F., Pagni, G., Pilipchuk, S.P., Gianni, A.B., Giannobile, W.V., Rasperini, G.: 3D-Printed scaffolds and biomaterials: review of alveolar bone augmentation and periodontal regeneration applications. Int. J. Dent. **2016** 1239842 (2016). https://doi.org/10.1155/2016/1239842
75. Rider, P., Kačarević, Ž.P., Alkildani, S., Retnasingh, S., Schnettler, R., Barbeck, M.: Additive manufacturing for guided bone regeneration: a perspective for alveolar ridge augmentation **19**, ISBN 4930206073 (2018)
76. Dodziuk, H.: Applications of 3D printing in healthcare. Kardiochir Torakochirurgia Pol **13**, 283–293 (2016). https://doi.org/10.5114/kitp.2016.62625
77. Ventola, C.L.: Medical applications for 3D printing: current and projected uses. P t **39**, 704–711 (2014)
78. Rankin, T.M., Giovinco, N.A., Cucher, D.J., Watts, G., Hurwitz, B., Armstrong, D.G.: Three-dimensional printing surgical instruments: are we there yet? J. Surg. Res. **189**, 193–197 (2014). https://doi.org/10.1016/j.jss.2014.02.020
79. Bose, S., Vahabzadeh, S., Bandyopadhyay, A.: Bone tissue engineering using 3D printing. Mater. Today **16**, 496–504 (2013)
80. Klammert, U., Gbureck, U., Vorndran, E., Rodiger, J., Meyer-, P., Kubler, A.C.: 3D powder printed calcium phosphate implants for reconstruction of cranial and maxillofacial defects. J. Craniomaxillofac Surg. **38**, 565–570 (2010). https://doi.org/10.1016/j.jcms.2010.01.009
81. Jariwala, S.H., Lewis, G.S., Bushman, Z.J., Adair, J.H., Donahue, H.J.: 3D Printing of personalized artificial bone scaffolds. 3D Print Addit. Manuf. **2**, 56–64 (2015). https://doi.org/10.1089/3dp.2015.0001

82. Perić, Ž, Rider, P., Alkildani, S., Retnasingh, S., Pejakić, M., Schnettler, R., Gosau, M., Smeets, R., Jung, O., Barbeck, M.: An introduction to bone tissue engineering. Int. J. Artif. Organs **43**, 69–86 (2020). https://doi.org/10.1177/0391398819876286
83. Konta, A.A., Garcia-Pina, M., Serrano, D.R.: Personalised 3D printed medicines: which techniques and polymers are more successful? Bioeng. **4** (2017). https://doi.org/10.3390/bioengineering4040079
84. Jin, F.L., Hu, R.R., Park, S.J.: Improvement of thermal behaviors of biodegradable poly (lactic acid) polymer. Compos. Part B Eng. **164**, 287–296 (2018)
85. Hamad, K., Kaseem, M., Yang, H.W., Deri, F., Ko, Y.G.: Properties and medical applications of polylactic acid: a review. eXPRESS Polym. Lett. **9**, 435–455 (2015) https://doi.org/10.3144/expresspolymlett.2015.42
86. Venkatesan, J., Kim, S.K.: Nano-hydroxyapatite composite biomaterials for bone tissue engineering–a review. J. Biomed. Nanotechnol. **10**, 3124–3140 (2014). https://doi.org/10.1166/jbn.2014.1893
87. Rasal, R.M., Janorkar, A.V., Hirt, D.E.: Poly(lactic acid) modifications. Prog. Polym. Sci. **35**, 338–356 (2010). https://doi.org/10.1016/j.progpolymsci.2009.12.003
88. Rao, M.G., Bharathi, P., Akila, R.M.: A comprehensive review on biopolymers. Sci. Rev. Chem. Commun. **4**(2), 61–68 (2014)
89. Ricard-blum, S.: The collagen family. Cold Spring Harb Perspect Biol. 1–19 (2011). https://doi.org/10.1101/cshperspect.a004978
90. Neiders, M.E., Andreana, S., Noble, B.: Collagen as an implantable material in medicine and dentistry. J. Oral Implantol. XXVIII (2002)
91. Lynn, A.K., Yannas, I.V., Bonfield, W.: Antigenicity and immunogenicity of collagen. J. Biomed. Res. 343–354 (2004). https://doi.org/10.1002/jbm.b.30096
92. Delmas, S.V.Æ.P.G.Æ.P.D.: The role of collagen in bone strength, 319–336 (2006). https://doi.org/10.1007/s00198-005-2035-9
93. Parenteau-, R., Gauvin, R., Berthod, F.: Collagen-based biomaterials for tissue engineering applications. Materials (Basel). **3**, 1863–1887 (2010). https://doi.org/10.3390/ma3031863
94. Rebelo, R., Fernandes, M., Fangueiro, R.: Biopolymers in medical implants: a brief review. Procedia Eng. **200**, 236–243 (2017)
95. Ghanaati, S., Unger, R.E., Webber, M.J., Barbeck, M., Orth, C., Kirkpatrick, J.A., Booms, P., Motta, A., Migliaresi, C., Sader, R.A., et al.: Scaffold vascularization in vivo driven by primary human osteoblasts in concert with host inflammatory cells. Biomaterials **32**, 8150–8160 (2011). https://doi.org/10.1016/j.biomaterials.2011.07.041
96. Kundu, B., Rajkhowa, R., Kundu, S.C., Wang, X.: Silk fibroin biomaterials for tissue regenerations. Adv Drug Deliv Rev **65**, 457–470 (2013). https://doi.org/10.1016/j.addr.2012.09.043
97. Barbeck, M., Booms, P., Unger, R., Hoffmann, V., Sader, R., Kirkpatrick, C.J., Ghanaati, S.: Multinucleated giant cells in the implant bed of bone substitutes are foreign body giant cells-New insights into the material-mediated healing process. J. Biomed. Mater. Res. A **105**, 1105–1111 (2017). https://doi.org/10.1002/jbm.a.36006
98. Nair, L.S., Laurencin, C.T.: Biodegradable polymers as biomaterials. Prog. Polym. Sci. **32**, 762–798 (2007). https://doi.org/10.1016/j.progpolymsci.2007.05.017
99. Santana, R.B., Miller, C.: Human intrabony defect regeneration with rhFGF-2 and hyaluronic acid—a randomized controlled clinical trial. Front. Bioeng. Biotechnol. **2** (2015). https://doi.org/10.1111/jcpe.12406
100. Lee, S.Y., Park, Y., Hwang, S.J.: Effect of bFGF and fibroblasts combined with hyaluronic acid-based hydrogels on soft tissue augmentation : an experimental study in rats. Maxillofac. Plast. Reconstr. Surg. 0 (2019)
101. Hickey, R.J., Pelling, A.E.: Cellulose biomaterials for. Tissue Eng. **7**, 1–15 (2019). https://doi.org/10.3389/fbioe.2019.00045
102. Miyamoto, T., Takahashi, S., Ito, H., Inagaki, H., Noishiki, Y.: Tissue biocompatibility of cellulose and its derivatives. J Biomed Mater Res **23**, 125–133 (1989). https://doi.org/10.1002/jbm.820230110

103. Yan, H., Jing, W., Fei, Y., Yingnan, S., Xiaoling, Z., Kerong, D.: Modification and evaluation of micro-nano structured porous bacterial cellulose scaffold for bone tissue engineering. Mater. Sci. Eng. C (2017). https://doi.org/10.1016/j.msec.2017.02.174
104. Venkatesan, J., Bhatnagar, I., Manivasagan, P., Kang, K., Kim, S.: Alginate composites for bone tissue engineering: a review. Int. J. Biol. Macromol. (2014). https://doi.org/10.1016/j.ijbiomac.2014.07.008
105. Hu, W.J., Eaton, J.W., Ugarova, T.P., Tang, L.: Molecular basis of biomaterial-mediated foreign body reactions. Blood **98**, 1231–1238 (2001). https://doi.org/10.1182/blood.v98.4.1231
106. Andrew, J.G., Andrew, S.M., Freemont, A.J., Marsh, D.R.: Inflammatory cells in normal human fracture healing. Acta. Orthop. Scand. **65**, 462–466 (1994). https://doi.org/10.3109/17453679408995493
107. Kalfas, I.H.: Principles of bone healing. Neurosurg. Focus. **10**, E1 (2001). https://doi.org/10.3171/foc.2001.10.4.2
108. Phillips, A.M.: Overview of the fracture healing cascade. Injury **36**(Suppl), S5-7 (2005). https://doi.org/10.1016/j.injury.2005.07.027
109. Little, N., Rogers, B., Flannery, M.: Bone formation, remodelling and healing. Surg **29**, 141–145 (2011). https://doi.org/10.1016/j.mpsur.2011.01.002
110. Schmidt-Bleek, K., Schell, H., Schulz, N., Hoff, P., Perka, C., Buttgereit, F., Volk, H.D., Lienau, J., Duda, G.N.: Inflammatory phase of bone healing initiates the regenerative healing cascade. Cell Tissue Res. **347**, 567–573 (2012). https://doi.org/10.1007/s00441-011-1205-7
111. Kolar, P., Schmidt-Bleek, K., Schell, H., Gaber, T., Toben, D., Schmidmaier, G., Perka, C., Buttgereit, F., Duda, G.N.: The early fracture hematoma and its potential role in fracture healing. Tissue Eng. Part B Rev. **16**, 427–434 (2010). https://doi.org/10.1089/ten.TEB.2009.0687
112. Bolander, M.E.: Regulation of fracture repair by growth factors. Proc. Soc. Exp. Biol. Med. **200**, 165–170 (1992). https://doi.org/10.3181/00379727-200-43410a
113. Vauhkonen, M., Peltonen, J., Karaharju, E., Aalto, K., Alitalo, I.: Collagen synthesis and mineralization in the early phase of distraction bone healing. Bone Min. **10**, 171–181 (1990). https://doi.org/10.1016/0169-6009(90)90260-m
114. Schlundt, C., El Khassawna, T., Serra, A., Dienelt, A., Wendler, S., Schell, H., van Rooijen, N., Radbruch, A., Lucius, R., Hartmann, S., et al.: Macrophages in bone fracture healing: their essential role in endochondral ossification. Bone **106**, 78–89 (2018). https://doi.org/10.1016/j.bone.2015.10.019
115. Remedios, A.: Bone and bone healing. Vet. Clin. North Am. Small. Anim. Pr. **29**, 1029–1044 (1999). https://doi.org/10.1016/s0195-5616(99)50101-0
116. Wu, A.C., Raggatt, L.J., Alexander, K.A., Pettit, A.R.: Unraveling macrophage contributions to bone repair. Bonekey Rep **2**, 373 (2013). https://doi.org/10.1038/bonekey.2013.107
117. Novosel, E.C., Kleinhans, C., Kluger, P.J.: Vascularization is the key challenge in tissue engineering. Adv. Drug. Deliv. Rev. **63**, 300–311 (2011). https://doi.org/10.1016/j.addr.2011.03.004
118. Almubarak, S., Nethercott, H., Freeberg, M., Beaudon, C., Jha, A., Jackson, W., Marcucio, R., Miclau, T., Healy, K., Bahney, C.: Tissue engineering strategies for promoting vascularized bone regeneration. Bone **83**, 197–209 (2016). https://doi.org/10.1016/j.bone.2015.11.011
119. Krishnan, L., Willett, N.J., Guldberg, R.E.: Vascularization strategies for bone regeneration. Ann. Biomed. Eng. **42**, 432–444 (2014). https://doi.org/10.1007/s10439-014-0969-9
120. Carano, R.A., Filvaroff, E.H.: Angiogenesis and bone repair. Drug. Discov. Today. **8**, 980–989 (2003). https://doi.org/10.1016/s1359-6446(03)02866-6
121. Keramaris, N.C., Calori, G.M., Nikolaou, V.S., Schemitsch, E.H., Giannoudis, P.: V Fracture vascularity and bone healing: a systematic review of the role of VEGF. Injury **39**(Suppl), S45-57 (2008). https://doi.org/10.1016/s0020-1383(08)70015-9
122. Anderson, J.M.: Mechanisms of inflammation and infection with implanted devices. Cardiovasc. Pathol. **2**, 33–41 (1993)

123. Ghanaati, S., Orth, C., Barbeck, M., Willershausen, I., Thimm, B.W., Booms, P., Stubinger, S., Landes, C., Sader, R.A., Kirkpatrick, C.J.: Histological and histomorphometrical analysis of a silica matrix embedded nanocrystalline hydroxyapatite bone substitute using the subcutaneous implantation model in Wistar rats. Biomed. Mater. **5**, 35005 (2010). https://doi.org/10.1088/1748-6041/5/3/035005
124. Ghanaati, S., Barbeck, M., Hilbig, U., Hoffmann, C., Unger, R.E., Sader, R.A., Peters, F., Kirkpatrick, C.J.: An injectable bone substitute composed of beta-tricalcium phosphate granules, methylcellulose and hyaluronic acid inhibits connective tissue influx into its implantation bed in vivo. Acta Biomater. **7**, 4018–4028 (2011). https://doi.org/10.1016/j.actbio.2011.07.003
125. Schaefer, S., Detsch, R., Uhl, F., Deisinger, U., Ziegler, G.: How degradation of calcium phosphate bone substitute materials is influenced by phase composition and porosity—Schaefer—2011—advanced engineering materials—Wiley online library. Adv. Eng. Mater. **13**, 342–350 (2011). https://doi.org/10.1002/adem.201000267
126. Hing, K.A.: Bioceramic bone graft substitutes: influence of porosity and chemistry—hing—international journal of applied ceramic technology—wiley online library. Appl. Ceram. Technol. **2005**(2), 84–199 (2005). https://doi.org/10.1111/j.1744-7402.2005.02020.x
127. Barbeck, M., Hoffmann, C., Sader, R., Peters, F., Hubner, W.D., Kirkpatrick, C.J., Ghanaati, S.: Injectable bone substitute based on beta-TCP combined with a hyaluronan-containing hydrogel contributes to regeneration of a critical bone size defect towards restitutio ad integrum. J. Oral. Implant. **42**, 127–137 (2016). https://doi.org/10.1563/aaid-joi-D-14-00203
128. Lorenz, J., Barbeck, M., Kirkpatrick, C.J., Sader, R., Lerner, H., Ghanaati, S.: Injectable bone substitute material on the basis of beta-TCP and hyaluronan achieves complete bone regeneration while undergoing nearly complete degradation. Int. J. Oral. Maxillofac Implant. **33**, 636–644 (2018). https://doi.org/10.11607/jomi.6026
129. Sieger, D., Korzinskas, T., Jung, O., Stojanovic, S.; Wenisch, S.; Smeets, R.; Gosau, M.; Schnettler, R., Najman, S., Barbeck, M.: The addition of high doses of hyaluronic acid to a biphasic bone substitute decreases the proinflammatory tissue response. Int. J. Mol. Sci. **20**, (2019). https://doi.org/10.3390/ijms20081969
130. Detsch, R., Schaefer, S., Deisinger, U., Ziegler, G., Seitz, H., Leukers, B.: In vitro: osteoclastic activity studies on surfaces of 3D printed calcium phosphate scaffolds. J. Biomater. Appl. **26**, 359–380 (2011). https://doi.org/10.1177/0885328210373285
131. Basle, M.F., Chappard, D., Grizon, F., Filmon, R., Delecrin, J., Daculsi, G., Rebel, A.: Osteoclastic resorption of Ca-P biomaterials implanted in rabbit bone. Calcif Tissue Int **53**, 348–356 (1993). https://doi.org/10.1007/bf01351842
132. Luttikhuizen, D.T., Harmsen, M.C., Van Luyn, M.J.: Cellular and molecular dynamics in the foreign body reaction. Tissue Eng. **12**, 1955–1970 (2006). https://doi.org/10.1089/ten.2006.12.1955
133. Ghanaati, S., Orth, C., Unger, R.E., Barbeck, M., Webber, M.J., Motta, A., Migliaresi, C., James Kirkpatrick, C.: Fine-tuning scaffolds for tissue regeneration: effects of formic acid processing on tissue reaction to silk fibroin. J. Tissue. Eng. Regen. Med. **4**, 464–472 (2010). https://doi.org/10.1002/term.257
134. Shen, Y., Redmond, S.L., Papadimitriou, J.M., Teh, B.M., Yan, S., Wang, Y., Atlas, M.D., Marano, R.J., Zheng, M., Dilley, R.J.: The biocompatibility of silk fibroin and acellular collagen scaffolds for tissue engineering in the ear. Biomed. Mater. **9**, 15015 (2014). https://doi.org/10.1088/1748-6041/9/1/015015
135. Stoppato, M., Stevens, H.Y., Carletti, E., Migliaresi, C., Motta, A., Guldberg, R.E.: Effects of silk fibroin fiber incorporation on mechanical properties, endothelial cell colonization and vascularization of PDLLA scaffolds. Biomaterials **34**, 4573–4581 (2013). https://doi.org/10.1016/j.biomaterials.2013.02.009
136. van Wachem, P.B., van Luyn, M.J., Nieuwenhuis, P., Koerten, H.K., Olde, L., Ten Hoopen, H., Feijen, J.: In vivo degradation of processed dermal sheep collagen evaluated with transmission electron microscopy. Biomaterials **12**, 215–223 (1991). https://doi.org/10.1016/0142-9612(91)90203-m

137. Ziats, N.P., Miller, K.M., Anderson, J.M.: In vitro and in vivo interactions of cells with biomaterials. Biomaterials **9**, 5–13 (1988). https://doi.org/10.1016/0142-9612(88)90063-4
138. Hernandez-Pando, R., Bornstein, Q.L., Aguilar Leon, D., Orozco, E.H., Madrigal, V.K., Martinez Cordero, E.: Inflammatory cytokine production by immunological and foreign body multinucleated giant cells. Immunology **100**, 352–358 (2000). https://doi.org/10.1046/j.1365-2567.2000.00025.x
139. Luttikhuizen, D.T., Dankers, P.Y., Harmsen, M.C., van Luyn, M.J.: Material dependent differences in inflammatory gene expression by giant cells during the foreign body reaction. J. Biomed. Mater Res. A **83**, 879–886 (2007). https://doi.org/10.1002/jbm.a.31420
140. Barbeck, M., Peric-Kacarevic, Z., Kavehei, F., Rider, P., Najman, S., Stojanovic, S., Rimashevskiy D., Wenisch, S., Schnettler, R.: The effect of temperature treatment of xenogeneic bone substitute on the tissue response–a mini review. Acta. Medica Median. **58**, 113–137 (2019)

Bioceramics in Orthopedic Surgery

Aleksandar Radunović, Ognjen Radunović, Maja Vulović, and Milan Aksić

Abstract Orthopedic surgery and traumatology is highly dependent on medical implants. Materials used in vivo must fulfill criteria as biocompatibility, ability to withstand mechanical load as well as chemical processes in organism. There is constant investigation of new materials and improving of existing ones, trying to achieve the ideal implant. Ceramics features as biocompatibility, inertness, smoothness make it very promising candidate for many orthopedic applications. At this moment majority of using of ceramics in orthopedic is for making bioactive coatings of the endoprosthesis surface achieving more rapid and stable fixation. Second is fabricating bearing surfaces from ceramics using it low friction coefficient, bioinertness and wettability properties. There are few generation of ceramics designed to improve its properties and lower the incidence of complication and failure. Majority of this occurs due to brittleness of ceramic implants. New generations show rapid decrease on incidence of complications and higher survival rates of implants. More improvements in ceramics are performed in order to lower the incidence of fractures.

Keywords Bioceramics · Implants · Orthopedic surgery

A. Radunović (✉)
Clinic for Orthopedic Surgery and Traumatology, Military Medical Academy, 11000 Belgrade, Serbia
e-mail: aradunovic@yahoo.com

O. Radunović
Faculty of Medicine, University of Belgrade, Dr Subotića 8, 11000 Belgrade, Serbia

M. Vulović
Department of Anatomy and Forensic Medicine, Faculty of Medical Sciences, University of Kragujevac, Kragujevac, Serbia

M. Aksić
Institute of Anatomy "Niko Miljanić", Faculty of Medicine, University of Belgrade, Dr Subotića 8, 11000 Belgrade, Serbia

S. Najman et al. (eds.), *Bioceramics, Biomimetic and Other Compatible Materials Features for Medical Applications*, Engineering Materials,
https://doi.org/10.1007/978-3-031-17269-4_3

1 Introduction

Orthopedic surgery and traumatology are probably part of medicine science that mostly relies on biomaterials for successful performing. It stands for osteosynthetic material used for trauma management as well as artificial joints and tissue substitutes. During past few decades there was a significant improvement in biomaterials used in orthopedic surgery including bioceramics. All those have prefix "bio" meaning intention of this implants to fulfill some special requirements desired for ideal implant.

- Biocompatibility—The term refers to the ability of a material to perform with an appropriate host response in a specific situation [1]. It is expected that any material implanted in organism will produce tissue reaction to a certain extent but it is important this changes doesn't jeopardize functionality and survival of the implant, as well as not to produce systemic immune response.
- Mechanical properties—implant is expected to have satisfactory mechanical and physical properties for successful replacement of nature tissue. This means as good as it possible balance of hardness, elasticity, yield stress, fatigue resistance, wear resistance, depending of implant type and purpose.
- Fabrication—it is expected for implants to be fabricated routinely, with consistent reproducibility, with capability of material to undergo sterilization process without affecting its properties. Frequently it's demanded to combine several materials in different parts of implant to achieve good function, so it is necessary to have materials that allows those combination.

At this moment, most frequently used materials in orthopedic surgery are metals, polymers and ceramics. Every single has its limitations and advantages that leads to further investigations searching ideal material or combination of materials, capable of fully mimicking bone tissue. Analyzing past decades of biomaterials research and engineering, classification can be made as following:

1. First generation—Bioinert materials
   Those materials were expected to have sufficient mechanical and physical properties without immune response and emitting toxic products.
2. Second generation—Bioactive and biodegradable materials
   Beginning of era of development of bioactive materials is since 1980. Those materials have additional feature of interacting with local tissue in order to produce response that will enhance the function of implant.
3. Third generation—Bioabsorbable materials
   More advances in bioengineering lead to materials able to stimulate cellular response at molecular level. Terms bioactivity and bioresorptivity should not be considered separately as they are often combined in materials to achieve better results. These tree also should not be observed as purely chronological classification, but more as conceptual as each generation denotes an evolution of the requirements and behavior of material [2].

2 Ceramics in Orthopedics and Traumatology

2.1 Basics of Bone Structure

Bone is natural composite material consisting of cells and bone matrix. Cells of bone tissue are: osteocytes, osteoclasts and osteoblasts. Osteoclasts are engaged in process of bone resorption. Osteoblasts synthetise bone matrix and have role in mineralization. Bone matrix consists of approximately 35% of organic matter (majority is type I collagen, and also proteoglycanes, matrix proteins, cytokinesand high stability. Alumina and growth factors) and 65% of inorganic matter (calcium phosphate in form of calcium hydroxyapatite, calcium carbonate, magnesium).

2.2 Ceramics

Increased interest in ceramics as biomaterial for orthopedic use started in 1960's. Initial use of ceramics was as alternative to metals to increase biocompatibility and avoid problems that occurred during use of purely metal components (inadequate integration, emission of toxic ions etc.).

Ceramics are defined as non-metallic inorganic materials and may have wide range of composition. According to their interaction with host bone they can be classified as in Fig. 1.

This classification is based upon interaction of ceramic material and local tissue.

Table 1 shows tissue response according to a type of implanted material.

Bioceramics used in orthopedics have to carry out some requirements:

1. Non-toxicity
2. Non-carcinogenic
3. Non-allergic
4. Non-inflammatory
5. Biocompatibility
6. Biofunctionality [3]

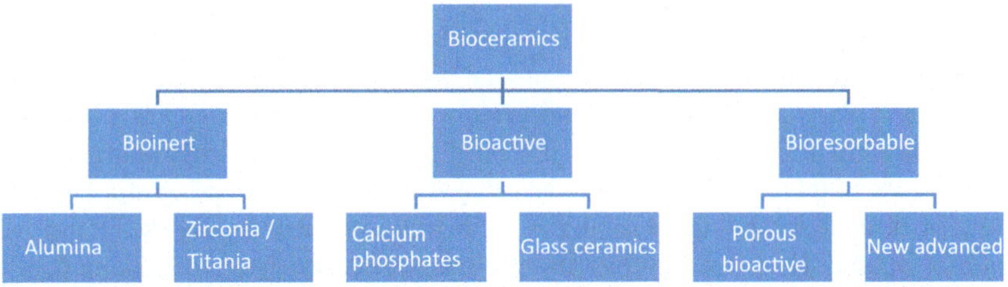

Fig. 1 Classification of bioceramics

Table 1 Response of tissue to different types of biomaterials

Type of ceramics	Local tissue reaction
Toxic	Death of surrounding tissue
Bioinert	Formation of fibrous tissue around implant
Bioactive	Formation of interfacial bond
Bioresorbable (biodegradable)	Replacement by surrounding tissue

There are certain properties of the material that strongly influence possibility of their biomedical application:

- Bioactivity—Ability of material to interact with host tissue
- Biodegradability—It is feature of material to be decomposed by biological processes in host tissue.
- Biocompatibility—usually is defined as ability of material to perform with an appropriate host response in specific application
- Physicochemical properties—including not only purely mechanical features of bulk implant (hardness, brittleness, elasticity, wear resistance) but also physicochemical properties of implant that produce favorable tissue response
- Osteoinductivity/Osteoconductivity—Osteoinductivity is capability of material to engage and induce undifferentiated cells or progenitor cells toward differentiation into osteoblasts. Osteoconduction is process by which bone is directed so as to conform to a material‘s surface.
- Porosity—capability of porosity along with pore distribution and size are pertinent parameters determining mechanical properties and biocompatibility. Porosity allows blood host blood vessels and surrounding bone ingrowth in implant and consequential deposition of cells.

At this moment, ceramics routinely used and fabricated are alumina and zirconia, calcium phosphate and bioactive glass.

Zirconia is metal dioxide of Zirconium (ZrO_2). It is suitable for using as biomaterial due to bioinertness and in orthopedic surgery for good mechanical features such as low wear and high stability. Alumina (Al_2O_3) is used in orthopedic surgery for more than 25 years, mostly for it manage to combine some excellent properties needed in this type of surgery: very low coefficient of friction, low wear rate, corrosion resistance. Zirconia has some advantages compared to alumina: lower Young modulus, higher tension resistance and higher fracture toughness. Thus, zirconia was designed for use as a bearing surface in total hip endoprosthesis.

Calcium phosphate (CaP) is the most frequently used bioceramics. It is produced by mixing calcium and phosphate in either acid or alkaline environment. Only compounds of this 2 with Ca/P ratio less than 1 are suitable for using as a biomaterial, because others are highly soluble. Calcium phosphate is usually used in form of hydroxyapatite (HA), due to similarity of synthetized HA to inorganic component of bone matrix. There are many forms of calcium phosphates but only few are used in orthopedic surgery due to its variability in solubility and toughness as well as ease of manufacturing: dicalcium phosphate dehydrate, dicalcium phosphate anhydrate, α and β tricalcium phosphate. Calcium phosphate based ceramics wield osteoconductive and osteoinductive attributes. There are some differences of various CaP regarding osteoconductivy/osteoinductivity and those are due to their physical and chemical properties. Roughness of materials used for covering implant surface can promote cells adhesion and protein adhesion too.

Bioglasses are specially designed materials consisting Na_2O–CaO–SiO_2 with P_2O_5, B_2O_3 and CaF_2 added. To enhance adhesion on the surface of this materials hydroxycalcium apatite layer is added. Possibility of adhesion is most important advantage if bioglasses, especially when using special procedures, it is possible to achieve adhesions even with soft tissue.

There are few principle aims of using ceramics in orthopedics:

- As a replacement for tissue
- For surface covering, making a layer that promotes osteointegration of the implant (mostly used in arthroplasties)
- As the bearing surface in joint arthroplasty

First Generation of Ceramics We already mentioned classification of biomaterials by different generations. First generation of ceramic biomaterials are alumina, zirconia and similar ceramics. At that time only limited number of formulations were available as well as porosity, purity and grain size of materials. All those lead to limits in biological, chemical and physical properties of first generation of ceramics. Nevertheless some of first generation ceramics are still widely used. Alumina has frequent use in orthopedic surgery mainly due to its good low friction and wear rate. Zirconia is still one of the strongest ceramics and is sometimes called steel ceramic, which make it very desirable for use in orthopedic surgery, especially for indications demanding high loads and repetitive movements (zirconia wear is less than 0.1 mm^3/million cycles).

Second Generation of Ceramics This generations was announced by research of bioactive materials at early 1980s. Ability of second generation materials to interact with surrounding tissue, producing biological response and promote rapid and stronger bonding of implant. Degradation of materials is mentioned as another important feature of second generation. Calcium phosphate in different variations is ceramics that represents second generation of biomaterials with those desirable features. Of course, due to its characteristics, it is used in specific orthopedic applications, with low demand for high load resistance and repetitive wear stresses.

Third Generation of Ceramics Those are materials capable of producing stimulation of the cellular response in molecular level. Deeper understanding of structure and improved manufacturing made possible combination of bioactivity and biodegradability. Materials belonging to this generation are often referred as biomimetic. Ceramic materials of this generations are mostly used for manufacturing ceramic or hybrid scaffolds.

2.3 Ceramics in Joint Arthroplasties

Total hip and knee arthroplasties are surgical procedures proven to hugely improve quality of life for majority of patients. Major indication for joint replacement is arthrosis—destruction of joint cartilage and consequential changes in surrounding tissues. All those leads to pain and loss of function of involved joint. There is a number of causes of arthritic changes in joints and according to them we can classify this as:

1. Primary arthrosis (idiopathic)—without known cause, but factors that probably influence occurrence are: overweight, hard labor, repetitive stresses, genetics, etc.
2. Secondary arthrosis—after intraarticular fracture, due to rheumatoid arthritis, systemic lupus, congenital and developmental abnormalities

Joint arthroplasty is performed by removing damaged cartilage tissue and replacing it with components of endoprosthesis. Different forms of arthroplasties are performed since the end of the 19 century, with huge number of failures in the beginning, mostly caused by lack of materials that will withstand repetitive stresses and have good biocompatibility. Aiming to make ideal implant, there was a great engineering effort to design new materials and implant geometries. At this moment there are following materials used in modern arthroplasties:

1. Metals and its alloys
2. Polyethylene
3. Ceramics
4. Polymethylmetacrilat (PMMA)
5. Hydroxyapatite coatings

All of this materials are required to have excellent biocompatibility and to perform with an appropriate host response in specific application. They also have to be non-allergenic, non-toxic and non-carcinogenic. For some applications it is desirable feature of the implant to have possibility of positive interaction with host tissue, promoting osteointegration of the implant.

They are also required having certain mechanical features: high compression, bending and torsional strength, wear resistance, fracture toughness, fatigue resistance during cyclic loading [4].

Metals and Alloys Mostly used in contemporary arthroplasties are Cobalt chrome (CoCr), Cobalt chrome Molybdene (CoCrMo), and Titanium (Ti) and its alloys ($Ti_6Al_{14}V$). Stainless steel is very rarely used in modern arthroplasties, mostly for its low biocompatibility.

Cobalt chrome and alloys have excellent strength, wear and corrosion characteristics, making them one of the most used materials for implants fabricating. They are mostly used for fabricating cemented femoral stems in hip arthroplasty (having better Young modulus comparing to titanium alloys) and for manufacturing of articulating heads (due to low friction coefficient).

Titanium and alloys are mostly used for manufacturing cementless femoral stems and acetabular components. Properties made them good choice for this purpose are: high mechanical strength, excellent corrosion resistance and biocompatibility [5].

Discussing using of metals in joint implants, we should mention some surface modifications of the metal implants, made to achieve more effective and rapid osteointegration. Titanium and tantalum are convenient for producing porous surfaces, making them more used in modern implant designs compared to other metals.

There are some problems arising from using metals as a materials for endoprosthesis. Metal implants have very high elastic modulus compared to a bone. Most of the load postoperatively is carried by the implant due to its higher stiffness and bone is left without adequate stress that is desirable for maintaining structural integrity and morphology of the bone. This phenomenon is known as a stress shielding, causing bone resorption and possible implant loosening.

Hydoxiapatite Coatings We already mentioned HA as a natural mineral, very similar to inorganic component of bone matrix. HA is ceramic with excellent biocompatibility, with slow resorption without emitting toxic materials. HA coatings on metallic implants in cementless joint arthroplasties enables direct strong bonding of the implant and bone in order to achieve stable fixation.

Polyethylene Polyethylene (PE) has been used in joint replacements for more than 50 years, and still is most widely used as articular surface as metal on polyethylene (MoP) articulation. PE is biologically inert material with low, but variable wear resistance that can be influenced by many factors as: type of sterilization, material used for articulation coupled with PE, etc. During PE wear debris is produced, which is proven to be responsible for osteolysis around implant component and loosening. Those induced research for PE with lower wear rates, improving it by creating cross-linked ultra-high molecular weight PE (UHMWPE) including addition of E vitamin to reduce oxidative stress damage. UHMWPE is one of the mostly used polymers as an orthopedic implant due to its high mechanical strength and biocompatibility [6]. Despite all modifications, wear debris is major concern using PE as bearing surface. New improvement is achieved producing X_3PE that is sequentially irradiated and annealed. This PE shows decreasing of wear rate up to 97% comparing to UHMWPE and also oxidation resistance with minimal free radicals emission and no delamination process [4].

Polymethylmethacrylate (PMMA) PMMA based bone cement is used for fixation of cemented components for joint arthroplasty, filling gap between implant and host bone. This forms interface that transfer forces from implant to bone and vice versa. PMMA bone cement is a two component system: polymer powder and monomer (methylmetacrilate) liquid are mixed together at the operating theater just before use.

Ceramics as Bearing Surfaces in Joint Arthroplasties Properties of ideal bearing surfaces:

- Biocompatibility
- Low coefficient of friction
- Small volume of wear particle generation

- Low tissue reaction to wear particles
- High resistance on third body wear
- Corrosion resistance in synovial fluid
- Shock absorber capacity

In hip arthroplasty there are several possible bearing couple combinations available:

- Polyethylene acetabulum- metallic femoral head (MoP)
- Polyethylene acetabulum- ceramic femoral head (CoP)
- Ceramic acetabulum- Ceramic femoral head (CoC)
- Metallic acetabulum- metallic femoral head (MoM)
- Metallic acetabulum- Ceramic femoral head

In knee arthroplasty, metal on polyethylene bearing couple is the most dominant option, although ceramic on polyethylene option is under reevaluation.

Metal on Highly Crosslinked Polyethylene Over the last five decades, the most widely used bearing surface couple in artificial hip joints is cobalt chrome femoral head articulating with a UHMWPE acetabular component achieving excellent long term results. This bearing surface couple remains the standard to which wear testing for other bearing articulations are compared.

UHMWPE was first used as a bearing surface for producing acetabulums since 1958. Several long chains of monomer ethylene constitute this polymer. The major issue of combining UHMWPE with metallic femoral heads was early wear which is related to following factors: sterilization, material properties, implant geometry and limited shelf life. The wear particles generated by metal on UHMWPE articulation cause a chronic inflammatory response to a foreign body which is mediated by macrophages with release of lytic enzymes, bone resorbing mediators and pro-inflammatory cytokines. This response ultimately leads to osteolysis in periprosthetic bone, causing fixation failure and aseptic loosening [7].

Metal on Metal Bearings Birmingham hip replacement was designed as a procedure with great expectations but high failure rates are an accepted fact. Anticipated advantages of MoM bearings are low wear, toughness, possibility of using very large heads, enabling stability and possibility of resurfacing procedures with bone sparing. The controversy remains about whether the cause of failure was poor component positioning, implant design or a combination of both.

Higher blood levels of cobalt and chromium that proven occurs, are arising concerns about intoxication effects of metallic ions and even increased cancer risk as well as occurrence of pseudotumors (named aseptic lymphocyte dominated vasculitis associated lesions-ALVAL). There was also some concerns about metal sensitivity caused by increase of metal ion levels in blood. New generations of MoM bearings applied in resurfacing hip arthroplasties are showing less problems and lower failure rates compared to older designs but different problems connected with emission of metallic ions are still noted. Majority of authors conclude there are no evidence for supporting MoM bearings as there is worrying increase in osteolysis, local soft tissue reactions, tissue and bone necrosis. There are also numerous reports showing significant affection of remote organs caused by toxicity of metallic ions [8].

Ceramic on Ceramic Bearings In the late 60s, CoC bearings were first introduced in total hip arthroplasty by Boutin as alternative bearing combination in order to improve wear characteristics and decrease rate of aseptic loosening. Those were made of pure alumina and were processed from industrial grade materials, resulting in impure alumina compared to modern ceramics. First generation of ceramics showed many problems including high failure rate, fractures, high wear rate. Second generation of ceramics was produced by adding molecules of calcium and magnesium oxide to reduce the grain size. Third generation of ceramics underwent additional changes in manufacturing in order to additionally minimize grain size with BIOLOX forte as example. Nascency of third generation of ceramics has hugely reduced the failure rate of fracture. Latest, fourth generation of ceramics is known as alumina matrix composite material. Major portion of material is alumina with nanosized, yttria stabilized zirconia particles stabilized in tetragonal phase within alumina. When fissures appear, zirconia undergoes phase change, increases volume and absorbs the energy of fissure. A small amount (<1%) of chromium oxide is added for hardening of ceramics weakened by adding of zirconia [9].

Properties of Ceramics as Bearing Surface

- Ceramics are very hard: on MOHS hardness scale current alumina products are classed 9 (diamond is classed 10). Ceramic hardness is measured in 3 ways. Scratch hardness is measured by the force needed to cut material. Indentation hardness is measured by the force required to cause plastic deformation. Rebound hardness is related to elasticity.
- Current bioceramics have fivefold lower fracture rate compared to former generation
- Ceramic surfaces are inert due to their stable molecular structure.
- They are lower density compared to metal so they weight less
- Can be polished to much lower surface roughness then other materials
- Have excellent resistance to third body wear and abrasions
- Very low debris generation (particle size 5–90 nm, mean 24 nm)
- Good tissue tolerance to particles
  - Weak inflammatory cascade
  - Small number of phagocytes
  - Minimal or nonexisting osteolysis
- Highly wettable. Ceramic surface allows bonding of hydrogen, creating a lubrication film that lower friction hugely.
- Low wear rate. Actual MoP bearing couples have wear rates of 0.137 mm/year. MoM wear rate is 0.005 mm/year while contemporary ceramics wear rate is 0.001–0.007 mm/year [10].

Though the ceramics are the new preferred bearing surface, especially for the young patients, they are not without their share of complications including squeaking noises, stripe wear, a rare bearing surface fracture or chipping during insertion

[11]. Complications have been more commonly associated with acetabular component malposition (verticalized cups), smaller femoral heads and non-adherence to meticulous surgical technique.

Technical Difficulties Titanium shell can deform up to 0.16 mm diametrically during cementless impaction, especially during impaction in good quality bone and press fit impaction (when impacted acetabular component is one size bigger compared to last used reamer). This can cause difficulties for insertion of ceramic liners as well as chipping of the liner during insertion. It was reported that failure to impact liner with sufficient force during assembly may also contribute to canting and dissociation.

Fractures All bearing surfaces and couples have the risk of possible fracture, but in ceramic on ceramic coupling the risk is highest. Modern generations of ceramics have much lower fracture rate compared to old ones, with some studies shown none fracture in 3 year follow up [12]. There are known factors that potentially favorize fracture: trauma, overweight, excessive physical activity, manufacturing process errors. Even when fracture occurs, majority of them are due to improper positioning of implant and consequential inadequate stress dispersion.

Dislocation There are no papers showing that ceramic on ceramic articulations can cause some material specific problems with dislocation of endoprosthesis. There are some generally known factors that increase incidence of dislocation and its good for some of them to be mentioned for future work on ceramic properties.

One of the major causes for hip dislocation is misorientation of endoprothesis components. It is necessary to have this in mind when planning new designs of components in future, allowing surgeon to have possibility of easy handling components in order to position them precisely.

It is also known for a long time that bigger femoral head diameter means bigger range of motion, prevention of impingement and lower rate of dislocations. For a long time, due to inadequate properties of ceramic, it was impossible to have large diameter ceramic heads. With new ceramic materials femoral heads in 36 mm diameters are widely available.

Squeaking Reported incidence of squeaking is 0–21%. It has received much attention but it doesn't decrease functionality of artificial joint and can be avoided by modification of activity [13]. Etiology of squeaking is not quite clear. As natural frequency of ceramics is above human threshold, there must be factors bringing it in audible range: insufficient lubrication, endoprosthesis design etc. Clinical investigations noticed connection of squeaking with few factors: patient characteristics, surgical technique and endoprosthesis design. Heavier and more active patients are at increased risk of squeaking due to increased mechanical load of implant. If components are positioned in manner that produces impidgement squeaking may occur. Finally, it is showed that some designs of implant have significantly more squeaking occurrence compared to other [14]. Some found that patients with smaller neck geometry are more likely to have this complication. Other authors found mismatch of components as cause of squeaking, others suggest changes of femoral head as possible cause for sound effect, while others think that lack of lubrication is causing this complication [15–18]. Having above mentioned in mind, it is most likely that

Table 2 Wear rates for different articulation couples

Femoral head	Acetabular liner	Wear rate (mm/year)
Third generation ceramic	UHMWP	0.11
Second generation metal	UHMWP	0.085
Second generation metal	Metal	0.0063
Third generation ceramic	Ceramic	0.004

squeaking is phenomenon with multiple causes and combination of implant, patient and surgery factors.

Ceramic on Crosslinked Polyethylene Use of ceramic head on HCLUHMWPE liners is gradually gaining wider acceptance, though it is still not very widely used. Clinical as well as laboratory data have shown that wear rates for CoP bearings are significantly lesser compared with MoP with studies showing 10–50% lesser wear (Table 2).

Various advantages of ceramic femoral heads over metal femoral heads articulating with crosslinked polyethylene are as follows:

1. The polished surface of ceramics have much lesser coefficient of friction as compared to metal
2. Better joint lubrication is achieved with use of ceramics
3. Metal ions are released from metal femoral heads causing oxidation and surface roughening whereas ceramics are chemically inert with no such issues
4. Ceramic heads have lower susceptibility to surface scratching

Future Directions

- Ceramic femoral head articulating with metal acetabular component. Its first described by Firkins et al. and likely advantage of this bearing combination is lower wear and generation of much lesser metal particles. It also allows use of larger ceramic heads, reducing the risk of ceramic fracture and increasing the number of femoral head opteions. Clinical studies are evaluating performance of this bearing coupling at selected centers
- Oxinium: oxidized zirconium has been developed and is in clinical usage for femoral heads for less than a decade. It is expected to provide wear resistance of ceramic without its fracture risk. However, long term clinical results are yet to prove its advantages.
- Silicone nitride bearings: ceramic (alumina/zirconium) fractures have remained a concern in ceramic bearings. An alternative bearing surface is being explored manufactured from powder of silicone nitride (Si_3Ni_4). This alternative ceramic has been used successfully in aerospace bearings as well as diesel engines. Silicone nitride pairings have a friction coefficient of 0.001 compared to 0.08 for Al_2O_3–Al_2O_3 pairings. Mechanical testing has shown higher fracture toughness, higher flexural strength and higher resistance to hydrothermal degradation. Biocompatibility tests have shown that silicone nitride does not produce any adverse reactions behaving similar to alumina. Clinical trials are currently underway and results of

same would decide clinical applicability and availability of this new alternative ceramic in the future. Clinical results have confirmed higher survivorship, lesser wear and low osteolysis producing, making this bearings excellent choice for young and active individuals.

- Alumina matrix composite: alumina has some very desirable properties such as: biocompatibility, low wear rate. In order to reach the growing requirements in orthopedic surgery alumina matrix composite was developed. In some commercially available products there is combination of alumina matrix and zirconia. Special methods of fabrication and chemical arrangements makes prevention of occurrence and propagation of cracks in this modern ceramics. Also some chromium oxide and strontium crystals are added to improve wear characteristics, hardness and toughness. Comparing this type of ceramics with old ones in movement simulator found extreme lowering in wear rate (from 1.84 mm^3 to 0.16 mm^3/million cycles) [19].

References

1. Black, J.: Biological Performance of Materials. ISBN 0-8493-3959-6 (2006)
2. Victor, S.P., Muthu, J.: Polymer ceramic composite materials for orthopedic applications—relevance and need for mechanical match and bone regeneration. J. Mechatronic **2**, 1–10 (2014). https://doi.org/10.1166/jom.2014.1030
3. Park, J.B., Bronzino, J.D. (eds.): Biomaterials Principles and Applications. CRC Press, Boca Raton (2003)
4. Nag, S., Banerjee, R.: Fundamentals of Medical Implant Materials. ASM Handbook, p. 23 (2012)
5. Head, W.C., Bauk, D.J., Emerson, R.H., Jr.: Titanium as the material of choice for cementless femoral components in total hip arthroplasty. Clin. Orthop. Relat. Res. **311**, 85–90 (1995)
6. Hosseinzadeh, H.R.S., Eajazi A., Shahi, A.S.: The bearing surfaces in total hip arthroplasty – options, material characteristics and selection. In: Fokter, S. (ed.), Recent Advances in Arthroplasty. ISBN: 978-953-307-990-5. InTech (2012)
7. Patel, S., Hossain, F.S., Haddad, F.S.: Bearing surfaces in lower limb total joint arthroplasty. In: British Editorial Society of Bone and Joint Surgery (2010)
8. Crawford, R., Ranawat, C.S., Rothman, R.H.: Metal on metal: is it worth a risk? J. Arthroplasty **25**(1), 1–2 (2010)
9. Masson, B.: Emergence of the alumina matrix composite in total hip arthroplasty. Int. Orthop. **33**(2), 359–363 (2009)
10. Higuchi, Y., Hasegawa, Y., Seki, T., Komatsu, D., Ishiguro, N.: Significantly lower wear of ceramic-on-ceramic bearings than metal-on-highly cross-linked polyethylene bearings: a 10- to 14-year follow-up study. J. Arthroplasty **31**(6), 1246–1250 (2016)
11. Scholes, S.C., Joyce, T.J.: Ceramic on ceramic joints: a suitable alternative material combination? In: Advances in Biomaterials Science and Biomedical Applications. Scholes and Joyce; InTech (2013)
12. Garino, J.P.: Modern ceramic-on-ceramic total hip systems in the United States: early results. Clin. Orthop. Relat. Res. **379**, 41–47 (2000)
13. Walter, W.L., O'Toole, G.C., Walter, W.K., Ellis, A., Zicat, B.A.: Squeaking in ceramic-onceramic hips: the importance of acetabular component orientation. J. Arthroplasty **22**, 496–503 (2007)

14. Parvizi, J., Bahar, A., Wong, J.C., Restrepo, C., Rothman, R.H.: A squeaky reputation: the problem may be design-dependant. Clin. Orthop. Relat. Res. **469**, 1589–1605 (2011)
15. Nevelos, J.E., Prudhommeaux, F., Hamadouche, M., et al.: Comparative analysis of two different types ofalumina-alumina hip prosthesis retrieved for asepticloosening. J. Bone Joint Surg. Br. **83**, 598–603 (2001)
16. Taylor, S., Manley, M.T., Sutton, K.: The role of stripe wearin causing acoustic emissions from alumina ceramicon-ceramic bearings. J. Arthroplasty **22**, 47–51 (2007)
17. Stewart, T.D., Tipper, J.L., Insley, G., et al.: Severe wear andfracture of zirconia heads against alumina inserts inhip simulator studies with microseparation. J. Arthroplasty **18**, 726–734 (2003)
18. White, S.P., Blom, A.W., Lee, M., et al.: The crescent sign:dissociation of the polyethylene liner from a modularacetabular component in total hip arthroplasty. Skeletal. Radiol. **34**, 620–624 (2005)
19. Streicher, R.M., Semlitsch, M., Schön, R., et al.: Metal-on metal articulation for artificial hip joints: laboratory study and clinical results. Proc. Inst. Mech. Eng. H. **210**, 223–232 (1996)

Materials in Biomedical Applications

Copper(II)-Loaded Polyphosphazenes as a Novel Detoxicant for Sarin

Jih Ru Hwu, Shui-Sheng Shiao, Ke-Yung King, Kuan-Miao Liu, Shwu-Chen Tsay, Wen-Chieh Huang, Chun-Shie Lin, Jen Luan Chen, Goran Lazović, and Vojislav Mitić

Abstract New copper(II)-loaded bifunctional phophazenes were developed for the hydrolysis of chemical warfare agents for nerve, such as notorious sarin. Synthesis of these target random copolyphosphazenes containing moieties of glycerol, *N*,*N*,*N′*-trimethyl-*N′*-(6-hydroxyhexyl)ethylenediamine, and Cu(II) was accomplished in seven steps. *p*-Nitrophenyl diphenylphosphate as a nerve-agent simulate of sarin was rapidly hydrolyzed by these copolyphosphazene complexes. Their skeleton underwent hydrolysis in aqueous media at 25 °C to yield glycerol, diamine, phosphoric acid, and ammonia. The self-degradability characteristic of the new copolymers is desirable in view of environmental protection.

Keyword Phosphazene copper(II) · Copolymer · Detoxicant · Sarin

1 Introduction

The sarin gas attacked the civilians in the Tokyo underground railway on 20 March 1995. This event grabbed the front pages of newspapers and horrified the world [1, 2]. Ten people were killed and more than 5000 were injured. Sarin (**1a**) was developed as a chemical weapon by the Nazis during the World War II although it was not used. Sarin has since been manufactured and stockpiled by many countries. Iraq used it

J. R. Hwu (✉) · S.-S. Shiao · K.-Y. King · K.-M. Liu · S.-C. Tsay · W.-C. Huang
Department of Chemistry, National Tsing Hua University, Hsinchu 300044, Taiwan
e-mail: jrhwu@mx.nthu.edu.tw

C.-S. Lin · J. L. Chen
Chemical System Research Division, National Chung-Shan Institute of Science and Technology, Taoyuan 325, Taiwan

G. Lazović
Faculty of Mechanical Engineering, University of Belgrade, Belgrade, Serbia

V. Mitić (Deceased)
Faculty of Electronic Engineering, University of Niš, Niš, Serbia

Institute of Technical Sciences of the Serbian Academy of Science and Arts, Belgrade, Serbia

S. Najman et al. (eds.), *Bioceramics, Biomimetic and Other Compatible Materials Features for Medical Applications*, Engineering Materials,
https://doi.org/10.1007/978-3-031-17269-4_4

against the Kurds in 1988 [2]. The main class of nerve agents used in chemical warfare belongs to toxic organophosphorous compounds represented by the structure **1**, in which R^1 and R^2 = OR, NR_2, or alkyl group; and X = leaving group, such as F and *p*-$OPhNO_2$ [3]. The ability of these organophosphorous compounds **1a–e** (i.e., sarin, soman, DFP, tabun, and VX) to inhibit enzymes (e.g., acetylcholinesterase) and thus to disrupt neurological function, forms their basic activities as chemical warfare agents. A number of studies have been undertaken to address the detoxification problems of such compounds [4–11]. As the awareness to protect the environment is greatly growing, it has become a necessity to develop new methods for the synthesis of degradable materials [12] to be used in warfare.

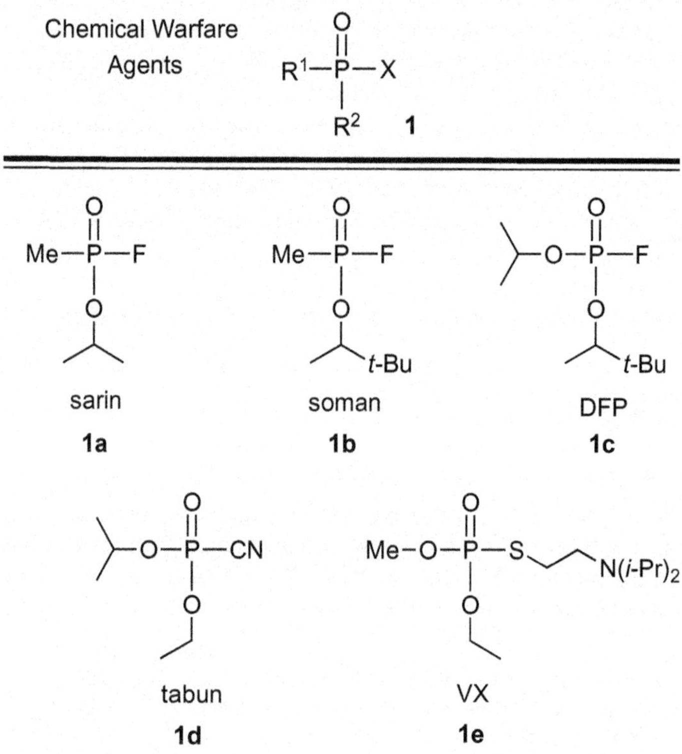

We report herein an unprecedented kind of copper (II)-loaded copolyphosphazenes **2**. The polymers were found to possess the capability of decomposing toxic organophosphorous nerve-agents. After acting as a detoxicant, the water-soluble random copolymers **2** gradually underwent hydrolytic breakdown in aqueous media.

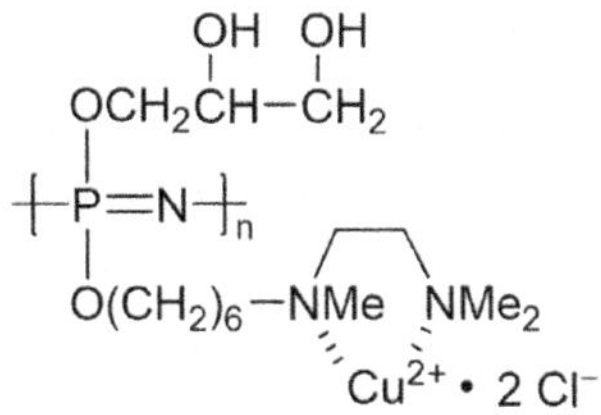

2

Design Menger et al. [10] reported that the copper complex of *N,N,N′*-trimethylethylenediamine group linked to a polystyrene moiety via a six-carbon spacer can render nerve-agent simulates inactive through catalytic hydrolysis. The polymers are implanted with copper on account of its ability to catalyze the hydrolysis of phosphorous (V) compounds [13]. The spacer is needed to provide the substrates a better access to the catalytic sites. One critical disadvantage associated with these polymers is their non-degradability. Polyphosphazenes containing ether or amino side chains were shown to be degradable [14, 15]. Accordingly, we designed and synthesized self-degradable copper-loaded random copolyphosphazenes **2** as nerve-agent detoxicants. Commercially available cyclic trimer **3**, *N,N,N′*-trimethylethylenediamine, and glycerol were used as the starting materials. Copper complex of *N,N,N′*-trimethylethylenediamine group was linked to the linear polydichlorophosphazene skeleton via a six-carbon spacer. Glyceryl units therein were added to increase the water solubility of copolymers **2**. Thus these new polymers could undergo hydrolytic breakdown in aqueous media to the innocuous glycerol and phosphoric acid with the concurrent release of ammonia [14].

2 Results and Discussion

Synthesis of the main-chain (Scheme 1) Linear polydichlorophosphazenes **4** were prepared by thermal polymerization of the cyclic trimer **3**. In the beginning, the process developed by Allcock [16–18] was applied and compound **3** was polymerized at 250 °C in a Pyrex combustion tube that was sealed under reduced pressure. Polyphosphazenes **4** were obtained in a relatively low yield (42%) although they had high molecular weights ($M_w \cong 2.1 \times 10^6$). Looking for a method to provide the desired polymers in a higher yield, we applied the Sennett's method [19] by using BCl_3 as a catalyst. Accordingly, polymers **4** were produced in 65% yield with $M_w \cong 1.0 \times 10^5$. Finally, use of S_8 as the catalyst, reported by Newman and Renoll, at 285 °C for 6.0 h led the monomer **3** to the desired polymers **4** in 81% with molecular weights $M_w = 3.8 \times 10^4$.

Synthesis of homopolyphosphazenes 6 with isopropylidene glycerol moieties in the side-chain (Scheme 2) Two of the three hydroxyl groups in glycerol were protected to prevent the possible cross-linking during the polymer preparation. Thus protection of glycerol with acetone was performed to give isopropylidene glycerol **5**

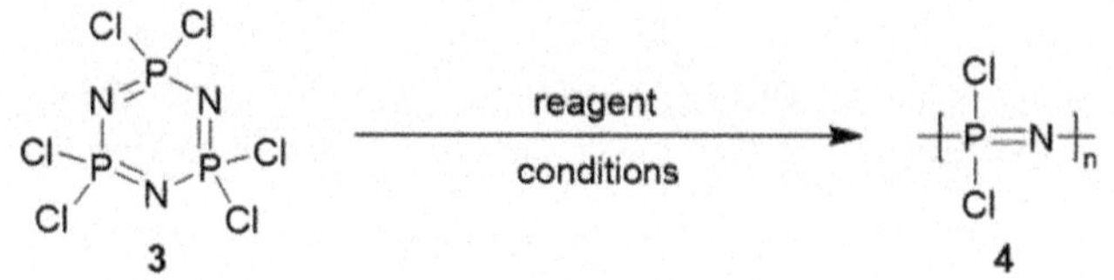

method		yield (%)	Mw
(a) Allcock	sealed combustion tube, 250 °C	42	2.1×10^6
(b) Sennett	BCl_3, 250 °C, 24 h	65	1.0×10^5
(c) Newman & Renoll	S_8, 285 °C, 6.0 h	81	3.8×10^4

Scheme 1 Three methods used for the preparation of polyphosphazenes **4**

(94% yield) [20]. Reaction of this protected glycerol **5** (2.2 equiv) with polymers **4** in the presence of NaH(s) (2.2 equiv) afforded the glycerol-containing homopolyphosphazenes **6** in 81% yield. The infrared spectrum revealed a P=N functional group at 1256 cm^{-1} and a C–O group at 1047 cm^{-1}. Its ^{31}P NMR spectrum displayed a singlet at –7.62 ppm; the ^1H NMR spectrum showed a multiplet at 4.36–4.82 ppm and two singlet at 1.64 and 1.80 ppm. These spectral data of polymers obtained by us are consistent with those of Allcock's [14] though the molecular weights of phosphazenes **6** ($M_w = 4.6 \times 10^4$) were relatively lower. The polymers **6** were non-crystalline and elastomeric at room temperature. They were soluble in THF but insoluble in water.

Synthesis of homopolyphosphazenes 10 with diamino groups in the side-chain (Scheme 3) 6-Iodo-1-hexanol (**8**) was prepared in 60% yield as a spacer by reaction of 1,6-hexanediol (**7**) with sodium iodide and chlorotrimethylsilane (1:1:1) in acetonitrile. Treatment of *N*,*N*,*N*′-trimethylethylenediamine with **8** in the presence of Na_2CO_3 in acetone at reflux for 12 h gave diamine **9** in 86% yield. Reaction of

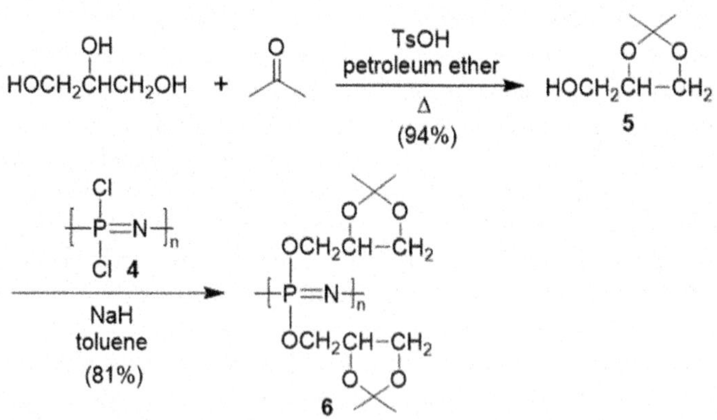

Scheme 2 Synthesis of glycerol-containing homopolyphosphazenes **6**

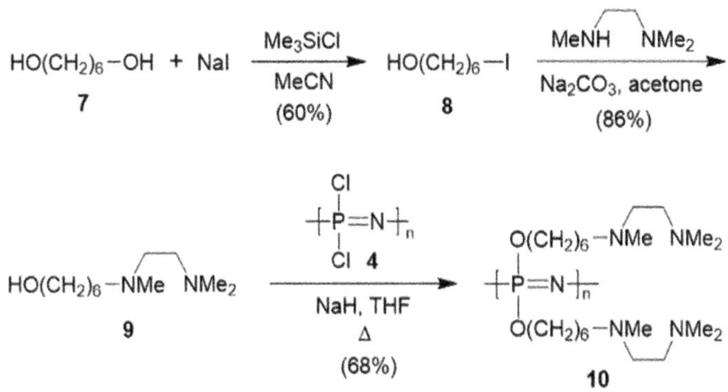

Scheme 3 Synthesis of ethylenediamine-containing homopolyphosphazenes **10**

diamine **9** with polymers **4** and NaH(s) by following the same method shown in Scheme 2 afforded the homopolyphosphazenes **10** in 68% yield. Its infrared spectrum revealed a P=N stretching at 1277 cm^{-1} and a C–O stretching at 1044 cm^{-1}. These polymers were soluble in aniline but almost insoluble in water.

Synthesis of bifunctional polyphosphazenes 12 and implantation of Copper(II) (Scheme 4) By modifying the homopolymerization reactions as shown in Schemes 2 and 3, we treated the protected glycerol **5**, diamine **9**, and polyphosphazenes **4** in a ratio of 1.1:1.1:1.0 with NaH(s) in THF and toluene. The solution was heated at reflux for 10 h to give random copolyphosphazenes **11** in 74% yield. The chlorine atoms in the starting polyphosphazenes **4** were replaced by the protected glycerol and the (diamino)alkoxyl moieties in a random fashion. Then the isopropylidene groups in polymers **11** were removed by use of 80% aqueous acetic acid at 25 °C for 7.0 h to give the desired random copolyphosphazenes **12** in 77% yield (Scheme 4). The ^{1}H NMR spectrum of **12** showed the ratio of glycerol to diamine group is 1.5:1.0.

Being soluble in water, the ^{31}P NMR spectrum of copolymers **12** showed a broad peak between –6.12 and –6.86 ppm. The molecular weights were determined to be $M_w = 9.91 \times 10^3$ by gel permeation chromatography (GPC) in an aqueous solution against poly(ethylene glycol) (PEG) standards.

Furthermore, copolymers **12** were treated with cupric chloride in ethanol at 25 °C. The desired nerve-agent detoxicant **2** was generated as a green elastomer in 98% yield (see the last step of Scheme 4).

Degradations of copolyphosphazenes 12 and 2 in aqueous media (Scheme 5) In order to test the stability of random copolymers **12** and **2**, we dissolved these new materials in water (10 mL). The solution was heated at 100 °C and stirred for 3 days. After the ^{31}P NMR spectrum of copolymer **12** changed to a singlet at 0.32 ppm, the solution was cooled down and the degraded products were characterized by ^{1}H NMR spectrometer. The same hydrolysis reaction was carried out in a buffer solution at pH 6.0–8.0 to simulate the pH range in nature. The broad peak between –6.12 and –6.86 ppm in the ^{31}P NMR spectrum of copolymers **12** slowly changed to a singlet

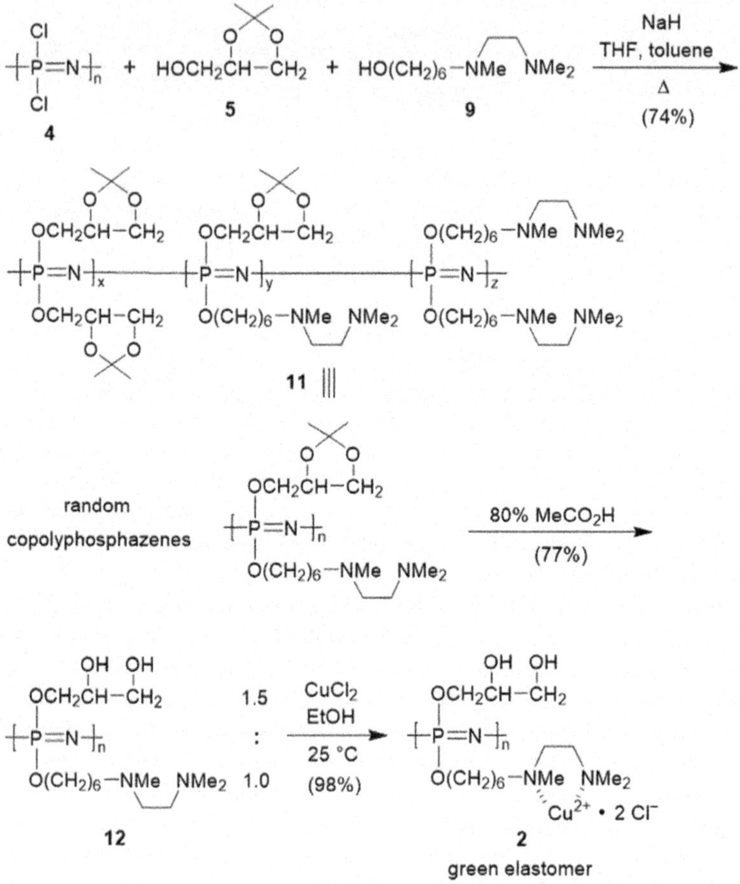

Scheme 4 Synthesis of glycerol- and ethylenediamine-containing random copolyphosphazenes **11**, **12**, and **2**

at 0.32 ppm. The copolymers **12** were gradually hydrolyzed to phosphoric acid in the buffer solution at 25 °C after 72 days. The same degradation also occurred to copolymer **2**.

Catalytic efficiency of Cu(II)-complexes (Scheme 6) To investigate efficiency of nerve-agent hydrolysis, the new copper-loaded random copolymers **2** were used. Moreover, *p*-nitrophenyl diphenylphosphate (PNDPP, **13**) was applied as a "simulant" that is relatively easy to handle in comparison with the relevant and more toxic nerve agents like sarin (**1a**) and soman (**1b**) [21]. The decrease of the UV intensity associated with PNDPP at $\lambda = 275$ nm or the increase of the intensity of 4-nitrophenol (**14**) at $\lambda = 317$ nm obeyed the pseudo-first order rate equation. It was used, along with the infinity absorbance, to calculate the rate constants.

We studied the efficiency of the hydrolysis of PNDPP (**13**) catalyzed by the copper-loaded copolyphosphazenes **2** and monomer **15**, respectively. The experiments were

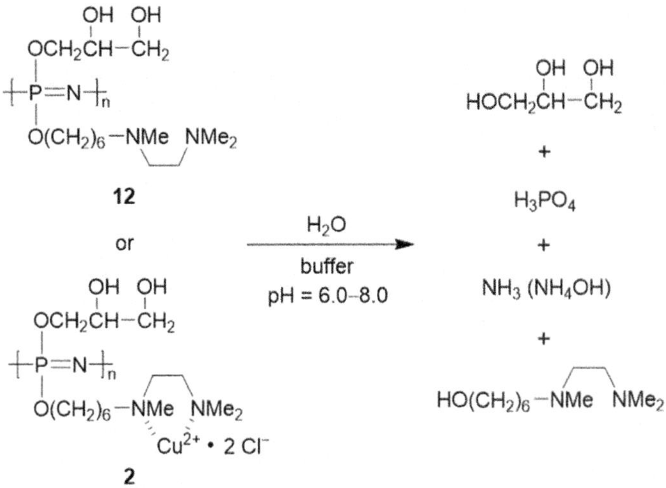

Scheme 5 Hydrolytic degradation of copolyphosphazenes **12** and **2** to give small fragments

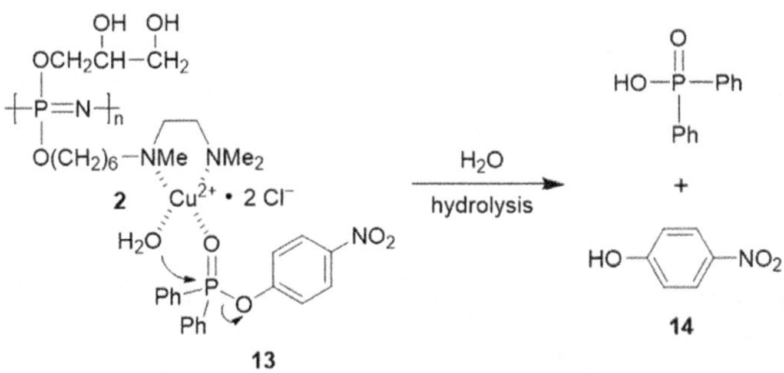

Scheme 6 Catalytic decomposition of PNDPP (**13**) by Cu(II)-copolyphosphazenes **2**

carried out in an aqueous solution with the reaction temperature kept at 25 °C. The observed rate constants for the hydrolysis of PNDPP (**13**) catalyzed by polymers **2** and the complex **15** are shown in Table 1.

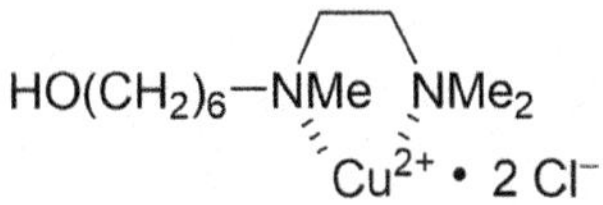

15

Both the random copolymers **2** and the monomer complex **15** were able to accelerate the hydrolysis of PNDPP (**13**) in comparison with an aqueous medium in the absence of any catalyst. For example, the rate of hydrolysis of PNDPP in the presence of Cu-loaded copolymers **2** with 8.00 mM was 258 times faster than that in

Table 1 Pseudo-first-order rate constant for hydrolysis of PNDPP (**13**) by use of copolymers **2** and the monomer complex **15** in an aqueous solution at 25 °C[a]

[Cu], mM	Cu(II) catalyst	k_{obsd}, $\times 10^{-4} s^{-1}$	$t_{1/2}$, min
0.55	Monomer **15**	8.56	13.5
0.55	Polymers **2**	2.67	43.3
1.00	Monomer **15**	13.5	8.56
1.00	Polymers **2**	3.58	32.3
2.00	Monomer **15**	31.2	3.70
2.00	Polymers **2**	7.82	14.8
4.00	Monomer **15**	42.6	2.71
4.00	Polymers **2**	13.8	8.37
8.00	Monomer **15**	96.3	1.19
8.00	Polymers **2**	31.7	3.64

[a]All reactions were carried out in the aqueous solution containing 10% dioxane (v/v) and monitored spectrophotometrically at 317 nm for the production of *p*-nitrophenol (**14**) from an initial [PNDPP] = 0.050 mM

the absence of a catalyst. The half-life time was 3.64 min for the detoxicant **2** to hydrolyze PNDPP. The half-life time, however, was 950 min without containing any catalyst. These data clearly indicate that the catalytic efficiency on the hydrolysis of phosphate agents (i.e., **13**) was greatly improved by two orders when being in the presence of the newly synthesized copper (II)-containing copolyphosphazenes **2**.

3 Conclusions

Copper (II)-containing random copolyphosphazenes **2** are developed as a new kind of detoxicants for efficient hydrolysis of a nerve-agent. These polymers have bifunctional characteristics: the glyceryl units therein increase water solubility and copper(II)-coordinated diamino groups can hydrolyze a phosphate agent. Meanwhile, their polyphosphazene skeleton possesses self-degradability, which is desirable for the concern related to environmental protection.

Synthesis of the bifunctional copolymers **2** has been accomplished in seven steps. The half-life time for the uncatalyzed hydrolysis of *p*-nitrophenyl diphenyl phosphate at 25 °C is 950 min. In the presence of the polymers **2**, the half-life time for the hydrolysis is reduced to 3.64 min, which is 261 times faster than the uncatalyzed process.

4 Experimental Procedures

General Procedure All reactions were carried out in oven-dried glassware (120 °C) under an atmosphere of nitrogen, unless as indicated otherwise. Acetone, hexanes, tetrahydrofuran, and toluene were purchased from Mallinckrodt Chemical Co. Hexanes and toluene were dried and distilled from CaH_2. Tetrahydrofuran was dried and distilled from sodium and benzophenone under an atmosphere of nitrogen. Chlorotrimethylsilane, copper (II) chloride, phosphonitrilic chloride trimer, sodium thiosulfate, and *N*,*N*,*N'*-trimethylethylenediamine were purchased from Aldrich Chemical Co. 1,6-Hexanediol, glycerol, sodium hydride, sodium iodide, and *p*-toluenesulfonic acid monohydrate were purchased from Merck Inc. *p*-Nitrophenyl diphenyl phosphate (PNDPP) was prepared according to the Gulick's procedure [22]. An explosion-proof oven from Blue M. Electric Co. and the Pyrex combustion tubes (10 × 200 mm) from Tung Kuang Glassware Industrial Co. were used to carry out experiments that required high temperatures.

Analytical thin layer chromatography (TLC) was performed on precoated plates (silica gel 60 F–254), purchased from Merck Inc. Gas chromatographic analyses were performed on a Hewlett–Packard 5890 Series II instrument equipped with a 25-m cross-linked methyl silicone gum capillary column (0.32-mm i.d.). Nitrogen gas was used as a carrier gas and the flow rate was kept constant at 14.0 mL/min. The retention time t_R was measured under the following conditions: injector temperature 260 °C, the initial temperature for column 70 °C, duration 2.00 min, increment rate 10 °C/min, and the final temperature for column 250 °C. Gas chromatography and low resolution mass spectral analyses were performed on a Hewlett–Packard 5890 Series II instrument equipped with a Hewlett–Packard 5971A Mass Selective Detector and a capillary HP-1 column. Purification by gravity column chromatography was carried out by use of Merck Reagents Silica Gel 60 (particle size 0.063–0.200 mm, 70–230 mesh ASTM).

Infrared (IR) spectra were measured on a Bomem Michelson Series FT–IR spectrometer. The wave numbers reported are referenced to the polystyrene 1601 cm^{-1} absorption. Absorption intensities are recorded by the following abbreviations: s, strong; m, medium; w, weak. Proton NMR spectra were obtained on a Varian Unity-400 (400 MHz) spectrometer or a Varian Gemini-300 (300 MHz) spectrometer by use of chloroform-*d* and D_2O as solvent and tetramethylsilane and 3-(trimethylsilyl)propionic acid sodium salt as internal standards. Carbon-13 NMR spectra were obtained on a Varian Unity-400 (100 MHz) spectrometer or a Varian Gemini-300 (75 MHz) spectrometer by used of chloroform-*d* and D_2O as solvent. Carbon-13 chemical shifts are referenced to the center of the $CDCl_3$ triplet (δ 77.0 ppm) and 3-(trimethylsilyl)propionic acid sodium salt (δ 0.0 ppm). Multiplicities are recorded by the following abbreviations: s, singlet; d, doublet; t, triplet; q, quartet; m, multiplet; *J*, coupling constant (hertz). Molecular weights of all synthesized polymers on the basis of polystyrene and poly(ethylene glycol) (PEG) standards were determined by gel permeation chromatography (GPC). Three columns packed with 10^3, 10^4, and 10^5 Å μ-styragel, respectively, were arranged in sequence onto a

Hewlett–Packard 1050 series HPLC instrument, which was equipped with ultraviolet and refractive index detectors. The flow rate was 1.5 mL/min for a sample containing 0.26% of the synthesized polymers in THF (g/mL) and D_2O (g/mL) at 45 °C.

Linear polydichlorophosphazenes (4) A mixture of hexachlorocyclotriphosphazene (**3**, 902 mg, 2.59 mmol, 1.0 equiv) and sulfur (30.1 mg, 0.941 mmol, 0.36 equiv) were added into a Pyrex combustion tube, which was then sealed by torch. The sealed tube was heated at 285 °C for 6.0 h. When the tube was cooled to 25 °C, the polymers were a transparent immobile material, in which crystallization of the residual trimer or other oligomers occurred slowly. The products were then cut into small pieces and then added to dry toluene. The polymers dissolved and became a viscous, colorless solution after continuous agitation for 24 h. The products were purified by re-precipitation from hexanes to give polymers **4** (0.732 g, 2.09 mmol) in 81% yield: ^{31}P NMR (THF, 122 MHz) δ –17.39 ppm; IR (neat) 2137 (w), 1291 (s, P=N), 755 (m, P–Cl), 577 (s), 522 (m) cm^{-1}; M_w 3.8×10^4. Their spectroscopic characteristics are consistent with those of the same materials reported [18].

Protected isopropylidene glycerol homopolyphosphazenes (6) To a dry toluene solution (150 mL) containing NaH (545 mg, 22.7 mmol, 2.2 equiv) and isopropylidene glycerol [20] (**5**, 3.49 g, 22.7 mmol, 2.2 equiv) was added polydichlorophosphazene (**4**, 1.21 g, 10.3 mmol, 1.0 equiv). After the reaction mixture was stirred at reflux for 6.1 h, it was cooled down and the resultant polymers were obtained by filtration. The products were purified by re-precipitation from THF into water and hexanes to give elastomeric polymers **6** (2.56 g, 8.34 mmol) in 81% yield: ^1H NMR (C_6D_6, 400 MHz) δ 1.64 (s, 3 H, CH_3), 1.80 (s, 3 H, CH_3), 4.36–4.82 (m, 5 H) ppm; ^{31}P NMR ($CDCl_3$, 122 MHz) δ –7.62 ppm; IR (neat) 2924 (s), 2857 (s), 1649 (m), 1256 (s), 1047 (s) cm^{-1}; M_w 4.6×10^4. Their spectroscopic characteristics are consistent with those of the same compound reported [14].

Diamino homopolyphosphazenes (10) To a dry THF solution (160 mL) containing NaH (483 mg, 20.1 mmol, 2.2 equiv) and *N,N,N*′-trimethyl-*N*′-(6-hydroxyhexyl)ethylenediamine [10] (**9**, 3.93 g, 20.1 mmol, 2.2 equiv) was added polydichlorophosphazenes (**4**, 1.21 g, 10.3 mmol, 1.0 equiv). After the reaction mixture was stirred at reflux for 10 h, it was cooled down and the resultant polymers were obtained by filtration. The products were washed with water and purified by re-precipitation from aniline into THF to give elastomeric polymers **10** (3.09 g, 7.02 mmol) in 68% yield: IR (neat) 2930 (s), 2861 (s), 1453 (s), 1277 (s), 1252 (s), 1044 (s) cm^{-1}.

Diamino–protected isopropylidene glycerol random copolyphosphazenes 11 To a dry toluene solution (100 mL) containing NaH (908 mg, 37.8 mmol, 2.2 equiv), isopropylidene glycerol [20] (**5**, 2.49 g, 18.9 mmol, 1.1 equiv), and *N,N,N*′-trimethyl-*N*′-(6-hydroxyhexyl)ethylenediamine [10] (**9**, 3.82 g, 18.9 mol, 1.1 equiv) was added polydichlorophosphazenes (**4**, 2.01 g, 17.2 mmol, 1.0 equiv). After the reaction mixture was stirred at reflux for 10 h, it was cooled down and the resultant polymers were obtained by filtration. The products were washed with water and purified by re-precipitation from aniline into THF to give elastomeric copolymers **11** (4.79 g, 12.7 mmol) as elastomeric polymers in 74% yield: IR (neat) 2930 (s), 2866 (s), 2692 (s), 1650 (s), 1470 (s), 1237 (s), 1052 (s), 973 (s) cm^{-1}.

Diamino–isopropylidene glycerol random copolyphosphazenes 12 Protected copolyphosphazenes **11** (435 mg, 1.15 mmol) were added to 80% aqueous CH_3CO_2H (15 mL) at room temperature. After the reaction mixture was stirred at 25 °C for 7.0 h, it was diluted with water, neutralized by aqueous sodium carbonate, extracted with ether, and dried over $MgSO_4$(s). Then the combined organic layers were concentrated by use of SpeedVac Systems to give random copolymers **12** (298 mg, 0.886 mmol) in 77% yield: ^{1}H NMR (D_2O, 400 MHz) δ 1.32–1.64 (br, 8 H, 4 × CH_2, 40%), 2.82 (s, 3 H, CH_3, 40%), 2.87 (s, 6 H, 2 × CH_3, 40%), 3.08–3.16 (m, 4 H, 2 × CH_2N, 40%), 3.53–4.22 (m, (5 H, 60% + 2 H, CH_2N, 40% + 2 H, 40%)) ppm; ^{31}P NMR (D_2O, 122 MHz) δ –6.12 to –6.86 (br) ppm; IR (neat) 3361 (s), 2940 (s), 1571 (s), 1419 (s), 1252 (s), 1045 (s) cm^{-1}; M_w 9.91 × 10^3.

Cu(II)-containing random copolyphosphazenes 2 A solution containing anhydrous $CuCl_2$ (554 mg, 4.11 mol, 1.0 equiv) in absolute ethanol (15 mL) was added to a solution containing polyphosphazenes **12** (1.32 g, 4.19 mmol, 1.0 equiv) in absolute ethanol (15 mL). After the reaction mixture was stirred at room temperature for 10 min, the resultant solids were washed with cold absolute ethanol and dried over P_2O_5(s) under reduced pressure overnight to give green elastomeric copolymers **2** (1.74 g, 4.11 mmol) in 98% yield: IR (neat) 3360 (s), 2938 (s), 1568 (s), 1422 (s), 1250 (s), 1041 (s) cm^{-1}; M_w 9.88 ×10^3.

Kinetics on the hydrolysis of PNDPP (13) A 1.00-cm cuvette containing water (3.0 mL) and copolymers **2** (1.59 mg, corresponding to 1.00 mM Cu^{2+}) was stoppered and placed on a magnetic stirrer. The reaction was initiated by addition of PNDPP (**13**, 20 μL of 7.50 mM) dissolved in spectral-grade acetonitrile (2.0 mL) and followed by stirring. After 5.0 min, the stirring was stopped and the solution was allowed to settle for 10 s. The UV spectrum was then secure. Subsequently, the cuvette was returned to stir for additional 5.0-min time segments. The decrease in the absorption of PNDPP (**13**) at $\lambda = 275$ nm and the increase in the absorption of 4-nitrophenol (**14**) at $\lambda = 317$ nm obeyed the pseudo-first order rate equation and were used, along with the infinity absorbance, to calculate the rate constants. For fast reactions, several cuvettes for a single rate determination were used.

Hydrolytic degradation of random copolyphosphazenes 12 Copolymers **12** (156 mg, 0.424 mmol) were dissolved in water (10 mL), which was heated at 100 °C for 72 h. The degradation was monitored by ^{31}P NMR spectrometer and GPC. After the ^{31}P NMR spectrum changed to a singlet at 0.32 ppm, the solution was cooled down and the degradation products were characterized by ^{1}H NMR spectroscopy. The same reaction was also carried out by use of copolyphosphazenes **2** in a buffer solution of pH 6.0–8.0.

Acknowledgements For financial support, we thank National Chung-Shan Institute of Science and Technology, Ministry of Science and Technology (Grant Nos. 109-2113-M-007-007 and 110-2634-F-007-023), and Ministry of Education (Grant Nos. 109QR001I5and 110QR001I5) of R.O.C. We also thank the MOST in Taiwan to support The Featured Areas Research Center Program within the framework of the Higher Education Sprout Project through the Frontier Research Center on Fundamental and Applied Sciences of Matters.

References

1. Nepovimova, E., Kuca, K.: The history of poisoning: from ancient times until modern ERA. Arch. Toxicol. **93**(1), 11–24 (2019); b) Ember, L.: Tokyo subway attack: chemical weapon possible terrorist tool. Chem. Eng. News. **73**(13), 6–7 (1995)
2. Fedarko, K., Desmond, E.W.: Shock to the system. Time **145**(15), 55 (1995)
3. Emsley, J., Hall, D.: The Chemistry of Phosphorous, pp. 494–509. Wiley, New York (1976)
4. Bigley, A.N., Harvey, S.P., Narindoshvili, T., Raushel, F.M.: Substrate analogues for the enzyme-catalyzed detoxification of the organophosphate nerve agents–sarin, soman, and cyclosarin. Biochemistry **60**(38), 2875–2887 (2021)
5. Imran, M., Singh, V.V., Garg, P., Mazumder, A., Pandey, L.K., Sharma, P.K., Ganesan, K.: In-situ detoxification of schedule-I chemical warfare agents utilizing $Zr(OH)_4$@W-ACF functional material for the development of next generation NBC protective gears. Sci. Rep. **11**(1), 1–21 (2021)
6. Dey, N., Kulhanek, J., Bureš, F., Bhattacharya, S.: Imidazole-functionalized Y-shaped push–pull dye for nerve agent sensing as well as a catalyst for their detoxification. J. Org. Chem. **86**(21), 14663–14671 (2021)
7. Manco, G., Porzio, E., Suzumoto, Y.: Enzymatic detoxification: a sustainable means of degrading toxic organophosphate pesticides and chemical warfare nerve agents. J. Chem. Technol. Biotechnol. **93**(8), 2064–2082 (2018)
8. Zhang, L., Murata, H., Amitai, G., Smith, P.N., Matyjaszewski, K., Russell, A.J.: Catalytic detoxification of organophosphorus nerve agents by butyrylcholinesterase-polymer-oxime bioscavengers. Biomacromol **21**(9), 3867–3877 (2020)
9. Hou, Y., An, H., Zhang, Y., Hu, T., Yang, W., Chang, S.: Rapid destruction of two types of chemical warfare agent simulants by hybrid polyoxomolybdates modified by carboxylic acid ligands. ACS Catal. **8**(7), 6062–6069 (2018)
10. Menger, F. M., Tsuno, T.: Organic reactions catalyzed by copper-loaded polymers. Reactivity vs polymer structure. J. Am. Chem. Soc. **111**(13), 4903–4907 (1989)
11. Kirlikovali, K.O., Chen, Z., Islamoglu, T., Hupp, J.T., Farha, O.K.: Zirconium-based metal–organic frameworks for the catalytic hydrolysis of organophosphorus nerve agents. ACS Appl. Mater. Interfaces **12**(13), 14702–14720 (2020)
12. Allcock, H.: Phosphorus-Nitrogen Compounds, 1st edn. Academic Press, New York (1972)
13. Gustafson, R.L., Martell, A.E.: A kinetic study of the copper(II) chelate-catalyzed hydrolysis of isopropyl methylphosphonofluoridate (sarin). J. Am. Chem. Soc. **84**(12), 2309–2316 (1962)
14. Allcock, H.R., Kwon, S.: Glyceryl polyphosphazenes: synthesis, properties, and hydrolysis. Macromolecules **21**(7), 1980–1985 (1988)
15. Zhou, N., Zhi, Z., Liu, D., Wang, D., Shao, Y., Yan, K., Meng, L., Yu, D.: Acid-responsive and biologically degradable polyphosphazene nanodrugs for efficient drug delivery. ACS Biomater. Sci. Eng. **6**(7), 4285–4293 (2020)
16. Allcock, H.R.: Polyphosphazene elastomers, gels, and other soft materials. Soft Matter **8**(29), 7521–7532 (2012)
17. a) Allcock, H.R., Reeves, S.D., Nelson, J.M., Crane, C.A., Manners, I.: Polyphosphazene block copolymers via the controlled cationic, ambient temperature polymerization of phosphoranimines. Macromolecules **30**(7), 2213–2215 (1997); b) Allcock, H.R., Kugel, R.L.: Phosphonitrilic compounds. V. cyclized products from the reactions of hexachlorocyclotriphosphazene (phosphonitrilic chloride trimer) with aromatic dihydroxy, dithiol, and diamino compounds. Inorg. Chem. **5**(6), 1016–1020 (1966)
18. Allcock, H.R., Morozowich, N.L.: Bioerodible polyphosphazenes and their medical potential. Polym. Chem. 3(3), 578–590 (2012); b) Allcock, H.R., Kugel, R.L., Valan, K.J.: Phosphonitrilic compounds. VI. High molecular weight poly(alkoxy- and aryloxyphosphazenes). Inorg. Chem. **5**(10), 1709–1715 (1966)
19. Sennett, M.S., Hagnauer, G.L., Singler, R.E., Davies, G.: Kinetics and mechanism of the boron trichloride-catalyzed thermal ring-opening polymerization of hexachlorocyclotriphosphazene in 1,2,4-trichlorobenzene solution. Macromolecules **19**(4), 959–964 (1986)

20. Newman, M.S., Renoll, M.: Improved preparation of isopropylidene glycerol. J. Am. Chem. Soc. **67**(9), 1621 (1945)
21. Ghosh, K.K., Sinha, D., Satnami, M.L., Dubey, D.K., Rodriguez-Dafonte, P., Mundhara, G.L.: Nucleophilic dephosphorylation of *p*-nitrophenyl diphenyl phosphate in cationic micellar media. Langmuir **21**(19), 8664–8669 (2005)
22. Gulick, W.M., Geske, D.H.: Examination of phosphorus hyperfine coupling constants in nitroaromatic anion radicals. J. Am. Chem. Soc. **88**(13), 2928–2934 (1966)

Biomaterials-Cells/Tissues Interactions

Stimuli-responsive Multilayers Based on Thiol Chemistry Controlling Adhesion and Growth of Fibroblasts

Christian Willems, Pegah Esmaeilzadeh, and Thomas Groth

Abstract Novel surface coatings for implants and scaffolds should not only be biocompatible but also stimuli-responsive so that they can be used versatilely in different applications by adapting to their specific surroundings. Multilayers composed of polysaccharides are biocompatible but lack an induced response to a change in the outer surroundings. Here a stimuli-responsive multilayer system based on chondroitin sulfate and chitosan was formed by modifying the polysaccharides with free thiol groups in a Steglich-analogous esterification to form redox-sensitive systems. These multilayers can reversibly change their mechanical, surface and chemical properties by crosslinking these thiol groups or subsequently cleaving the disulfide bond. Treatment of these multilayers with the oxidizing agent chloramine-T leads to the formation of disulfide bonds, which can promote the adhesion of proteins like fibronectin or human fibroblasts onto the surface, while the usage of the reducing agent tris(2-carboxyethyl) phosphine (TCEP) can cleave the disulfide bond again which leads to a low FN and fibroblast adhesion. This demonstrates the usefulness of applying switchable multilayer systems in the field of tissue engineering as this technique can be used to either promote or restrict specific cell growth. It could be shown that this process can be repeatedly carried out and reversed so that the surface properties are multiple times switchable.

Keyword Thiomers · Stimuli-responsive · Bioactive surfaces · Implants · Fibroblast adhesion

---

C. Willems · P. Esmaeilzadeh · T. Groth (✉)
Department of Biomedical Materials, Martin-Luther University Halle-Wittenberg, 06120 Halle (Saale), Germany
e-mail: thomas.groth@pharmazie.uni-halle.de

T. Groth
Interdisciplinary Center of Materials Science, Martin-Luther University Halle-Wittenberg, 06099 Halle (Saale), Germany

S. Najman et al. (eds.), *Bioceramics, Biomimetic and Other Compatible Materials Features for Medical Applications*, Engineering Materials,
https://doi.org/10.1007/978-3-031-17269-4_5

1 Introduction

Surface modification of implants and scaffolds for tissue engineering is a promising approach to adjust surface properties of specific biomaterials to a variety of applications. For example, bone implants require tight bonding to surrounding tissue, which requires it to promote adhesion and the growth of osteoblasts, while coatings of sensor surfaces shall reduce colonization with fibroblast and fibrous capsule formation to permit a continuous exchange of solutes required for the function of the device. Specifically chemical and physical properties have to be controlled. The latter like wetting [1] and electrical surface potential [2] may directly affect the adsorption of proteins that promote or suppress adhesion of cells. For example, surfaces with moderate wettability and positive surface charge aid in the adsorption of proteins and adhesion of cells, while those of high wettability and negative charge may suppress it [3–5]. Also mechanical properties of coating can be used to affect cell adhesion, growth and differentiation, as softer substrata generally suppress adhesion of cells, while stiffer, harder surfaces have a promoting effect [6, 7]. A further progress in surface coatings and biomaterials is achieved when such physical properties can be regulated on demand by responding to certain stimuli, such as a change in pH [8], temperature [9], ionic strength [10] or bio-chemical environment [10, 11]. Such responsive materials can be used to precisely control the release of bioactive substances [12] and also the behaviour of cells [13].

A method of surface modification that has found widespread recognition for biomedical applications are polyelectrolyte multilayers, which are formed by the layer-by-layer techniques [14]. By repeatedly immersing a substrate in oppositely charged polyelectrolyte solutions, multi-layered systems are formed, which are held together through ionic and other types of interactions [14, 15]. Because of a continuing search for more biocompatible materials, the usage of glycosaminoglycans as building blocks for multilayer systems has come into focus, since GAG's represent polyelectrolytes that are biocompatible and degradable [16]. Cross-linking of polysaccharide based multilayers by different chemical means has been also suggested to improve stability and has also shown advantages regarding to bioactivity of multilayer coatings by changes in the mechanical properties of coatings [17] and controlled release of growth factors [18]. Hence, GAG's and other polysaccharides like alginate, chitosan, etc. have found widespread use in making biogenic and bioactive coatings and freestanding films for application in in bone replacement, wound healing, tissue engineering of skin, etc. [16, 18–20].

A reversible cross-linking process of polyelectrolyte multilayers may be also an attractive means to generate coatings that can change their physical intrinsic and surface properties in response to the environmental stimuli, like the formation and breaking of imine bonds depending on pH of environment [21]. Another example is based on the formation of disulfide bonds from adjacent thiol groups in the presence of an oxidizing agent and which can be cleaved again in a reducing environment [22, 23]. Such systems may permit repeated cycles of bond formation and splitting, representing entirely reversible systems that may change their properties depending on the environment in the body or pathological conditions like inflammation [13]. Hence, multilayer systems that possess an additional opportunity for intrinsic crosslinking of thiols may not only increase the stability of the system, but permit also a change of properties towards the biological system depending on the redox state of the multilayers [13].

In this article, we describe the synthesis of thiolated chitosan and chondroitin sulfate that were used for the formation of polyelectrolyte multilayers based primarily on their opposite charge. Formation of disulfide bonds was achieved by exposure of multilayers to basic pH or chloramine-T [22] with the latter being more effective. Splitting i.e. reduction of disulifde bonds was achieved by exposure to tris(2-carboxyethyl)phosphine (TCEP) [24]. We can show here not only that the redox state of multilayers affects their physical properties and subsequent adsorption of fibronectin and adhesion of fibroblasts, but also demonstrate that the redox state is completely reversible regarding physical properties and biological response.

2 Materials and Methods

2.1 Materials

3,3′-dithiodipropionic acid (DTPA, 99%), 11-mercaptoundecanoic acid (MUDA, 95%) and native chondroitin sulfate A sodium salt (obtained from bovine trachea, Mw ~ 25 kDa, degree of sulfation: 0.8) were received from Sigma–Aldrich [Steinheim, Germany]. Native low molecular weight (LMW) chitosan (10–50 kDa, 82.6–87.5% degree of deacetylation) was provided by Heppe Medical Chitosan GmbH [Halle (Saale), Germany]. 1-(3-dimethyl-aminopropyl)—3-ethylcarbodiimide hydrochloride (EDC, 98+%) was purchased from Alfa Aesar [Karlsruhe, Germany], and Dithiothreitol (DTT) from VWR International GmbH [Poole, England]. Dialysis bags (Spectra/Por membrane, Mw cutoff = 3500 kDa), tris(2-carboxyethyl)-phosphine-hydrochloride (TCEP), 5,5′-dithiobis-(2-nitrobenzoic acid) (DTNB, Ellman's reagent), 1,4-diazabicyclo [2.2.2] octane, deuterium oxide (D_2O), disposable polystyrene cuvettes and organic solvents were all purchased from Carl Roth GmbH [Karlsruhe, Germany]. Tris(hydroxymethyl) aminomethane (TRIS) was purchased from Merck KGaA [Karlsruhe, Germany]. Poly(2-vinylpyridine) was purchased from PSS [Mainz, Germany]. Glass cover slips (diameter: 15 mm) were purchased from Menzel GmbH & Co KG [Braunschweig, Germany]. Silicon wafers with an area of 16 * 16 mm^2 were purchased from Silico Materials [Kaufering, Germany]. Gold-coated glass sensors (16 * 16 mm^2) were purchased from Ssens [Enschede, Netherlands]. Syringe filters consisting of cellulose acetate with a pore size of 0.2 μm were purchased from Diagonal GmbH & Co KG [Münster, Germany]. Dulbeccos modified Eagle medium (DMEM) as well as fetal bovine serum (FBS), Penicillin, streptomycin and fungizone were purchased from Biochrom GmbH

[Berlin, Germany]. Human plasma fibronectin, labelled with fluorescein isothiocyanate (FITC) was purchased from Yo-Proteins [Ronninge, Swede]. Phalloidin CruzFluor™ 555 was purchased from Santa Cruz Biotechnologies [Santa Cruz, United States]. TO-PRO™-3was purchased from Invitrogen [Darmstadt, Germany]. Mowiol 4-88 was purchased from Calbiochem [Darmstadt, Germany]. 3, 3′-dithiobis (propanoic hydrazide) (DTPHY) was synthesized according to a method described elsewhere [23]. Phosphate buffered saline (PBS) was prepared by dissolving 0.20 g (2.7 mmol) KCl, 8.01 g (137.0 mmol) NaCl, 0.19 g (1.4 mmol) KH_2PO_4 and 0.76 g (4.3 mmol) Na_2HPO_4 in 1 L of H_2O at a pH of 7.4. Unless mentioned otherwise, the used water is ultrapure deionized Milli-Q water with a conductivity of 0.055 mS/cm.

2.2 *Synthesis of Thiolated Components*

Synthesis of Thiolated Chondroitin Sulfate Chondroitin sulfate (CS) was partially thiolated with the aim of functionalizing 25% of the polymer. CS (1 g) was dissolved in 125 mL H_2O under stirring at room temperature after which DTPHY (0.14 g) was slowly added to the solution. The pH of the solution was adjusted to 4.75 with HCl and EDC (0.20 g) was subsequently added to the solution. It was stirred for 2.5 h, while the pH was continually kept at 4.75. Afterwards the pH was increased to 7.0 with NaOH to stop the reaction. The reduction of the disulfide bond was accomplished by gradually adding DTT (0.60 g) to the stirred solution. After changing the pH of the solution to 8.5 with NaOH, it was stirred over night, after which the pH was adjusted to 3.5. The solution was dialyzed against a 100 mM NaCl solution at pH 3.5 for 2 days and diluted HCl with a pH of 3.5 for 2 further days. Freeze drying the product produced a white powder, which was stored at 4 °C.

Synthesis of Thiolated Chitosan Chitosan (Chi) was partially thiolated with the aim of functionalizing 25% of the polymer. Low molecular weight (LMW) Chi (0.50 g) was dissolved in a mixture of 150 mL H_2O and 4 mL 2 M HCl under stirring at room temperature for 1 day. DTPA (132.00 mg) was dissolved in 3 mL methanol. The pH of the chitosan solution was adjusted to 4.75 and the DTPA solution was added dropwise. EDC (0.36 g) was dissolved in 1 mL H_2O. The pH of the reaction solution was again adjusted to 4.75 and the EDC solution was added. The reaction was stirred for 4 h, while the pH was kept at 4.75. The reduction of the disulfide bond was accomplished by gradually adding DTT (0.40 g) to the stirred solution. It was stirred for 1 h and the pH was subsequently changed to 3.5. The solution was dialyzed against a 100 mM NaCl solution at pH 3.5 for 2 days and diluted HCl with a pH of 3.5 for 2 further days. Freeze drying the product gave a white powder, which was stored at 4 °C.

2.3 *Characterization of Thiolated Polysaccharides*

Gel Permeation Chromatography The average molecular weight of the native and thiolated polysaccharides was determined using gel permeation chromatography (GPC) using an Agilent 1200 system from Agilent Technologies equipped with Novema columns (2 × 10,000 Å, 1 × 30 Å, 300 mm × 8 mm, 10 μm) from the company PSS [Mainz, Germany] and a refractive index detector to monitor the luting fraction. 0.3 M formic acid was used as mobile phase at a flow rate of 0.5 mL/min and a temperature of 35 °C. As a standard, poly(2-vinylpyridine) was used.

Fourier Transform Infrared Spectroscopy IR spectroscopy was performed with a TENSOR 27 Fourier transform infrared spectrometer from Bruker Optics GmbH [Ettlingen, Germany]. The measurement takes place in a range of 400–4000 cm^{-1} with a resolution of 4 cm^{-1} steps and 16 scans per sample. The samples were pressed together with KBr to form a pellet.

Raman Spectroscopy Raman spectroscopy was performer with a Bruker Raman spectrometer from Bruker Optics GmbH, equipped with a ND:YAG laser (excitation wavelength: 1024 nm; laser output: 150 mW). The measurement takes place in a Raman shift range of 0–3500 cm^{-1} with a resolution of 4 cm^{-1} steps.

UV/VIS Spectroscopy The thiol content was quantified by performing the Ellman's test using a Specord 200 UV–VIS spectrometer from Analytik Jena [Jena, Germany] [25]. The sample was mixed with 5-thio-2-nitrobenzoic acid (molar absorption coefficient at 412 nm: 14,150 M^{-1} cm^{-1}) and UV–VIS measurements at 412 nm were recorded [26]. The thiol content is given as a ratio of the actual thiol concentration (c_{SH}) to the theoretical one ($c_{SH}{}^{th}$), which is calculated for a concentration of 2 mg/mL and an expected molecular weight of the thiolated polysaccharide per repeating unit (Mw^{th}) (Formula 1) [23].

$$C_{SH}^{th} = 2\ mg/\left(Mw^{th} \times 1\ mL\right). \quad (1)$$

2.4 *Formation of Multilayers from Native and Thiolated Polysaccharides*

Substrate Preparation Glass cover slips were cleaned by immersing them in a solution of 0.5 M NaOH in 96% ethanol for 2 h at room temperature. Afterwards they were washed 10 times with H_2O (immersion time: 5 min), dried in a nitrogen stream and stored in H_2O. Silicon wafers were cleaned according to the "RCA-1" cleaning protocol. 65 mL of an aqueous 27 vol% NH_4OH solution were mixed with 65 mL of an aqueous 30 vol% H_2O_2 solution and 325 mL of H_2O (volume ratio: 1:1:5) and heated to 75 °C. The wafers were immersed in the solution for 15 min and washed 10 times in H_2O (immersion time: 5 min). After drying in a nitrogen stream, they were stored in H_2O [27]. Gold-coated glass sensors were cleaned by immersing them first in 99.8% ethanol and then in H_2O. The cleaned sensors were coated with a monolayer of 11-mercaptoundecanoic acid (MUDA) by incubating them over night at room temperature in a solution of MUDA in 99.8% ethanol (c = 2 mM). Afterwards they were washed with ethanol and H_2O and dried under a nitrogen stream.

Formation of Polyelectrolyte Multilayers The preparation of each PEM system was identical with the type of used substrate being the only difference. Either native chondroitin sulfate (n-CS), thiolated chondroitin sulfate (t-CS) native chitosan (n-Chi) or thiolated chitosan (t-Chi) were dissolved in a 150 mM NaCl solution, which was subsequently adjusted to pH 4, using 0.05 M acetic acid. The final polyelectrolyte concentration is 1 mg/mL. All solutions were filtered through a syringe filter with a pore size of 0.2 μm. The synthesis of the multilayer systems was performed at room temperature. The substrates were immersed in the polycation solution (either n-chi or t-Chi) and incubated for 20 min. They were subsequently washed by incubating them 3 times for 5 min in a 150 mM NaCl solution with a pH of 4. Following the washing step, the substrates were immersed in the polyanion solution (either n-CS or t-CS) and incubated for 20 min. They were subsequently washed by incubating them 3 times for 5 min in a 150 mM NaCl solution with a pH of 4. This cycle was repeated 5 times, so that the final PEM composition consists of 10 layers.

Oxidation and Reduction of Thiol Groups in PEMs Two different methods of oxidation were applied: one caused by a change in the pH and one facilitated by the usage of the oxidizing agent chloramine-T, as published recently [28]. All used solutions were filtered through a syringe filter with a pore size of 0.2 μm. The oxidation and reduction steps are respectively labelled Oxi and Red. If the steps are repeated several times, the systems are accordingly labelled $(Oxi/Red)_n$ or $(Red/Oxi)_n$ where n stands for the number of repeated cycles and the order indicates which process was performed first.

Oxidation by pH Change Multilayers were incubated in a 150 mM NaCl solution with a pH of 9.3 for either 1.5 or 4.5 h. To wash the PEM's, they were subsequently incubated in a 150 mM NaCl solution with a pH of 4 two times for 5 min and one time in H_2O. This method is further known as pH 9 method throughout this article.

Oxidation Through Treatment with Chloramine-T (ChT) ChT was dissolved in a 150 mM NaCl solution with a pH of 4 and a ChT concentration of 5 mmol/L. The multilayers were incubated in the ChT solution for 90 s and subsequently incubated in a 150 mM NaCl solution with a pH of 4 five times for 5 min and one time in H_2O. This method is further known as ChT method throughout this article.

To perform the reduction, tris-(2-carboxyethyl)-phosphine hydrochloride (TCEP) was dissolved in a 150 mM NaCl solution with a pH of 4 and a TCEP concentration of 5 mmol/L. The multilayers were incubated in the TCEP solution for 30 min and subsequently washed by incubating the PEM's in a 150 mM NaCl solution with a pH of 4 five times for 5 min and one time in H_2O.

2.5 Characterization of Polyelectrolyte Multilayers

Surface Plasmon Resonance (SPR) SPR analysis was performed using the*i*SPR—SPR-imaging equipment from IBIS Technologies [Enschede, Netherlands]. Cleaned gold sensors were used as a substrate for the multilayer systems and placed in the flow chamber. First, the flow chamber was equilibrated by purging it with a 150 mM NaCl solution with a pH of 4. Then 10 different regions of interest on the substrate surface were selected. The measurements were performed at a temperature of 25 °C and a flow rate of 3 μL/min. The polycation solutions were prepared as mentioned above and alternately injected in 20-min intervals into the flow chamber, followed by a washing step with a 150 mM NaCl solution (pH 4). 10 values were measured at each injection and washing step and samples were tested in duplicates.

Ellipsometry The thickness of multilayers and their stability over time was measured with an M-2000V ellipsometer from the J. A. Woollam Company [Lincoln, NE, USA], equipped with a WVase32 software. Silicon wafers were used as substrates for the multilayer systems. Wafers without multilayers were used as a reference and a thickness of 1.6 nm was determined for those. Thiolated and native PEM systems with 5 bilayers and a polyanion as a terminal layer were used for the measurements. Directly after their synthesis, the samples were measured to determine their initial thickness. Then they were incubated in a 150 mM NaCl solution with a pH of 9.3 for 90 min. After washing them with H_2O, they were dried in a nitrogen stream. All samples were incubated in a 1% penicillin/streptomycin/fungizone solution in PBS. They were incubated for 1, 7, 14 and 21 days, washed and dried as described above and measured with the ellipsometer under dry conditions. The wavelength range was chosen as 400–1000 nm and the angle range was chosen as 55–70°. On each surface, 5 different spots were chosen for a measurement. Each sample was measured in triplicate. The Cauchy model was used to calculate the refractive index as a function of wavelength as seen in Formula 2:

$$n(\lambda) = A_n + B_n/\lambda^2 + C_n/\lambda^4 \tag{2}$$

The values or A_n, B_n, and C_n were determined by using the mean value of the fitted parameters of thiolated multilayer systems with 20 and 30 layers as systems with a lower number of layers did not yield any reliable values, which is in accordance to results reported elsewhere [29]. The values, which are valid for all multilayer systems, are listed in Table 1.

UV/Vis Spectroscopy The multilayer samples were formed in disposable polystyrene cuvettes according to the formation of polyelectrolyte multilayers mentioned above with a bilayer number of n = 20 for increased sensitivity. The

Table 1 Values for the Cauchy model

A_n	B_n	C_n
1.50	0	0

thiol content was determined via Ellman's assay as stated above. 5,5′-dithiobis-(2-nitrobenzoic acid) (DTNB) was dissolved in PBS with a concentration of 0.1 mol/L and a pH of 7.5. The so called Ellman's reagent was added to the cuvettes, which were gently shaken for 1 h in the dark at room temperature. The thiol concentration was determined by UV/Vis-spectroscopy at a wavelength of 412 nm. All tests were performed in triplicate [25].

Water Contact Angle The PEM surface wettability was determined by measuring the static water contact angle (WCA) of a Milli-Q water droplet on the surface at room temperature. Glass wafers were used as substrates and the samples were equilibrated for 24–48 h at ambient conditions prior to testing. The WCA was measured with a OCQ15+ device from Dataphysics GmbH [Filderstadt, Germany]. The sessile drop method was used and each sample was analyzed with 5 different droplets with a volume of 0.5 μL using the Ellipse fitting method. For this, 10 consecutive values were considered. Each test was performed in triplicate.

Surface Potential Measurements The pH-dependent zeta-potential of multilayers was measured with the SurPASS electrokinetic analyzer from Anton Paar [Graz, Austria]. Glass wafers were used as substrates. 1 mM KCl solution was used as a model electrolyte and 0.1 M NaOH solution was used to change the pH from 3.0 to 10.0. A flow rate of 100–150 mL/min at a maximum pressure of 300 mbar was chosen. Each test was performed in triplicate.

Atomic Force Microscopy The surface topography and elastic modulus were determined with the atomic force microscope AFM Nanowizard II from JPK Instruments [Berlin, Germany]. Glass wafers were used as substrates. Standard silicon nitride cantilevers (MLCT) from Bruker [Santa Barbara, USA] were used for force map spectroscopy experiments and silicon nitride cantilevers (SNL) from Bruker were used for intermittent contact mode measurements. The intermittent contact mode measurements were performed in a 150 mM NaCl solution with a pH of 4. All experiments were performed in a standard liquid cell from JPK Instruments. The force-constant calibration was carried out by the thermal noise method [30]. The elastic moduli were calculated from each single force curve according to an advanced Hertzian model for spherical indenter geometry [31]. The programs JPK Data Processing V5.0.85 and Gwyddion software V2.49 were used for data post-processing, to calculate the Young's modulus and to determine roughness parameters according to DIN EN ISO 4287/4288.

2.6 Biological Experiments

Measurement of Fibronectin Adsorption on Polyelectrolyte Multilayers For the determination of fibronectin adsorption, different multilayer systems were directly synthesized in black well plates (Greiner). Human plasma fibronectin, labelled with FITC was dissolved in PBS at a pH of 7.4 with the final concentration of 20 μg/mL. 100 μL were added to each well and incubated at 37 °C for 4 h in the dark [22]. Afterwards, the supernatant was removed and the fluorescence intensity was measured with a FLUOStar Optima plate reader from BMG Labtech [Offenburg, Germany] (excitation filter: 485 nm; emission filter: 520 nm; gain: 1300) with PBS as a blank. Each sample was measured 8 times.

Cell Adhesion Studies For cell adhesion studies, human dermal fibroblasts from Promocell [Heidelberg, Germany] were used at a density of 25,000 cells/mL. Glass was used as a substrate for the multilayer systems. Before seeding the cells, half of the samples were coated with fibronectin. For this, FN was dissolved in PBS at a pH of 7.4 and a concentration of 20 μg/mL. The samples were then incubated with the FN solution at 37 °C for 4 h. Cells, seeded on uncoated multilayers were incubated with DMEM, containing 10% FBS, while cells seeded on coated systems were incubated with DMEM without FBS. The cells were incubated for 24 h in a humidified atmosphere of 5% CO_2 and 95% air at 37 °C.

After 24 h of incubation, the medium was removed and the cells were washed with PBS. A 4% paraformaldehyde solution in PBS was added and the cells were fixed at room temperature for 15 min. After washing the samples 3 times with PBS for 5 min, a 0.1 vol% triton X-100 solution was added for 10 min. After washing the samples 3 times with PBS for 5 min, a 1 wt% bovine serum albumin solution was added to block nonspecific binding sites and the system was incubated for 2.5 h. The filamentous actin was stained with Phalloidin CruzFluor™ 555 conjugate and the cell nuclei were stained with TO-PRO™-3. Each reagent was diluted in a 1 wt% BSA solution in PBS (dilution of Phalloidin CruzFluor™: 1:1000; dilution of TO-PRO™-3: 1:4000). The cells were incubated in the Phalloidin solution for 30 min and subsequently immersed in PBS 3 times for 5 min. Afterwards the cells were incubated in the TO-PRO solution for 30 min and subsequently immersed in PBS 3 times for 5 min. After washing the samples with H_2O, they were fixed with to object holders with Mowiol 4-88 containing 25 mg/mL 1,4-diazabicyclo [2.2.2]-octane. The cell samples were analyzed using a confocal laser scanning microscope LSM 710 equipped with the ZEN 2011 software from Carl Zeiss [Oberkochen, Germany]. The evaluation of the images was performed using the ImageJ software (version 1.50e). Each sample was measured in triplicate.

Cell Proliferation Studies For cell proliferation studies, human dermal fibroblasts from Promocell [Heidelberg, Germany] were seeded at a density of 25,000 cells/mL. Glass was used as a substrate for the multilayer systems. The samples were incubated with DMEM, containing 10% FBS and 1% Pen/Strep/Amphotericin B. The cells were incubated for 72 h in a humidified atmosphere of 5% CO_2 and 95% air at 37 °C. The samples were analyzed using a EC3 phase-contrast microscope from Leica [Wetzlar, Germany], equipped with a DMIL camera and the software LAS EZ (V. 2.0.0, Leica) for image analysis. Each sample was measured in triplicate.

Statistical Analysis The statistical analysis of the data was performed using Origin software with a Kruskal-Wallis ANOVA calculator. The statistical significance was determined for an error probability $p \leq 0.05$ and marked by asterisks in the figures.

3 Results and Discussion

3.1 Synthesis and Analysis of Thiolated Compounds

The thiolation of CS and Chi was accomplished by functionalizing the polymer backbone with DTPHY for CS and DTPA for chitosan in an EDC-mediated reaction, analogous to a Steglich esterification with a subsequent reduction of the disulfide bond (see Fig. 1).

The EDC links with the carboxy groups of the chondroitin sulfate to form an active ester-intermediate, which subsequently reacts with the hydrazide group of the DTPHY [23]. For the functionalization of chitosan, EDC conversely forms an active ester-intermediate with the carboxy group of the DTPA, which reacts with the primary amine group of the chitosan. A reduction of the disulfide compound results in the generation of thiol groups. The presence of thiol groups in both compounds was verified by FTIR- and Raman spectroscopy, which are shown in Figs. 2 and 3.

In the FTIR spectrum of t-CS, characteristic peaks for the C–S stretching, C–H bending, N–H bending and CH_2 group stretching vibrations of the CH_2-S group could be found at 601–730 cm^{-1}, 879–914 cm^{-1}, 1490–1558 cm^{-1} and 2839–2877 cm^{-1} respectively. A new signal at 1716–1760 cm^{-1} corresponds to the C=O stretching vibrations, stemming from the amide, which suggests that the carboxyl groups partly reacted with the hydrazide groups. The weak signal at 2526–2594 cm^{-1} might be assigned to the weak S–H stretching vibrations. The FTIR spectrum of t-Chi showed results comparable to t-CS. In comparison with the spectrum of the unmodified chitosan, new peaks can be seen at 615–725 cm^{-1} (C–S stretching vibration), 873–918 cm^{-1} (C–H bending), 1504–1579 cm^{-1} (N–H vibration (amide I)), 2821–2879 cm^{-1} (sym. CH_2 group stretching in –CH_2–S–) and 2526–2594 cm^{-1} (S–H stretching vibration), which indicate a successful functionalization with DTPA [32].

To confirm the successful cleavage of the disulfide bond and the presence of free thiol groups in the polysaccharides, Raman spectra of the substances were recorded, as the C–S vibration of thiol groups shows up in a finger print region without the interference of other groups (Fig. 3) [33].

The spectra shown in Fig. 3 show peaks at 2571 cm^{-1} and 673–677 cm^{-1}, which coincide with the S–H and C–S vibrations respectively according to literature [34]. The successful grafting of both polysaccharides with the linker to obtain free thiol groups was confirmed. The degree of thiolation was also determined quantitatively via the reaction with Ellmans reagent and subsequent analysis by UV–Vis spectrometry. Furthermore, the molecular weights of the products were analyzed with gel permeation chromatography. The results are listed in Table 2.

In general, for both molecules, a degree of thiolation of 25% was expected. However, the Ellman's assay determined a degree of thiolation of 32.5% for chondroitin sulfate and 13.7% for chitosan. A higher degree of functionalization was considered as beneficial for CS because the thiol groups are required to crosslink CS with its t-Chi counterpart. On the other hand, a lower degree of functionalization for chitosan may also be advantageous because a charge density can be kept, which is

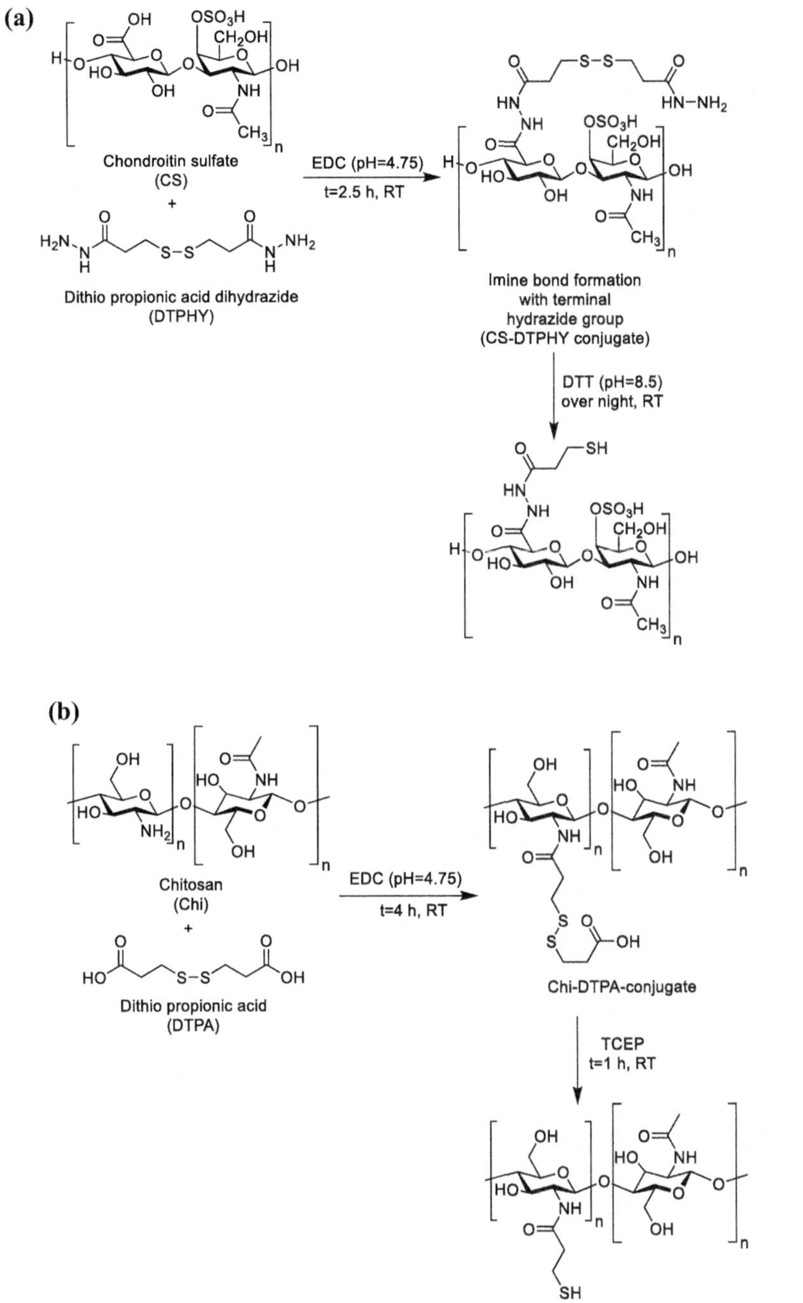

Fig. 1 **a** The thiolation of chondroitin sulfate (t-CS) with a disulfide-containing hydrazide crosslinker DTPHY, mediated by EDC and subsequent reduction of the disulfide bond with DTT. **b** The thiolation of chitosan (t-Chi) with a disulfide-containing crosslinker DTPA, mediated by EDC and subsequent reduction of the disulfide bond with TCEP

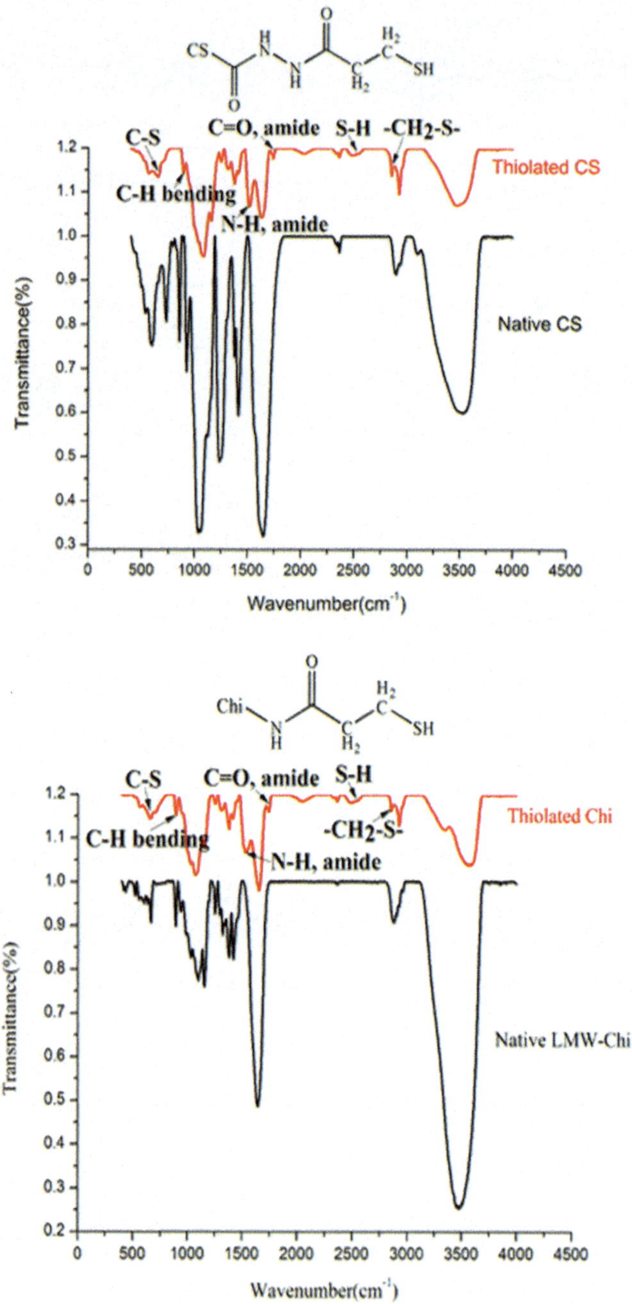

Fig. 2 FTIR spectra of native and thiol-functionalized chondroitin sulfate (CS) and chitosan (Chi). Reprinted with permission from Ref. [32]. Copyright 2017

high enough for the required Coulomb interactions as the thiol functionalization of chitosan consumes free amine groups, which are responsible for the positive charge of the polysaccharide [35]. Hence, both polysaccharides shall still have a sufficient number of charged groups that are required for Coulomb attraction and ion pairing during the multilayer formation process. This is also in accordance to other publications, where the degree of thiolation is in a similar range (under 50%) [23, 36]. This is advantageous, as the original properties of the polysaccharides should be preserved.

The GPC measurements show that the molecular weight of t-CS molecules is higher than that of the native CS, which is presumably because the higher degree

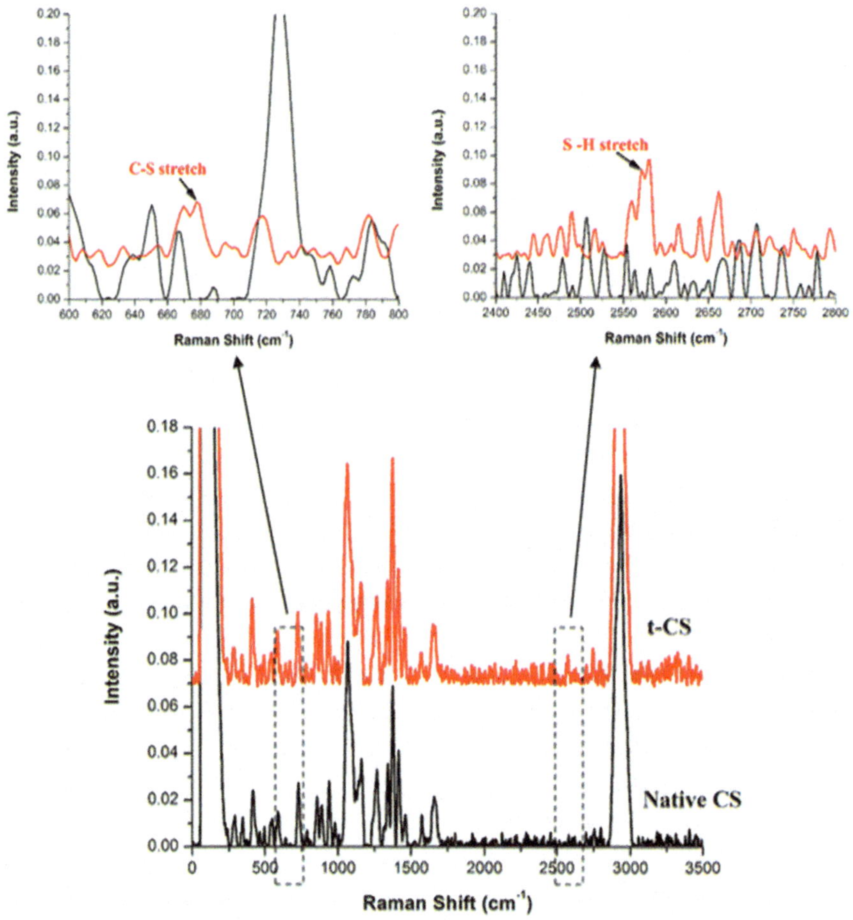

Fig. 3 Raman spectra of native and thiol-functionalized chondroitin sulfate (CS) and chitosan (Chi) (upper figure: Raman spectra of chondroitin sulfate and thiolated chondroitin sulfate (t-CS); lower figure: Raman spectra of chitosan and thiolated chitosan, t-Chi). Reprinted with permission from Ref. [32]. Copyright 2017

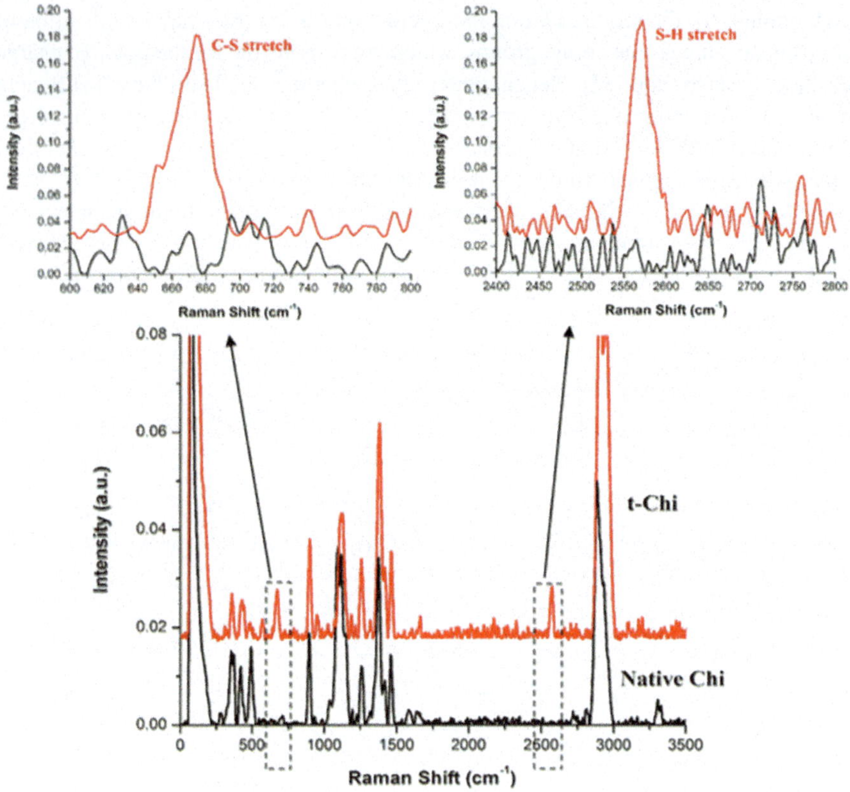

Fig. 3 (continued)

Table 2 GPC Molecular weight distribution analysis and degree of thiolation

Sample polymer	M_n (kDa)	M_w (kDa)	PDI (M_w/M_n)	Degree of thiolation
n-CS	25.00	35.00	1.40	/
t-CS	30.00	45.00	1.50	32.53%
n-Chi	20.00	61.92	3.09	/
t-Chi	20.55	65.28	3.18	13.70%

Reprinted with permission from Ref. [32]. Copyright 2017

of functionalization leads to a higher molecular weight of the polymer chain. The comparison between native and thiolated chitosan shows only a small increase in the molecular weight and polydispersity index after the functionalization, which suggests that the thiolation does not influence the size of the polymer through unwanted crosslinking by disulfide bonds. Because the thiolation degree is not very high, the increase in molecular weight of t-Chi was low as well.

3.2 Formation and Analysis Multilayers

The multilayers were formed by alternating deposition of the positively charged chitosan (pH 4 of solution protonates the amino groups of Chi [37]) and the negatively charged chondroitin sulfate onto the different type of model surfaces, such as glass, gold and silicone. Multilayers consisting of native polysaccharides were compared with multilayers consisting of thiolated polysaccharides to determine the influence of thiolation and potential covalent bonding that happens between two layers through the reaction of two thiols with each other. Surface plasmon resonance was used to study the formation process of the multilayers (Fig. 4).

It can be observed, that the increase in angle shift for thiolated polysaccharides is higher than for native precursors. One possibility for this occurrence is the presence of hydrophobic methylene group, which is introduced through grafting the DTPHY or DTPA into the polysaccharides backbone, which can lead to additional hydrophobic interactions between the layers. This might increase the adsorption of the polysaccharides during the multilayer formation in addition to ion pairing [38]. The growth behaviour of both types of multilayers with increasing layer number seems to be exponential, which is consistent with results of studies with other polysaccharide-based multilayer systems [39].

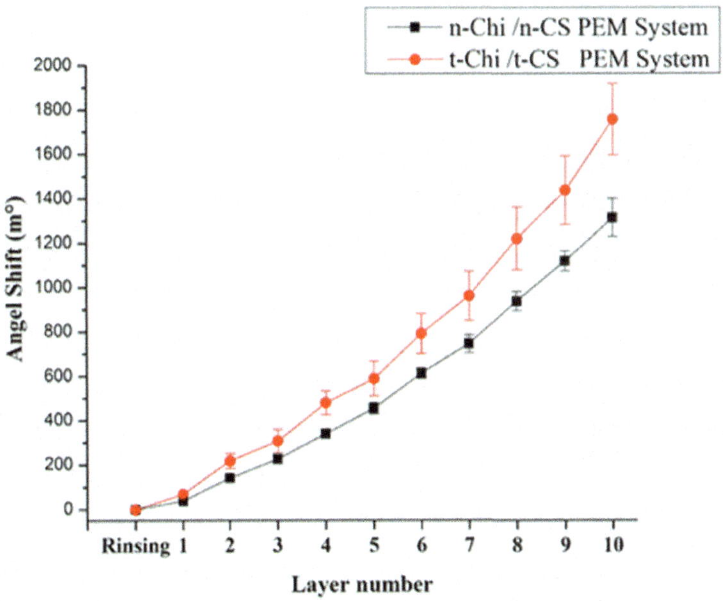

Fig. 4 Growth of multilayers of either thiolated or native polysaccharides measured by surface plasmon resonance angle shifts (odd layers are thiolated (t-Chi) of native chitosan (n-Chi) and even layers are thiolated (t-CS) or native chondroitin sulfate (n-CS)). Reprinted with permission from Ref. [31]. Copyright 2017

Ellman's reagent was used to determine the quantity of the thiol groups in the multilayers, which was done after formation of multilayers from t-CS and t-Chi on glass slides by a dip rinsing process. Figure 5 shows the results of these studies, which included also different ways to oxidize the thiol groups so that disulfide bonds are formed inside the multilayers. Indeed, the maximum content in free thiol groups is seen after the formation of [t-CS/t-Chi] multilayers, indicated by the highest absorbance. Two different strategies are employed here to achieve oxidation of thiols. The first is based on increasing pH value to achieve deprotonation of sulfur in thiol to obtain an unpaired electron that promotes the formation of disulfide bond with adjacent thiol groups [40]. The second is to use the oxidizing agent chloramine-T that has been employed by other groups [28]. Figure 5 shows the results of the Ellman's test for the layers immediately after the synthesis and after several hours of incubation at a high pH value or the exposure to the oxidizing agent chloramine-T.

An increase in the incubation time at basic pH leads to a decrease of the absorbance intensity at 412 nm indicating a significant loss of free thiols with time with this oxidation procedure. Hence, it can be assumed that the longer the incubation time, the higher the number of thiol groups that form disulfide bonds and crosslink the

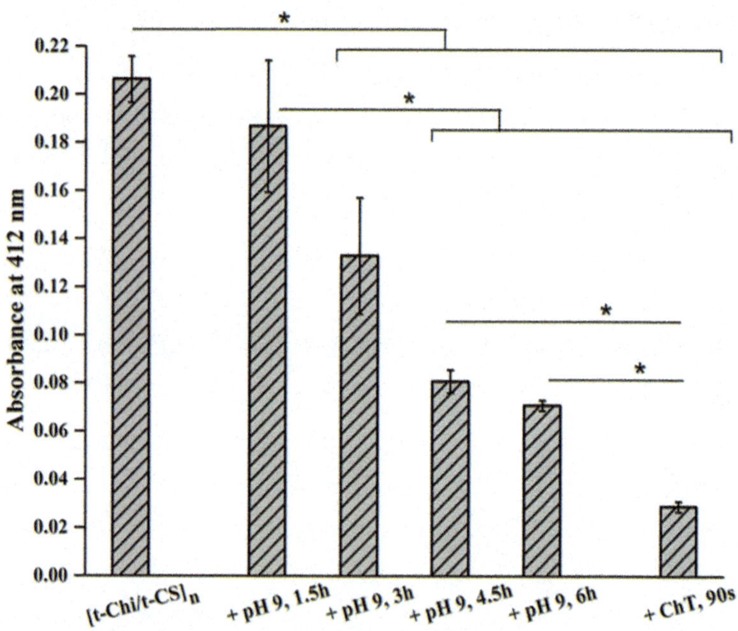

Fig. 5 Absorbance analysis of Ellman's test to determine the amount of free thiols in multilayer systems comprised of thiolated chitosan (t-Chi) and thiolated chondroitin sulfate (t-CS) with a number of layers n = 20. $[\text{t-Chi/t-CS}]_n$ shows the absorbance intensity of untouched multilayers, while the other columns show the absorbance intensity after their treatment with a 150 mM NaCl solution at a pH of 9 (incubation times of 1.5, 3, 4.5 and 6 h) or with chloramine-T (ChT) for 90 s. Error bars represent ±SD. (*): statistically significant difference ($p \leq 0.05$). Reprinted with permission from Ref. [22]. Copyright 2018 American Chemical Society

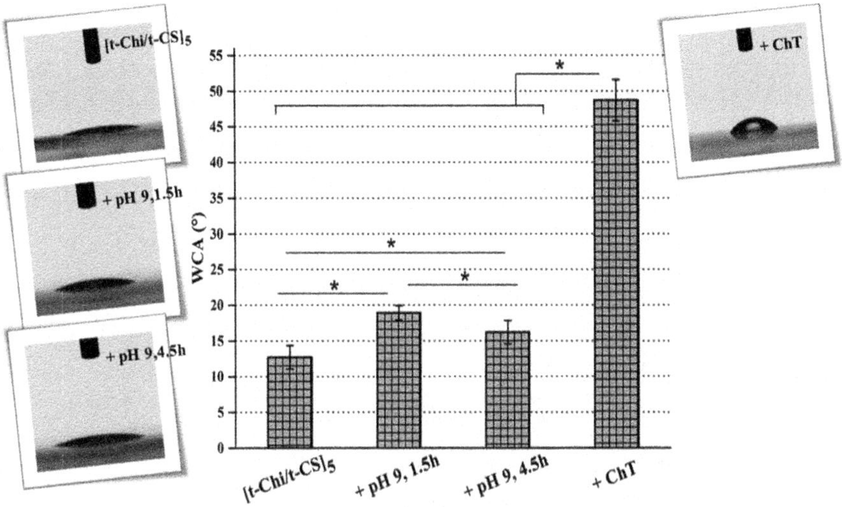

Fig. 6 Water contact angles (°) of initial [t-Chi/t-CS]$_5$ multilayers and after oxidation at pH 9, monitored at 1.5 h and 4.5 h and 90 s oxidation with chloramine-T (ChT). Photographs show the shape of 0.5 μL droplet of ultrapure water on the multilayer films. t: thiolated; Chi: chitosan. CS: chondroitin sulfate Means ± SD. (*): statistically significant ($p \leq 0.05$). Reprinted with permission from Ref. [22]. Copyright 2018 American Chemical Society

multilayer. The highest conversion rate is seen for chloramine-T as oxidizing reagent. Since no significant difference is seen between incubation times of 4.5 and 6 h, the incubation times of 1.5 and 4.5 h at pH 9 and ChT were chosen for the oxidation of thiols in subsequent experiments.

Wetting properties of biomaterials are an indicator for the adsorption of proteins and attachment and spreading of cells as regulators of cell fate [3, 5]. Therefore, water contact angles of the multilayers were measured before and after the treatment with oxidizing agents. Figure 6 shows the water contact angles of the different multilayers.

The multilayer [t-Chi/t-CS]$_5$ has a very hydrophilic surface, which is due to the presence of hydrophilic and polar groups in both polysaccharides such as amine, carboxy, hydroxyl and sulfate groups. After the incubation in a basic environment, the WCA of the surface slightly but significantly increases, which indicates that a change of the surface, relating to the oxidation of thiol groups has taken place. Since the thiol groups only make up a relatively small part of the surface, no bigger changes were expected. By contrast, the WCA changes drastically after the incubation in ChT and the surface becomes more hydrophobic, which may have a promoting effect on protein adsorption and cell adhesion.

Beside wetting properties, the surface potential of biomaterials is another regulator of protein adsorption and cell adhesion [4]. Therefore the zeta potential of multilayers was measured at different pH values, which is shown in Fig. 7.

The zeta potential is determined by the presence of charged groups at the interface between multilayers and outer electrolyte solutions. However, since streaming

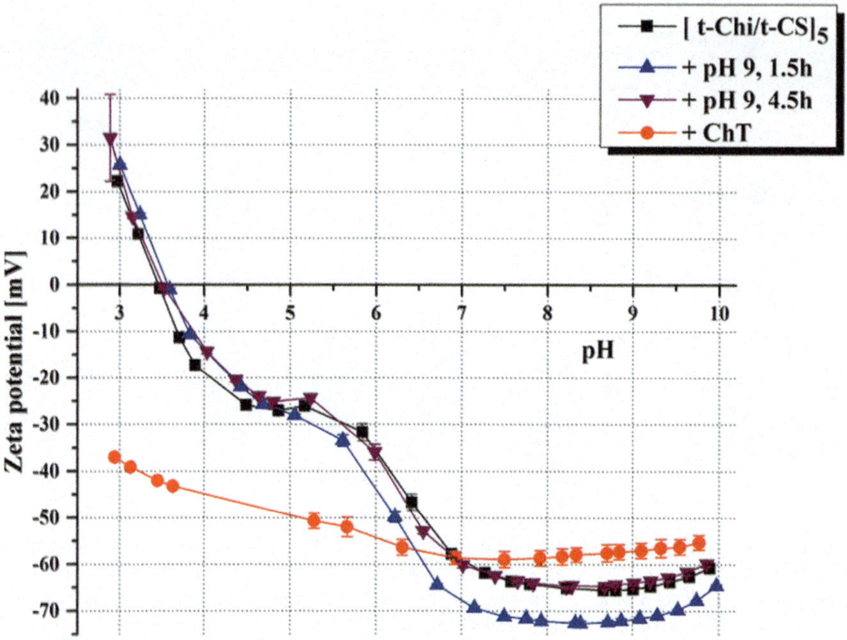

Fig. 7 Zeta potential of the [t-Chi/t-CS]$_5$ multilayer upon oxidation by pH 9, 1.5 h and pH 9, 4.5 h versus chloramine-T(ChT). Measurements were performed in 1 mmol/L KCl electrolyte via an acid-to-based pH titration. t: thiolated. Chi: chitosan. CS: chondroitin sulphate. Reprinted with permission from Ref. [22]. Copyright 2018 American Chemical Society

potential is not only determined by the outermost layer of polyelectrolytes [41], but adjacent layers, titration from acidic to basic pH shows typically changes that are related to the presence of basic groups like amino groups in chitosan and acidic like carboxylic and sulfate groups in chondroitin sulfate [17]. Figure 7 shows that longer or shorter incubation of thiolated multilayers at basic pH 9 did not lead to any significant changes in zeta potential, though some moderate changes were observed in wetting properties. Since the crosslinking of the thiol groups does not interfere with the ionic groups present in both layers, no significant change is expected. By contrast, ChT-treated multilayers show a significantly lower zeta potential at low pH values, which indicates that some of the amino groups of chitosan are no longer available to generate a positive charge on the surface. It is probable that the chloramine T is not only promoting disulfide bond formation, but undergoes also some side reactions amine groups in a nucleophilic substitution to form a less polar compound [42, 43].

Atomic force microscopy was used to analyse the surface topography and the mechanical properties of the different multilayers, which may also have some effect on cell adhesion [44]. The AFM pictures and corresponding mechanical measurements can be found in Fig. 8.

The images show that untreated multilayers in a swollen state are represented by globular structures covering the surface. It is also visible that they look similar to

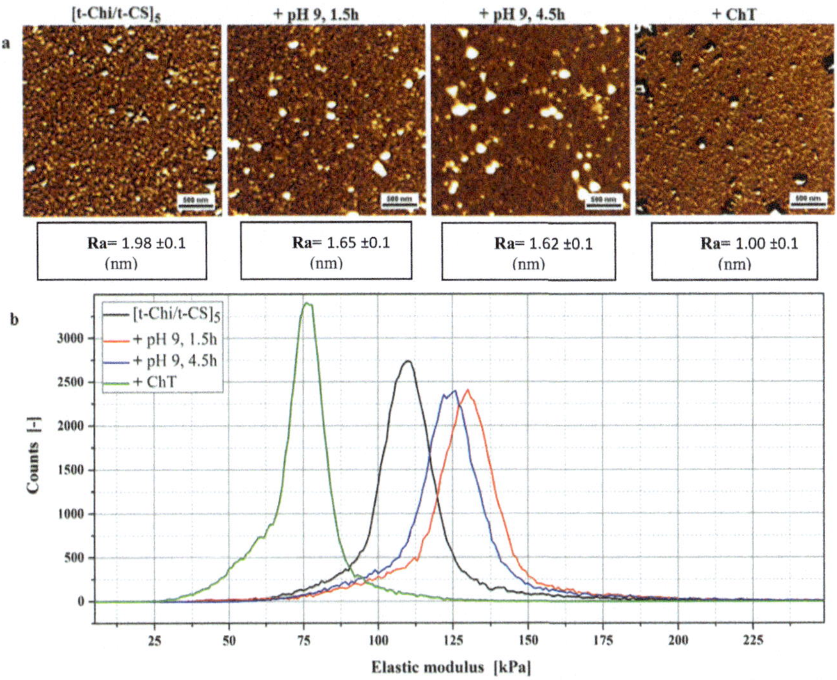

Fig. 8 **a** Topographical images of multilayers using intermittent contact mode in 150 mM NaCl solution. **b** Distribution curves of Young's moduli (E) were calculated from each single force curve in a force-map of 256 × 256 pi^2 within an area of 3 × 3 μm^2. t: thiolated. Chi: chitosan. CS: chondroitin sulfate. ChT: chloramine-T. Reprinted with permission from Ref. [22]. Copyright 2018 American Chemical Society

those exposed to pH 9 for 1.5 and 4.5 h. This is also represented by similar roughness values as shown in Table 3. However, AFM images of multilayers treated with ChT seem to have smaller, more vermiculate-like structures on the surfaces, which corresponds also to lower roughness values. The surface roughness was quantified and the roughness average (Ra) as well as the root mean squared roughness (Rq) are listed in Table 3.

Table 3 Surface roughness of [t-Chi/t-CS]$_5$ multilayers treated under different conditions

Sample	Ra (nm)^a	Rq (nm)^a
[t-Chi/t-CS]$_5$	1.98 ± 0.10	2.56 ± 0.20
+ pH 9 (1.5 h)	1.65 ± 0.10	2.07 ± 0.10
+pH 9 (4.5 h)	1.62 ± 0.10	2.18 ± 0.10
+ ChT	1.00 ± 0.10	1.25 ± 0.10

^{a}Roughness average (Ra) and root mean square roughness (Rq) for multilayers derived from atomic force microscopy in 150 mM NaCl solution

Table 4 Elastic modulus of multilayers treated under different conditions

Sample	E modulus (kPa)
[t-Chi/t-CS]$_5$	110
+ pH 9 (1.5 h)	124
+ pH 9 (4.5 h)	130
+ ChT	76

The elastic modulus was determined in a NaCl solution (150 mmol/L, pH 4) as well, which represents the stiffness of the multilayers that shall be influenced by the degree of crosslinking between singular layers [45]. The graphical representation of measurements is shown in Fig. 8a and mean E moduli in Table 4.

It is expected that a higher degree of disulfide bond formation lead to stiffer multilayers and thus a higher E modulus. Indeed, such changes are observed after the treatment of multilayers with pH 9 showing also that a longer exposure leads to slightly increased E modulus (Table 4). However, a significant drop was observed for the ChT-treated [t-Chi/t-CS]$_5$ multilayers, although the Ellman's test confirmed a significant drop in the concentration of free thiol groups. This is a further indicator of a potential side reaction of the ChT with amino groups, as already indicated with the lower zeta potential. As the number of available amino groups decreases, the number of ionic interactions between the oppositely charged layers decreases as well, which should lead to a lower degree of ionic crosslinking that cannot be compensated by the formation of new disulfide bonds. Hence, the multilayers become softer here.

3.3 Cyclic Redox-Mediated Switching of Multilayer Cross-Linking and Biological Response

The treatment of [t-Chi/t-CS]$_5$ multilayer with oxidizing agents should lead to the formation of disulfide bonds as it has been detected indirectly by the decrease of free thiols shown in the previous section (see Fig. 5 again). The newly formed disulfide bonds can be broken again to reform free thiol groups by using a reducing agent. We selected here Tris-(2-carboxyethyl)-phosphine hydrochloride (TCEP) as effective reducing agent that permits the formation of free thiol groups [24]. Because with ChT we have a strong oxidizing and with TCEP a strong reducing agent, we were interested to see if we are able to test the possibility to repeatedly switch the multilayers between cross-linked and non-cross-linked states. In Fig. 9 the Ellman's test after the treatment with either TCEP or ChT is shown, which corresponds to concentration of free thiol groups in the multilayers. Higher absorbance represents here higher concentration of thiols [25].

Figure 9 shows in the upper part together with the chemical formulas of oxidizing and reducing agents that after treatment of [t-Chi/t-CS]$_5$ multilayers with ChT a marked decrease in the absorbance can be seen, which means a large part of thiol groups is oxidized and may be consumed by disulfide bond formation. After treatment

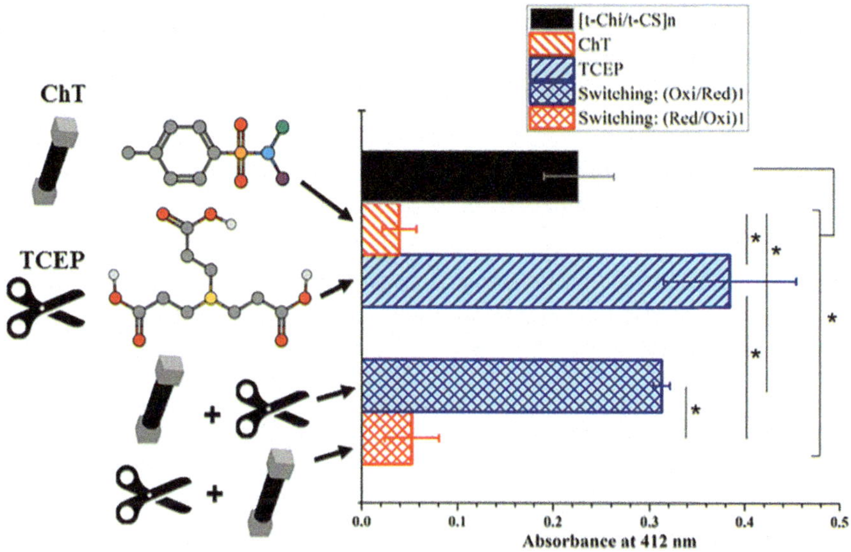

Fig. 9 UV–Vis absorbance analysis following the Ellman's test for quantification of thiols in multilayers. The $[\text{t-Chi/t-CS}]_n$ multilayers were subjected to ChT oxidation and TCEP reduction. t-Chi: thiolated chitosan. t-CS: thiolated chondroitin sulfate. n = 10: number of double layers. ChT: Chloramine-T. TCEP: tris(2-carboxyethyl) phosphine. Error bars express ±SD, for triplicate samples. (*): statistically significant, where statistically non-significant differences correspond to reversibility of the redox reactions distinguished from the results in the early TCEP and ChT states. Molecular structure illustrations include: C: gray atoms, O: red atoms, S: orange atom, N: blue atom, Na: green atom, Cl: violet atom, H: white atoms and P: yellow atom. Reprinted with permission from Ref. [13]. Copyright 2018 American Chemical Society

of these oxidized multilayers with the reducing agent TCEP a high absorbance at 412 nm can be seen again, which indicates reformation of free thiol groups detected by Ellmans reagent. It is also remarkable that absorbance after treatment with TCEP is higher than that of the original $[\text{t-Chi/t-CS}]_5$ which indicated that a higher quantity of free thiols can be found after reduction with TCEP. Figure 9 shows in the lower part that a cyclic oxidation and reduction of the multilayers is possible by both reagents showing that after previous oxidation with ChT a subsequent reduction with TCEP (oxi/red) leads to a quantity of thiols that is higher than that of the original $[\text{t-Chi/t-CS}]_5$ multilayer. In addition, the opposite step from prior reduction with TCEP to oxidation by ChT leads to a thiol content that is comparable to the first oxidation step. Hence, this indicates that the whole system is cyclable, which means that the disulfide bonds can be broken and reformed repeatedly. These subsequent oxidation and reduction steps affect also wetting properties, zeta potential and E modulus leading to values that corresponds well to that of oxidized and reduced multilayers shown here before. More details can be found in a previous article from our group [13]. Since the oxidation and reduction of thiol groups leads to changes in the mechanical and surface properties, it is assumed that these multilayers can specifically control the adsorption of proteins and adhesion of cells depending on the redox state of the multilayers.

3.4 *Effect of Redox State on Adsorption of Fibronectin and Adhesion of Fibroblasts*

The adsorption of the extracellular matrix proteins is a prerequisite for cell adhesion and integrin ligation, which in turn leads to the survival, growth and differentiation of cells. The adsorption of the protein fibronectin (FN) that is recognized by cellular integrin, such as the a5b1 integrin in fibroblasts [3], was used as an indicator for the biocompatibility of the multilayers. FN was labelled with a fluorescent dye and its intensity was measured on the [t-Chi/t-CS]$_5$ multilayers in dependence on the redox state (Fig. 10).

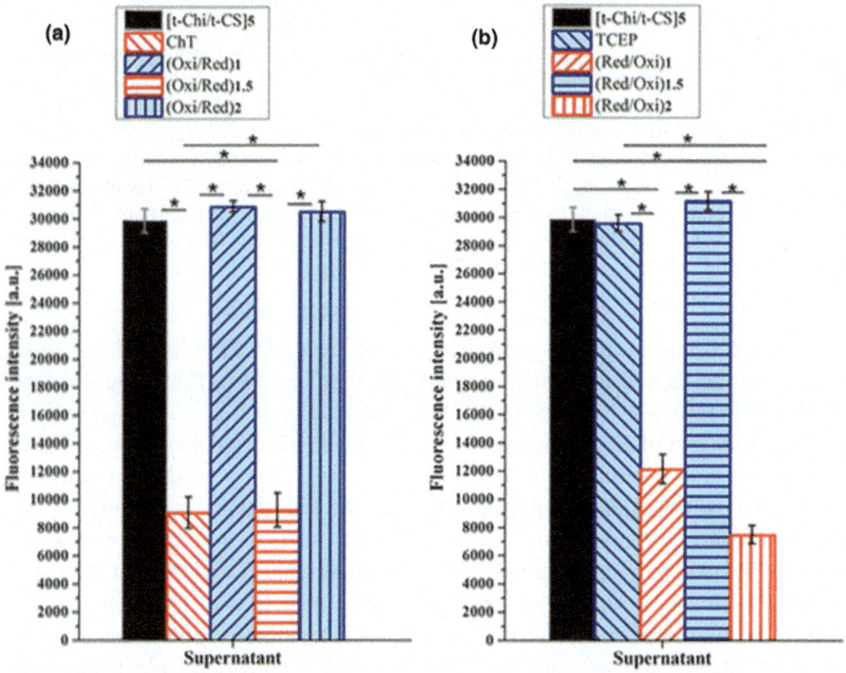

Fig. 10 The average fluorescence intensity of FITC-conjugated fibronectin (FN) exposed to 4 sequences of serial redox reactions (**a**) and its reverse (**b**) of chloramine-T (ChT) as oxidizing and tris(2-carboxyethyl) phosphine (TCEP) as reducing agent. The multilayer supernatant was analyzed after exposure to FITC-FN representing the fraction of FN that was not absorbed and thus found in supernatant solution. Means ± SD of eight replicates from each condition. (*): statistically significant ($p \leq 0.05$). Reprinted with permission from Ref. [13]. Copyright 2018 American Chemical Society

The fluorescence intensity (FI) of the supernatants was measured after incubation of multilayers with the fluorescent FITC-FN solution. Here, a high fluorescence intensity in the supernatant indicates a low level of protein adsorption, while a low intensity indicates adsorption of FITC-FN on the multilayer surface. Several steps of oxidation-reduction cycles were done starting either with the oxidation by ChT and subsequent cycles of reduction/oxidation (Fig. 10a), while in Fig. 10b the process starts first with the reduction of multilayers followed by oxidation and so on. It is visible in Fig. 10 that in each case of oxidation a lower FI is observed, which corresponds to higher protein adsorption, while the subsequent treatment with the reducing agent TCEP leads to a drastic reduction in the adsorption capability of the $[\text{t-Chi/t-CS}]_5$ multilayers. This is regardless of the order of treatments, which means that the multilayer system is completely reversible regarding the redox state and the corresponding adsorption of protein FN. This behaviour is probably controlled by the wetting properties since the treatment with ChT leads to a more hydrophobic surface, while the initial or reduced state of $[\text{t-Chi/t-CS}]_5$ multilayers is related to lower water contact angles as shown in the WCA measurements. Previous studies have shown that hydrophobic and moderate wettable surfaces tend to adsorb more proteins than hydrophilic surfaces [46]. Comparing the first and second oxidizing treatment, it is obvious that the adsorption capabilities of the surface are similar, which means that the multilayer can be returned to its oxidized or reduced state even after several cycles. That represents a perfect stimuli-responsive system that can easily be switched between to two different states as reviewed previously by us [10].

As a high FN concentration on the surface is also beneficial to the adhesion of cells, studies were performed with human fibroblast. Figure 11 shows images of the immunefluorescent staining of fixed human dermal fibroblasts (HDF) that were stained against filamentous F-Actin (red) and nuclei (blue) at lower magnification (a) and higher magnification (b) either in presence (i) or absence of 10% bovine serum with pre-coating of multilayers with 20 μg/ml FN (ii).

Figure 11a provides a survey on the effect of redox state of thiolated multilayers on fibroblast adhesion showing that oxidation with chloramine-T provides surfaces with high adhesiveness for cells (ChT), which is also effective when these multilayers were subsequently reduced by TCEP and oxidized again by ChT ($(\text{Oxi/Red})_{1.5}$). On the contrary, the reduction of multilayers by TCEP ($(\text{Oxi/Red})_1$) and subsequent oxidation and reduction ($(\text{Oxi/Red})_2$) generates multilayers of very low adhesiveness for fibroblasts. Figure 11b shows a higher magnification of cells adhering on the same $[\text{t-Chi/t-CS}]_5$ multilayers as described above. It is obvious that oxidated and reduced state of multilayers go along different phenotypes of fibroblasts. Fibroblasts adhering on oxidized $[\text{t-Chi/t-CS}]_5$ multilayers (ChT, $(\text{Oxi/Red})_{1.5}$) are characterized by an elongated, polarized phenotype with longitudinal organization of actin stress fibres, while cells on reduced ($(\text{Oxi/Red})_1$; $(\text{Oxi/Red})_2$) surfaces are not well spread with little signs of actin polymerization. The stained nuclei were used to quantify fibroblast adhesion on the surfaces, which is shown in Fig. 12. Quantitative analysis of cell adhesions shows that number of adhering fibroblasts was higher on all surfaces pre-coated with FN when compared to their culture in the presence of 10% serum, which

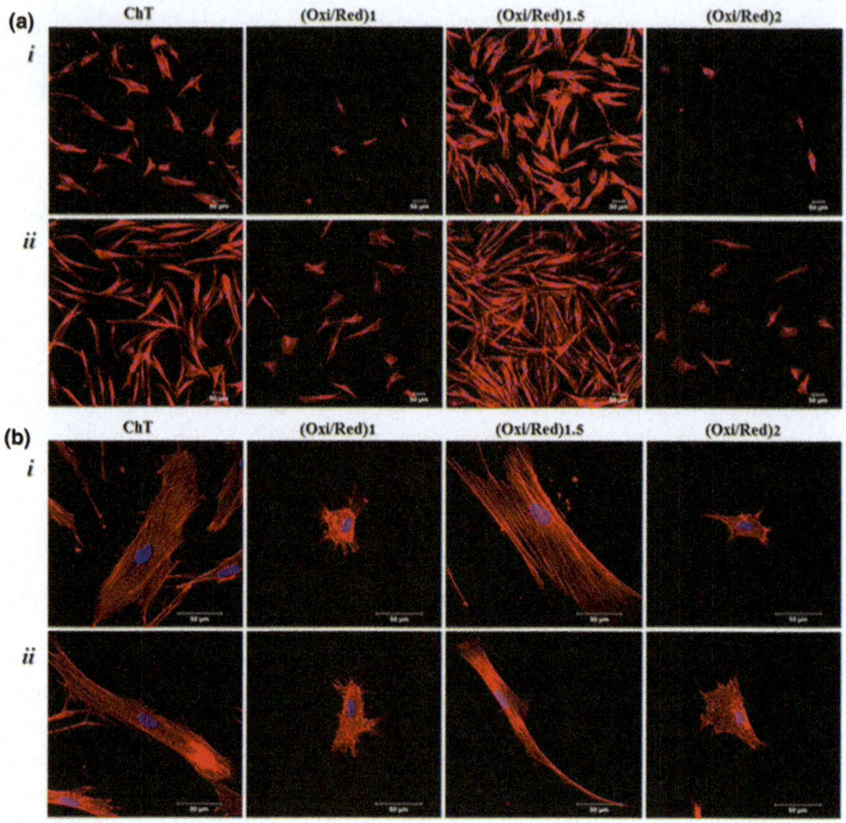

Fig. 11 Representative images of immunefluorescent staining studies (**a** at low and **b** at high magnifications, scale bar: 50 μm) of fibroblast cells using confocal laser scanning microscopy (CLSM) after 24 h of cultivation on triggered multilayers, (i) incubation in the presence of 10% fetal bovine serum and (ii) precoating with 20 μg mL^{-1} fibronectin. Cells were stained with red-fluorescent Phalloidin CruzFluor™ 555 conjugate for labeling actin, and with blue-fluorescent TO-PRO™-3 for staining nuclei. 4 sequences of the reversible consecutive switching, serve here as an example. The results stand for triplicate sets. Reprinted with permission from Ref. [13]. Copyright 2018 American Chemical Society

is due to the high concentration of FN during pre-adsorption process compared to traces of adhesion promoting proteins, such as vitronectin and fibronectin in serum [47]. Quantitative analysis demonstrates also that oxidized state of multilayers is causing a significantly higher adhesion of fibroblasts in comparison to the reduced state.

Since cell spreading is a modulator of signal transduction via mitogen-activated protein kinases (MAPK) linked through ligation of integrins to extracellular matrix ligands like FN [48], effects of redox state on cell growth were expected, too. In Fig. 13a qualitative analysis of fibroblast growth after 72 h is provided by phase contrast images of the fibroblasts. The micrographs illustrate again the reversibility

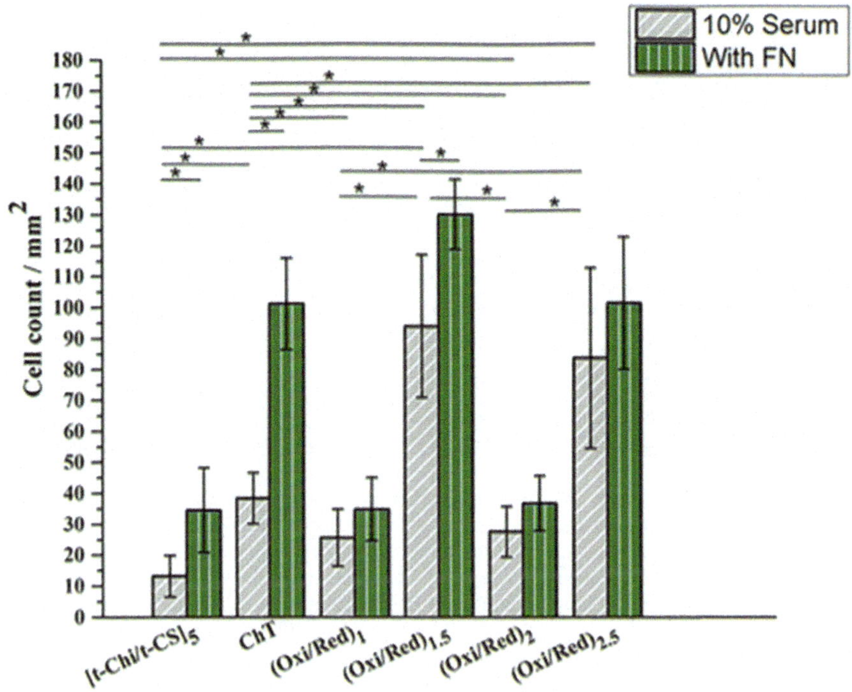

Fig. 12 The effects of sequential oxidation-reduction cycles of multilayers on fibroblast adhesion in the presence of 10% fetal bovine serum (FBS) or after fibronectin pre-coating (FN, 20 μg mL^{-1}) on cell count. 5 sequences of switching reactions of original [t-Chi/t-CS]$_5$ multilayer serve here as an example. Reprinted with permission from Ref. [13]. Copyright 2018 American Chemical Society

of the redox process that started with oxidation of multilayers and subsequent reduction/oxidation cycles in the upper and reduction with subsequent oxidation-reduction cycles in the lower row. All states when [t-Chi/t-CS]$_5$ multilayers are in an oxidized state are providing conditions that promote cell growth leading to the establishment of confluent monolayers of fibroblasts, while the reduced state is suppressing cell growth permitting only the presence of few cells of very elongated phenotype. Results of fibroblast adhesion and growth studies reflect changes in the multilayer properties depending on the redox state, which are either permitting or suppressing protein adsorption that provides the basis for ligation of cell adhesion receptors to matrix proteins like fibronectin. It is also obvious that the aforementioned reversibility of the redox status of the multilayers is not only related to their physical properties, but also to their bioactivity towards human fibroblasts.

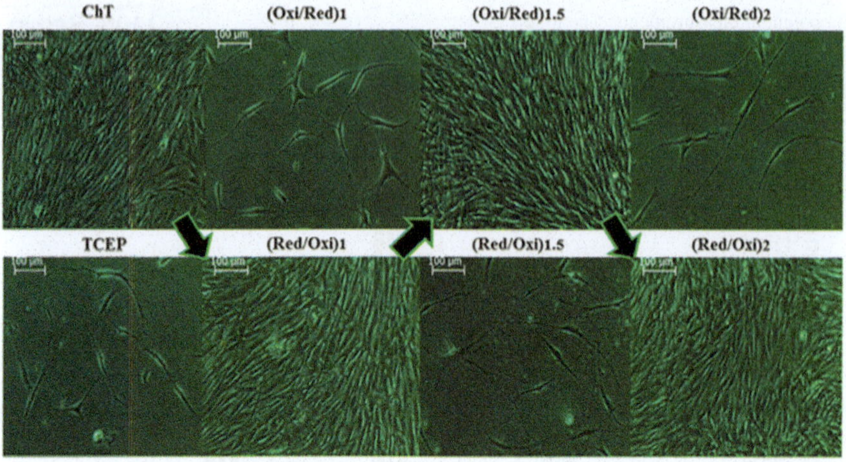

Fig. 13 Representative phase-contrast images of fibroblasts after 72 h having cultured on 8 redox-models of responsive multilayers. The first row representing 4 sequencing steps of chloramine-T (ChT)-initiated switching stands parallel to second row for TCEP-initiated switching. The black arrows follow each of the sequences ended to the oxidized states. Low magnification, scale bar: 100 μm. Reprinted with permission from Ref. [13]. Copyright 2018 American Chemical Society

4 Conclusion

This article demonstrates that the functionalization of polysaccharides with thiol groups can lead to a new type of stimuli responsive multilayer system. It could be shown that polysaccharides can be modified with a significant share of thiol groups in a Steglich-analogous esterification between the polysaccharide and a disulfide-carrying compound and a subsequent reduction of said compound to form free thiol groups. The usage of thiolated chondroitin sulfate and chitosan in the synthesis of surface coatings with the layer-by-layer technique leads to redox sensitive multilayers as their properties such as the wettability, zeta potential and elastic modulus can be modulated by applying either an oxidizing or a reducing agent to the surface to crosslink the thiol groups or cleave the disulfide bonds. It could be demonstrated that the crosslinking process is reversible and repeatable. It was also found that the oxidation with chloramine-T provided surfaces with a high adhesiveness for proteins like fibronectin and human dermal fibroblasts, which was significantly lower on surfaces, which were reduced by TCEP. These findings show that the incorporation of redox sensitive cross-linkable groups can lead to a stimuli-responsive surface that can be readily change its mechanical and surface properties and is able to selectively promote or inhibit cell adhesion.

Acknowledgements The authors acknowledge the excellent support by Alexander Köwitsch in guiding P.E. in synthesis and analysis of thiolated polysaccharides, Steffen Fischer for his kind support of analysis by Raman spectroscopy, Matthias Menzel for doing the atomic force microscopy, Wolfgang Fuhrmann for guidance in ellipsometry measurements and Marlis Porobin for supporting zeta potential measurements. The financial support from Deutsche Forschungsgemeinschaft in the frame of the project Gr 1290/12-1 is greatly acknowledged.

References

1. Li, Y., Wei, Y., Liao, J., Hao, Y., Ning, C., Jiang, L., Wang, S.: Surface wettability switched cell adhesion and detachment on conducting polymer nanoarray. Adv. Mater. Interfaces **3**, 1600598 (2016)
2. Kaneko, S., Yamaguchi, K., Nakanishi, J.: Dynamic substrate based on photocleavable poly (ethylene glycol): zeta potential determines the capability of geometrical cell confinement. Langmuir **29**, 7300–7308 (2013)
3. Altankov, G., Grinnell, F., Groth, T.: Studies on the biocompatibility of materials: fibroblast reorganization of substratum-bound fibronectin on surfaces varying in wettability. J. Biomed. Mater. Res. Official J. Soc. Biomater. Jpn. Soc. Biomater. **30**, 385–391 (1996)
4. Altankov, G., Richau, K., Groth, T.: The role of surface zeta potential and substratum chemistry for regulation of dermal fibroblasts interaction. Materialwiss. Werkstofftech. Entwicklung Fertigung Prüfung Eigenschaften Anwendungen Technischer Werkst. **34**, 1120–1128 (2003)
5. Faucheux, N., Schweiss, R., Lützow, K., Werner, C., Groth, T.: Self-assembled monolayers with different terminating groups as model substrates for cell adhesion studies. Biomaterials **25**, 2721–2730 (2004)
6. Discher, D.E., Janmey, P., Wang, Y.-L.: Tissue cells feel and respond to the stiffness of their substrate. Science **310**, 1139–1143 (2005)
7. Engler, A.J., Richert, L., Wong, J.Y., Picart, C., Discher, D.E.: Surface probe measurements of the elasticity of sectioned tissue, thin gels and polyelectrolyte multilayer films: correlations between substrate stiffness and cell adhesion. Surf. Sci. **570**, 142–154 (2004)
8. Chen, Y.-H., Chung, Y.-C., Wang, I.-J., Young, T.-H.: Control of cell attachment on pH-responsive chitosan surface by precise adjustment of medium pH. Biomaterials **33**, 1336–1342 (2012)
9. Tekin H., Sanchez J.G., Tsinman, T., Langer, R., Khademhosseini, A.: Thermoresponsive platforms for tissue engineering and regenerative medicine. AIChE J. Am. Inst. Chem. Eng. **57**, 3249 (2011)
10. Esmaeilzadeh, P., Groth, T.: Switchable and obedient interfacial properties that grant new biomedical applications. ACS Appl. Mater. Interfaces **11**, 25637–25653 (2019)
11. Roberts, J.N., Sahoo, J.K., McNamara, L.E., Burgess, K.V., Yang, J., Alakpa, E.V., Anderson, H.J., Hay, J., Turner, L.-A., Yarwood, S.J.: Dynamic surfaces for the study of mesenchymal stem cell growth through adhesion regulation. ACS Nano **10**, 6667–6679 (2016)
12. Zhu, Y., Shi, J., Shen, W., Dong, X., Feng, J., Ruan, M., Li, Y.: Stimuli-responsive controlled drug release from a hollow mesoporous silica sphere/polyelectrolyte multilayer core–shell structure. Angew. Chem. **117**, 5213–5217 (2005)
13. Esmaeilzadeh, P., Menzel, M., Groth, T.: Cyclic redox-mediated switching of surface properties of thiolated polysaccharide multilayers and its effect on fibroblast adhesion. ACS Appl. Mater. Interfaces **10**, 31168–31177 (2018)
14. Silva, J.M., Reis, R.L., Mano, J.F.: Biomimetic extracellular environment based on natural origin polyelectrolyte multilayers. Small **12**, 4308–4342 (2016)
15. Hong, J., Lowack, K., Schmitt, J., Decher, G.: Layer-by-layer deposited multilayer assemblies of polyelectrolytes and proteins: from ultrathin films to protein arrays. In: Trends in Colloid and Interface Science VII. Springer, Berlin (1993)
16. Köwitsch, A., Zhou, G., Groth, T.: Medical application of glycosaminoglycans: a review. J. Tissue Eng. Regen. Med. **12**, e23–e41 (2018)

17. Zhao, M., Li, L., Zhou, C., Heyroth, F., Fuhrmann, B., Maeder, K., Groth, T.: Improved stability and cell response by intrinsic cross-linking of multilayers from collagen I and oxidized glycosaminoglycans. Biomacromolecules **15**, 4272–4280 (2014)
18. Anouz, R., Repanas, A., Schwarz, E., Groth, T.: Novel surface coatings using oxidized glycosaminoglycans as delivery systems of bone morphogenetic protein 2 (BMP-2) for bone regeneration. Macromol. Biosci. **18**, 1800283 (2018)
19. Apte, G., Repanas, A., Willems, C., Mujtaba, A., Schmelzer, C.E., Raichur, A., Syrowatka, F., Groth, T.: Effect of different crosslinking strategies on physical properties and biocompatibility of freestanding multilayer films made of alginate and chitosan. Macromol. Biosci. **19**, 1900181 (2019)
20. Yuvarani, I., Kumar, S.S., Venkatesan, J., Kim, S.-K., Sudha, P.: Preparation and characterization of curcumin coated chitosan-alginate blend for wound dressing application. J. Biomater. Tissue Eng. **2**, 54–60 (2012)
21. Tao, Y., Liu, S., Zhang, Y., Chi, Z., Xu, J.: A pH-responsive polymer based on dynamic imine bonds as a drug delivery material with pseudo target release behavior. Polym. Chem. **9**, 878–884 (2018)
22. Esmaeilzadeh, P., Köwitsch, A., Liedmann, A., Menzel, M., Fuhrmann, B., Schmidt, G., Klehm, J., Groth, T.: Stimuli-responsive multilayers based on thiolated polysaccharides that affect fibroblast cell adhesion. ACS Appl. Mater. Interfaces **10**, 8507–8518 (2018)
23. Köwitsch, A., Abreu, M.J., Chhalotre, A., Hielscher, M., Fischer, S., Mäder, K., Groth, T.: Synthesis of thiolated glycosaminoglycans and grafting to solid surfaces. Carbohyd. Polym. **114**, 344–351 (2014)
24. Krel, A., Latajka, R., Bujacz, G., Bal, W.: Coordination properties of tris(2-carboxyethyl) phosphine. Inorg. Chem **42**, 1994–2003 (2003)
25. Ellman, G.L.: Tissue sulfhydryl groups. Arch. Biochem. Biophys. **82**, 70–77 (1959)
26. Riddles, P.W., Blakeley, R.L., Zerner, B.: Ellman's reagent: 5, 5′-dithiobis (2-nitrobenzoic acid)—a reexamination. Anal. Biochem. **94**, 75–81 (1979)
27. Gale, G.W., Cui, H., Reinhardt, K.A.: Aqueous cleaning and surface conditioning processes. In: Handbook of Silicon Wafer Cleaning Technology. Elsevier, Amsterdam (2018)
28. Wang, L.-M., Chang, H., Zhang, H., Ren, K.-F., Li, H., Hu, M., Li, B.-C., Martins, M.C.L., Barbosa, M.A., Ji, J.: Dynamic stiffness of polyelectrolyte multilayer films based on disulfide bonds for in situ control of cell adhesion. J. Mater. Chem. B **3**, 7546–7553 (2015)
29. Almodóvar, J., Place, L.W., Gogolski, J., Erickson, K., Kipper, M.J.: Layer-by-layer assembly of polysaccharide-based polyelectrolyte multilayers: a spectroscopic study of hydrophilicity, composition, and ion pairing. Biomacromolecules **12**, 2755–2765 (2011)
30. Sader, J., Chon, J., Mulvaney, P.: Rev. Sci. Instrum. (1999)
31. Johnson, K.: Contact Mechanics, vol. 95, p. 365. Cambridge University Press, Cambridge (1985)
32. Esmaeilzadeh, P., Köwitsch, A., Heyroth, F., Schmidt, G., Fischer, S., Richter, K., Groth, T.: Synthesis of thiolated polysaccharides for formation of polyelectrolyte multilayers with improved cellular adhesion. Carbohyd. Polym. **157**, 1205–1214 (2017)
33. Socrates, G.: Infrared and Raman Characteristic Group Frequencies: Tables and Charts. Wiley, Hoboken (2004)
34. Bandyopadhyay, S., Dey, A.: Convenient detection of the thiol functional group using H/D isotope sensitive Raman spectroscopy. Analyst **139**, 2118–2121 (2014)
35. López-León, T., Carvalho, E., Seijo, B., Ortega-Vinuesa, J., Bastos-González, D.: Physicochemical characterization of chitosan nanoparticles: electrokinetic and stability behavior. J. Colloid Interface Sci. **283**, 344–351 (2005)
36. Bravo-Osuna, I., Schmitz, T., Bernkop-Schnürch, A., Vauthier, C., Ponchel, G.: Elaboration and characterization of thiolated chitosan-coated acrylic nanoparticles. Int. J. Pharm. **316**, 170–175 (2006)
37. Denuziere, A., Ferrier, D., Domard, A.: Chitosan-chondroitin sulfate and chitosan-hyaluronate polyelectrolyte complexes. Physico-chemical aspects. Carbohydr. Polym. **29**, 317–323 (1996)

38. Borges, J., Mano, J.F.: Molecular interactions driving the layer-by-layer assembly of multilayers. Chem. Rev. **114**, 8883–8942 (2014)
39. Crouzier, T., Picart, C.: Ion pairing and hydration in polyelectrolyte multilayer films containing polysaccharides. Biomacromolecules **10**, 433–442 (2009)
40. Monahan, F.J., German, J.B., Kinsella, J.E.: Effect of pH and temperature on protein unfolding and thiol/disulfide interchange reactions during heat-induced gelation of whey proteins. J. Agric. Food Chem. **43**, 46–52 (1995)
41. Werner, C., Zimmermann, R., Kratzmüller, T.: Streaming potential and streaming current measurements at planar solid/liquid interfaces for simultaneous determination of zeta potential and surface conductivity. Colloids Surf., A Physicochem. Eng. Aspects **192**, 205–213 (2001)
42. Gowda, B.K., Prashanth, P., Gowda, S., Ananda, S.: Kinetics of oxidation of aliphatic primary amines by CAB in alkaline medium catalyzed by β-cyclodextrine. Int. J. Chem. Res. 8–13 (2011)
43. Dannan, H., Crooks, P.A., Dittert, L.W., Hussain, A.: Kinetics and mechanism of chlorine exchange between chloramine-T and secondary amines. J. Pharm. Sci. **81**, 652–656 (1992)
44. Schneider, A., Francius, G., Obeid, R., Schwinté, P., Hemmerlé, J., Frisch, B., Schaaf, P., Voegel, J.-C., Senger, B., Picart, C.: Polyelectrolyte multilayers with a tunable Young's modulus: influence of film stiffness on cell adhesion. Langmuir **22**, 1193–1200 (2006)
45. Caridade, S.G., Monge, C., Almodóvar, J., Guillot, R., Lavaud, J., Josserand, V., Coll, J.-L., Mano, J.F., Picart, C.: Myoconductive and osteoinductive free-standing polysaccharide membranes. Acta Biomater. **15**, 139–149 (2015)
46. Xu, L.-C., Siedlecki, C.A.: Effects of surface wettability and contact time on protein adhesion to biomaterial surfaces. Biomaterials **28**, 3273–3283 (2007)
47. Steele, J.G., Johnson, G., Underwood, P.A.: Role of serum vitronectin and fibronectin in adhesion of fibroblasts following seeding onto tissue culture polystyrene. J. Biomed. Mater. Res. **26**, 861–884 (1992)
48. Juliano, R.L., Haskill, S.: Signal transduction from the extracellular matrix. J. Cell Biol. **120**, 577–585 (1993)

Properties of Hydroxyapatite-Based Biomaterials Important for Interactions with Cells and Tissues

Jelena M. Živković, Nenad Ignjatović, and Stevo Najman

Abstract Mammal bone tissue is mainly composed of an inorganic component consisting of calcium phosphate (CaP) ceramics, predominantly calcium hydroxyapatite (HAp), in addition to the organic component. Properties of HAp enable the modification of its structure, surface, design of particle size at the micro and the macro levels, hybridization with polymers, metals, etc., which makes it a very important biomaterial in the future as well. The properties of HAp can be improved by combination with a large number of therapeutic and/or diagnostic agents. CaP and HAp occupy a significant place in the research of different types of multifunctional and hybrid materials for potential application in diagnostic, preventive, oncological, reconstructive and regenerative medicine. There are numerous data on the properties of HAp and HAp-based biomaterials relevant to their use, such as composition, particle size, material shape, porosity, surface charge, topography, etc. This chapter also discusses the different properties of hydroxyapatite and hydroxyapatite-based biomaterials important for interaction with cells and tissues. In addition to references to literature data, the results of our research with different hydroxyapatite-based biomaterials in different in vitro and in vivo experimental models in the field of bone tissue engineering and regenerative medicine are presented.

J. M. Živković and N. Ignjatović are contributed equally.

J. M. Živković · S. Najman (✉)
Department of Biology and Human Genetics, Faculty of Medicine, University of Niš, 18000 Niš, Serbia
e-mail: stevo.najman@medfak.ni.ac.rs

J. M. Živković
e-mail: jelena.zivkovic.biologija@medfak.ni.ac.rs

N. Ignjatović
Institute of Technical Sciences of the Serbian Academy of Science and Arts, Knez Mihailova 35/IV, P.O. Box 377, 11000 Belgrade, Serbia
e-mail: nenad.ignjatovic@itn.sanu.ac.rs

S. Najman
Department for Cell and Tissue Engineering, Scientific Research Center for Biomedicine, Faculty of Medicine, University of Niš, 18000 Niš, Serbia

S. Najman et al. (eds.), *Bioceramics, Biomimetic and Other Compatible Materials Features for Medical Applications*, Engineering Materials,
https://doi.org/10.1007/978-3-031-17269-4_6

Keywords Hydroxyapatite · Nanomaterial · Surface characteristics · Porosity · Scaffold · Tissue engineering

1 Introduction

Hydroxyapatite (HAp) is a widespread natural mineral, which is the main mineral of mammalian bones, it is significantly present in dentin and enamel in teeth, and it can be found in other mammalian tissues to some extent. In nature, it is also found in other solid structures (clam, eggshell, shrimps, corals, marine algae, etc.). The natural structural role of hydroxyapatite has determined the application to both natural and synthetic HAp are widely used for bone repair and regeneration either alone or as composite biomaterials designed in the form of blocks, granules, scaffolds or orthopedic and dental implant coatings. For these reasons HAp is the main component of large number of biomaterials that are nowadays in use in bone tissue engineering. Design of novel hydroxyapatite-based biomaterials is a major goal of the scientist in this field that will lead to an ideal biomaterial used for successful bone regeneration.

For decades, there has been a tendency for researchers to find a way to replace a damaged organ of the body with a new one. A special problem in orthopedic surgery is finding a way to compensate for large bone defects. Tissue engineering offers an approach that involves the use of bone replacement materials in combination with cells. These biomaterials must be biocompatible and be able to induce the formation of new bone tissue with optimal vascularization.

Exactly, physicochemical and biological properties and spatial organization of hydroxyapatite biomaterials enable adhesion, migration, proliferation and differentiation of cells. The biological properties of biomaterials are directly correlated with their physicochemical properties, such as such as composition, particle size, material form, porosity, internal architecture, topography and surface characteristics and electrical charge. The use of nanomaterials for this purpose is being investigated in a whole range of ceramic biomaterials based on hydroxyapatite that mimic bone structure, because bone is also made of nanostructures.

Important properties of HAp materials are the ability to modify structure and surface, design particle size at micro and macro level, hybridization with polymers, metals, etc., which makes this biomaterials interesting for future research and various applications, except in reconstructive and regenerative, also in diagnostic, preventive, oncological medicine, and other areas of biomedicine.

2 General Characteristics and Application of Hydroxyapatite-Based Biomaterials

2.1 Hydroxyapatite Ceramics—Research History and Chemical Characteristics

Human bone is made mostly of an inorganic component consisting of calcium-phosphate (CaP) ceramics, predominantly calcium hydroxyapatite (HAp), organic collagen components, and water. The earliest references to CaP appeared around 1770, and since 1950 there has been a growing number of scientific publications directly or indirectly related to CaP and HAp [1]. Natural mammalian bone tissue is organized in such a way that HAp crystals (10–50 nm in length) are finely distributed along collagen fibers [2].

Synthesized in the laboratory, but very similar in composition and structure to natural tissue, HAp ($Ca_5(PO_4)_3(OH)$) has become a challenge for many researchers in materials science due to its good biocompatibility. HAp is a mineral from the broad apatite family with a general formula $M_5(ZO_4)_3X$, where M can be a rare earth metal and X: OH^-, F^-, Cl^- or CO_3^{2-}. The formula of HAp is $Ca_5(PO_4)_3(OH)$, whereas $Ca_{10}(PO_4)_6(OH)_2$ is the formula of the unit cell thereof. The most common structure of HAp belongs to the hexagonal system with the space group $P6_3/m$. HAp is a ceramic material in which most bonds are a mixture of ionic and covalent types. The solubility of HAp at 25 °C is 0.0003 g/L, ($-\log(Ks) = 116.8$), and it is stable in the pH range of 9.5–12 [1].

The basic properties of HAp enable the modification of its structure, surface, design of size at the micro and the macro levels, hybridization with polymers, metals, etc., which is why some researchers rightly call it the material for the future [3]. In addition to chemical modification, which involves doping with various elements [4], the properties of HAp can be enhanced by combining it with a large number of therapeutic and/or diagnostic agents [5].

Since the beginning of the twenty-first century, CaP and HAp have assumed an important place in the research of different types of multifunctional and hybrid materials based on them [6] for potential applications in preventive, cancer, reconstructive and regenerative medicine. Figure 1 shows a global scheme of the field of research and potential application of multifunctional and hybrid materials based on CaP and HAp.

2.2 HAp-Based Materials—Medical Applications

In recent years, CaP and HAp-based materials have been strategically integrated with contrast agents and therapeutic agents for various molecular imaging modalities,

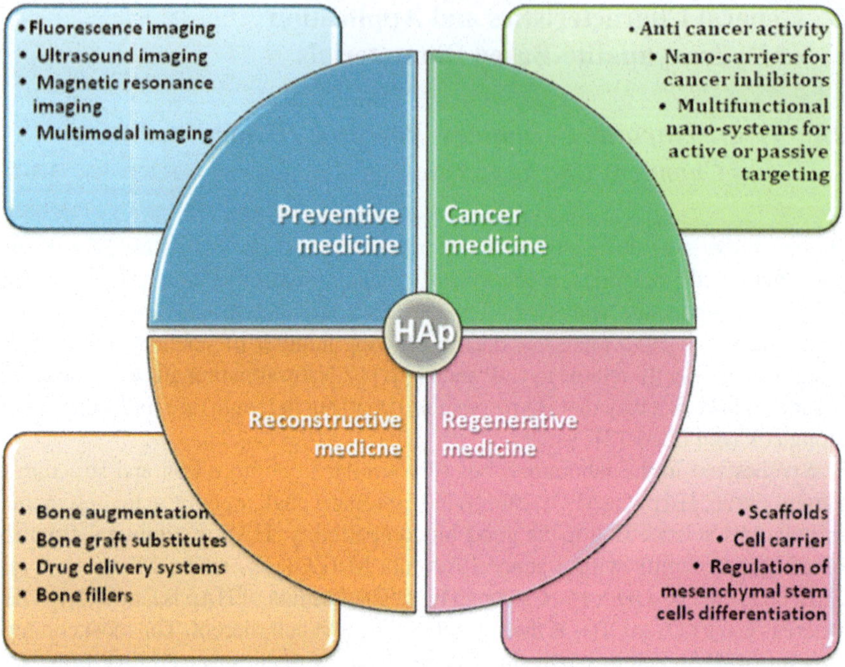

Fig. 1 Biomaterials based on calcium phosphate in medical sciences

including fluorescence imaging, magnetic resonance imaging, ultrasound imaging or multimodal imaging [5].

Applications in diagnostics and preventive medicine. The doping of the basic structure of hydroxyapatite (Fig. 2) with various rare earth elements enables its potential application in PREVENTIVE medicine as a contrast agent in multi-modal imaging techniques. Lanthanide-doped HAp particles have been created and they are suitable for lumino-magnetic agents for use in multimodal imaging that allows simultaneous use of computed tomography, photoluminescence and magnetic resonance imaging. By emulsification and hydrothermal processing, particles of pure HAp ($Ca_5(PO_4)_3(OH)$) have been synthesized, as well as magnetic HAp (gadolinium doped HAp, $Ca_{4.775}Gd_{0.15}(PO_4)_3(OH)$) and lumino magnetic HAp (ytterbium, thulium and europium doped HAp, $Ca_{4.775}Gd_{0.03}Yb_{0.1}Tm_{0.02}(PO_4)_3(OH)$, $Ca_{4.91}Gd_{0.02}Eu_{0.04}(PO_4)_3(OH)$). The biocompatibility of these systems has been investigated and confirmed in vitro using dental pulp stem cells isolated from a human patient [7]. A novel in situ procedure has resulted in successful radio labeling of HAp nanoparticles with iodine (^{125}Iodine) [8]. The procedure makes it possible to obtain stable ^{125}I-HAp particles whose biodistribution following intravenous administration, in vivo, can be determined and quantified in a simple and easy manner. The use of a low-energy gamma emitter ^{125}I for radio labeling can make the diagnostic procedure safe to a great extent.

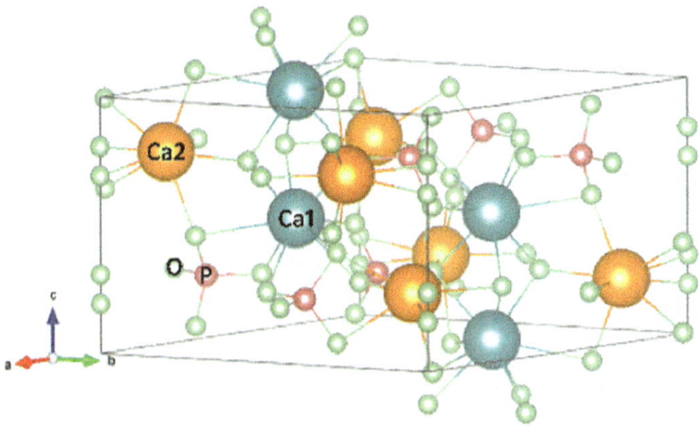

Fig. 2 Schematic structure of the HAp

HAp-based and other materials with applications in oncology. HAp particles have shown mild inhibitory properties against human glioma cells and they also induce their apoptosis [9]. Of particular importance are studies that indicate the possibility of targeting the mitochondria of malignant lung cells with nano HAp particles, causing their apoptosis [10]. This type of research has outlined the new fields of application of HAp-based systems, such as CANCER medicine, one of the areas with many challenges not only for oncologists but also for researchers. The capacity and efficiency of HAp-based anti-cancer systems have been improved by designing high-capacity carriers for the delivery of anti-cancer inhibitors. HAp particles are coated with a bioresorbable and biocompatible polymer, which acts as a reservoir for the delivery of selected drug (Fig. 3).

Fig. 3 SEM image of nano HAp coated with a bioresorbable polymer

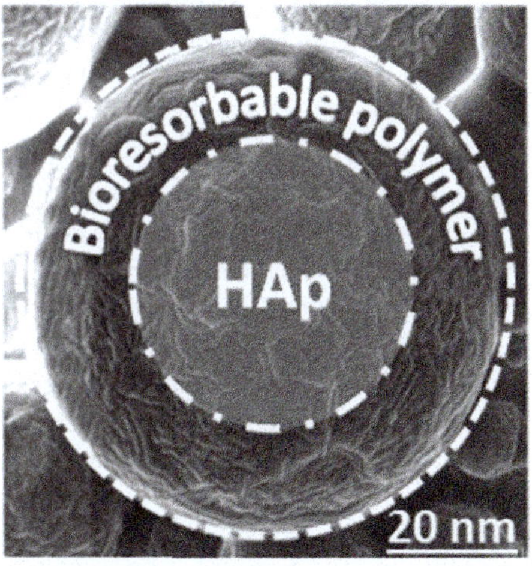

After application, the bioresorbable polymer is resorbed simultaneously with the release of the anti-cancer drug. For these purposes, bioresorbable and biocompatible polymers are used, including poly-DL-lactide-co-glycolide (PLGA), poly-1-lactide (PLLA), chitosan (Ch), chitosan oligosaccharide lactate (ChL), etc. Following intravenous administration, in vivo, HAp particles coated with the polymer blend PLGA-Ch accumulate in the lungs [8]. That is why the HAp/PLGA-Ch particle system is used to deliver androstane-based cancer inhibitors in potential lung cancer treatments [11]. One of the major challenges in the treatment of cancer today is to make the applied treatment and the used drug as cytotoxic as possible to cancer cells and, at the same time, as non-toxic as possible to the healthy ones. During the treatment, it is necessary to achieve a high selectivity of the drug in order to reduce the undesirable side effects that diminish the success of the treatment. Androstane (A)-based cancer inhibitors, A-loaded HAp coated with PLGA-Ch [11], were created and their selectivity was examined towards lung cancer cells (A549) was examined. The generated spherical particles A-HAp/PLGA-Ch were uniformly distributed with a diameter of d50 = 168 nm [12]. The forces on the materials–bio interfaces in the first interactions were electrostatic in nature. The zeta potential value (ξ) is of particular importance in solid–liquid interfaces and interactions. The zeta potential of A-HAp/Ch-PLGA particles (-8.7 ± 0.5 mV) was significantly more negative than that of A-free HAp/Ch-PLGA particles (-2.8 ± 0.8 mV). MTT and trypan blue dye exclusion assays confirmed that the A-HAp/PLGA-Ch system had a selective activity against lung cancer cells (A549), accompanied with a high viability ($83 \pm 3\%$) of regular MRC5 human lung fibroblasts, and it caused no harm to primary mouse lung fibroblasts. Systems were designed based on chitosan oligosaccharide lactate (ChL)-coated HAp nanoparticles as a vehicle for the delivery of steroid drugs to target breast cancer cells [13]. Various steroid derivatives (3β-hydroxy-16-hydroxymino-androst-5-en-17-one (B) and 3β, 17β-dihydroxy-16-hydroxymino-androst-5-ene (C)) were captured in a carrier composed of HAp nanoparticles coated with ChL. Significant changes in zeta potential were registered, in general. The zeta potential of C-HAp/ChL particles (32.3 ± 0.7 mV) was significantly more positive than that of drug-free HAp/ChL (13.80 ± 0.82 mV). The cell-selective toxicity of the B-HAp/ChL and C-HAp/ChL systems was confirmed using the MTT—colorimetric test with tetrazolium salt, DET—dye exclusion test, and FC—flow cytometry. The tests confirmed the fourfold cytotoxicity of B-HAp/ChL particles to breast cancer cells (MDA-MB-231) compared to healthy cells (MRC-5). Particularly pronounced selectivity was observed in C-HAp/ChL particles, which showed six times higher cytotoxicity to breast cancer cells than to the healthy ones. The low selectivity of pure B and C derivatives towards cancer cells was drastically increased when they were delivered using a spherical carrier based on polymer-coated HAp, which is a promising new concept for the application of anti-cancer drugs in oncology.

Applications of HAp-based materials in reconstructive medicine. So far, hybrid systems based on HAp have been the most widely used systems in RECONSTRUCTIVE medicine. HAp particles were doped with cobalt (Co) ions, and XRD and ICP techniques confirmed the stable structure of the apatite crystal lattice after doping. Spherical particles of Co-doped HAp (Co-HAp) with sizes smaller than

100 nm and cobalt content of 5–12 wt% were obtained [14]. During antimicrobial activity testing, all types of Co-HAp particles exhibited significant activity against *Escherichia coli* and *Staphylococcus aureus* [13]. Bone defects caused by osteoporosis were reconstructed with nanoparticulate Co-HAp. During an in vitro assay performed on cell lines (MC3T3-E1 and Caco-2), Co-HAp particles exhibited moderate cytotoxicity [15]. After the reconstruction of animal bone defects, in vivo, the obtained histomorphometric and histopathological results were not consistent with previous in vitro tests. In vivo results indicated accelerated osteogenesis and the formation of newly formed high-quality bone tissue in a defect with high-quality blood vessels, when the defect was filled with Co-HAp particles. The reason for this might be mild hypoxia caused by Co-HAp particles during in vitro tests. In real, living and dynamic systems, in vivo, mild hypoxia induces the expression of VEGF and EPO genes which improve vascularization and angiogenesis. After 24 weeks, bone defects reconstructed with a Co-HAp particulate filler were filled with a new tissue matrix composed of dense collagen fibers containing centers of mineralization [16].

Bone tissue engineering with multifunctional and hybrid synthetic materials. Bone tissue engineering (BTE) is constantly developing new ways of synthesis towards obtaining multifunctional and hybrid synthetic materials, which are expected to support damaged bone tissue, to act as a temporary substrate, to play the role of a matrix for cell growth and differentiation, but also to have the ability to control the rate of drug release into the surrounding tissue. Systems based on HAp coated with bioresorbable polymers (Fig. 3) have been designed as multifunctional carriers of antibiotics [17], vitamins [18], etc. After filling a bone defect with multifunctional particles of HAp/polymer, in the initial phase, the biodegradable polymer is resorbed and antibiotics or vitamins are simultaneously released. After the polymer is completely resorbed, HAp particles remain in the defect and take the role of an active filler. The resorption time of the polymer depends on many factors, such as the molecular weight, crystallinity, porosity, the free volume of the polymer, etc. The obtained results indicate that this type of carrier/filler enables simultaneous bone regeneration and the local delivery of antibiotics or vitamins.

The composition, structure and properties of the basic unit of a multifunctional system consisting of HAp phases and a bioresorbable polymer were designed in detail with end use in mind [19]. The degree of crystallinity of the HAp phase also plays a significant role in the formation of the properties of hybrid systems based on HAp and bioresorbable polymers. In addition to different physical and chemical properties, highly crystalline HAp exhibits different interactions in the biological environment than poorly crystalline HAp [20, 21]. The influence of the degree of crystallinity of HAp cannot be analyzed individually but in relation to the composition, shape and size of HAp particles.

The shape, size and particle size distribution (PSD) of HAp determine not only the properties of the material but also its interactions with the biological environment. Particular attention was given to HAp/bioresorbable polymer systems whose primary particles were < 100 nm in size, because this type of particles shows superior properties, compared to other types [21]. Reconstructions of various bone defects were performed using particulate HAp/bioresorbable polymer systems and the success of reconstruction and the creation of new bone tissue was confirmed not only by histopathological analysis but also by other physicochemical techniques [22]. This type of system is practical and easy to use as a filler for bone defects with no limitation imposed on the size of the defect [23]. In addition to bone defect reconstruction with particulate HAp/bioresorbable polymer systems, special attention is paid to the safety of this material and its impact on distant organs and tissues. Kidney and liver tissues are chosen because potential degradation products of this material can be transported there by body fluids. After the successful reconstruction of mandibular bones with particulate HAp/bioresorbable polymer, no pathological changes in liver and kidney tissues have been detected [24].

3D scaffolds based on granules of HAp. 3D scaffolds based on granules of HAp and a bioresorbable polymer (PLLA) have been obtained by cold and hot pressing (Fig. 4). The obtained 3D scaffolds have a compressive strength of up to 140 MPa and the elasticity module of up to 10 GPa, which is close to the values of strength and modulus of human bones. The thermodynamic properties of macroporous crosslinked PLLA and HAp/PLLA, such as the Flory-Huggins interaction parameters χ_{12}^{∞}, the partial molar free energy ΔG_1^{∞}, the partial molar heat of mixing, the free energy ΔG_1^{S}, the enthalpy ΔH_1^{S} and the entropy ΔS_1^{S} sorption with the sorbates of different chemical nature and polarity have been analyzed [25]. The phenomena in the interphase area between HAp and PLLA are of great importance for the complete understanding of the exploitation of biomaterials during and after application.

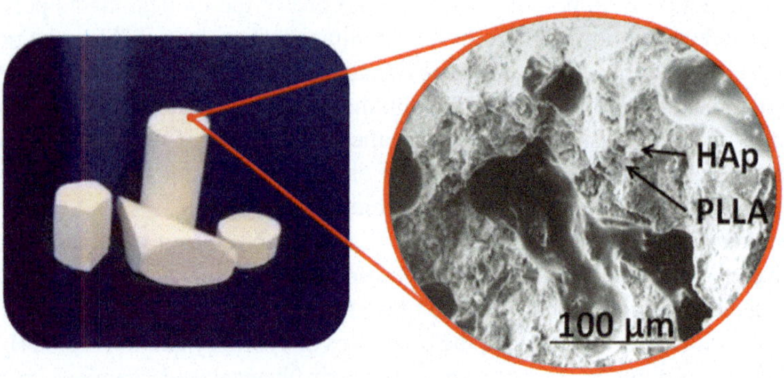

Fig. 4 3D scaffolds of HAp/PLLA obtained by hot pressing

3 Properties of Hydroxyapatite-Based Biomaterials Important for Interactions with Cells

3.1 *Porosity*

Porosity of biomaterial represents the ratio of all its pores' volume to the total volume of biomaterial. It is, so called, total porosity. Together with pore size and pore interconnectivity, porosity greatly affects application of biomaterials [26].

Porosity percentage. Since natural bone consists of cortical and trabecular bone tissue, which are characterized by porosity of 5–10% and 75–90% respectively, it would be ideal for the biomaterial to be porous as well [27]. One of the researches in which the importance of HAp porosity has been shown is the research of Dawson et al. [28] who have compared porous and non-porous HAp granules combined with autologous bone marrow aspirate containing mesenchymal stem cells, in critical size femoral chondyle defect model in adult rabbits. They have determined that in bone defects filled with porous HAp regeneration was significantly greater and less dependent on mesenchymal stem cells' concentration, compared with non-porous HAp [28]. In one clinical trial porous HAp loaded with bone marrow stromal cells was used in treatment of human large bone diaphysis defects. Fusion between implant and the host bone was observed 5–7 months after surgery, while 6–7 years after surgery integration of the implants was preserved [29]. One of the parameters of favorable scaffold-assisted bone regeneration is the penetration of surrounding tissue rich in cells and blood vessels. It has been shown that a higher percentage of HAp porosity, similar to that in trabecular bone, positively affects tissue ingrowth. This is related to the fact that a higher percentage of porosity affects the increase of biomaterial surface area and this leads to increased protein absorption and ion exchange [30–32]. Likewise, porosity also facilitates tissue ingrowth by increasing the resorption rate of otherwise slowly degradable HAp. For example, superporous hydroxyapatite Apaceram-ax® (HOYA Co. Ltd, Tokyo, Japan) with 85% porosity implanted in rabbits' femoral critical size defects, during 12 weeks of observation showed balanced resorption with ingrowth of new bone tissue, which has improved its mechanical properties [33]. Study with highly porous HAp performed on rats has shown that HAp porous blocks with 77% porosity, seeded with bone marrow-derived osteoblasts, induced mature bone formation 4 weeks after subcutaneous implantation [34]. Cylindrical HAp foams with 80–85% porosity implanted in rabbit tibia, after 8 weeks were partly or completely filled with new mature bone tissue [35].

Pore size. Ideal pore size in bioceramics should be also the same as one in trabecular bone tissue. It is considered that minimal pore size optimal for bone regeneration and mineralization is around 100 μm, although some studies indicates that 50 μm pore size is enough for osteoconduction [36, 37]. This conclusion is also supported by the results of Galois and Mainard [38] who have conducted the experiment in which porous HAp cylinders were implanted in rabbits' femoral defects. During 12 month period bone ingrowth into HAp ceramic through 45–80 μm pore size was delayed compared to the higher pore size, and the optimum pore size for bone ingrowth was between 80 and 250 μm [38]. In another experiment with HAp blocks combined with BMP-2, subcutaneously implanted in rats, the highest production of new bone was in implants with pore size of 300–400 μm, while bone formation decreased in HAp blocks with pore size smaller or higher than 300–400 μm [39]. In some studies, HAp scaffolds with pores significantly larger were used, for example in the study of Li et al. [40], in which scaffolds with 750–900 μm sized pores had the fastest angiogenesis and osteogenesis, compared to scaffolds with smaller or higher pore sizes [40].

Still, it might be the best for HAp scaffolds to contain pores of different sizes, when we talk about multi-scale porosity, which is again in accordance with the structure of natural bone [41, 42]. In this respect, pores are generally divided in macropores (pores bigger than 50 μm) and micropores (pores smaller than 10 μm) [43]. Multi-scale porosity is important because pores of different sizes have different roles in interacting with cells and tissues. Thus, small-diameter pores lead to enlargement of the surface area and thus increase protein adsorption and ion exchange, enhancing cell adhesion, likewise greater concentrations of diluted ions from scaffold can regulate osteogenesis and angiogenesis. Large-diameter pores sustain cell migration and colonization, as well as vascularization through scaffold [44–47]. Bone ingrowth and mechanical properties similar to those in trabecular bone were observed in HAp scaffolds with multi-scale porosity (250–350 μm for macropores and 2–8 μm for micropores) and incorporated recombinant human bone morphogenetic protein-2 (rhBMP-2) whose role was to initiate bone formation, given intramuscular scaffold's implantation [48]. HAp blocks with macropores sized around 350 μm and with around 40 vol% microporosity, implanted in bone defects of New Zealand White rabbits, showed more new bone tissue ingrowth in regard to implants without microporosity [49]. Human osteoblast-like cells seeded on porous HAp with micro- and macroporosity protrude filopodia through micropores, while forming multilayers in macropores, so micropores could play a role in cell attachment to biomaterial [50]. Micropores can also be populated with cells, as it has been shown in experiments with biphasic calcium phosphate scaffolds implanted in pig mandibles [51]. It is believed that microporosity enables creation of capillary forces that pull cells toward scaffold micropores in vitro after contact of microporous substrate and cell suspension, as well as in vivo after contact of scaffold with the physiological fluid at defect site [51, 52].

Benefits of multiscale porosity and pore interconnections in HAp scaffolds, that favorably influence cellular events after implantation, are shown in Fig. 5.

Pore interconnectivity. At last but not least, pore interconnectivity trough scaffolds is critical factor for bone formation. In some cases, even when pores are of corresponding size, scaffolds cannot support new bone formation due to lack or poor interconnection between pores. Pore interconnection is necessary for fluid circulation through scaffolds, which facilitates cell migration and equal cell distribution [53]. In porous HAp implants with fully interconnected pores (interpore connections from 10 to 80 μm in diameter) implanted into a rabbit femoral condyle, bone, bone marrow and blood vessels could be seen, while implant strength increased 9 weeks after

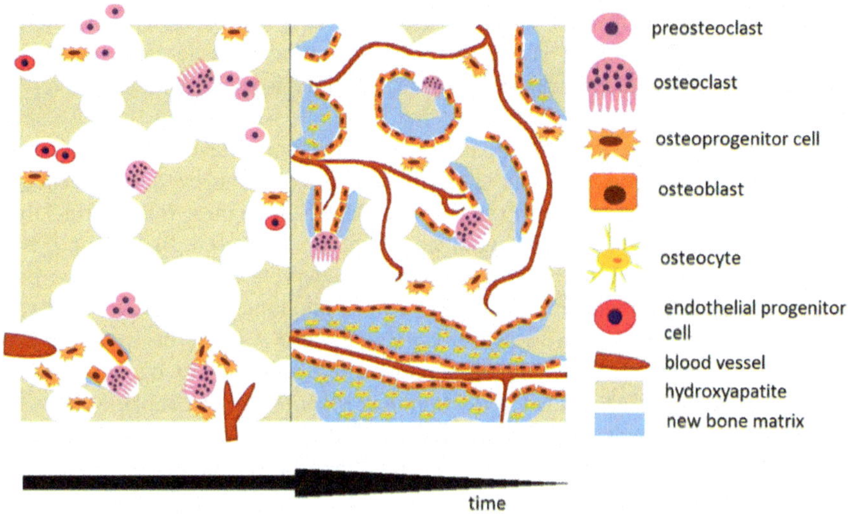

Fig. 5 Cellular events in HAp scaffold with multiscale porosity and fully interconnected pores after implantation

implantation [54]. Through interconnections blood vessels can also pass, whereby their diameter depends directly on interconnection size [55].

Regardless of the difference in particle size between nano-HAp and micro-HAp, interaction with cells depends on the same parameters, which are porosity, pore size and pore interconnectivity.

In investigation of the ability to repair bone defects of rabbits' radii, with assistance of nano-HAp (with pores 50–150 μm, 100–250 μm, 300–500 μm in size), it was found that nano-HAp with 100–250 μm pores after 12 weeks had the biggest potential for complete defects' reparation [56]. The lotus-type nano-hydroxyapatite/polyurethane (n-HAp/PU) scaffolds with 84% porosity and highly connected macropores close to 600 μm have been relieved as a suitable scaffold for osteoblast-like MG-63 cells proliferation and attachment [57].

3.2 *Particles*

HAp is an inert and biocompatible material. However, the size and shape of HAp granules greatly affects the viability and behavior of the cells with which they interact, because in the form of small particles and needle-shaped particles it can be cytotoxic.

Particle size. It has been observed that small HAp particles can cause cell damage in vitro. For example, HAp particles 0.5–3.0 μm in size, among the different particle sizes examined (0.5–3.0 μm, 37–63 μm, 177–250 μm, and 420–841 μm), have led to a decrease in the number of osteoblasts in culture, decrease in Transforming growth factor beta 1 (TGF-β1) synthesis and an increase in Prostaglandin E2 (PGE2) concentration [58]. TGF-β1 is important for normal bone tissue development and homeostasis [59], while increased PGE2 concentration is sign of inflammation [60]. Although inflammatory reaction is the first stage in tissue healing [61, 62], small micro-sized HAp particles appear to induce a stronger and unfavorable inflammatory response, as it has been shown in a study on murine bone marrow derived dendritic cells, where HAp particles 1–6 μm in size induced the highest Interleukin-1 beta (IL-1β) secretion [63]. Bio-Oss® (Geistlich-Pharma, Wolhusen, Switzerland) with particles 0.25 mm to 1 mm in size, obtained by deproteinization of bovine bone in a subcutaneous implantation model has shown good interaction with blood cells (from blood clot), bone marrow cells, macrophages and Adipose-derived stem cells (ADSCs), supporting in these combinations the angiogenic and osteogenic processes [64–70]. Algipore® (AP, DENTSPLY Implants Manufacturing GmbH, Mannheim, Germany), with particles 0.3–2 mm and pores 5–10 μm in size, is a natural apatite from red algae. The results of experiments that involved subcutaneous implantation of this material in mice with or without blood, showed the ingrowth of microvessels through the channels of these particles [71].

Great attention is also paid to nano-sized HAp particles because the natural bone itself is composed of nano-sized elements. MC3T3-E1 osteoblast proliferation was better on HAp scaffolds made of nano-HAp powder in relation to HAp scaffolds made of micro-HAp powder [72]. Webster and colleagues have investigated effects of nanosized particles on osteoblast adhesion [73]. They showed that 67 nm HAp particles improved osteoblast function, compared to 179 nm HAp particles, in culture conditions. This result was attributed to the fact that nanophase ceramics had the higher absorption of vitronectin, protein which promotes osteoblast adhesion and function, in comparison to conventional ceramics [73]. HAp nanoparticles sized around 20, 40 and 80 nm act on the bone marrow mesenchymal stem cells in vitro in such a way that those of the smallest size have the most favorable effect on cell viability and proliferation [74]. HAp particles with diameters of 20 and 80 nm, as well as micro-HAp, were studied on human osteoblast-like MG-63 cells in vitro. Results of this study have shown that 20 nm HAp particles promote cell growth and inhibit cell apoptosis, suggesting that they could be suitable for clinical applications [75]. In another study, osteogenic effect of HAp with particles sized 50, 100 and 150 nm was investigated on human mesenchymal stem cells. Although all particles' types could promote stem cells' differentiation into osteoblasts, smaller-sized nano-HAp (50 and 100 nm) had the best effect [76]. Experiment with implants made of nano calcium phosphate coated with poly(DL-lactide-co-glycolide), or abbreviated N-CP/DLPLG, combined with blood cells (from blood clot) and bone marrow cells, subcutaneously implanted into mice, has shown that this biomaterial can be supporting scaffold for these cells in order to improve the osteoreparative process [77].

Particle shape. The shape of HAp particles has a significant effect on the cellular response. Comparison of three HAp particle forms (spherical, irregular and needle-shaped), has revealed that needle-shaped particles induced production of cytokines (TNF-a, IL-6 and IL-10) by human monocytes, announcing inflammatory reaction [78]. In another study, a comparison was made in the strength of inflammatory response to HAp particles of different sizes (0.1, 5, 20, 100 μm), shapes (needle-shaped/spherical) and surface topography (smooth/rough surface). Needle-shaped particles have provoked a strong inflammatory response, unlike smooth, spherical particles and larger particles. Cytotoxicity of needle-shaped HAp particles have been linked to release of reactive oxygen species during the process of phagocytosis [63]. Also, in experiment with sphere shaped, rod shaped, needle shaped and plate shaped nano-HAp, the highest cytotoxic effect was in culture of BEAS-2B cells with needle shaped and plate shaped nano-HAp [79].

It is important to draw attention to whether HAp particles will be cytotoxic or not, depends not only on their shape and size, but also on the method of their preparation, likewise concentration [80].

3.3 Surface Topography

After implantation, cells first come into contact with the surface of biomaterial. For that reason, three-dimensional structure of biomaterial surface, i.e. its surface topography is one of the important parameters that influence the further fate of attached cells [81]. However, it is important to note that the biomaterial, in either in vivo or in vitro conditions, comes into contact with body fluids or medium and the proteins from them bind to the biomaterial surface, which is called protein absorption. In this way, the qualitative composition of the biomaterial surface changes. This process occurs during the entire stay in the organism, and is characterized by the succession of different molecules on the surface of the biomaterial over time. Along with changes in the composition of bound ions, minerals, water, proteins and other molecules, the composition of bound cells, their shape and behavior also change [82, 83].

Surface roughness of the HAp matrix affects cell attachment. Yang and colleagues have examined osteoblasts behavior on three hydroxyapatite two dimensional films with different topological roughness. Their results showed that with increase of surface roughness, protein adsorption increased, as well as proliferation of osteoblasts [84]. Deligianni and coworkers have investigated the effect of three HAp types with different surface roughness on human bone marrow cells response. Results have shown that cell adhesion and proliferation increase with the increase of HAp roughness [85]. Experiments with human bone-marrow mesenchymal stem cells cultured on HAp discs with various micro size roughnesses have shown that rough surfaces with average roughness from 0.77 to 1.09 μm and mean distance between peaks ranging from 53.9 to 39.3 μm topography supports osteogenic differentiation. The proposed mechanism by which surface topography affects the osteogenic process is through affecting cell attachment and cytoskeletal tension [86]. In another study, plasma-sprayed HAp-coated titanium (HAp-Ti) surface and the titanium substrate were examined. HAp-Ti had larger micro-scale roughness, and could absorb larger amount of recombinant human bone morphogenetic protein 2 (BMP-2). This property influenced bone marrow mesenchymal stem cells cultured on the HAp-Ti, which have showed more pronounced ability of osteogenic differentiation [87]. Rat osteosarcoma ROS 17/2.8 cells have attached and proliferated better on rougher surfaces probably because cells that have been attached on rough surfaces have had better availability of the medium and serum proteins which flowed through the material grooves under attached cells [88]. Experiments with human osteoblasts cultivated on HAp substrates with rough and smooth surfaces immersed in fibronectin solution, have shown that fibronectin increased number of attached cells on both surfaces types, while osteoblasts have attached better on rough HAp substratum [89]. In controlling the osteogenic process, it is not only important that cells that will differentiate into osteoblasts bind to the surface of biomaterial, but also is important the binding, differentiation and function of phagocytic cells such as osteoclasts. Macrophages, as cells also with phagocytic ability, create inflammatory microenvironment which is prerequisite for normal tissue reparation [64, 69] and release cytokines and growth factors important for osteogenesis. It seems that nanoscale surfaces are less suitable for osteoclasts formation and function compared to the HAp microsized topography [90]. It is believed that one of the reasons may be the inability to maintain the resorption apparatus of osteoclasts on smooth surfaces [91]. Lin and coworkers pointed out HAp with micro-nanohybrid structured surface, because it was shown that it attracts a larger amount of fibronectin and vitronectin, proteins necessary for osteoblast adhesion, growth, and differentiation, compared to the nanosurfaces [92]. HAp with nanostructured topography has beneficial effects on cell attachment and spreading. HAp with microstructured topography enhances cell adhesion, proliferation, and osteogenic differentiation. So, micro-nanohybrid structured HAp surface could be most similar to the bone structure, in which there are also structures from nano to micro sizes, and thus the environment closest to the natural one [92, 93].

4 Conclusion

The important properties of HAp is the ability to modify the structure and surface, design of particle size at the micro and the macro levels, hybridization with polymers, metals, etc., which makes this biomaterial interesting for future research and applications, also. The properties of HAp can be improved by combining it with a large number of therapeutic and/or diagnostic agents. Therefore, different types of multifunctional and hybrid materials based on CaP and HAp are being investigated for potential applications in diagnostic, preventive, oncological, reconstructive and regenerative medicine.

The doping of the basic structure of hydroxyapatite with various rare earth elements enables its potential application as a contrast agent in multi-modal imaging techniques.

HAp particles have shown mild inhibitory properties against cancer cells, and the capacity and efficiency of HAp-based anti-cancer systems are improved by designing high-capacity carriers to deliver anti-cancer inhibitors. HAp particles coated with a bioresorbable polymer can act as a reservoir for the delivery of the selected drug.

HAp-based materials are applicable in many ways in reconstructive medicine. There are results showing that osteoporosis can be repaired with Co-HAp nanoparticles, as well as that there is accelerated osteogenesis and the formation of newly formed high-quality bone tissue in a defect with high-quality blood vessels, when the defect is filled with Co-HAp particles.

Bone tissue engineering with multifunctional and hybrid synthetic materials is constantly developing to provide support damaged bone tissue, act as a temporary substrate, play a matrix role for cell growth and differentiation, but also to have the ability to control the drug release rate into surrounding tissue. For this purpose, HAp-based systems coated with bioresorbable polymers are designed as multifunctional carriers of antibiotics, vitamins, etc. The degree of crystallinity of the HAp phase also plays a significant role in the formation of the properties of hybrid systems based on HAp and bioresorbable polymers. BTE also constructs 3D scaffolds based on Hap granules, which have compressive strength, which is close to the strength values and other characteristics of human bones.

Although HAp is an inert material, the size and shape of HAp granules greatly affect the vitality and behavior of the cells with which they interact, because in the form of small particles and needle particles it can be cytotoxic. Also, small HAp particles appear to elicit a stronger and more unfavorable inflammatory response. Great attention in research is also paid to nano-sized HAp particles, which mimics natural bone composed of nano-sized elements.

The porosity and interconnected network of pores and channels in the BTE construct are essential for cell nutrition, migration and proliferation, as well as for vascularization and new tissue formation. On the other hand, the porous surface is important to facilitate the mechanical connection of the scaffold and the surrounding tissue in order to improve the mechanical stability of the implanted BTE construct and the implant.

Surface topography of biomaterials is one of the important parameters that influence the further fate of bound cells. So cell adhesion and proliferation increase with increasing HAp roughness. In the regulation of the osteogenic process, it is important that in addition to the cells that will differentiate into osteoblasts, phagocytic cells such as osteoclasts bind to and function on the surface of the biomaterial.

HAp with nanostructured and microstructured topography improves cell adhesion and cell proliferation and differentiation. It is important to note that the micro-nanohybrid structured HAp surface is most similar to the bone structure, which contains structures from nano to micro sizes, and thus makes the cell environment closest to natural.

Acknowledgements The authors would like to thank the Ministry of Education, Science and Technological Development of Republic of Serbia (Grants No: 451-03-9/2021-14/200113 and III41017) for support.

References

1. Dorozhkin, S.V.: A detailed history of calcium orthophosphates from 1770s till 1950. Mater. Sci. Eng. C Mater. Biol. Appl. **33**(6), 3085–3110 (2013)
2. Taton, T.A.: Nanotechnology. Boning up on biology. Nature **412**, 491–492 (2001)
3. Habraken, W., Habibovic, P., Epple, M., Bohner, M.: Calcium phosphates in biomedical applications: materials for the future? Mater. Today **19**, 69–87 (2016)
4. Uskoković, V.: Ion-doped hydroxyapatite: an impasse or the road to follow? Ceram. Int. **46**, 11443–11465 (2020)
5. Qi, C., Lin, J., Fu, L.H., Huang, P.: Calcium-based biomaterials for diagnosis, treatment, and theranostics. Chem. Soc. Rev. **47**(2), 357–403 (2018)
6. Haider, A., Haider, S., Soo, H.S., Kang, I.K.: Recent advances in the synthesis, functionalization and biomedical applications of hydroxyapatite: a review. RSC Adv. **7**, 7442–7458 (2017)
7. Ignjatović, N.L., Mančić, L., Vuković, M., Stojanović, Z., Nikolić, M.G., Škapin, S., Jovanović, S., Veselinović, Lj., Uskoković, V., Lazić, S., Marković, S., Lazarević, M.M., Uskoković, D.P.: Rare-earth (Gd3+, Yb3+/Tm3+, Eu3+) co-doped hydroxyapatite as magnetic, up-conversion and down-conversion materials for multimodal imaging. Sci. Rep. **9**(1), 1–15 (2019)
8. Ignjatović, N., Vranješ Djurić, S., Mitić, Ž, Janković, D., Uskoković, D.: Investigating an organ-targeting platform based on hydroxyapatite nanoparticles using a novel in situ method of radioactive ^{125}Iodine labeling. Mater. Sci. Eng., C Mater. Biol. Appl. **43**, 439–446 (2014)
9. Chu, S.H., Feng, D.F., Ma, Y.B., Li, Z.Q.: Hydroxyapatite nanoparticles inhibit the growth of human glioma cells in vitro and in vivo. Int. J. Nanomed. **7**, 3659–3666 (2012)
10. Sun, Y., Chen, Y., Ma, X., Yuan, Y., Liu, C., Kohn, J., Qian, J.: Mitochondria-targeted hydroxyapatite nanoparticles for selective growth inhibition of lung cancer in vitro and in vivo. ACS Appl. Mater. Interfaces **8**(39), 25680–25690 (2016)
11. Ignjatović, N., Penov-Gaši, K., Wu, V., Ajduković, J., Kojić, V., Vasiljević-Radović, D., Kuzmanović, M., Uskoković, V., Uskoković, D.: Selective anticancer activity of hydroxyapatite/chitosan-poly(D, L)-lactide-co-glycolide particles loaded with an androstane-based cancer inhibitor. Colloids Surf., B Biointerfaces **148**, 629–639 (2016)
12. Ignjatović, N.L., Penov-Gaši, K.M., Ajduković, J.J., Kojić, V.V., Marković, S.B., Uskoković, D.P.: The effect of the androstane lung cancer inhibitor content on the cell-selective toxicity of hydroxyapatite-chitosan-PLGA nanocomposites. Mater. Sci. Eng., C Mater. Biol. Appl. **89**, 371–377 (2018)
13. Ignjatović, N.L., Sakač, M., Kuzminac, I., Kojić, V., Marković, S., Vasiljević-Radović, D., Wu, V., Uskoković, V., Uskoković, D.: Chitosan oligosaccharide lactate coated hydroxyapatite nanoparticles as a vehicle for the delivery of steroid drugs and the targeting of breast cancer cells. J. Mater. Chem. B **6**, 6957–6968 (2018)
14. Ajduković, Z., Mladenović-Antić, S., Ignjatović, N., Stojanovic, Z., Kocić, B., Najman, S., Petrović, N., Uskoković, D.: In vitro evaluation of nanoscale hydroxyapatite-based bone reconstructive materials with antimicrobial properties. J. Nanosci. Nanotechnol. **16**, 1420–1428 (2016)
15. Ignjatović, N., Ajduković, Z., Savić, V., Najman, S., Mihailović, D., Vasiljević, P., Stojanović, Z., Uskoković, V., Uskoković, D.: Nanoparticles of cobalt-substituted hydroxyapatite in regeneration of mandibular osteoporotic bones. J. Mater. Sci. Mater. Med. **24**, 343–354 (2013)
16. Ignjatovic, N., Ajdukovic, Z., Rajkovic, J., Najman, S., Mihailovic, D., Uskokovic, D.: Enhanced osteogenesis of the nanosize cobalt substituted hydroxyapatite. J. Bionic Eng. **12**, 604–612 (2015)
17. Ignjatovic, N., Ninkov, P., Sabetrasekh, R., Uskokovic, D.: A novel nano drug delivery system based on tigecycline-loaded calciumphosphate coated with poly-DL-lactide-co-glycolide. J. Mater. Sci. Mater. Med. **21**, 231–239 (2010)
18. Ignjatović, N., Uskoković, V., Ajduković, Z., Uskoković, D.: Multifunctional hydroxyapatite and poly(D,L-lactide-co-glycolide) nanoparticles for the local delivery of cholecalciferol. Mater. Sci. Eng., C Mater. Biol. Appl. **33**, 943–950 (2013)

19. Ignjatovic, N., Tomic, S., Dakic, M., Miljkovic, M., Plavsic, M., Uskokovic, D.: Synthesis and properties of hydroxyapatite/poly-L-lactide composite biomaterials. Biomaterials **20**, 809–816 (1999)
20. Ignjatovic, N.L., Liu, C.Z., Czernuszka, J.T., Uskokovic, D.P.: Micro and nano/injectable composite biomaterials of calcium phosphate coated with poly(dl-lactide-co-glycolide). Acta Biomater. **3**, 927–935 (2007)
21. Ignjatovic, N., Ajdukovic, Z., Savic, V., Uskokovic, D.: Size effect of calcium phosphate coated with poly-DL-lactide-co-glycolide on healing processes in bone reconstruction. J. Biomed. Mater. Res. B Appl. Biomater. **94**(1), 108–117 (2010)
22. Ignjatovic, N., Savic, V., Najman, S., Plavsic, M., Uskokovic, D.: A study of HAp/PLLA composite as a substitute for bone powder, using FT-IR spectroscopy. Biomaterials **22**, 571–575 (2001)
23. Ignjatović, N., Wu, V., Ajduković, Z., Mihajilov-Krstev, T., Uskoković, V., Uskoković, D.: Chitosan-PLGA polymer blends as coatings for hydroxyapatite nanoparticles and their effect on antimicrobial properties, osteoconductivity and regeneration of osseous tissues. Mater. Sci. Eng., C Mater. Biol. Appl. **60**, 357–364 (2016)
24. Ignjatovic, N.L., Janković, R., Uskokovic, V., Uskoković, D.: Effects of hydroxyapatite@poly-lactide-co-glycolide nanoparticles combined with Pb and Cd on liver and kidney parenchyma after the reconstruction of mandibular bone defects. Toxicol. Res. **8**(2), 287–296 (2019)
25. Nastasović, A.B., Ignjatović, N.L., Uskoković, D.P., Marković, D.D., Ekmeščić, B.M., Maksin, D.D., Onjia, A.E.: Determination of thermodynamic interactions of poly(l-lactide) and biphasic calcium phosphate/poly(l-lactide) composite by inverse gas chromatography at infinite dilution. J. Mater. Sci. **49**, 5076–5086 (2014)
26. Sampath, U.G.T.M., Ching, Y.C., Chuah, C.H., Sabariah, J.J., Lin, P.C.: Fabrication of porous materials from natural/synthetic biopolymers and their composites. Materials (Basel, Switzerland) **9**(12), 991 (2016). https://doi.org/10.3390/ma9120991
27. Polo-Corrales, L., Latorre-Esteves, M., Ramirez-Vick, J.E.: Scaffold design for bone regeneration. J. Nanosci. Nanotechnol. **14**(1), 15–56 (2014). https://doi.org/10.1166/jnn.2014.9127
28. Dawson, E.R., Suzuki, R.K., Samano, M.A., Murphy, M.B.: Increased internal porosity and surface area of hydroxyapatite accelerates healing and compensates for low bone marrow mesenchymal stem cell concentrations in critically-sized bone defects. Appl. Sci. **8**(8), 1366 (2018). https://doi.org/10.3390/app8081366
29. Marcacci, M., Kon, E., Moukhachev, V., Lavroukov, A., Kutepov. S., Quarto, R., Mastrogiacomo, M., Cancedda, R.: Stem cells associated with macroporous bioceramics for long bone repair: 6- to 7-year outcome of a pilot clinical study. Tissue Eng. **13**(5), 947–955 (2007). https://doi.org/10.1089/ten.2006.0271
30. Hannink, G., Arts, J.J.: Bioresorbability, porosity and mechanical strength of bone substitutes: what is optimal for bone regeneration? Injury **42**(Suppl 2), S22–S25 (2011). https://doi.org/10.1016/j.injury.2011.06.008
31. Hing, K.A.: Bone repair in the twenty-first century: biology, chemistry or engineering? Philos. Trans. A Math. Phys. Eng. Sci. **362**, 2821–2850 (2004). https://doi.org/10.1098/rsta.2004.1466
32. Hing, K.A.: Bioceramic bone graft substitutes: influence of porosity and chemistry. Int. J. Appl. Ceram. Technol. **2**, 184–199 (2005). https://doi.org/10.1111/j.1744-7402.2005.02020.x
33. Okanoue, Y., Ikeuchi, M., Takemasa, R., Tani, T., Matsumoto, T., Sakamoto, M., Nakasu, M.: Comparison of in vivo bioactivity and compressive strength of a novel superporous hydroxyapatite with beta-tricalcium phosphates. Arch. Orthop. Trauma Surg. **132**(11), 1603–1610 (2012). https://doi.org/10.1007/s00402-012-1578-4
34. Dong, J., Kojima, H., Uemura, T., Kikuchi, M., Tateishi, T., Tanaka, J.: In vivo evaluation of a novel porous hydroxyapatite to sustain osteogenesis of transplanted bone marrow-derived osteoblastic cells. J. Biomed. Mater. Res. **57**(2), 208–216 (2001). https://doi.org/10.1002/1097-4636(200111)57:2<208::aid-jbm1160>3.0.co;2-n
35. Sepulveda, P., Bressiani, A.H., Bressiani, J.C., Meseguer, L., König, B., Jr.: In vivo evaluation of hydroxyapatite foams. J. Biomed. Mater. Res. **62**(4), 587–592 (2002). https://doi.org/10.1002/jbm.10173

36. Hulbert, S.F., Morrison, S.J., Klawitter, J.J.: Tissue reaction to three ceramics of porous and non-porous structures. J. Biomed. Mater. Res. **6**(5), 347–374 (1972). https://doi.org/10.1002/jbm.820060505
37. Chang, B.S., Lee, C.K., Hong, K.S., Youn, H.J., Ryu, H.S., Chung, S.S., Park, K.W.: Osteoconduction at porous hydroxyapatite with various pore configurations. Biomaterials **21**(12), 1291–1298 (2000). https://doi.org/10.1016/s0142-9612(00)00030-2
38. Galois, L., Mainard, D.: Bone ingrowth into two porous ceramics with different pore sizes: an experimental study. Acta Orthop. Belg. **70**(6), 598–603 (2004)
39. Tsuruga, E., Takita, H., Itoh, H., Wakisaka, Y., Kuboki, Y.: Pore size of porous hydroxyapatite as the cell-substratum controls BMP-induced osteogenesis. J. Biochem. **121**(2), 317–324 (1997). https://doi.org/10.1093/oxfordjournals.jbchem.a021589
40. Li, J., Zhi, W., Xu, T., Shi, F., Duan, K., Wang, J., Mu, Y., Weng, J.: Ectopic osteogenesis and angiogenesis regulated by porous architecture of hydroxyapatite scaffolds with similar interconnecting structure in vivo. Regenerative Biomater. **3**(5), 285–297 (2016). https://doi.org/10.1093/rb/rbw031
41. Gao, C., Peng, S., Feng, P., Shuai, C.: Bone biomaterials and interactions with stem cells. Bone Res. **5**, 17059–17059 (2017). https://doi.org/10.1038/boneres.2017.59
42. Elias, C.N., Meyers, M.A., Valiev, R.Z., et al.: Ultrafine grained titanium for biomedical applications: an overview of performance. J. Mater. Res. Technol. **2**, 340–350 (2013)
43. Miao, X., Sun, D.: Graded/gradient porous biomaterials. Materials (Basel) **3**(1), 26–47 (2010). https://doi.org/10.3390/ma3010026
44. Xing, F., Li, L., Zhou, C., Long, C., Wu, L., Lei, H., Kong, Q., Fan, Y., Xiang, Z., Zhang, X.: Regulation and directing stem cell fate by tissue engineering functional microenvironments: scaffold physical and chemical cues. Stem Cells Int. **2019**, 2180925 (2019). https://doi.org/10.1155/2019/2180925
45. Henkel, J., Woodruff, M.A., Epari, D.R., Steck, R., Glatt, V., Dickinson, I.C., Choong, P.F., Schuetz, M.A., Hutmacher, D.W.: Bone regeneration based on tissue engineering conceptions—a 21st century perspective. Bone Res. **1**(3), 216–248 (2013). https://doi.org/10.4248/BR201303002
46. LeGeros, R.Z.: Properties of osteoconductive biomaterials: calcium phosphates. Clin. Orthop. Relat. Res. **395**, 81–98 (2002). https://doi.org/10.1097/00003086-200202000-00009
47. Hing, K.A., Annaz, B., Saeed, S., Revell, P.A., Buckland, T.: Microporosity enhances bioactivity of synthetic bone graft substitutes. J. Mater. Sci. Mater. Med. **16**(5), 467–475 (2005). https://doi.org/10.1007/s10856-005-6988-1
48. Woodard, J.R., Hilldore, A,J., Lan, S,K., Park, C.J., Morgan, A.W., Eurell, J.A., Clark, S.G., Wheeler, M.B., Jamison, R.D., Wagoner Johnson, A.J.: The mechanical properties and osteoconductivity of hydroxyapatite bone scaffolds with multi-scale porosity. Biomaterials **28**(1), 45–54 (2007). https://doi.org/10.1016/j.biomaterials.2006.08.021
49. Malmström, J., Adolfsson, E., Arvidsson, A., Thomsen, P.: Bone response inside free-form fabricated macroporous hydroxyapatite scaffolds with and without an open microporosity. Clin. Implant Dent. Relat. Res. **9**(2), 79–88 (2007). https://doi.org/10.1111/j.1708-8208.2007.00031.x
50. Annaz, B., Hing, K.A., Kayser, M., Buckland, T., Di Silvio, L.: Porosity variation in hydroxyapatite and osteoblast morphology: a scanning electron microscopy study. J. Microsc. **215**(Pt 1), 100–110 (2004). https://doi.org/10.1111/j.0022-2720.2004.01354.x
51. Rustom, L.E., Boudou, T., Lou, S., Pignot-Paintrand, I., Nemke, B.W., Lu, Y., Markel, M.D., Picart, C., Wagoner Johnson, A.J.: Micropore-induced capillarity enhances bone distribution in vivo in biphasic calcium phosphate scaffolds. Acta Biomater. **44**, 144–154 (2016). https://doi.org/10.1016/j.actbio.2016.08.025
52. Polak, S.J., Rustom, L.E., Genin, G.M., Talcott, M., Wagoner Johnson, A.J.: A mechanism for effective cell-seeding in rigid, microporous substrates. Acta Biomater. **9**(8), 7977–7986 (2013). https://doi.org/10.1016/j.actbio.2013.04.040
53. Reinwald, Y., Johal, R.K., Ghaemmaghami, A.M., Rose, F.R.A.J., Howdle, S.M., Shakeshef, K.M.: Interconnectivity and permeability of supercritical fluid-foamed scaffolds and the effect

of their structural properties on cell distribution. Polymer **55**, 435–444 (2014). https://doi.org/10.1016/j.polymer.2013.09.041
54. Tamai, N., Myoui, A., Tomita, T., Nakase, T., Tanaka, J., Ochi, T., Yoshikawa, H.: Novel hydroxyapatite ceramics with an interconnective porous structure exhibit superior osteoconduction in vivo. J. Biomed. Mater. Res. **59**(1), 110–117 (2002). https://doi.org/10.1002/jbm.1222
55. Mastrogiacomo, M., Scaglione, S., Martinetti, R., Dolcini, L., Beltrame, F., Cancedda, R., Quarto, R.: Role of scaffold internal structure on in vivo bone formation in macroporous calcium phosphate bioceramics. Biomaterials **27**(17), 3230–3237 (2006). https://doi.org/10.1016/j.biomaterials.2006.01.031
56. Zhu, W., Xiao, J., Wang, D., Liu, J., Xiong, J., Liu, L., Zhang, X., Zeng, Y.: Experimental study of nano-HA artificial bone with different pore sizes for repairing the radial defect. Int. Orthop. **33**(2), 567–571 (2009). https://doi.org/10.1007/s00264-008-0572-5
57. Li, L., Zhao, M., Li, J., Zuo, Y., Zou, Q., Li, Y.: Preparation and cell infiltration of lotus-type porous nano-hydroxyapatite/polyurethane scaffold for bone tissue regeneration. Mater. Lett. **149**, 25–28 (2015). https://doi.org/10.1016/J.MATLET.2015.02.106
58. Sun, J.S., Liu, H.C., Chang, W.H., Li, J., Lin, F.H., Tai, H.C.: Influence of hydroxyapatite particle size on bone cell activities: an in vitro study. J. Biomed. Mater. Res. **39**(3), 390–397 (1998). https://doi.org/10.1002/(sici)1097-4636(19980305)39:3<390::aid-jbm7>3.0.co;2-e
59. Wu, M., Chen, G., Li, Y.P.: TGF-β and BMP signaling in osteoblast, skeletal development, and bone formation, homeostasis and disease. Bone Res. **4**, 16009–16009 (2016). https://doi.org/10.1038/boneres.2016.9
60. Park, J.Y., Pillinger, M.H., Abramson, S.B.: Prostaglandin E2 synthesis and secretion: the role of PGE2 synthases. Clin. Immunol. **119**(3), 229–240 (2006). https://doi.org/10.1016/j.clim.2006.01.016
61. Živković, J.M., Najman, S.J., Stojanović, S., Najdanović, J.G.: Interactions between skeletal system and macrophages in homeostasis and bone injury. FU Med. Biol. **18**(1), 6–11 (2016)
62. Vasiljević, P.J., Živković, J., Vukelić-Nikolić, M., Najman, S.: Determining the biological properties of biomaterials in vivo. In: Zivic, F., Affatato, S., Trajanovic, M., Schnabelrauch, M., Grujovic, N., Choy, K. (eds.) Biomaterials in Clinical Practice, pp. 477–499. Springer, Cham (2018). https://doi.org/10.1007/978-3-319-68025-5_17
63. Lebre, F., Sridharan, R., Sawkins, M.J., Kelly, D.J., O'Brien, F.J., Lavelle, E.C.: The shape and size of hydroxyapatite particles dictate inflammatory responses following implantation. Sci. Rep. **7**(1), 2922 (2017). https://doi.org/10.1038/s41598-017-03086-0
64. Živković, J.M., Najman, S.J., Vukelić, M.Đ, Stojanović, S., Aleksić, M.V., Stanisavljević, M.N., Najdanović, J.G.: Osteogenic effect of inflammatory macrophages loaded onto mineral bone substitute in subcutaneous implants. Arch. Biol. Sci. **67**(1), 173–186 (2015). https://doi.org/10.2298/ABS140915020Z
65. Najdanović, J.G., Cvetković, V.J., Stojanović, S., Vukelić-Nikolić, M.Đ., Stanisavljević, M.N., Živković, J.M., Najman, S.J.: The influence of adipose-derived stem cells induced into endothelial cells on ectopic vasculogenesis and osteogenesis. Cell Mol. Bioeng. **8**(4), 577–590 (2015). https://doi.org/10.1007/s12195-015-0403-x
66. Cvetković, V.J., Najdanović, J.G., Vukelić-Nikolić, M.Đ, Stojanović, S., Najman, S.J.: Osteogenic potential of in vitro osteo-induced adipose-derived mesenchymal stem cells combined with platelet-rich plasma in an ectopic model. Int. Orthop. (SICOT) **39**(11), 2173–2180 (2015). https://doi.org/10.1007/s00264-015-2929-x
67. Najman, S.J., Cvetković, V.J., Najdanović, J.G., Stojanović, S., Vukelić-Nikolić, M.Đ, Vučković, I., Petrović, D.: Ectopic osteogenic capacity of freshly isolated adipose-derived stromal vascular fraction cells supported with platelet-rich plasma: a simulation of intraoperative procedure. J. Craniomaxillofac. Surg. **44**(10), 1750–1760 (2016). https://doi.org/10.1016/j.jcms.2016.08.011
68. Najdanović, J., Cvetković, V., Stojanović, S., Vukelić-Nikolić, M., Čakić-Milošević, M., Živković, J., Najman, S.: Effects of bone tissue engineering triad components on vascularisation process: comparative gene expression and histological evaluation in ectopic bone forming

model. Biotechnol. Biotech. Eq. **30**(6), 1122–1131 (2016). https://doi.org/10.1080/13102818.2016.1213662
69. Živković, J.M., Vukelić-Nikolić, M.Đ., Najdanović, J.G., Stojanović, S., Vitorović, J.S., Radenković, M.B., Najman, S.J.: Bone tissue engineering based on bone marrow in blood clot loaded on mineral matrix carrier: experimental study in subcutaneous mice model. Acta Med. Median **56**(3), 5–11 (2016). https://doi.org/10.5633/amm.2017.0301
70. Najdanović, J., Cvetković, V., Vukelić-Nikolić, M., Stojanović, S., Živković, J., Najman, S.: Vasculogenic potential of adipose-derived mesenchymal stem cells in vitro induced into osteoblasts applied with platelet-rich plasma in an ectopic osteogenic model. Acta Med. Median **58**(4), 57–65 (2019). https://doi.org/10.5633/amm.2019.0408
71. Barbeck, M., Najman, S.J., Stojanović, S.T., Mitić, ŽJ., Živković, J.M., Choukroun, J., Kovačević, P.T., Sader, R., Kirkpatrick, C.J., Ghanaati, S.: Addition of blood to a phycogenic bone substitute leads to increased in vivo vascularization. Biomed. Mater. **10**(5), 055007 (2015). https://doi.org/10.1088/1748-6041/10/5/055007
72. Smith, I.O., McCabe, L.R., Baumann, M.J.: MC3T3-E1 osteoblast attachment and proliferation on porous hydroxyapatite scaffolds fabricated with nanophase powder. Int. J. Nanomed. **1**(2), 189–194 (2006). https://doi.org/10.2147/nano.2006.1.2.189
73. Webster, T.J., Ergun, C., Doremus, R.H., Siegel, R.W., Bizios, R.: Specific proteins mediate enhanced osteoblast adhesion on nanophase ceramics. J. Biomed. Mater. Res. **51**(3), 475–483 (2000). https://doi.org/10.1002/1097-4636(20000905)51:3%3c475::aid-jbm23%3e3.0.co;2-9
74. Cai, Y., Liu, Y., Yan, W., Hu, Q., Tao, J., Zhang, M., Shi, Z., Tang, R.: Role of hydroxyapatite nanoparticle size in bone cell proliferation. J. Mater. Chem. **17**, 3780–3787 (2007). https://doi.org/10.1039/B705129H
75. Shi, Z., Huang, X., Cai, Y., Tang, R., Yang, D.: Size effect of hydroxyapatite nanoparticles on proliferation and apoptosis of osteoblast-like cells. Acta Biomater. **5**(1), 338–345 (2009). https://doi.org/10.1016/j.actbio.2008.07.023
76. Yang, X., Li, Y., Liu, X., Zhang, R., Feng, Q.: In vitro uptake of hydroxyapatite nanoparticles and their effect on osteogenic differentiation of human mesenchymal stem cells. Stem Cells Int. 2036176 (2018). https://doi.org/10.1155/2018/2036176
77. Janićijević, J.M., Najman, S.J., Ignjatović, N.L., Savić, V.P., Kocić, J.S., Vasiljević, P.J., Vukelić, M.Đ., Uskoković, D.P.: Nanomaterial NCP/DLPLG as potentional tissue graft in osteoreparation in combination with bone marrow cells on subcutaneous implantation model. Hem. Ind. **62**(3), 205–210 (2008). https://doi.org/10.2298/HEMIND0803205J
78. Laquerriere, P., Grandjean-Laquerriere, A., Jallot, E., Balossier, G., Frayssinet, P., Guenounou, M.: Importance of hydroxyapatite particles characteristics on cytokines production by human monocytes in vitro. Biomaterials **24**(16), 2739–2747 (2003). https://doi.org/10.1016/s0142-9612(03)00089-9
79. Zhao, X., Ng, S., Heng, B.C., Guo, J., Ma, L., Tan, T.T., Ng, K.W., Loo, S.C.: Cytotoxicity of hydroxyapatite nanoparticles is shape and cell dependent. Arch. Toxicol. **87**(6), 1037–1052 (2013). https://doi.org/10.1007/s00204-012-0827-1
80. Motskin, M., Wright, D.M., Muller, K., Kyle, N., Gard, T.G., Porter, A.E., Skepper, J.N.: Hydroxyapatite nano and microparticles: correlation of particle properties with cytotoxicity and biostability. Biomaterials **30**(19), 3307–3317 (2009). https://doi.org/10.1016/j.biomaterials.2009.02.044
81. Rabel, K., Kohal, R.J., Steinberg, T., Tomakidi, P., Rolauffs, B., Adolfsson, E., Palmero, P., Fürderer, T., Altmann, B.: Controlling osteoblast morphology and proliferation via surface micro-topographies of implant biomaterials. Sci. Rep. **10**(1), 12810 (2020). https://doi.org/10.1038/s41598-020-69685-6
82. Elwing, H.: Protein absorption and ellipsometry in biomaterial research. Biomaterials **19**(4–5), 397–406 (1998). https://doi.org/10.1016/s0142-9612(97)00112-9
83. Thevenot, P., Hu, W., Tang, L.: Surface chemistry influences implant biocompatibility. Curr. Top. Med. Chem. **8**(4), 270–280 (2008). https://doi.org/10.2174/156802608783790901.PMID:18393890;PMCID:PMC3230929

84. Yang, G., Liu, Z., Guo, Y., Zhang, J., Li, H., Shi, W., Feng, J., Wang, K., Yang, L.: Osteoblast response to the surface topography of hydroxyapatite two-dimensional films. J. Biomed. Mater. Res. A **105**(4), 991–999 (2017). https://doi.org/10.1002/jbm.a.35967
85. Deligianni, D.D., Katsala, N.D., Koutsoukos, P.G., Missirlis, Y.F.: Effect of surface roughness of hydroxyapatite on human bone marrow cell adhesion, proliferation, differentiation and detachment strength. Biomaterials **22**(1), 87–96 (2001). https://doi.org/10.1016/s0142-9612(00)00174-5
86. Yang, W., Han, W., He, W., Li, J., Wang, J., Feng, H., Qian, Y.: Surface topography of hydroxyapatite promotes osteogenic differentiation of human bone marrow mesenchymal stem cells. Mater. Sci. Eng. C Mater. Biol. Appl. **60**, 45–53 (2016). https://doi.org/10.1016/j.msec.2015.11.012
87. Wu, S., Liu, X., Gao, C.: Role of adsorbed proteins on hydroxyapatite-coated titanium in osteoblast adhesion and osteogenic differentiation. Sci. Bull. **60**, 691–700 (2015). https://doi.org/10.1007/s11434-015-0753-8
88. Li, L., Crosby, K., Sawicki, M., Shaw, L.L., Wang, Y.: Effects of surface roughness of hydroxyapatite on cell attachment and proliferation. J. Biotechnol. Biomater. **2**, 150 (2012). https://doi.org/10.4172/2155-952X.1000150
89. Deligianni, D., Korovessis, P., Porte-Derrieu, M.C., Amedee, J.: Fibronectin preadsorbed on hydroxyapatite together with rough surface structure increases osteoblasts' adhesion "in vitro": the theoretical usefulness of fibronectin preadsorption on hydroxyapatite to increase permanent stability and longevity in spine implants. J. Spinal Disord. Tech. **18**(3), 257–262 (2005)
90. Costa-Rodrigues, J., Carmo, S., Perpétuo, I.P., Monteiro, F.J., Fernandes, M.H.: Osteoclastogenic differentiation of human precursor cells over micro- and nanostructured hydroxyapatite topography. Biochim. Biophys. Acta **1860**(4), 825–835 (2016). https://doi.org/10.1016/j.bbagen.2016.01.014
91. Geblinger, D., Addadi, L., Geiger, B.: Nano-topography sensing by osteoclasts [published correction appears in J. Cell Sci. **123**(10), 1814]. J. Cell Sci. **123**(Pt 9), 1503–1510 (2010). https://doi.org/10.1242/jcs.060954
92. Lin, K., Xia, L., Gan, J., Zhang, Z., Chen, H., Jiang, X., Chang, J.: Tailoring the nanostructured surfaces of hydroxyapatite bioceramics to promote protein adsorption, osteoblast growth, and osteogenic differentiation. ACS Appl. Mater. Interfaces **5**(16), 8008–8017 (2013). https://doi.org/10.1021/am402089w
93. Ranella, A., Barberoglou, M., Bakogianni, S., Fotakis, C., Stratakis, E.: Tuning cell adhesion by controlling the roughness and wettability of 3D micro/nano silicon structures. Acta Biomater. **6**(7), 2711–2720 (2010). https://doi.org/10.1016/j.actbio.2010.01.016

Comparative in Vitro Study on Anti-inflammatory Activity of Covalent Versus Layer-by-Layer-Bound Heparin and Hyaluronan Including Signal Transduction Through Transcription Factor NF-κB

Guoying Zhou, Hala Al Khoury, Adrian Hautmann, Haitong Wan, and Thomas Groth

Abstract Chronic inflammation and subsequent fibrotic encapsulation are the major factors that can hamper the function of biomaterials following implantation. Our work aimed to develop novel anti-inflammatory coatings to enhance biocompatibility of the biomaterials, but also to unravel the mechanism of their anti-inflammatory activity for guiding the design of more biocompatible materials. Here, we present two methods for immobilization of glycosaminoglycans (GAGs), namely hyaluronan (HA) and heparin (Hep) on model substrates either through chemical bonding of a GAG monolayer or through physical adsorption via the layer-by-layer (LBL) technique as GAG-chitosan (Chi) multilayers. We then show a comparative study of the covalent- vs. LBL-bound GAGs on physical properties, anti-inflammatory effects and the potential anti-inflammatory mechanism. It was found that both covalent- and LBL-bound GAG coatings can generate great anti-inflammatory effects regarding cellular responses of THP-1 macrophages. A higher inflammation-inhibiting potential of the LBL system was observed compared to covalent system with Hep-Chi multilayer showing the highest inhibitory activity. Furthermore, the mechanism investigations revealed that the anti-inflammatory activities of the GAG-immobilized coatings are not only related to increased hydrophilicity, but also caused by their active involvement in signal transduction on the NF-κB pathway at macrophage cellular level during inflammation.

G. Zhou · H. Wan
College of Life Science, Zhejiang Chinese Medical University, Hangzhou 310053, China

G. Zhou · H. Al Khoury · A. Hautmann · T. Groth (✉)
Department Biomedical Materials, Institute of Pharmacy, Martin-Luther-University Halle-Wittenberg, 06099 Halle (Saale), Germany
e-mail: thomas.groth@pharmazie.uni-halle.de

S. Najman et al. (eds.), *Bioceramics, Biomimetic and Other Compatible Materials Features for Medical Applications*, Engineering Materials,
https://doi.org/10.1007/978-3-031-17269-4_7

Keywords Inflammation · Glycosaminoglycans · Hyaluronan · Heparin · THP-1 macrophages · Layer-by-layer technique · Foreign body giant cells (FBGCs) · IL-1β · NF-κB

1 General Introduction

When a biomaterial is implanted inside a living tissue, the surgical procedure and the material can trigger a series of events with undesired host responses. This includes injury, blood-biomaterial contact, protein adsorption on the material surface and subsequent onset of acute and chronic inflammation, granulation tissue development, fibrotic encapsulation of the biomaterial, ending in the failure of implantation [1, 2]. Therefore, it is of great importance to design biomaterials with enhanced anti-inflammatory activity and thus can better guide host responses towards a successful tissue integration of the biomaterial, i.e. the medical device.

It is well known that surface properties of biomaterials can modulate the protein adsorption and with that the cellular activation and inflammatory response towards the implants [3, 4]. We and others showed in previous studies that hydrophobic CH_3- and moderately hydrophilic NH_2-terminated model surfaces bind more adhesion-promoting proteins like fibronectin and vitronectin, which then promote macrophage adhesion and subsequent inflammatory actions in vitro, followed by a thicker fibrous capsule formation in vivo [5–7]. By contrast, it was found that hydrophilic and anionic COOH-terminated surfaces had a lower potential to induce inflammatory responses both in vitro and in vivo [7]. Therefore, a strategy based on covering biomaterial surfaces with a hydrophilic/anionic, bioactive layer might be a quite promising solution to inhibit inflammation [8]. On the other hand, surface modification with intrinsic anti-inflammatory compounds has been proven as another useful approach for improving the biocompatibility of materials [9–11]. Among the various anti-inflammatory compounds, glycosaminoglycans (GAGs) like hyaluronan (HA) and heparin (Hep) have been suggested, due to their binding ability of a wide range of extracellular matrix (ECM) proteins, cytokines and enzymes which are associated with inflammation [12, 13]. In particular, high molecule weight HA (HMw-HA) was reported to decrease pro-inflammatory cytokine production, macrophage adhesion and formation of multi-nucleated giant cells in vitro as well as fibrotic encapsulation in vivo [14]. The anti-inflammatory activities of HMw-HA have been attributed to the cross-linking of the CD44 cell receptor, which can mediate clues from HA to pathways that supress the pro-inflammatory response and promote wound healing [15, 16]. On the other hand, Hep can bind selectins, cytokines and chemokines that inhibit leukocyte activation and infiltration, which further lowers pro-inflammatory cytokine release [17]. Furthermore, it is worth noting that both HA and Hep possess hydrophilic/anionic character by the presence of carboxyl (HA and Hep) and sulfate (Hep only) groups that allow the tuning of material surface properties towards increased hydrophilicity [18]. Therefore, the immobilization of GAGs on biomaterial surfaces might generate promising anti-inflammatory coatings, by the twofold action of increasing hydrophilicity of surfaces as well as their direct intrinsic anti-inflammatory activities.

A more detailed understanding of the anti-inflammatory mechanism of GAGs immobilized on biomaterials might pave the way for future biomaterial design with improved biocompatibility. The NF-κB signalling pathway has been reported to play essential roles in regulation of the immune system, cell proliferation, cell differentiation and cell death, but has been also identified as key factor in modulation of inflammatory responses through exerting a direct influence on the regulation of inflammation-related gene activation, gene expression and cytokine production [19]. It has been suggested that the anti-inflammatory activity of Hep and HA relies on their binding to receptors or subunits of nuclear factor-κB (NF-κB), leading to a down-regulation of NF-κB translocation to nucleus, which further lowers the following inflammatory response [20].

Here, two types of GAGs, namely HA and Hep were immobilized on model substrate by either chemical covalent or physical adsorptive binding to develop anti-inflammatory coatings. THP-1 monocytes were stimulated by phorbol-12-myristate-13-acetate (PMA) to obtain macrophage-like cells [21, 22]. The anti-inflammatory activities of the GAG-modified surfaces were then investigated regarding THP-1-derived macrophage adhesion, spreading, foreign body giant cells (FBGCs) formation, as well as pro-inflammatory cytokine production, which can all represent the pro-inflammatory potential of a given material [16, 23, 24]. We could show that the inflammatory responses were largely reduced after immobilization of HA and Hep by both methods, but to a different extent by the respective immobilization methods and types of GAGs. In addition, we shed light on the potential mechanism of their anti-inflammatory action, by studying their effect on NF-κB signal transduction [25]. Results are reported herein.

1.1 Immobilization Methods of GAGs for Anti-inflammatory Targeting

Owing to the various advantages and functions of glycosaminoglycans (GAGs) including good biocompatibility, great anticoagulation and anti-inflammatory potentials, GAGs like hyaluronan (HA) and heparin (Hep) are widely used in many medical applications as coatings for implants and scaffolds for anti-inflammatory targeting [12].

In general, the immobilization methods can be subdivided into two classes, namely chemical bonding and physical adsorption. The chemical modification can form stable covalent bonds, which highly depends on the available functional groups of the substances [26]. In this regard, both HA and Hep possess multiple chemically reactive groups such as carboxyl, vicinal hydroxyl groups and reducing ends of the hemiacetal of polysaccharide molecules, which can be utilized to immobilize them on material surfaces by different chemical methods [27]. For example, in previous studies of our group, chemically activated aldehyde-GAGs were immobilized on amino- or hydrazide-modified substrata through reductive amination, while thiol-GAGs could be either directly immobilized on gold or indirectly immobilized on vinyl-functionalized surfaces through thiol-ene reaction [28, 29]. Additionally, 1-ethyl-3-(3-dimethylaminopropyl)carbodiimide (EDC), or EDC/N-hydroxysuccinimide (NHS) mediated reactions are also used for the covalent linkage of GAGs onto amino-functionalized scaffolds or matrices, through the reaction of activated carboxyl and amine groups [30]. Such chemically GAG-immobilized surfaces are well defined model systems to study protein-surface, cell-surface interactions but are also used as anti-inflammatory coatings for improving the biocompatibility of biomaterials [31, 32].

On the other hand, the layer-by-layer (LBL) technique has attracted a lot of attention for various biomedical applications since it is a highly flexible and cost-effective method to design multilayer architectures [33]. Factors influencing the properties of the multilayers include the adsorption conditions like pH, temperature, ionic strength of solution, the molecular weight and concentration of polyelectrolytes (PEL). Electrostatic forces and van der Waals forces are some of the intrinsic driving forces to multilayer formation [34, 35]. Such variation of factors allows the build up of a broad range of surface coatings with different physicochemical and biological properties [36]. Biomacromolecules like polypeptides, proteins and GAGs that have charged groups represent PEL and thus can be easily applied by LBL technique [37, 38]. Particularly, it was found recently that Hep and chitosan (Chi) multilayer systems possess synergic effects on the inhibition of inflammation and immune reactions, when used as coatings for Langerhans islet implantation in rats [39]. Therefore, the LBL technique might be a useful tool to make materials with enhanced anti-inflammatory activity.

In this study, we employed two different methods for immobilization of HA and Hep on model substrates for anti-inflammatory targeting. HA or Hep were covalently immobilized on amino-functionalized self-assembling monolayers (NH2-SAM) to form HA or Hep monolayers by EDC/NHS crosslinking chemistry, which can be defined as covalent-bound coatings. The LBL-bound coatings were formed by the alternating deposition of HA or Hep as polyanions and Chi as polycation on a primary poly(ethylenimine) (PEI) substrate to generate HA-Chi or Hep-Chi multilayers through the LBL technique. The more detailed procedure for preparation of these surfaces was described in our previous papers [16, 40]. A schematic diagram of the formed GAG-immobilized surfaces using the two techniques is shown in Fig. 1. The prepared surfaces were then characterized by water contact angle (WCA) measurements, zeta potential measurements and atomic force microscopy (AFM) to confirm their successful immobilization on the control substrates.

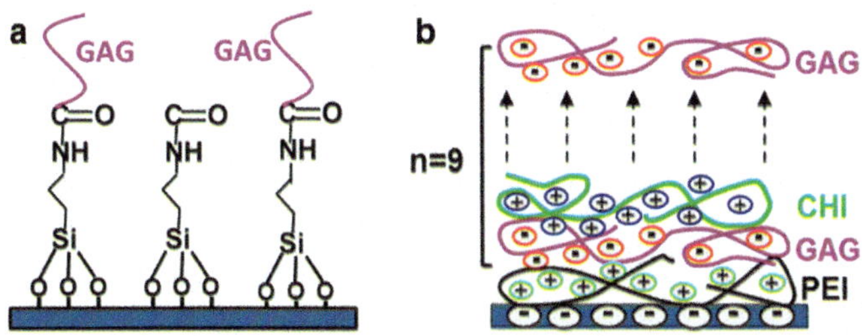

Fig. 1 Schematic diagram of GAG-immobilized surfaces using covalent bonding (**a**) and layer-by-layer (LBL) technique (**b**) GAG-Glycosaminoglycan; Chi-chitosan; PEI-poly(ethyleneimine). Reproduced with permission [2]. Copyright 2018, John Wiley and Sons

2 Results

2.1 Physical Characterization of GAG-Modified Surfaces

Wettability of Surfaces by WCA Measurement Static water contact angle (WCA) is a simple technique to measure the wetting abilities of the surfaces. The static WCA measurements were conducted with an OCA 15+ device (DataPhysics, Filderstadt, Germany) using the sessile drop method. It was shown in Fig. 2 that the original amino-terminated SAM (NH_2) and poly(ethylenimine) (PEI) substrates generated moderately wettable surfaces while the immobilization of GAGs resulted in more hydrophilic surfaces regardless of immobilization method. Furthermore, Hep-modified surfaces had higher wettability, as indicated by the smaller WCA, compared to HA-modified surfaces with both immobilization methods. Moreover, the same type of GAG (HA or Hep)-modified surfaces generated similar wettability with both methods, indicating that the WCA of the specific GAG-coated surfaces is not affected by the immobilization methods here.

Zeta Potential of Surfaces Zeta potential measurements can provide information about surface charge properties and are used here as a method for the indirect monitoring of GAG immobilization. Figure 3 shows the zeta potentials of primary substrates and GAG-modified surfaces by covalent-bound monolayers (Fig. 3a) and LBL-bound multilayers (Fig. 3b) as a function of pH. A typical decline of zeta potential with increasing pH value was observed for all surfaces. At physiological pH, the zeta potential of NH_2 (Fig. 3a) and PEI surfaces (Fig. 3b) had the least negative charges, with PEI even exhibiting a positive zeta potential. In comparison, the zeta potentials decreased significantly for both covalent-(Fig. 3a) and LBL-(Fig. 3b) bound GAGs. Furthermore, clear differences can be found between each HA- and Hep- modified surfaces. Moreover, the point-of-zero-charge (PZC) of HA- and Hep-based multilayers are much greater than that of their corresponding covalent monolayers, indicating an effect of the immobilization method on the zeta potential curves.

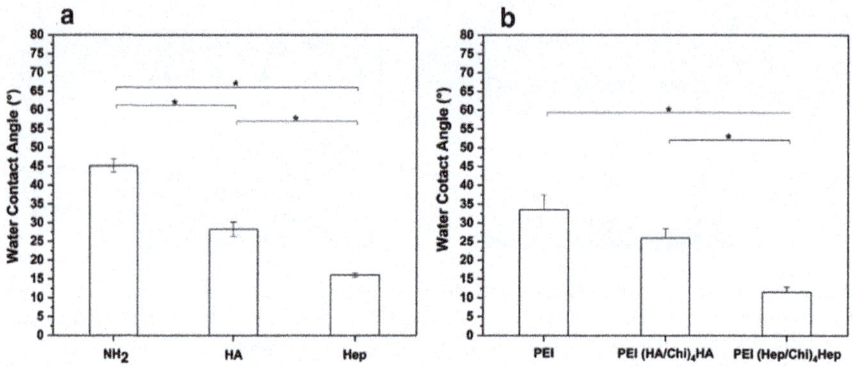

Fig. 2 Static water contact angles (WCA) for covalent-(**a**) and LBL-(**b**) bound hyaluronan (HA) and heparin (Hep) on amino-terminated SAM (NH_2) and poly(ethylenimine) (PEI) substrates, respectively. HA-surfaces after immobilization of HA on amino-terminated SAM; Hep-surfaces after immobilization of Hep on amino-terminated SAM; PEI(HA-Chi)$_4$HA-up to nine layers on top of PEI with HA as polyanion and outer layer; PEI(Hep-Chi)$_4$Hep-up to nine layers on top of PEI with Hep as polyanion and outer layer. Results represent means ± SD of two independent experiments (n = 6), $*p \leq 0.05$. Reproduced with permission [25]. Copyright 2020, John Wiley and Sons

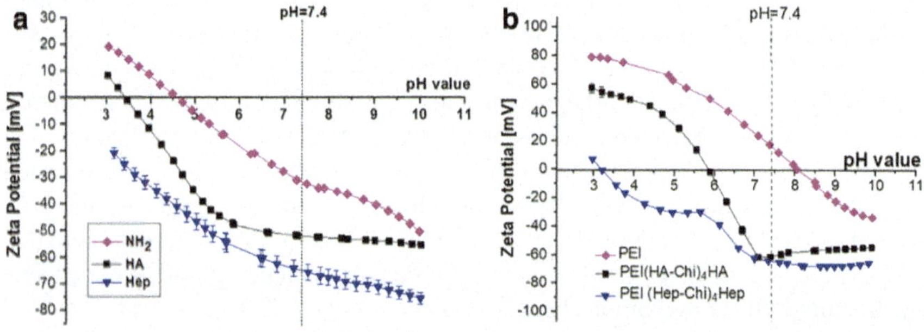

Fig. 3 Zeta potential measurements of covalent-(**a**) and LBL-(**b**) bound hyaluronan (HA) and heparin (Hep) on amino-terminated SAM (NH_2) and poly(ethylenimine) (PEI)substrates, respectively. HA-surfaces after immobilization of HA on amino-terminated SAM; Hep-surfaces after immobilization of Hep on amino-terminated SAM; PEI(HA/Chi)$_4$HA- up to nine layers on top of PEI with HA as polyanion. PEI(Hep/Chi)$_4$Hep-up to nine layers on top of PEI with Hep as polyanion. Reproduced with permission [25]. Copyright 2020, John Wiley and Sons

Topography of Surfaces by Atomic Force Microscopy The surfaces modified with both methods were investigated towards surface topography by using Nano-R2 atomic force microscopy (Pacific Technologies, Santa Clara, CA). Figure 4a shows a slight change of the topography together with smoother surfaces after the covalent immobilization of HA and Hep compared to the primary NH_2-terminated substrate. By contrast, the topography of LBL-bound HA and Hep shown in Fig. 4b indicates smaller differences between both GAGs with a similar range of 40–60 nm in the z

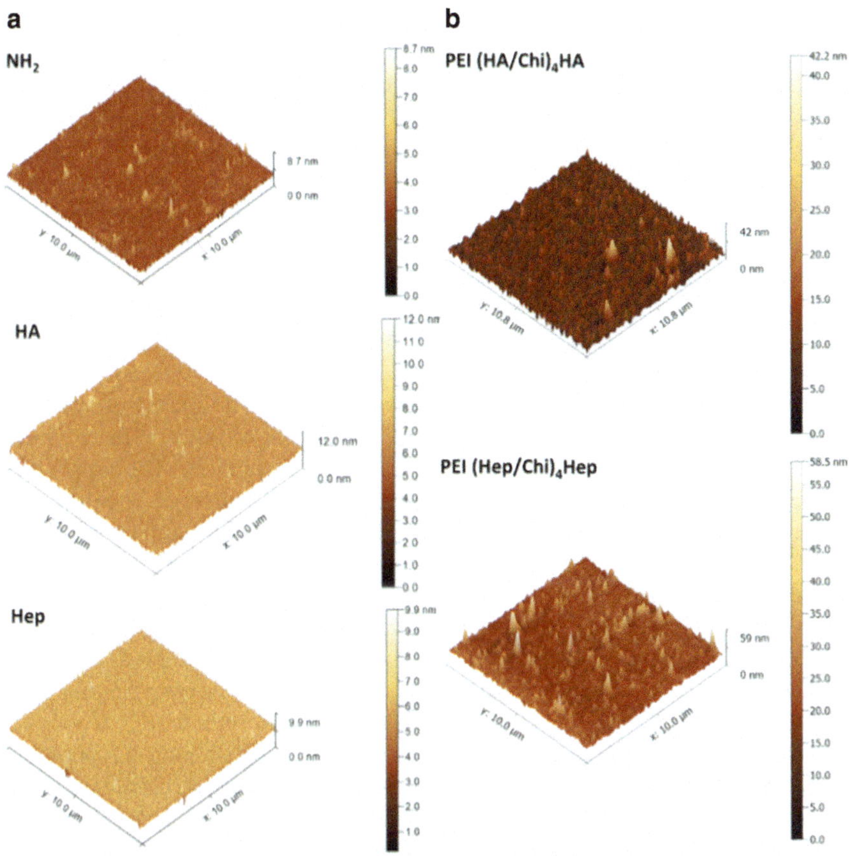

Fig. 4 Atomic force microscopy (AFM) images of covalent-(**a**) and LBL-(**b**) bound hyaluronan (HA) and heparin (Hep) on amino-terminated SAM (NH_2) and poly(ethylenimine) (PEI) substrates, respectively. Reproduced with permission [25]. Copyright 2020, John Wiley and Sons

dimension. Moreover, a more homogenous surface topography was observed with multilayers containing HA as a terminal layer in comparison to Hep. Additionally, it can be seen that the LBL-coating had a higher thickness as illustrated by the higher range in the z axis in comparison to the covalent-bound monolayers of both GAGs.

2.2 *Anti-inflammatory Activity of GAG-Modified Surfaces*

As macrophages are one of the key effector cell types in inflammatory responses after a biomaterial is implanted, their responses on a biomaterial can reflect the pro- or anti-inflammatory potential of a given material [16, 41]. Hence, the anti-inflammatory activity of the GAG-modified surfaces by both covalent and LBL immobilization methods were investigated by THP-1-derived macrophages in terms of macrophage adhesion, spreading, fusion into foreign body giant cells (FBGCs) and the pro-inflammatory cytokine IL-1β production in vitro.

Adhesion of Macrophages on GAG-modified Surfaces Adhesion of macrophages on GAG-modified surfaces was investigated by cultivation of cells in serum-free RPMI 1640 medium for 24 h followed by staining of adherent macrophages using histochemical giemsa staining as shown in Fig. 5a, b. It was shown that the control NH_2 and PEI surfaces resulted in the highest adherence of macrophages with more spread and elongated phenotypes of cells. By contrast, the cell number and cell area were much reduced with an apparent rounded cell shape on all GAG-modified surfaces, except the covalent-bound Hep surface. Beside the morphological studies, a quantitative estimation of cell adhesion (cell count, Fig. 5c, d) and cell spreading (aspect ratio, Fig. 5e, f) was conducted by image analysis of the microscopy images. Figure 5c, d display that the number of adherent macrophages was much higher in comparison to all GAG-modified surfaces. The aspect ratio of adherent macrophages, shown in Fig. 5e, f, depicts an enhanced polarization of macrophages on NH_2 and PEI surfaces as reflected by a higher aspect ratio value when compared to either covalent- or LBL-bound HA or Hep surface. Furthermore, both cell count and aspect ratio results illustrated that the type of GAGs exerted great effects on the cell adhesion and spreading behavior but in a different way for the two immobilization methods. There, the HA surface had the highest suppressive effects on macrophage adhesion and spreading in covalent system, however the Hep-based $PEI(Hep/Chi)_4Hep$ surface was more effective in the LBL system.

Apart from the histological studies, immunofluorescence staining was applied to investigate the macrophage adhesion and spreading morphology on different surfaces by visualization of actin cytoskeleton (red) and vinculin (green) for focal adhesion after 24-h incubation using a Zeiss LSM 710 confocal light scanning microscope (CLSM; Zeiss, Oberkochen, Germany). It can be seen from Fig. 6 that macrophages on the original NH2 and PEI surfaces adhered more strongly with a larger cell spreading area and enhanced expression of actin (red) and vinculin (green), when compared to the GAG-modified surfaces. However, there was no actin stress fibers observed even for NH2 and PEI surfaces. Instead, spot like actin structures were found at the periphery of macrophages for NH2 and covalent-bound HA and Hep monolayers (Fig. 6a) while plenty of filopodia were found at the periphery of macrophages cultured on PEI surface (Fig. 6b). Furthermore, a clustered distribution of vinculin rather than focal adhesion plaques was observed for all surfaces. Moreover, the type of GAGs once again affected the cell morphology in a different way for the two immobilization methods. Thereby, the covalent HA monolayer was more successful than the Heparin monolayer in inhibiting macrophage spreading, while the Hep-based $PEI(Hep/Chi)_4Hep$ multilayer had a higher inhibiting effect than the HA-based $PEI(HA/Chi)_4HA$ multilayer.

Fusion of Macrophages on GAG-modified Surfaces It has been well known that the fusion of macrophages to form foreign body giant cells (FBGCs) represents a hallmark of chronic inflammation and the extent of FBGC formation can reflect the pro- or anti-inflammatory potential of biomaterials [2]. Therefore, the fusion of

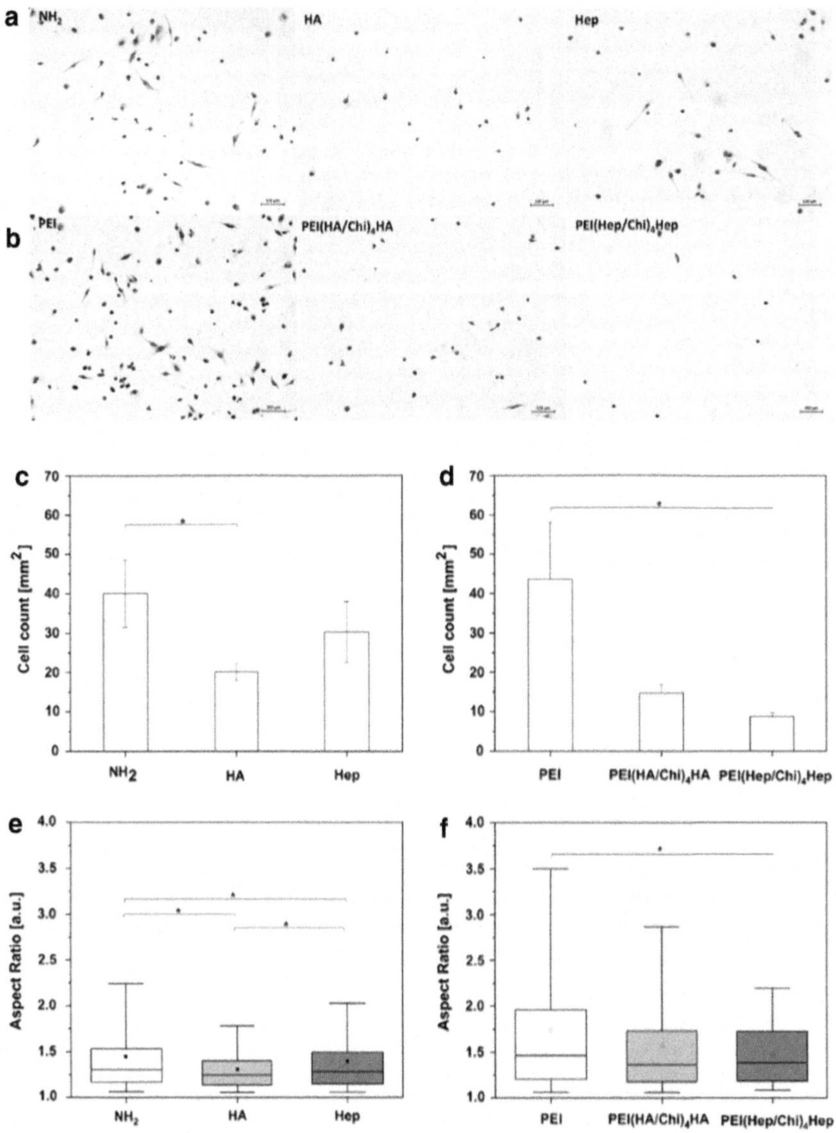

Fig. 5 Transmitted light microscopic images of macrophage adhesion (**a**, **b**), quantitative cell count per area (**c**, **d**), cell aspect ratio (**e**, **f**) of macrophage adhesion on covalent-(**a**, **c**, **e**) and LBL-(**b**, **d**, **f**) bound hyaluronan (HA) and heparin (Hep) on amino-terminated SAM (NH_2) and poly(ethyleneimine) (PEI) substrates, respectively. [Scale bar: 100 μm]. THP-1-derived macrophages were cultured in serum-free RPMI 1640 medium for 24 h and stained by 10% (v/v) giemsa solution. Data represent mean ± SD, n = 4, $*p \leq 0.05$. Reproduced with permission [25]. Copyright 2020, John Wiley and Sons

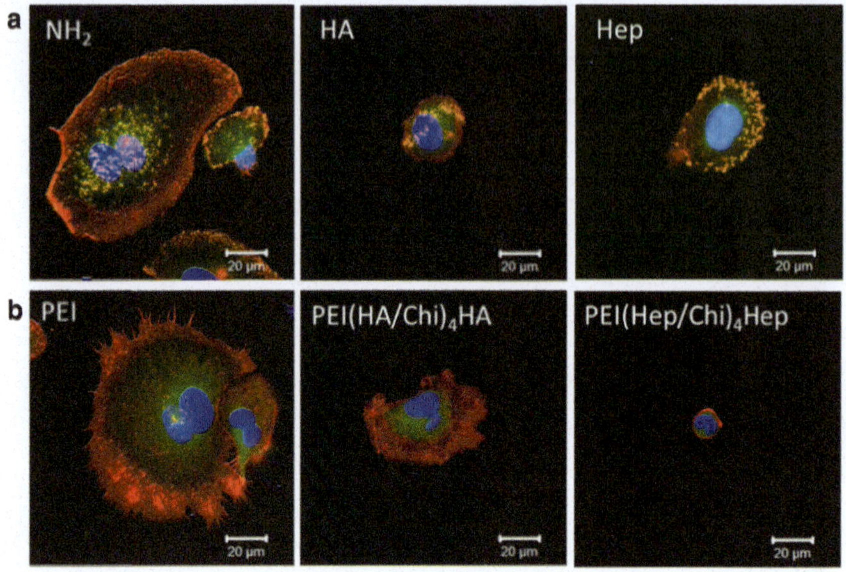

Fig. 6 The representative CLSM images of macrophages after incubation for 24 h in serum-free RPMI medium on covalent-(**a**) and LBL-(**b**) bound hyaluronan (HA) and heparin (Hep) on amino-terminated SAM (NH_2) and poly(ethylenimine) (PEI) substrates, respectively. The cells were stained for actin (red), vinculin (green) and nucleus (blue). [63X, scale bar: 20 μm]. Reproduced with permission [16]. Copyright 2015, John Wiley and Sons

macrophages and FBGC formation on the different surfaces was studied with giemsa staining of cells after 10 days culture in presence of serum in RPMI-1640 medium. FBGCs are defined as multinucleated giant cells, characterized by multiple nuclei ($n \geq 2$) in one cell body and an extended cytoplasm compared to single macrophages. The yellow arrows in Fig. 7 depict that there was FBGC formation on all surfaces, especially on the control NH2 and PEI surfaces. The quantitative analysis of FBGC formation area was conducted by image analysis. The results are shown in Fig. 7c, d. Generally, the FBGC formation data followed the similar trend as observed in macrophage adhesion and spreading experiments. Namely, the control NH2 and PEI surfaces showed the highest degree of FBGC formation in comparison to all GAG-modified surfaces. Moreover, it was found the degree of FBGC formation was lowest on HA and PEI(Hep-Chi)4Hep surface for covalent and LBL system, respectively.

β1 integrin expression can play important roles in regulating the process of macrophage fusion and FBGC formation [42]. Therefore, the expression of β1 integrin in macrophages adhering on different GAG-modified surfaces was monitored here and served as another parameter for possible anti-inflammatory activity. Figure 8 depicts that the expression of β1 integrin (green color) was mostly detected around the nuclei of macrophages. In addition, it was observed that the β1 integrin expression was much stronger on the NH2 and PEI surfaces and much weaker on GAG-modified surfaces either by covalent or LBL immobilization. Furthermore, the

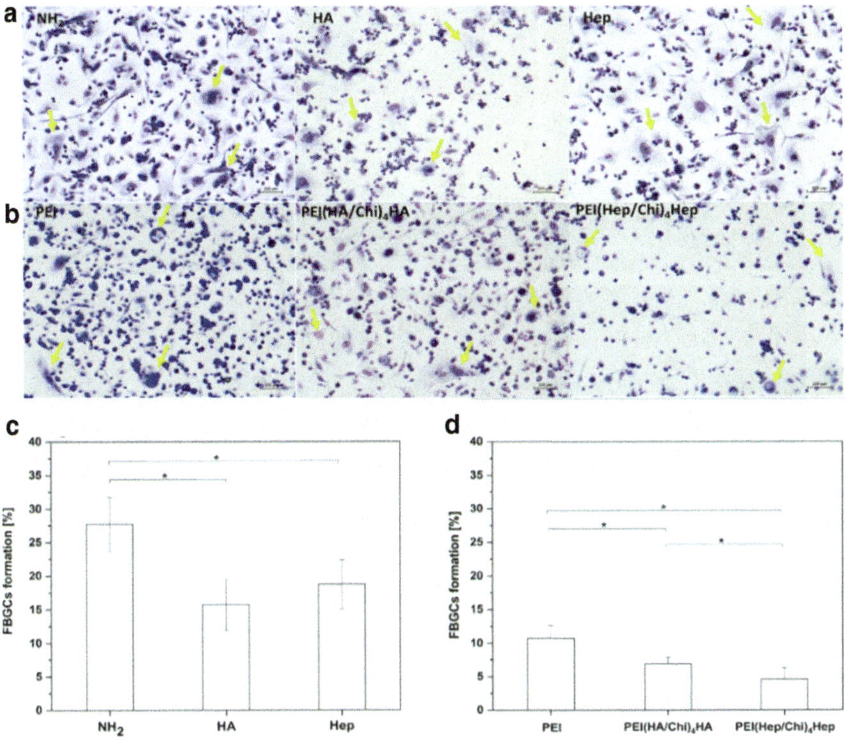

Fig. 7 Giemsa staining of foreign body giant cells (FBGCs) (**a**, **b**) after 10 day-incubation and quantified area percentage of FBGCs (**c**, **d**) formed on covalent-(**a**, **c**) and LBL-(**b**, **d**) bound hyaluronan (HA) and heparin (Hep) on amino-terminated SAM (NH_2) and poly(ethylenimine) (PEI) substrates, respectively. Data represent mean ± SD, n = 10, $^*p \leq 0.05$. Reproduced with permission [25]. Copyright 2020, John Wiley and Sons

covalent-bound HA monolayer and PEI(Hep/Chi)$_4$Hep multilayer had the lowest expression of β1 integrin, which is in line with the macrophage adhesion, spreading and FBGC formation results.

Pro-inflammatory Cytokine Production The production of pro-inflammatory cytokines like interleukin-6 (IL-6) and interleukin-1β (IL-1β) from macrophages cultured on biomaterial surfaces can reflect the pro-inflammatory potential of a given material [43]. Besides, lipopolysaccharides (LPS), a major component of the cell wall of gram-negative bacteria, can activate macrophages and upregulate the pro-inflammatory cytokine production [44]. Therefore, the anti-inflammatory activities of the GAG-modified surfaces were investigated in terms of the typical pro-inflammatory cytokine IL-1β production after 24 h incubation in both presence (black bars) and absence (white bars) of LPS treatment using an enzyme-linked immunosorbent assay (Elisa) kit. Additionally, the cell viability was evaluated by a Qblue (resazurin) test to normalize the cytokine IL-1β expression to the quantity of living cells represented by relative fluorescence units (RFU). Figure 9 displays that

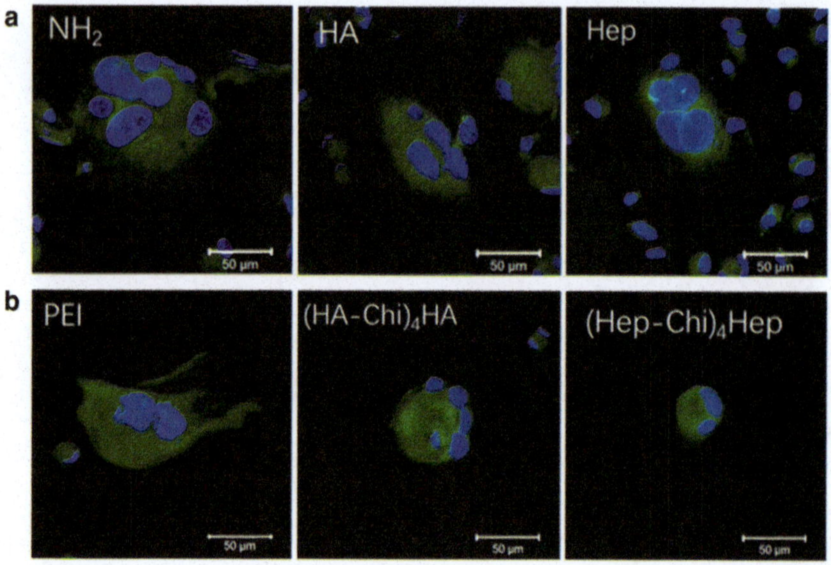

Fig. 8 The representative CLSM images of β1 integrin expression in fusing macrophages/FBGCs after 10 day-incubation on covalent-(**a**) and LBL-(**b**) bound hyaluronan (HA) and heparin (Hep) on amino-terminated SAM (NH_2) and poly(ethylenimine) (PEI) substrates, respectively. Cells were stained for β1 integrin (green) and nuclei (blue) [Scale bar: 50 μm]. Reproduced with permission [16]. Copyright 2015, John Wiley and Sons

the IL-1β production was upregulated on all surfaces upon LPS stimulation, indicating the responsiveness and functionality of the THP-1 derived macrophages. Additionally, it was found that cells on PEI surface produced the highest amount of IL-1β both with and without LPS stimulation. Cultures of macrophages on GAGs in multilayer systems showed that cells on PEI(Hep/Chi)$_4$Hep multilayers produced lower quantities of IL-1β compared to PEI(HA/Chi)$_4$HA multilayers (Fig. 9b). However, covalent immobilization of HA provoked also a downregulation of the IL-1β production, which was not significant (Fig. 9b). Indeed, the effect was significant for HA before normalization by RFU (Data not shown).

2.3 *Potential Mechanism of Anti-inflammatory Activity of GAG-Modified Surfaces*

Immunofluorescence Staining of NF-κB in Macrophages The activation of the canonical NF-κB pathway results in the translocation of the p65 subunit into the nucleus of macrophages where it can bind to promoter and enhancer regions associated with the inflammatory response [45]. Thus, the level of p65 translocation can reflect the extent of NF-κB activation and was evaluated here by immunofluorescence

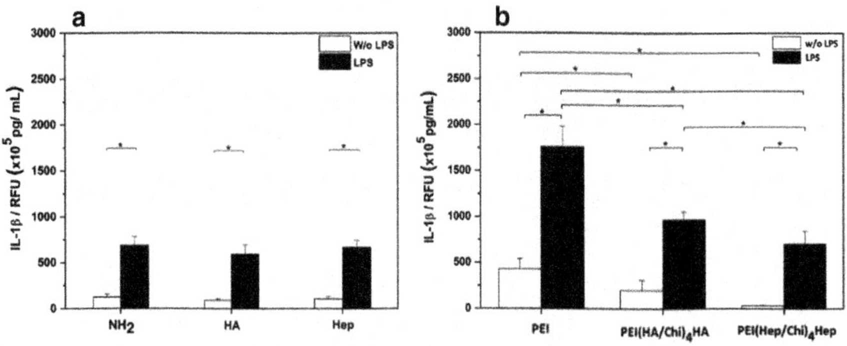

Fig. 9 Pro-inflammatory cytokine IL-1β secretion in macrophages after 24-h incubation in absence (white bars) and presence (black bars) of lipopolysaccharide (LPS) on covalent-(**a**) and LBL-(**b**) bound hyaluronan (HA) and heparin (Hep) on amino-terminated SAM (NH_2) and poly(ethylenimine) (PEI) substrates, respectively. Data represent mean ± SD, n = 6, $^*p \leq 0.05$

staining. As shown in Fig. 10, the p65 subunit of NF-κB (green colour) can be found in the cell cytoplasm as well as in the nuclei, upon activation of the NF-κB-pathway. The nuclear area was assessed by staining with TO-PRO-3 (blue colour). Thereafter, a quantitative analysis of the ratio of nuclear to cytoplasmatic staining of the p65 subunit was used as an indicator for translocation of NF-κB. It can be seen from Fig. 10c, d that the highest extent of p65 translocation was found on the control NH2 and PEI surfaces either with or without LPS stimulation. By contrast, immobilization of GAGs by both methods significantly reduced the p65 translocation as illustrated by the smaller value of the nuclear/cytoplasmic ratio. Additionally, it was found that Hep-modified surfaces possessed a significantly higher inhibitory activity towards p65 translocation with both immobilization methods in comparison to HA-modified.

Association of FITC-labelled GAGs with Macrophages Studied by CLSM and Flow Cytometry The association of immobilized GAGs with macrophages was firstly investigated by visualization of the cell membrane (red color) and FITC-labelled GAGs (green color) in macrophages cultured on covalent-(Fig. 11a) and LBL-(Fig. 11b) bound FITC-labelled HA or Hep surfaces. Figure 11a, b show that only a red staining of DID of the cell membrane was observed on the control NH_2 and PEI surfaces, since there were no FITC-labelled GAGs on these substrates. By contrast, the immobilization of the FITC-labelled HA or Hep with both methods showed an association of FITC-labelled HA or Hep (green color) with DID-stained cells (red color). Furthermore, a different localization of the two types of GAGs was found. A co-localization with the cell surface was noticed for FITC-labelled HA while an intracellular localization with apparent presence in the nuclear area was seen for FITC-labelled Hep with both immobilization methods.

Flow cytometry measurements were also performed to estimate the ability of macrophages to take up the immobilized FITC-labelled GAGs. Results are shown in Fig. 12a, c with dot blots of the side scatter (SSC, y axis) versus the FITC fluorescence (x axis). All samples were thresholded to their corresponding background

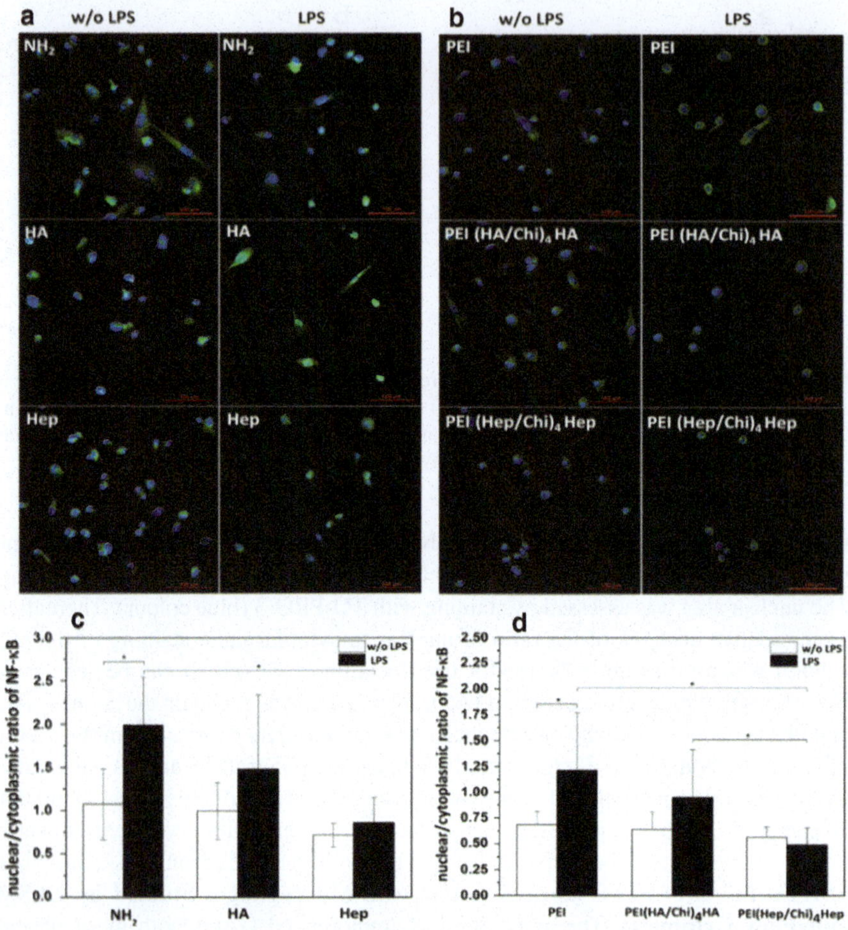

Fig. 10 Immunofluorescence staining of the nucleus with TO-PRO-3 (blue color) and the cytoplasm with monoclonal antibody detection of p65 subunit of NF-κB (green color) in unstimulated (left column) and Lipopolysaccharide (LPS) stimulated macrophages (right column) on covalent-(**a**) and LBL-(**b**) bound HA or Hep surfaces(Scale bar: 100 μm).The quantified data of nuclear/cytoplasmic ratio of macrophages on covalent-(**c**) and LBL-(**d**) bound HA or Hep surfaces and their substrates (NH_2 and PEI) were analyzed by ImageJ in the absence (white bars) and presence (black bars) of LPS. Data represent mean ± SD, n = 10, *$p \leq 0.05$. Reproduced with permission [25]. Copyright 2020, John Wiley and Sons

(NH2 without FITC staining for covalent samples and PEI without FITC staining for multilayer samples), and the remaining signal was considered as an indicator for association of FITC-labelled GAG with macrophages. Moreover, quantitative evaluation of macrophages positive for FITC-labelled GAGs is shown in Fig. 12b, d. A significant difference between HA- and Hep-modified samples was found, but acted in an opposite manner for the two immobilization methods. It was observed a

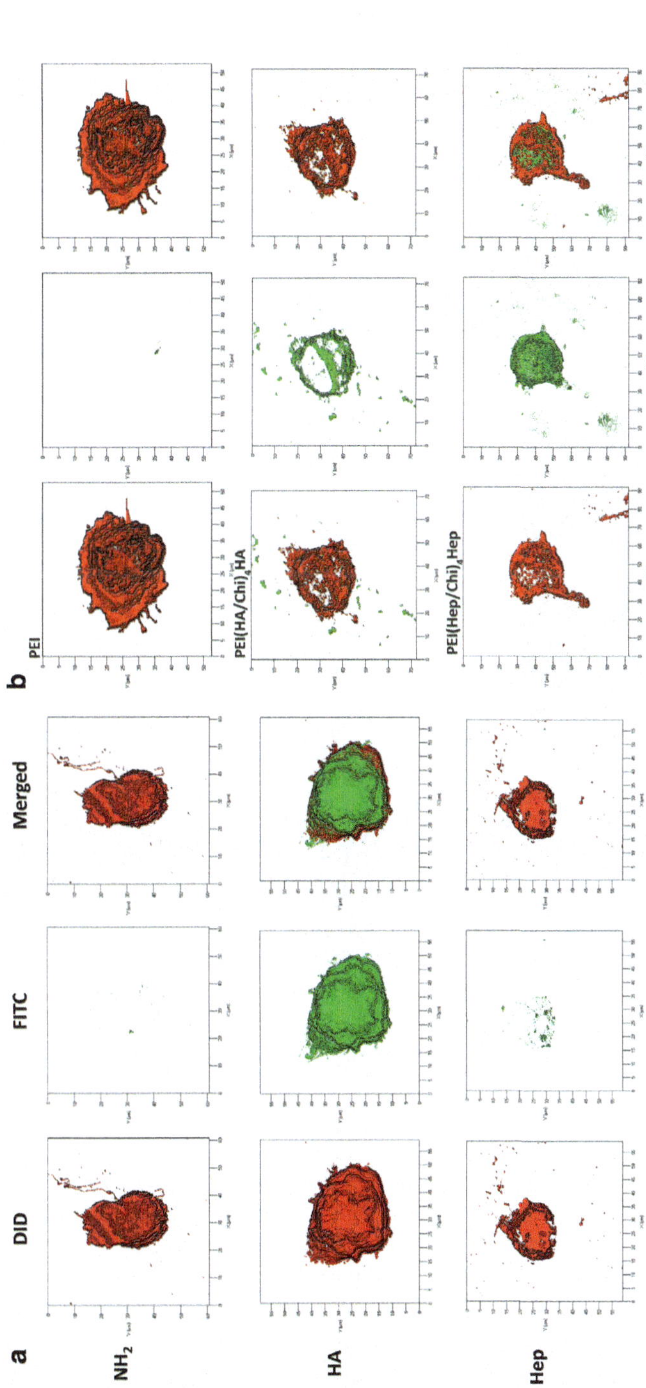

Fig. 11 Representative CLSM 3D view of macrophages on covalent-(**a**) and LBL-(**b**) bound HA or Hep surfaces and their substrata (NH_2 and PEI) in z-stack model by surface projection. The cells were stained by DID (red, membrane staining) and FITC-labelled GAGs (green) (63X, scale bar: 20 μm). Reproduced with permission [25]. Copyright 2020, John Wiley and Sons

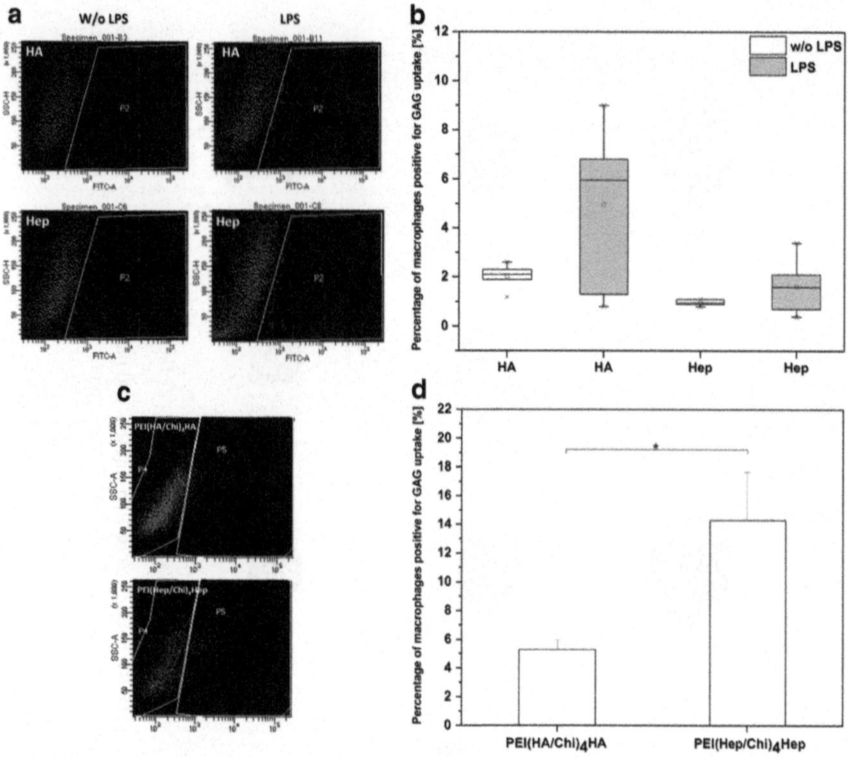

Fig. 12 Representative flow cytometry images of macrophages (**a**, **c**) and the quantified percentage of macrophages positive for GAG uptake after 48-h culture on covalent-(**b**) and LBL-(**d**) bound HA or Hep surfaces. Data represent mean ± SD, n = 6, $*p \leq 0.05$. Reproduced with permission [25]. Copyright 2020, John Wiley and Sons

higher uptake capacity of FITC-labelled HA as covalent coating, but a lower uptake capacity as LBL coating compared to the Hep-modified surfaces.

3 Discussion

Two facile ways for immobilization of the anti-inflammatory GAGs HA and Hep by either covalent or LBL bonding for development of novel anti-inflammatory coatings of biomedical devices and implants were shown here, including first studies on the potential mechanism of their anti-inflammatory activity. The anti-inflammatory effects of HA- and Hep-modified surfaces were evident by significantly reduced macrophage adhesion, spreading, FBGC formation, integrin β1 expression and IL-1β production, but to a different extent and in a different way between the two respective immobilization methods, which was related to the NF-κB signal transduction pathway.

Physicochemical studies were performed to monitor the successful immobilization of GAGs on the control substrates and at the same time to characterize the resulting surface properties like wettability, surface potential and topography. Here, the wettability and charge properties were closely related to the molecular composition and charge density of the GAGs. Hence, HA- and Hep-modified surfaces resulted in more hydrophilic and negatively charged surfaces compared to the amino terminated controls of NH_2 [46] and PEI [47] surfaces, owing to the presence of carboxyl and sulfate groups in HA and Hep [12]. Indeed, the Hep-based surfaces possessed a higher wettability and more negative charges than HA-based surfaces with both immobilization methods. This can be attributed to the high content of sulfate monoesters and sulfamido groups in Hep compared to the lesser quantity of negatively charged carboxyl groups in HA [48, 49]. Furthermore, although no significant differences between both GAGs in zeta potential values at pH 7.4 were seen, strong shifts on the point-of-zero-charge (PZC) of the zeta potential curves for the same GAG using different immobilization methods were observed. Transition from negative to positive zeta potentials were found at lower pH values for covalent coatings compared to LBL adsorbed GAGs, which is related to the presence of chitosan as polycation in multilayers. This is because, the streaming zeta potential measurements of polyelectrolyte multilayers takes also the layers underneath the top layer into account, which in this case is consisting of chitosan in the LBL systems [50], while covalent coatings represent only the surface potential of the pure non-swollen surface. Hence, also the PCZ of Hep was found at lower pH value than for HA. Overall, the wettability and surface charge properties together with the topography studied by AFM proved the successful immobilization of GAGs on top of the NH_2 and PEI surfaces and reflected the hydrophilic and anionic nature of both GAG coatings.

The anti-inflammatory activity of GAG-modified surfaces prepared by both methods were investigated towards a THP-1-derived macrophage response. As expected, the pro-inflammatory control NH_2 and PEI surfaces caused the highest extent of macrophage adhesion and spreading, which is based on the presence of a high number of amino groups, making these substrates moderately wettable and more positively charged, which in return promotes protein adsorption and cell adhesion [51]. By contrast, all GAG-modified surfaces showed significantly suppressive effects on cell adhesion and spreading, which are partially due to the hydrophilicity of these surfaces [52]. Here, the type of GAG obviously plays a pivotal role, but surprisingly in a different way for the two respective immobilization methods. The HA monolayer in the covalent system and the Hep-based $PEI(Hep/Chi)_4Hep$ multilayer in LBL system showed higher inhibition of macrophage adhesion and spreading compared to the other types of GAG-based surfaces. The subsequent FBGC formation and integrin β1 expression studies yielded a similar trend as observed with adhesion and spreading results. NH_2 and PEI surfaces provoked the highest and the HA monolayer and $PEI(Hep/Chi)_4Hep$ multilayers the lowest FBGC formation and integrin β1 expression. This is reasonable, because a certain number of macrophage adhesion is necessary for the macrophages to fuse with others to form FBGCs. The formation of FBGCs is normally accompanied by an increased integrin β1 expression [53, 54]. Nevertheless, besides the initial macrophage adhesion number, the motility of macrophages, which could be driven by cytokine release, might also account for the FBGC formation and integrin β1 expression [55]. Finally, the downregulation of the pro-inflammatory cytokine IL-1β production on the LBL GAG multilayers confirmed their superior potential to inhibit an inflammatory response. It was also seen that PEI(Hep/Chi)$_4$Hep multilayer was more efficient than the PEI(HA/Chi)$_4$HA multilayer, which cannot be only attributed to the highest wettability and most negative charges, but also to the multiple physiological effects of Hep [9, 11, 12]. On the other hand, no significant reduction of IL-1β production was found on either HA- or Hep-based covalent monolayers, indicating a lower efficiency in inhibiting pro-inflammatory cytokine production of the covalent system compared to the LBL system.

Hence, the potential mechanism of the anti-inflammatory action of GAGs was studied focusing on NF-κB signalling pathway to understand the differences between the efficacy of covalent and LBL system. As expected, GAG-modified surfaces showed a significantly lower translocation of p65 subunit of NF-κB to the nuclear area compared to control surfaces, with Hep-based coatings showing the highest inhibition in p65 subunit translocation for both covalent and LBL methods. These results are consistent with other findings that HA and Hep can affect NF-κB signalling pathways leading to a downregulation of NF-κB translocation to the nucleus, which inhibits the subsequent inflammatory responses [56]. In addition, the observed highest inhibitory effects on Hep-based multilayer may be attributed to the physical adsorption, allowing Hep to be released and subsequently uptaken by macrophages, resulting in increased inhibition of NF-κB translocation [57]. Indeed, the association and internalization of HA and Hep by macrophages were confirmed by confocal images with visualization of cell membrane and FITC-labelled GAGs, as well as flow cytometry by analysis of macrophages positive for FITC-labelled GAGs. It was reported that endocytosis or anionic transporters might be the main reasons for the presence of anionic Hep inside macrophages [57], while the intracellular presence of FITC-HA might be due to CD44 receptor endocytosis with the bound ligand [58]. Hence, Hep effects may be superior compared to that of HA. The observed mobilisation of HA and Hep in the covalent system seen by association and uptake of GAG through macrophages might be caused by partial release of GAG molecules from the samples through the secretion of reactive oxygen species (ROS), hyaluronidases and heparinases by macrophages [25, 59, 60].

4 Conclusions and Perspectives

The study presented here shows the type of GAGs (HA and Hep) and the immobilization method (covalent- vs. LBL-bonding) affect not only physical surface properties but also biological responses of macrophage in terms of adhesion, spreading, FBGC formation, integrin β1 expression and pro-inflammatory cytokine IL-1β production. Besides, the studies on mechanism of anti-inflammatory effects of GAG-modified surfaces revealed that pharmaceutical effects of GAGs contributed largely to their activity based on the suppression of NF-κB signalling pathway. It demonstrates the potential of immobilization of HA and Hep on material surfaces to inhibit inflammatory responses by both covalent and LBL immobilization of these GAGs. Indeed, the GAG-Chi multilayers assembled by LBL technique, particularly the Hep-Chi multilayer displayed a higher anti-inflammatory activity than the covalent-bound monolayers of both GAGs, as illustrated by the suppression of IL-1β release. However, both methods of immobilization have their distinct advantages. The LBL technique based on physical adsorption is more flexible and does not require prior chemical activation of surfaces, while the covalent immobilization based on chemical bonding is more stable and can be used possibly in long-term in vivo applications [56]. Moreover, because of their ease and applicability to a wide range of different biomaterials such as polymers, metals and ceramics, etc., both methods can be widely used as versatile tools for improving the biocompatibility of materials [61]. Overall, one can conclude that HA and Hep coatings have great potentials in reducing the adverse inflammatory responses of biomaterials for a variety of biomedical applications such as implants and tissue engineering scaffolds.

Acknowledgements This work was supported by Zhejiang Provincial Natural Science Foundation of China (No. LQ21H180004), National Natural Science Foundation of China (No.81930111), the Scientific Research Starting Foundation from Zhejiang Chinese Medical University, and bilateral cooperation funded by DAAD and Ministry of Education, Science and Technological Development of the Republic of Serbia (period 531 2019–2020).

References

1. Anderson, J.M., Rodriguez, A., Chang, D.T.: Foreign body reaction to biomaterials. Semin. Immunol. **20**(2), 86–100 (2008)
2. Zhou, G., Groth, T.: Host Responses to Biomaterials and anti-inflammatory design-a brief review. Macromol. Biosci. **18**(8), 1800112 (2018)
3. Thevenot, P., Hu, W., Tang, L.: Surface chemistry influences implant biocompatibility. Curr. Top. Med. Chem. **8**(4), 270–280 (2008)
4. Bulbul, E., Hegemann, D., Geue, T., Heuberger, M.: How the dynamics of subsurface hydration regulates protein-surface interactions. Colloids Surfaces B-Biointerfaces **190**, 110908 (2020)
5. Zhou, G., Loppnow, H., Groth, T.: A macrophage/fibroblast co-culture system using a cell migration chamber to study inflammatory effects of biomaterials. Acta Biomater. **26**, 54–63 (2015)
6. Zhou, G., Liedmann, A., Chatterjee, C., Groth, T.: In vitro study of the host responses to model biomaterials via a fibroblast/macrophage co-culture system. Biomater. Sci. **5**(1), 141–152 (2017)
7. Barbosa, J.N., Madureira, P., Barbosa, M.A., Aguas, A.P.: The influence of functional groups of self-assembled monolayers on fibrous capsule formation and cell recruitment. J. Biomed. Mater. Res., Part A **76**(4), 737–743 (2006)

8. Lv, L., Xie, Y. T., Li, K., Hu, T., Lu, X., Cao, Y. Z., Zheng, X. B.: Unveiling the mechanism of surface hydrophilicity-modulated macrophage polarization. Adv. Healthc. Mater. **7**(19), (2018)
9. Proudfoot, A.: Glycosaminoglycan analogs as a novel anti-inflammatory strategy. Front. Immunol. **3**(293), 293 (2012)
10. Taylor, K.R., Gallo, R.L.: Glycosaminoglycans and their proteoglycans: host-associated molecular patterns for initiation and modulation of inflammation. FASEB J. **20**(1), 9–22 (2006)
11. Kim, D.H., Smith, J.T., Chilkoti, A., Reichert, W.M.: The effect of covalently immobilized rhIL-1ra-ELP fusion protein on the inflammatory profile of LPS-stimulated human monocytes. Biomaterials **28**(23), 3369–3377 (2007)
12. Kowitsch, A., Zhou, G.Y., Groth, T.: Medical application of glycosaminoglycans: a review. J. Tissue Eng. Regen. Med. **12**(1), E23–E41 (2018)
13. Mousavi, S., Moradi, M., Khorshidahmad, T., Motamedi, M.: Anti-inflammatory effects of heparin and its derivatives: a systematic review. Adv. Pharmacol. Sci. **2015**, 507151 (2015)
14. Hsieh, C.Y.C., Hu, F.-W., Chen, W.-S., Tsai, W.-B.: Reducing the foreign body reaction by surface modification with collagen/hyaluronic acid multilayered films. ISRN Biomater. **2014**, 718432 (2014)
15. Ruppert, S.M., Hawn, T.R., Arrigoni, A., Wight, T.N., Bollyky, P.L.: Tissue integrity signals communicated by high-molecular weight hyaluronan and the resolution of inflammation. Immunol. Res. **58**(2–3), 186–192 (2014)
16. Zhou, G., Niepel, M.S., Saretia, S., Groth, T.: Reducing the inflammatory responses of biomaterials by surface modification with glycosaminoglycan multilayers. J. Biomed. Mater. Res., Part A **104**(2), 493–502 (2016)
17. Young, E.: The anti-inflammatory effects of heparin and related compounds. Thromb Res **122**(6), 743–752 (2008)
18. Morla, S.: Glycosaminoglycans and glycosaminoglycan mimetics in cancer and inflammation. Int. J. Mol. Sci. **20**(8), 1963 (2019)
19. Hayden, M.S., Ghosh, S.: Signaling to NF-κB. Genes Develop. **18**(18), 2195–2224 (2004)
20. Li, X., Zheng, Z., Li, X., Ma, X.C.: Unfractionated heparin inhibits lipopolysaccharide-induced inflammatory response through blocking p38 MAPK and NF-kappa B activation on endothelial cell. Cytokine **60**(1), 114–121 (2012)
21. Theus, S.A., Cave, M.D., Eisenach, K.D.: Activated THP-1 cells: an attractive model for the assessment of intracellular growth rates of Mycobacterium tuberculosis isolates. Infect. Immun. **72**(2), 1169–1173 (2004)
22. Park, E.K., Jung, H.S., Yang, H.I., Yoo, M.C., Kim, C., Kim, K.S.: Optimized THP-1 differentiation is required for the detection of responses to weak stimuli. Inflamm. Res. **56**(1), 45–50 (2007)
23. Sheikh, Z., Brooks, P.J., Barzilay, O., Fine, N., Glogauer, M.: Macrophages, foreign body giant cells and their response to implantable biomaterials. Materials **8**, 5671–5701 (2015)
24. Xia, Z., Triffitt, J.T.: A review on macrophage responses to biomaterials. Biomed. Mater. **1**(1), R1–R9 (2006)
25. AlKhoury, H., Hautmann, A., Erdmann, F., Zhou, G., Stojanović, S., Najman, S., Groth, T.: Study on the potential mechanism of anti-inflammatory activity of covalently immobilized hyaluronan and heparin. J. Biomed. Mater. Res., Part A **108**(5), 1099–1111 (2020)
26. Husar, G.M., Anziano, D.J., Leuck, M., Sebesta, D.P.: Covalent modification and surface immobilization of nucleic acids via the Diels-Alder bioconjugation method. Nucleosides, Nucleotides Nucleic Acids **20**(4–7), 559–566 (2001)
27. Sun, Z.C., Wei, Z., Wei, K.M.: Heparan sulfate: Structure, function, modification and synthesis. Prog. Chem. **20**(7–8), 1136–1142 (2008)
28. Yang, Y., Koewitsch, A., Ma, N., Maeder, K., Pashkuleva, I., Reis, R.L., Groth, T.: Functionality of surface-coupled oxidised glycosaminoglycans towards fibroblast adhesion. J. Bioact. Compat. Polym. **31**(2), 191–207 (2016)
29. Kowitsch, A., Niepel, M.S., Michanetzis, G.P.A., Missirlis, Y.F., Groth, T.: Effect of immobilized thiolated glycosaminoglycans on fibronectin adsorption and behavior of fibroblasts. Macromol. Biosci. **16**(3), 381–394 (2016)

30. Daamen, W.F., van Moerkerk, H.T.B., Hafmans, T., Buttafoco, L., Poot, A.A., Veerkamp, J.H., van Kuppevelt, T.H.: Preparation and evaluation of molecularly-defined collagen-elastin-glycosaminoglycan scaffolds for tissue engineering. Biomaterials **24**(22), 4001–4009 (2003)
31. Wang, K., Luo, Y.: Defined surface immobilization of glycosaminoglycan molecules for probing and modulation of cell-material interactions. Biomacromol **14**(7), 2373–2382 (2013)
32. Koewitsch, A., Yang, Y., Ma, N., Kuntsche, J., Maeder, K., Groth, T.: Bioactivity of immobilized hyaluronic acid derivatives regarding protein adsorption and cell adhesion. Biotechnol. Appl. Biochem. **58**(5), 376–389 (2011)
33. Hammond, P.T.: Building biomedical materials layer-by-layer. Mater. Today **15**(5), 196–206 (2012)
34. Richardson, J.J., Bjoernmalm, M., Caruso, F.: Technology-driven layer-by-layer assembly of nanofilms. Science **348**(6233), aaa2491 (2015)
35. Niepel, M., Köwitsch, A., Yang, Y., Ma, N., Aggarwal, N., Guduru, D., Groth, T.: Generic methods of surface modification to control adhesion of cells and beyond. In: Biomater. Surface Sci. 441–467
36. Nishiguchi, A., Matsusaki, M., Akashi, M.: Cell-cell crosslinking by bio-molecular recognition of heparin-based layer-by-layer nanofilms. Macromol. Biosci. **15**(3), 312–317 (2015)
37. Almodovar, J., Place, L.W., Gogolski, J., Erickson, K., Kipper, M.J.: Layer-by-layer assembly of polysaccharide-based polyelectrolyte multilayers: a spectroscopic study of hydrophilicity, composition, and ion pairing. Biomacromol **12**(7), 2755–2765 (2011)
38. Richert, L., Lavalle, P., Payan, E., Shu, X.Z., Prestwich, G.D., Stoltz, J.-F., Schaaf, P., Voegel, J.-C., Picart, C.: Layer by layer buildup of polysaccharide films: physical chemistry and cellular adhesion aspects. Langmuir: The ACS J. Surfaces Coll. **20**(2), 448–458 (2004)
39. Hong, S.W., Jeong, J.H., Lee, D.Y., Byun, Y.: Layer-by-layer building up of heparin and glycol chitosan for rat pancreatic islet xenotransplantation to mouse. Macromol. Res. **21**(8), 911–915 (2013)
40. Zhou, G., Al-Khoury, H., Groth, T.: Covalent immobilization of glycosaminoglycans to reduce the inflammatory effects of biomaterials. Int. J. Artif. Organs **39**(1), 37–44 (2016)
41. Rayahin, J.E., Gemeinhart, R.A.: Activation of macrophages in response to biomaterials. Results Probl. Cell Differ. **62**, 317–351 (2017)
42. McNally, A.K., Macewan, S.R., Anderson, J.M.: alpha subunit partners to beta1 and beta2 integrins during IL-4-induced foreign body giant cell formation. J. Biomed. Mater. Res., Part A **82**(3), 568–574 (2007)
43. Schmidt, D.R., Kao, W.J.: The interrelated role of fibronectin and interleukin-1 in biomaterial-modulated macrophage function. Biomaterials **28**(3), 371–382 (2007)
44. Zhang, H., Peterson, J.W., Niesel, D.W., Klimpel, G.R.: Bacterial lipoprotein and lipopolysaccharide act synergistically to induce lethal shock and proinflammatory cytokine production. J. Immunol. (Baltimore, Md. : 1950) **159**(10), 4868–78 (1997)
45. Liu, T., Zhang, L., Joo, D., Sun, S.-C.: NF-κB signaling in inflammation. Signal Transduct. Target. Ther. **2**, 17023 (2017)
46. Zeng, X.X., Xu, G.H., Gao, Y.A., An, Y.: Surface Wettability of (3-Aminopropyl)triethoxysilane Self-Assembled Monolayers. J. Phys. Chem. B **115**(3), 450–454 (2011)
47. Chen, Z.H., Lv, Z.Y., Sun, Y.F., Chi, Z.G., Qing, G.Y.: Recent advancements in polyethyleneimine-based materials and their biomedical, biotechnology, and biomaterial applications. J. Mat. Chem. B **8**(15), 2951–2973 (2020)
48. Shriver, Z., Capila, I., Venkataraman, G., Sasisekharan, R.: Heparin and heparan sulfate: analyzing structure and microheterogeneity. Handb. Exp. Pharmacol. **207**, 159–176 (2012)
49. Garantziotis, S., Savani, R.C.: Hyaluronan biology: a complex balancing act of structure, function, location and context. Matrix Biol. **78–79**, 1–10 (2019)
50. Duval, J.F.L., Kuttner, D., Werner, C., Zimmermann, R.: Electrohydrodynamics of soft polyelectrolyte multilayers: point of zero-streaming current. Langmuir **27**(17), 10739–10752 (2011)

51. Faucheux, N., Tzoneva, R., Nagel, M.-D., Groth, T.: The dependence of fibrillar adhesions in human fibroblasts on substratum chemistry. Biomaterials **27**(2), 234–245 (2006)
52. Bacakova, L., Filova, E., Parizek, M., Ruml, T., Svorcik, V.: Modulation of cell adhesion, proliferation and differentiation on materials designed for body implants. Biotechnol. Adv. **29**(6), 739–767 (2011)
53. Vignery, A.: Osteoclasts and giant cells: macrophage-macrophage fusion mechanism. Int. J. Exp. Pathol. **81**(5), 291–304 (2000)
54. McNally, A.K., Anderson, J.M.: Beta1 and beta2 integrins mediate adhesion during macrophage fusion and multinucleated foreign body giant cell formation. Am. J. Pathol. **160**(2), 621–630 (2002)
55. Kyriakides, T.R., Foster, M.J., Keeney, G.E., Tsai, A., Giachelli, C.M., Clark-Lewis, I., Rollins, B.J., Bornstein, P.: The CC chemokine ligand, CCL2/MCP1, participates in macrophage fusion and foreign body giant cell formation. Am. J. Pathol. **165**(6), 2157–2166 (2004)
56. Biran, R., Pond, D.: Heparin coatings for improving blood compatibility of medical devices. Adv. Drug Deliv. Rev. **112**, 12–23 (2017)
57. Young, E.: The anti-inflammatory effects of heparin and related compounds. Thromb. Res. **122**(6), 743–752 (2008)
58. Knudson, W., Chow, G., Knudson, C.B.: CD44-mediated uptake and degradation of hyaluronan. Matrix Biol. **21**(1), 15–23 (2002)
59. Li, J.-P., Vlodavsky, I.: Heparin, heparan sulfate and heparanase in inflammatory reactions. Thromb. Haemost. **102**(11), 823–828 (2009)
60. Puissant, E., Boonen, M.: Monocytes/macrophages upregulate the hyaluronidase HYAL1 and adapt its subcellular trafficking to promote extracellular residency upon differentiation into osteoclasts. PLoS ONE **11**(10), e0165004 (2016)
61. Murugesan, S., Xie, J., Linhardt, R.J.: Immobilization of heparin: approaches and applications. Curr. Top. Med. Chem. **8**(2), 80–100 (2008)

Biomimetics in Orthopedic Surgery and Traumatology

Aleksandar Radunović, Ognjen Radunović, Maja Vulović, and Milan Aksić

Abstract Biomimetics is considered producing materials in manner that imitate natural tissues and their properties. There is increased need for artificial tissue replacement as autografts that are routinely used have limited resources. There are few different types of tissues in orthopedic surgery and traumatology that frequently need substitution for restoring satisfactory function of locomotory system, thus different kind of biomimetics are developed to fulfill this gap. There are many materials used for this purpose, none of them completely fulfill expected criteria. Basically all biomimetics can be classified as elastic, soft and hard. Elastic are designed for replacing menisci, tendons, ligaments. Soft biomimetics are used as a replacement for skin, muscles and cartilage tissue. Hard biomimetics are replacement for bone tissue. There are some completely synthetic biomimetics but modern approaches tend to combine them with natural materials tending to get best of both worlds. Hybrid materials are expected to combine properties of its ingredients and successfully mimic natural tissues.

Keywords Biomimetics · Orthopedics · Tissue engineering

A. Radunović (✉)
Clinic for Orthopedic Surgery and Traumatology, Military Medical Academy, Belgrade, Serbia
e-mail: aradunovic@yahoo.com

O. Radunović
Faculty of Medicine, University of Belgrade, Dr Subotića 8, 11000, Belgrade, Serbia

M. Vulović
Department of Anatomy and Forensic Medicine, Faculty of Medical Sciences, University of Kragujevac, Kragujevac, Serbia

M. Aksić
Institute of Anatomy "Niko Miljanić", Faculty of Medicine, University of Belgrade, Dr Subotića 8, 11000 Belgrade, Serbia

S. Najman et al. (eds.), *Bioceramics, Biomimetic and Other Compatible Materials Features for Medical Applications*, Engineering Materials,
https://doi.org/10.1007/978-3-031-17269-4_8

1 Introduction

Biomimetics or **biomimicry** is the emulation of the models, systems, and elements of nature for the purpose of solving complex human problems [1]. The terms "biomimetics" and "biomimicry" are derived from Ancient Greek: βίος (*bios*), life, and μίμησις (*mīmēsis*), imitation, from μιμεῖσθαι (*mīmeisthai*), to imitate, from μῖμος (*mimos*), actor.

Living beings have adapted to a constantly changing environment during evolution through mutation, recombination, and selection [2]. The core idea of the biomimetic philosophy is that nature's inhabitants including animals, plants, and microbes have the most experience in solving problems and have already found the most appropriate ways to last on planet Earth [3].

1.1 Biomimetics in Orthopedic

During routine orthopedic work, there are many indications for replacements of soft and hard tissues. Majority of those are due to trauma, malignant diseases and congenital defects. As human body itself has many regenerative potentials its possible, for minor to medium size defects, to be managed by natural healing or combination of reconstructive surgery and natural healing, while huge defects always need additional material for management. At this moment medicine relies on biological scaffolds for managing these problems. Biological scaffold is provided when part of tissue has been harvested with specific technique and transferred on a host patient in order to replace missing tissue and serve as a scaffold for hosts regenerative processes. The term routinely used for this kind of substitute is graft. According to graft origin we are talking about autografts, allografts and xenografts.

Table 1 shows advantages and disadvantages of different graft types.

Autografts are harvested from a patient and used on his organism to manage the tissue defect (tissue transplanted from one part of the body to another).

Allografts are harvested from another patient and transferred to a host patient (same species but different genotype - human to human transplantation).

Xenografts are parts of a tissues harvested from one species and transferred to other species (animals to human). Typically are used porcine dermis and small intestine or bovine pericardium and dermis, sometimes equine tissue.

The key to as good imitation of biological tissues as possible is to achieve physical and chemical properties of target tissue. Therefore, available biomimetics used in musculoskeletal pathology can be roughly divided in educational purposes as elastic, soft and hard.

Elastic Biomimetics Those are ment to substitute tissues that are naturally elastic such as tendons, ligaments and menisci in the knee as well as glenoid labrum in the shoulder.

Table 1 Advantages and disadvantages of different graft types

Graft type	Autograft	Allograft	Xenograft
Advantages	• Provides cells and healing factors that are significant for tissue regeneration • No risk of transmissive diseases • No risk of graft rejection due to immune reaction of the host	• No need for additional surgery • Structural support is provided from the positioning of the graft • In case of bony grafts there is osteoconductivity (but poor osteoinductivity) • No donor site morbidity	• Available in greater amount • Available in larger sizes
Disadvantages	• Availability is limited (especially when in need for substantial graft size) • Donor site pain and morbidity • Need for additional surgery	• Can cause host immunological response • Slower integration compared to autografts • Limited availability • Risk of transferable disease • While restructuring in organism mechanical strength is significantly decreased	• Risk of contamination with animal microorganisms • Can cause host immunological response • Slower integration compared to autografts

Those tissues consist of different kind of cells and extracellular matrix (ECM). ECM is composed of nonfibrous part (glycosaminoglycans) and fibrous part (elastin and collagen). Elastin has huge half life so there is a need for it in organism only when there is trauma to elastic tissue and reparation process demands elastin. Although, it is necessary to know that newly formed tissue have much poorer performance due to inadequate organization of fibers in freshly produced reparatory elastin and limited production of elastin in adult cells. Therefore, elasticity must be incorporated in synthetic scaffold itself.

There are few methods for acquiring elastin in laboratory. Animal derived elastin is challenging for production. By producing elastin with recombinant techniques, mostly on bacteria, it is possible to achieve good results in protein synthesis but the crosslinks and topography of such elastin fibers will produce elastin with lower mechanical quality compared to native one. Purely synthetic elastomers have advantage of possible producing in variety of dimensions and forms. Additionally they can be modified by changing a part of their structure or way they are crosslinked. Polyglycerol co-sebacate (PGS), poly-1,8-octanediol co-citrate (POC), polyurethanes (PU), polyhydroalkanoate (PHA) are frequently used in research. In order to achieve desired biocompatible and mechanical properties it is often necessary to combine different materials and produce hybrid tissue replacements. There is vast number of combinations with some authors grouping it as: synthetic polymer-polymer hybrid, protein-protein hybrid and synthetic polymer-protein hybrid [4].

Menisci are notorious for its almost nonexisting healing potential due to low vascularization in majority of meniscal body. Situation is somewhat better with tendons and ligaments. Using of allografts and meniscal transplantation are pretty demanding procedure mostly for problems with providing sufficient amounts of allografts. For obtaining good functional results with this procedure proper patient selection should be performed as well as good preoperative planning and especially templating of meniscal size which implies need for considerable stock of allografts for successful surgery. Some papers show high rate of complications and need for revision surgery [5]. Those are reasons for conducting research towards bioengineered materials for those purposes. Materials with most promising properties for use as elastic biomimetics in meniscal pathology are collagen, native elastin, elastin-like polypeptides, synthetic elastomers and elastic hybrid materials [4].

Soft Biomimetics Primary idea of developing those materials is to make substitutes for skin, muscles and cartilage tissue. AT this moment majority of techniques for soft tissue reconstruction rely on tissue grafts. Application of synthetic implants are limited by few factors and most noticeable are implant tearing or deformation and tissue resorption. Natural biomaterials can be used as synthetic replacement for soft tissues separately or combined with synthetic materials that reinforce them. Most widely used in this manner are collagen, hyaluron, fibrin, cryopreserved amniotic membrane, chitosan, acellular dermal matrix etc. In commercially available products they are often combined with stem cells or differentiated cells (fibroblasts and keratinocytes mostly). Natural polymers are very demanding for manipulation so there are attempts of using synthetic polymers as base for constructing scaffolds of different mechanical and chemical properties. Unfortunately there are some problems associated with this concept, typical for almost every synthetic materials in vivo: over time there is deterioration of materials and subsequent emission of degradational products of material as well as issues with biocompatibility [6].

Cartilage tissue is specific for its minor self-repair capacity. It is an avascular tissue and oxygen and nutritive substances necessary for its normal functioning are provided by direct diffusion from synovial fluid and repetitive moving of the joints enhances this process. This means that any degree of injury may cause significant degenerative changes in joint due to repetitive stresses, especially on bear loading joints. When in need for managing chondral defect, nowadays surgeon will routinely use one of the following techniques, depending on the defect size:

- Microfracture: usually used for managing of smaller defects or eventually moderate size when patient expect lower activity level. It is performed by creating few minor holes that reaches subchondral bone marrow expecting to form fibrous clot that will cover defect and afterwards be transformed in fibrocartilage tissue.
- Autologous chondral transplantation for moderate size defects. Donor area can be non weight bearing part of the joint cartilage tissue and graft can be harvested as a solitary one or as few minor grafts when using a mosaicplasty technique.
- When defects exceed 2.5–3 cm^2 osteochondral allografts or autologous chondrocyte implantation are used.

For few decades it is well known there is possibility for engineering cartilage tissue using autologous adult chondrocytes. This method has limitations in everyday surgical work so there are many attempts of using different progenitor cell sources [7]. It was shown there are significant potentials of cells from adipose and other tissues as well as use progenitors from embryonic stem cells. A beginning of 1990 is period of uprising of biomaterials with nowadays present concept of commercially available materials based on hybrid natural-synthetic platforms. Due to specific histological organization of hyaline cartilage tissue it becomes stiffer as the rate of loading increases [8].

Aiming to imitate this characteristic, researchers found materials for hyaline cartilage substitution have to be designed with nonlinear, inhomogeneous and viscoelastic properties [9]. Ideal scaffold should have adequate architecture and mechanical properties, as mentioned, biodegradability, biocompatibility, to enable cell adhesion, porosity and permeability. At this moment in commercial use are the scaffolds that serves as a temporary matrix for implanted cells, giving mechanical support for new tissue formation. Those scaffolds are made from type I/III collagen and hydroxyapatite based materials [10]. Natural material based scaffolds have advantages being similar to local tissue (biocompatibility, bioactivity, biodegradability), but their principle disadvantages are: mechanical weakness (especially in moist environment) and nonresistance to many processing conditions (high pressure and temperature). Next instance are hydrogels that have similar nonresistance to aquatic environment as natural scaffolds. Thus research are going toward synthetic scaffolds that can provide mechanical strength alongside with biocompatibility and biodegradability by virtue of hardiness to physical and chemical challenges of surrounding tissue. Synthetic materials currently most frequently used are: polyethylene glycol (PEG), polylactic acid (PLA), polycaprolactone (PCL), polyglycolic acid (PGA) and copolymers as polylactic coglycolic acid (PLGA). They have very promising results, but still remains huge disadvantage of releasing acid products during biodegradation, with possibility of consequential inflammatory reaction in organism. Analyzing current literature, hybrid scaffolds seems to be most promising one, with combining synthetic polymers (mostly PLGA and PLA) with natural materials (collagen and chitosan).

Hard Biomimetics They are designed as an attempt to substitute bone when necessary. Bone itself is highly specialized form of connective tissue with multiple functions: provide hard framework for the body, protects internal organs, enables motion serving as attachment for muscles, enabling lever mechanism for tendons and maintenance of mineral homeostasis. Another property of bone of paramount importance is possibility of constant remodeling. In this process parts of old bone are resorbed by bone resorbing cells (osteoclasts) and gradually replaced with new bone produced by bone forming cells (osteoblasts). This constant remodeling enables bone to adapt to mechanical loads. This is defined as Wolf‘s law, developed by German surgeon Julius Wolf in nineteenth century. According to it, bone in healthy person will adapt to the loads under which it is placed. When loading on bone or part of bone increases it will be remodeled and become stronger to resist load. The same stands for reverse process: if load is decreased, the bone becomes less dense and weaker due to lower stimulus needed for remodeling process. Whole remodeling process is performed through mechanism called mechanotransduction when mechanical signals are converted in biochemical signals and cellular signaling. When reduction in bone structure occurs it is named osteopenia. Sometimes it is consequence of generally lower activity (older people), treating of fractured bone, when load is not permitted while fracture is healed. Special form of osteopenia is stress shielding, phenomenon known in hip arthroplasty with some endoprosthesis design. It occurs in situation when implant take overload instead of bone, so parts of bone around implant underwent process of osteolysis that ultimately can produce implant loosening.

Bone is natural composite consisting of organic, inorganic part and water. Organic component of bone consists of more than 30 proteins with collagen type 1 making more than 90% and rest are noncollagenous proteins. Those different proteins have various functions, although not completely cleared. Majority of them have significant roles in mineralization of bone matrix. They also take part in regulation of osteoclasts and osteoblasts function and differentiation of bone cell by supporting their attachments to bone. Inorganic component is primarily crystalline hydroxyapatite. Organic component makes approximately 30% and organic 60% of weight while 10% is water weight. As about volume, inorganic component occupy40%, organic 35% and water 25%.

It is also important to have basic knowledge of macroscopic bone architecture.

Long bones are composed of cortical and cancellous bone tissue. Those are differently presented in various areas of bone. Diaphysis or the bone shaft is the central part of long bones and it has walls made of cortical bone. Metaphyses are widening of the bone at its ends and these areas are mostly made from cancellous bone with cortical bone forms the outer shell. Cortical bone is very resistant to a one way directioned loads while cancellous bone and its trabecular structure are capable for withstand loads in different directions.

Due to increased incidence of traumatism in last decades, there is great need for bone graft materials. There is also huge increase in number of implanted artificial joints in degenerative and rheumatic diseases, so there is always search for new materials that would enable longer survival of implants. In adequate functioning of musculoskeletal system there is huge role of soft tissues (muscles, ligaments, tendons, menisci, etc.) that are very frequently injured and very often there is need for artificial replacements of those tissues.

In routine work in majority of health facilities, when substitution for host bone is needed, surgeons use bone autografts (bone harvested from patient) or bone allografts (bone that is harvested from other patient, controlled for infective agents and frozen on −60 to −80 °C). The most important advantage of using those bone grafts is mechanical similarity to a host bone. Principle disadvantages are: possibility of transmission of infective agents (when using allografts) from host and limited amounts of auto- and allografts. Those leaded to investigations for engineering biomaterials with properties and structure similar to those in live organism. Biomaterials are used in orthopedic surgery for more than 50 years but still there is none that has mechanical properties of natural bone and such resistance and adaptation to repetitive stresses. There are many reasons for biomaterial implant failure but majority of them are due to artificial materials acting as a passive scaffold without possibility of remodeling and adapt to biomechanical circumstances in organism. At this moment most widely used substitutes for auto- and allografts are demineralized bone matrix (DBM) and synthetic bone graft substitutes (calcium sulfate and phosphate in majority of cases with addition of collagen, or polymers).

Calcium phosphates are minerals consisting of calcium cations and phosphate anions. Its existence in bones is discovered in 1769 and from beginning of twentieth century it is studied as material for clinical use having a wide range of potential utilization. There is spectrum of features making them excellent biomaterials: acting as bioactive scaffold that enables attachment of bone cells, their stimulation to grow, multiply and form a new bone. It also forms excellent bond with bone tissue without interposition of fibrous layer and facilitate growth of bone tissue and rapid early fixation. Thus the increase in use of CaP as biocompatible and bioactive material in orthopedic surgery. During research in this area many variants of calcium phosphates are considered for orthopedic use in different forms such as: coatings, cement and scaffold based on this material. There are also attempts to improve performance of calcium phosphates in combination with different agents.

Degradation and releasing of ions are crucial for good bioactive properties of calcium phosphate. Increasing of concentration of Ca and P ions stimulates formation of bone minerals on the surface of CaP and also influence expression of various osteoblast differentiation markers. Calcium ions influence many cascades important in bone healing process. They cause bone formation and ripening through calcification, stimulates mature bone cells forming nitric oxide and inducing bone growth precursors cells for bone regeneration [11]. Phosphate ions also influence processes of bone growth in many ways. They regulate proliferation and differentiation of osteoblasts and promotes expression of bone morphogenetic protein [12]. Calcium phosphates have rough surface enabling attachment of proteins and cells on it. Porosity of CaP enables contact with body fluid on larger area and promotes ingrowth of blood vessels.

Types of Calcium Phosphates

Nanodimensional Calcium Phosphates Nanometer size of particles provide maximum strength, better interaction with cells and can be considered as a storage for minerals needed for bone remodelation process. It is found that nano structure decreases percentage of mechanical failure, improves friction and wear characteristics and increases density [13]. As there is significant increase in surface area, there is also improvement in biological and cellular reaction. Due to mentioned properties of nano sized CaP applications are mostly in hybrid biocomposites for enhancing bioactivity and manufacturing of scaffolds. This type of calcium phosphates is also used as a career for drugs providing them safety from degradation, promoting local delivery and control their release [14]. Nano sized calcium phosphates have large surface compared to volume and are able to be loaded with much higher quantity of drugs.

Cements Calcium phosphate cements (CPC) are used for bone augmentation and substitution for a long time. Since 1980 there is increased interest for their improvement which resulted in many commercially available products at this moment. All of them are produced as a result of interaction between liquid and solid phase. Mixing of those produces paste that gradually hardens and become solid mass. Solid phase is made from different calcium phosphate compounds while liquid part are different aqueous solutions (sodium orthophosphate, H3PO4 or citric acid). Mixing liquid and solid phase produces viscous paste that can be manipulated very well manually or injected into a bone and form desired shape. It hardens on body temperature but has an excellent property of hardening with slightly exothermic reaction. For example PMMA (polymethylmethacrylate bone cement) has similar physical properties but hardens with highly exotermic reaction that can cause local tissue necrosis. Although there are numerous available formulations of CaP cement components there are only two possible final products: brushite (dicalcium phosphate dehydrate) or apatite (hydroxyapatite). In vivo settings brushite can transform to apatite.

Calcium phosphates cement seems like very promising material for bone substitution, regeneration and other mentioned applications, still there are some issues that limits application. Pure CPC, without additives is prone to liquid–solid components separation. Without additives it also have low strength, high brittleness, low impact resistance and low tensile strength, so the application is limited mostly to non weight bearing indications in orthopedic surgery [15]. In majority of clinical applications CaP cements are injected in trabecular bone to avoid failures. Once when hardened CaP cement resembles to trabecular bone mostly. In order to enhance mechanical properties of CaP cement various types of fibers, fillers and additives are used: bioactive glass, collagen fibers, carbon nanotube etc. It is preferable to use biodegradable fillers and additives that does not impact porosity of CaP cement thus keeping best properties of CaP unaffected.

Majority of clinical applications of CaP cements are for bone augmentation and bone defect management in appropriate indications. They are used for augmentation of osteoporotic vertebral bodies augmentation and also for treatment of vertebral fractures. They are used for bone defect healing in surgeries that doesn't demand high pressure resistance of implants (maxillofacial, oral surgery). CaP cements are also used as drug delivery systems providing incorporation of drugs as well as gradual emission. There are multiple ongoing research with CaP as delivery agent for antibiotics, anticancer drugs and anti-inflammatory agents with promising results.

Coatings Metallic materials are widely used in orthopedic surgery for different purposes. Biocompatible metals have good mechanical properties in terms of mechanical strength and torque resistance but don't fulfill criteria regarding bioactivity. Surface of orthopedical implants is crucial while trying to achieve stable osteointegration performing joint arthroplasties. Surface optimization with adequate coating is found to be the best way to optimize implant for specific orthopedic application. Calcium phosphate showed good results when applied as a biomaterial in human organism so there are various attempts of using it as a coating on different metallic implants used in joint arthroplasties. Different types of CaP are used as coating materials with good osteoconductive properties enabling stable and rapid osteointegration

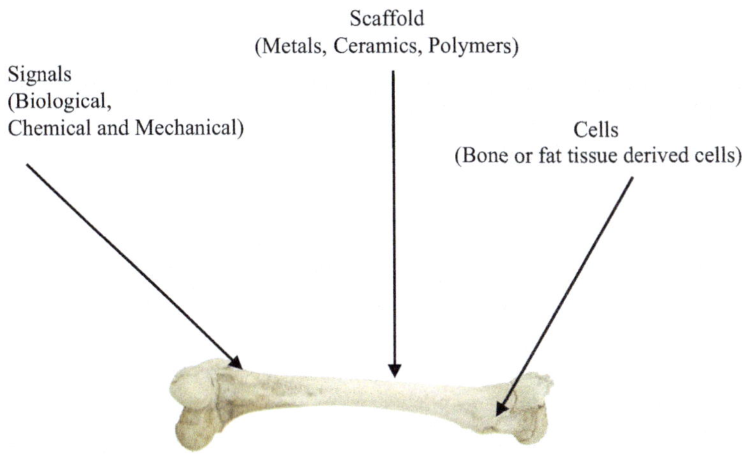

Fig. 1 Basic constituents of bone tissue engineering [16]

of implant compared to non coated implants. Osteoconductive properties of different CaP's vary depending on surface porosity, pore size, geometry. There are several CaP coatings methods, commercially most widely used is plasma spray. Beside physical deposition techniques some other techniques are used: wet chemical techniques (sol-gel method, biomimetic precipitation, cathodic electrodeposition etc.). Deposition method hugely depends on metal that is used as an implant main part.

Basic Constituents of Bone Tissue Engineering Basic constituents for bone tissue engineering (Fig. 1) are scaffolds, cells and signals [16].

Scaffolds serves as replacements/reinforcements in order to provide favorable conditions for production of native tissue. Scaffolds used in bone surgery are expected to be bioactive, biodegradable and porous. Bioactivity means promotion of interaction of cells and biomaterial, enhancing adhesion of cells and later proliferation, migration and differentiation. Biodegradability is the feature enabling replacement of scaffold with native tissue during desirable time period, without emitting toxic products during that process. Additionally scaffolds in orthopedic surgery and traumatology of musculoskeletal system are expected to be durable and capable of withstanding significant mechanical loads. Principle problem is not only to achieve desired mechanical sustainability but to preserve it through process of biodegradation, at least sufficiently long for tissue to recover. Some materials (ceramics) can withstand great amount of compressive loads, they are prone to failure on tensile forces and such facts should be considered while choosing ideal material for scaffold.

Based on materials used for fabrication, scaffolds can be: Metals, ceramics and polymers. They also can be observed as naturally derived or synthetically manufactured; resorbable and nonresorbable; with or without osteoconductivity and osteoinductivity. None of those are ideal and choice hugely depends on anticipated use. For example naturally derived scaffolds have excellent biomechanical properties but are in lack of mechanical strength and have high degradation rate. Scaffolds with low degradation rate may not integrate properly into a tissue and start to act as foreign body.

Cells are necessary for tissue origination as well for integration with host organism. Cells are integrated in implied scaffold in different manners and most frequently used in orthopedic regenerative surgery are mesenchymal stem cells (MSC). They are very convenient for this purpose as have ability to differentiate into various types of cells (osteoblasts, myoblasts, chondroblasts, tenocytes) [17]. Another huge advantage of MSC is simple process of harvesting. MSC from bone marrow aspirate are considered gold standard at this moment but MSC derived from adipose tissue are gaining in popularity, primarily for increased availability and easier harvesting. Other sources of MSC are periosteum, skin, umbilical cord blood and amniotic fluid. It is shown that MSC harvested from different tissues have various differentiation potentials [17]. Implanted MSC doesn't have only structural effect in host organism. When implanted they also make modulation of immune response, making less possible tissue rejection by host organism [18].

By signals we consider intrinsic or extrinsic factors that may affect tissue regeneration process. Those signals can be biological (growth factors and platelets rich plasma), chemical (statins, biphosphonates), mechanical (pressure or distraction).

Indications for Using Biomimetics in Orthopedic Surgery and Traumatology As already mentioned all research dealing with bioengineering of hard, soft and elastic tissues are more frequent because there is increased need for substitution of those tissues in routine work. Most frequent indications for using these materials are:

- Acute fractures of long bones
- Delayed unions and nonunions of long bones
- Osteonecrosis (avascular necrosis)
- Osteochondral defects

Majority of acute fractures doesn't require any additional treatment beside surgical stabilization. Many factors influence bone healing process. Age of patient is one of the most important as cell and signal activity decreases rapidly with aging. Comorbidity, as diabetes and osteoporosis, can notably jeopardize bone healing. Life habits as smoking and chronic alcoholism are also risk factors known for decades. There are some other conditions that can influence formation of satisfactory callus at fracture site: nutritional status of patient (intake of proteins and calcium), hypovitaminosis (especially D and C). And last, but not least, fracture related factors are of huge importance while estimating need for additional means of enhancing bone healing (open or closed fracture, degree of comminution, segmental fractures with double impaired vascularization of bone, large devitalized bone fragments). Decision for applying proper enhancement method demands excellent knowledge of bone histophysiology, methods of surgical stabilization and knowledge of characteristics of available bone substitutes materials.

References

1. Vincent, J.F.V., et al.: Biomimetics: its practice and theory. J. Roy. Soc. Interface **3**(9), 471–482 (2006). https://doi.org/10.1098/rsif.2006.0127. PMC 1664643. PMID 16849244
2. Knippers J, Nickel KG, Speck TC (2016) Biomimetic research for architecture and building construction: biological design and integrative structures. Springer. ISBN 978-3-319-46374-2. OCLC 967523159
3. Collins, G.R., Gaudi, A.: Structure and form. Perspecta **8**, 63–90 (1963). https://doi.org/10.2307/1566905. ISSN 0079-0958. JSTOR 1566905
4. Coenen, A.M.J., et al.: Elastic materials for tissue engineering applications: natural, synthetic, and hybrid polymers. Acta Biomater. **79**, 60–82 (2018)
5. González-Lucena, G., Gelber, P.E., Pelfort, X., Tey, M., Monllau, J.C.: Meniscal allograft transplantation without bone blocks: a 5- to 8-year follow-up of 33 patients. J. Arthrosc. Relat. Surg. **26**(12), 1633–1640 (2010)
6. Hacker, M.C., Krieghoff, J., Mikos, A.G.: Synthetic polymers. In: Principles of Regenerative Medicine, p. 559–590. Elsevier (2019)
7. Langer, R., Vacanti, J.P.: Tissue engineering. Science **260**, 920–926 (1993)
8. Park, S., Hung, C.T., Ateshian, G.A.: Mechanical response of bovine articular cartilage under dynamic unconfined compression loading at physiological stress levels. Osteoarthritis Cartilage **12**, 65–73 (2004)
9. Guilak, F., Butler, D.L., Goldstein, S.A.: Functional tissue engineering: the role of biomechanics in articular cartilage repair. Clin. Orthop. Relat. Res. **391**, S295–S305 (2001)
10. Bistolfi, A., Ferracini, R., Galletta, C., Tosto, F., Sgarminato, V., Digo, E., Vernè, E., Massè, A.: Regeneration of articular cartilage: scaffold used in orthopedic surgery. A short handbook of available products for regenerative joints surgery. Clin. Sci. Res. Rep. **1**, 1–7 (2017)
11. Riddle, R.C., et al.: MAP kinase and calcium signaling mediate fluid flow-induced human mesenchymal stem cell proliferation. Am. J. Physiol. Cell Physiol. **290**, C776–C784 (2006)
12. Tada, H., et al.: Phosphate increases bone morphogenetic protein-2 expression through cAMP-dependent protein kinase and ERK1/2 pathways in human dental pulp cells. Bone **48**, 1409–1416 (2011)
13. Lin, K., Chang, J., Lu, J., Wu, W., Zeng, Y.: Properties of β-$Ca_3(PO_4)_2$ bioceramics prepared using nano-size powders. Ceram. Int. **33**(6), 979–985 (2007)
14. Palazzo, B., Iafisco, M., Laforgia, M., Margiotta, N., Natile, G., Bianchi, C.L., Walsh, D., Mann, S., Roveri, N.: Biomimetichydroxyapatite-drug nanocrystals as potential bonesubstitutes with antitumor drug delivery properties. Adv. Funct. Mater. **17**(13), 2180–2188 (2007)
15. Kruger, R., Groll, J.: Fiber reinforced calcium phosphate cements—on the way to degradable load bearing bone substitutes? Biomaterials **33**, 5887–5900 (2012)
16. Tatara, A.M., Mikos, A.G.: Tissue engineering in orthopaedics. J. Bone Joint Surg. Am. **98**, 1132–1139 (2016)
17. Al-Nbaheen, M., Vishnubalaji, R., Ali, D., Bouslimi, A., Al-Jassir, F., Megges, M., Prigione, A., Adjaye, J., Kassem, M., Aldahmash, A.: Human stromal (mesenchymal) stem cells from bone marrow, adipose tissue and skin exhibit differences in molecular phenotype and differentiation potential. Stem Cell Rev. **9**(1), 32–43 (2013)
18. Caplan, A.I., Correa, D.: The MSC: an injury drugstore. Cell Stem Cell **9**(1), 11–15 (2011)

Production Methods and Testing of Materials for Medical Applications

Multifunctional Bio-ceramic Scaffolds and Composites Fabricated by the Freeze Casting Techniques

Po-Yu Chen and Haw-Kai Chang

Abstract Freeze-casting is a solidification technique for fabricating scaffolds with tunable micro-scale porous structures. In this chapter, the processing principles, theories, and experimental parameters of freeze casting technique are introduced. Two selected natural bio-ceramics, namely silica-based diatomite and fish scale-extracted hydroxyapatite, are utilized as raw materials to fabricated scaffolds and composites. The intrinsic nano-porous features of diatomites are well preserved and integrated with the aligned micro-channels formed by ice dendrites during freezing. The hierarchical porous scaffolds exhibit ultra-lightweight, high porosity, superhydrophilicity and can be applied in the fields of filtration, water absorption and retention, oil–water separation, and thermal insulation. Fish scale-extracted hydroxyapatite scaffolds and composites are eco-friendly and cost-effective and can be heavy metal ion adsorption from wastewater and biomedical fields, such as bone grafting or dental materials. Future perspectives and applications of freeze casting technique are discussed.

Keywords Solidification · Freeze casting · Scaffolds · Composites · Silica · Hydroxyapatite

1 Freeze Casting

1.1 Introduction

The first observation on the freezing of solution and suspension can be dated back to 1908, when Lottermoser [1] observed the formation of materials with honeycomb structures under freezing. In 1954, Maxwell et al. [2] first used the term "freeze casting" to describe the process of forming refractory powders through casting, freezing, liquid sublimation, followed by sintering. It was not until the early 2000s when freeze casting technique received increasing attention and was utilized to fabricate

P.-Y. Chen (✉) · H.-K. Chang
National Tsing Hua University, Hsinchu 300044, Taiwan (R.O.C.)
e-mail: poyuchen@mx.nthu.edu.tw

S. Najman et al. (eds.), *Bioceramics, Biomimetic and Other Compatible Materials Features for Medical Applications*, Engineering Materials,
https://doi.org/10.1007/978-3-031-17269-4_9

ceramic materials with unidirectionally aligned porous structures. Freeze casting has become a popular research field owing to several advantages, such as relatively simple and low cost, wide material selectivity, scalability, eco-friendly, flexibility of processes and controllability of microstructures. The number of freeze-casting related journal papers published per year increased significantly from less than 10 in the early 2000s to over 150 in 2016. Deville et al. [3, 4] and Scotti and Dunand [5] have comprehensively collected and reviewed over 800 freeze-casting papers and summarized in an open data repository (freezecasting.net). The diversity of materials selection and corresponding applications of freeze-casting techniques also grew considerably, expanding from ceramics and polymers to metals, alloys, and their composites (ceramic/polymer, ceramic/metal, metal/polymer).

1.2 Processing Principles

A freeze casting system is shown in Fig. 1. The slurry or suspension of particles is poured into a mold surrounded by a thermally insulating Teflon wall and connected to a thermally conductive copper stick at the bottom, which is immersed in a liquid nitrogen bath. The PID controller connected with heating tape and thermocouple at the top of the copper stick is utilized to carefully control the cooling rate of the slurry.

Typical freeze casting process of ceramic materials consists of four steps: slurry preparation, solidification, sublimation, and sintering. Figure 2 shows the illustrations of the four processing steps along with the liquid–solid-gas phase diagram of water [4]. The ceramic particles are first uniformly dispersed in water and form slurry. During the solidification process, the solvent (water) starts to freeze from the cold

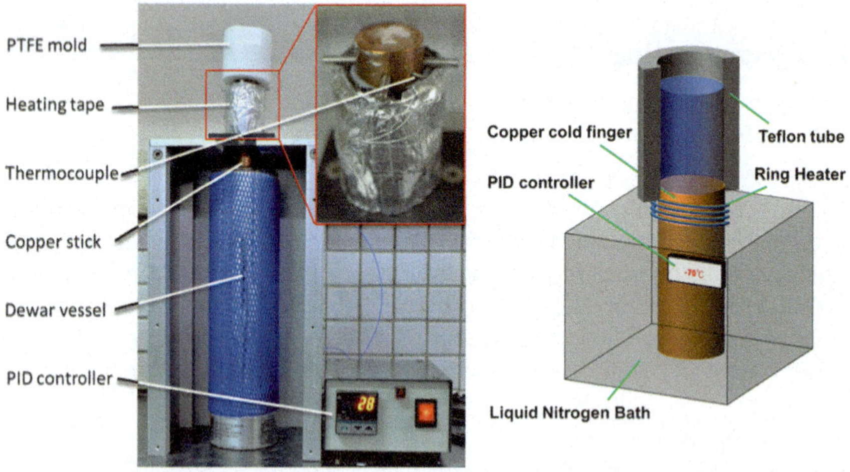

Fig. 1 The freeze-casting system and the main components: a Dewar vessel containing liquid nitrogen, a Teflon-covered mold, a copper stick, a thermal couple, a heating tape, and a PID controller

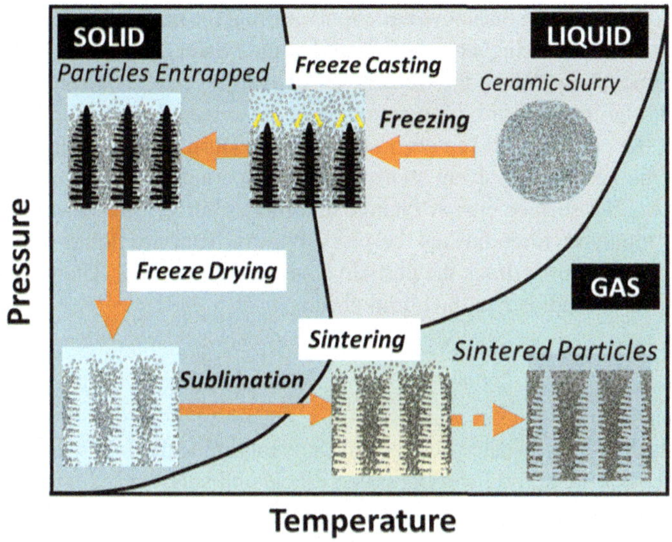

Fig. 2 Schematic illustrations shows the freeze casting, sublimation, and sintering and phase diagram of water [4]

end of the slurry and lamellar ice dendrites grow along the cooling direction. Under proper solidification conditions, the ceramic particles are repelled by ice dendrites and accumulated within space between adjacent ice dendrites, forming a ceramic-ice two phase lamellar structure. After solidification, the ice dendrites are removed by sublimation (or freeze drying process) under reduced pressure at low temperature, resulting in a green body where the vertically aligned porous structures are the direct replica of the ice crystals. Finally, the green body is sintered at high temperature to strengthen and consolidate the structure. Observable shrinkage may occur after sintering process.

1.3 Theories

The most critical step of the freeze casting process is the freezing step, where the particles are rejected by ice dendrites, forming directional lamellar microstructure. The theories and mechanisms related to the freezing step have been reviewed by Zhang et al. [6] and Wegst et al. [7]. Based on thermodynamic theory, the free energy of a particle in the slurry can be expressed as:

$$\Delta\sigma_0 = \sigma_{ps} - \left(\sigma_{pl} + \sigma_{sl}\right)$$

where σ_{ps}, σ_{pl} and σ_{sl} in the above equation represent the surface free energy between particle and solid (freezing ice), particle and liquid (water), and solid (ice) and liquid (water), respectively. When the free energy of system ($\Delta\sigma_0$) is lower than zero, the particle will be trapped and disappeared from the system [6]. On the other hand, if $\Delta\sigma_0 > 0$, the particle will remain in the solvent. During the freezing process, the particle remained in the solvent receives two competing forces: the repulsive force which resists the surface energy change and the attractive force owing by viscous drag. The repulsive force pushes the particle away from the liquid–solid interface and the attractive force drags the particle close to the interface. The repulsive force of a particle with radius r in the liquid phase is

$$F_R = 2\pi\,\Delta\sigma = 2\pi\,\Delta\sigma_0\left(\frac{a_0}{d}\right)^n$$

where a_0 is the mean distance between the solvent molecules in the liquid layer, d is the thickness of the liquid layer between particle and solid–liquid interface, and the exponent n is the correction factor of the repulsive force, typically range from 1 to 4. Assuming $n = 1$ (neglect the correction factor), the repulsive force becomes

$$F_R = 2\pi\,\Delta\sigma = 2\pi\,\Delta\sigma_0\frac{a_0}{d}$$

The attractive force from viscous drag derived by the Stoke's law can be described as:

$$F_\eta = \frac{6\pi\eta v r^2}{d}$$

This condition corresponds to a thin film of liquid solvent fills the gap between particle and solid–liquid interface. By balancing the two forces, the critical velocity of the freezing front can be derived as:

$$v_{cr} = \frac{\Delta\sigma_0 a_0}{3\eta r}$$

If the velocity exceeds this critical value ($v > v_{cr}$), the particle will be encapsulated by the solid phase and the liquid film between the particle and the freezing front will disappear. On the contrary, if $v < v_{cr}$, the particle will be rejected by the freezing front. Therefore, critical requirements for successful freeze casting process are proper solid loading (with particle–particle interactions) and freezing front velocity ($v < v_{cr}$).

1.4 Tunable Microstructures

The major advantage of freeze casting technique is the controllability of microstructures by tuning processing parameters. The processing-microstructure relationships of freeze casting have been comprehensively reviewed. [4, 5] Common experimental parameters for freeze castings are material selections (solutes, solvents, binders, dispersants), solid fraction, solidification parameters (solidification velocity, cooling rate, cooling techniques, undercooling) and applying extrinsic driving forces (gravity, electrical, magnetic fields, rotation). Ceramics have been widely utilized as raw materials for freeze casting compared to metals and polymers. Metals and alloys are denser than solvents and often encounter sediment problem and polymers may dissolve or interact with solvents. The porous structures in freeze-casted materials are intrinsically determined by the morphologies of the solidified solvents. Despite the water/ice system has been commonly applied, various solvents such as camphene, cyclohexane, dioxane, tert-butyl alcohol (TBA), which can generate different porous morphologies (isotropic, honeycomb, etc.).

The porosity of scaffolds is related to initial solid fraction, which can be expressed by the following linear relationship:

$$\emptyset_p = a \cdot \emptyset_s + b$$

where Φ_p is the porosity, Φ_s is the solid volume fraction in the suspension, a and b are the slope and intercept, respectively. There are upper and lower limits for solid volume fractions. If the solid volume fraction is too low, the suspension is too dilute to form scaffold with structural integrity and proper mechanical stability. If the solid volume fraction is too high, the suspension may be too viscous and the solidified solvent cannot repel the particles.

The solidification velocity plays a critical role in freeze casting. An empirical power law correlates solidification velocity and microstructural characteristic:

$$\lambda = C \cdot \upsilon^k$$

where λ is the structure wavelength defined as the average width of a pore plus the width of its adjacent solid wall, v is the solidification velocity (freeze front velocity), C and k are constants. The exponent k typically varies from -0.03 to -1.3. Therefore, the characteristic structure wavelength decreases with increasing solidification velocity. Practically, the cooling rate in the freeze casting system is the experimental factor that determines the microstructure of scaffolds. Higher the cooling rate, finer the solidified solvent (ice dendrite), and finer the pore size or inter-lamellae spacing, and vice versa. Freeze casting can be modified or integrated with various methods, such as sol–gel process, cross-linking, polymer infiltration, 3D printing, and templating techniques to fabricate scaffolds or composites with controllable and more complex structures.

2 Diatomite-Based Silica Scaffolds

2.1 Introduction

Diatomite, also known as diatomaceous earth, is the silica-based micro-sized fossils formed after the death of diatoms (Fig. 3). Diatoms are unicellular algae characterized by their rigid hydrated silicon dioxide ($SiO_2 \cdot nH_2O$) exoskeletons called "frustules". There are known to be over 100,000 species of diatoms with diverse morphologies and shapes which can be found abundantly in aqueous environments. The frustules of diatoms have unique, nano-porous structure and superior physical and chemical properties (diverse morphology and architecture, high porosity, high permeability, large surface area, low thermal conductivity, chemical inertness, super-hydrophilicity, biocompatibility and eco-friendly) which lead to a variety of applications, such as filter, abrasive, paint filler, pesticide carrier, insulating and water absorbing materials. Several techniques, such as shape-preserving chemical conversion, atomic layer deposition and sonochemistry can template the hierarchical porous structure with different materials and further lead to broader applications in catalysts, sensors, batteries, solar cells, MEMS/NEMS devices, microcapsules for controlled drug delivery, etc. In this section, we introduce diatomite-based silica scaffolds with hierarchically micro-/nano-porous structures fabricated by freeze casting and their properties, functionalities and applications [8].

2.2 Fabrication Methods

Food-grade diatomite powder (Fossil Shell Flour®, USA) was mixed with 1wt% of PVA (98–99% hydrolyzed, high molecular weight, Alfa Aesar, USA) and PEG (average molecular weight: 6000, Alfa Aesar, USA) binders, 3% sodium polyacrylate

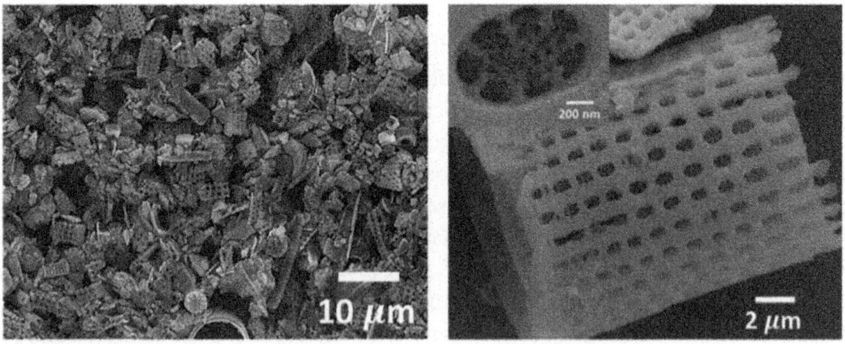

Fig. 3 SEM image of the raw diatomite powder and high magnification micrographs of an individual diatomite showing nano-sized porous feature

anionic dispersant (DARVAN® 811, Vanderbilt Minerals, USA), and water to form slurries of 15 wt%, 20 wt%, 25wt% diatomite solid contents. The slurries were placed in the PTFE mold in the above-mentioned freeze casting system and frozen from 10 °C to −140 °C with adjustable cooling rates (2, 5, 10, and 15 °C/min). After the freeze casting process, the frozen slurries were then placed into the freeze dryer (FD4.5/-80, Firstek, Taiwan) at low temperature (< −80 °C) under reduced pressure (50 mTorr) for 48 h to sublimate the ice while maintain the porous channels of the green bodies, which were further sintered at 1050 °C or 1100 °C for 4 h in a box furnace (Lindberg/Blue M™, Thermal Product Solutions, USA).

2.3 Structural Characterization

Figure 4 shows the macroscopic appearance of the as-synthesized diatomite scaffolds along with a series of SEM images revealing three distinctive zones, namely dense, cellular, and lamellar zones, from the bottom toward the top of the scaffolds. The diatomite particles in the initial dense and cellular zones are randomly and isotropically oriented while those in the major lamellar zones are parallelly aligned. In the lamellar zone, diatomite lamellae gradually transform from tilted orientation to aligned orientation along the growth direction of ice dendrites (the cooling direction).

Figure 5 are SEM micrographs at higher magnification of diatomite scaffolds freeze-casted with cooling rates of (a) 2 °C/min, (b) 5 °C/min, (c) 10 °C/min, and (d) 15 °C/min, respectively. The nano-sized pores in the diatomite are well preserved after sintering and the diatomite particles are aligned along the cooling direction. The cannel widths and lamellae thicknesses decrease with increasing cooling rates, as shown in Fig. 5. The average channel widths decrease from 29.26 ± 3.00 μm, 19.88 ± 1.56 μm, 15.78 ± 2.43 μm, to 12.12 ± 1.25 μm as the cooling rates increase from 2 °C/min, 5 °C/min, 10 °C/min, to 15 °C/min, respectively. The average lamellae thicknesses show the similar trend, decreasing from 11.79 ± 2.84 μm, 6.32 ± 1.63 μm, 3.38 ± 0.46 μm, to 3.06 ± 0.62 μm with increasing cooling rates. The diatomite scaffolds possess micro-sized channels and nano-sized pores and the hierarchically porous features lead to superior properties and functionalities, such as high porosity, ultra-lightweight, water absorption/retention, thermal insulating, and effective oil/water separation capabilities.

2.4 Mechanical Properties

Mechanical properties of diatomite scaffolds with 30 vol% solid loading were measured under compression by a universal testing system (Instron 3343, Instron, USA) equipped with a 1 kN load cell at a strain rate of 10^{-3} s^{-1}. Representative compressive stress–strain curves of diatomite scaffolds freeze-casted at cooling rates of 2 °C/min, 5 °C/min, and 10 °C/min are shown in Fig. 6. The porosity values of

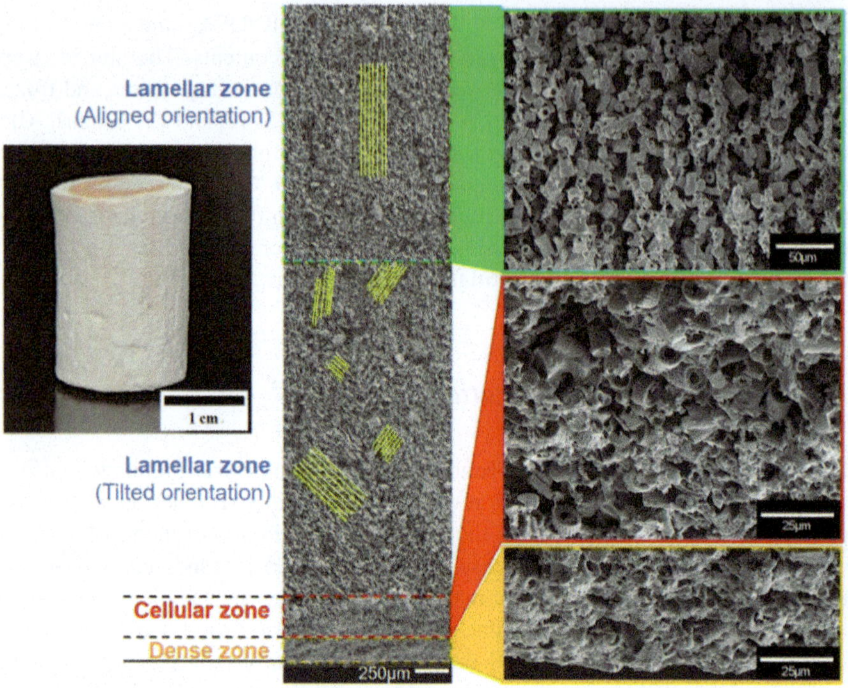

Fig. 4 Photograph of the as-synthesized diatomite scaffold and SEM images showing three distinctive regions: dense, cellular and lamellar zones

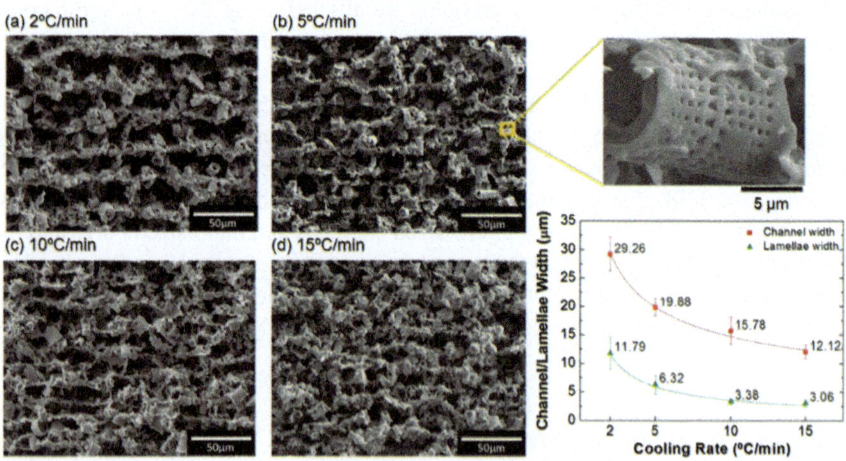

Fig. 5 SEM micrographs of the diatomite scaffolds synthesized with cooling rates of **a** 2 °C/min, **b** 5 °C/min, **c** 10 °C/min, and **d** 15 °C/min. Channel and lamellae widths decrease with increasing cooling rates [8]

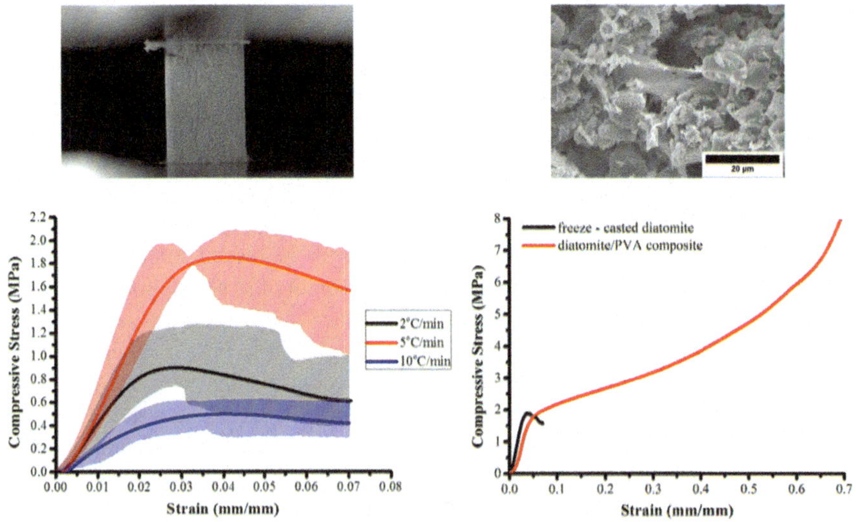

Fig. 6 Representative stress–strain curves of diatomite scaffolds synthesized at different cooling rates and diatomite/PVA composite scaffold

2 °C/min, 5 °C/min, and 10 °C/min scaffolds are 87.74 ± 0.36%, 83.45 ± 0.32%, and 83.96 ± 0.44%, respectively, and the average compressive strengths are 0.96 ± 0.22 MPa, 1.99 ± 0.09 MPa, and 0.53 ± 0.08 MPa, correspondingly. The hierarchically porous structured diatomite scaffolds can maintain structural integrity under proper compressive loads. Results indicate that 5 °C/min scaffolds exhibit superior compressive strength than the other two groups and the specific compressive strengths reach ~5.2×10^{-3} MPa/kg·m^{-3}.

The compressive mechanical properties of the diatomite scaffolds can be further improved by introducing various types of organic polymers, such as polyvinyl acetate (PVA), polydimethylsiloxane (PDMS), alginate, chitosan, silica aerogel, etc. Typically, freeze-casted diatomite scaffolds are immersed in the polymeric solution at elevated temperature which enables proper cross-linking or gel formation. For example, the compressive strength and elastic modulus of diatomite scaffold infiltrated with 5 wt% PVA can reach 2.4 MPa and 78 MPa, respectively. More importantly, the PVA-infiltrated diatomite scaffolds exhibit plastic deformation and ductile behavior compared to relatively brittle diatomite scaffolds. The compressive stress–strain curve of diatomite/PVA composite scaffolds shows linear elasticity, plastic plateau, and final densification which are representative for cellular solids with plastic buckling behavior. The inset SEM image shows that the PVA forms ductile, stretchable membrane which reinforces the diatomite-based lamellae. The micro-scale channels formed from ice dendrites during freeze casting and nano-scale pores on the diatomites are still remained after PVA infiltration. By adopting this approach, various ceramic/polymer composite scaffolds can be fabricated to enhance mechanical properties and fulfill different functionalities.

2.5 Water Absorption and Retention

The water absorption and water retention capabilities of hierarchically porous diatomite scaffolds were evaluated and compared to silica scaffolds made of solid SiO_2 powders. Diatomite and silica scaffolds were placed in a closed system with controlled 90% relative humidity at 23 °C. The water absorption was determined by the ratio of increased weight due to water absorption divided by the original weight of scaffold and the water retention was obtained from the instantaneous weight after varying durations up to 8 h divided by the initial weight of scaffolds soaked in water for 24 h.

The water absorption and retention results are shown in Fig. 7. After one hour, diatomite and silica scaffolds started to obviously uptake water with the absorption rates of 72 wt%/hr and 29 wt%/hr, respectively. After 4 to 4.5 h, the water absorption of silica scaffolds saturated at ~75 wt%. The water absorption of diatomite scaffolds can further increase up to ~280 wt% and saturate after 5.5 h. The water absorption performance of diatomite scaffolds is much better than commonly used commercial ceramic materials, such as porcelain tiles (≤0.5), ceramic tiles (10–60), and ceramic coasters (~16). The superior water absorption capability of diatomite scaffolds may result from the hierarchical micro/nano-porous structures and high specific surface area. The water retention capability is presented in term of the time required for half of the initially absorbed water evaporated ($t_{1/2}$). As shown in Fig. 7, water evaporated more rapidly from silica scaffolds than diatomite scaffolds. The half-time ($t_{1/2}$) for diatomite scaffolds was ~6 h and that of silica scaffolds was ~4 h. The diatomite scaffolds possess superior water retention capability. The water absorption and water retention capabilities of diatomite scaffolds can be further improved by introducing hydrophilic alginate and fabricating diatomite/alginate composite scaffolds. The water absorption of diatomite/alginate composite scaffolds can reach ~375 wt% with much better water retention capability. The half-time for diatomite/alginate composite scaffolds can last for ~24 h.

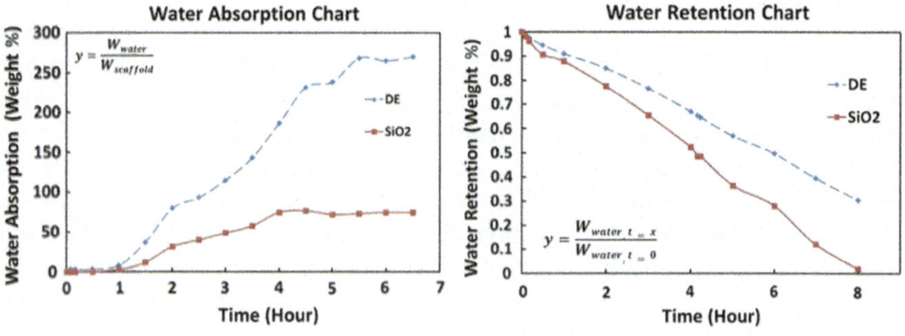

Fig. 7 Water absorption and water retention (wt%) of silica (SiO_2) and diatomaceous earth (D.E.) scaffolds are plotted versus time duration (hour)

2.6 Thermal Properties

Thermal conductivities of scaffolds were measured along the axial (freezing direction) and the radial (across adjacent lamellae) directions. Figure 8 shows the thermal conductivity of diatomite scaffold, diatomite/PVA scaffold, diatomite/alginate scaffold, and alginate scaffold compared to that of selected thermal insulation materials. The thermal conductivity (0.32 W/mK) of freeze-casted diatomite scaffolds along the axial direction is considerably higher than that along the radial direction (0.11 W/mK). The strong orientation dependence is the consequence of the anisotropic lamellar microstructure of freeze-casted scaffolds. The thermal insulation performance can be further improved by incorporating various polymers with diatomites and forming diatomite/PVA and diatomite/alginate composite scaffolds. The thermal conductivity value of freeze-casted diatomite/PVA composite scaffolds in the radial direction (~0.05 W/mK) are lower than conventional thermal insulation materials, such as polytetrafluoroethylene (PTFE) (0.25 W/mK), light weight concrete (0.1–0.3 W/mK), and insulating brick (0.15 W/mK) and comparable to commercial insulation materials, such as expanded polystyrene (0.03 W/mK), polyurethane (0.02–0.03 W/mK), and fibreglass (0.033–0.044 W/mK). Additionally, diatomite-based composite scaffolds synthesized by freeze casting possess competitive advantages, including good mechanical properties, low cost and eco-friendly, fireproof and flame retardancy which can be potentially applied as thermal insulating or building materials.

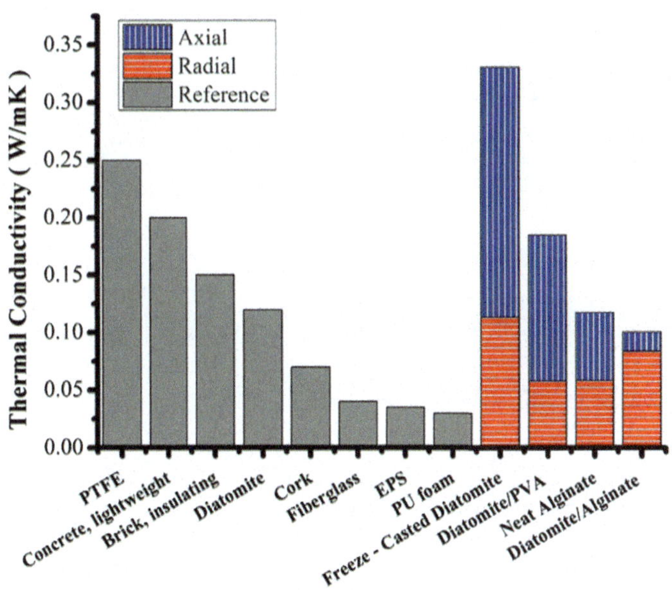

Fig. 8 Thermal conductivity values of freeze-casted diatomite scaffolds and diatomite/polymer composites along axial and radial directions compared with commercial insulation materials

2.7 Oil–Water Separation

The intrinsically hydrophilic diatomite scaffolds with anisotropically aligned micro-channels and nano-porous features can be applied to filtrate oily-contaminated water. Lo et al. [8] The diatomite scaffolds were sectioned into 2 mm thin plates. Contact angle measurements reveal that the freeze-casted diatomite plates exhibit superhydrophilicity and superoleophilicity in air with contact angles ~0° (Fig. 9). Water and soybean oil droplets penetrate into porous diatomite plates within 14 ms. Remarkably, the diatomite plates exhibit superoleophobicity underwater. The underwater contact angles of soybean oil, hexane, hexadecane, dodecane are 169.42°, 167.08°, 166.95° and 168.3°, respectively (Fig. 9). The oil–water separation process is schematically illustrated in Fig. 10. The hierarchically porous diatomite plates trap water in the micro-channels and nano-pores, forming a stable oil/water interface and repelling oil or other organic solvents. The underwater superoleophobicity of diatomite plates leads to high separation efficiency, reaching 99.7%, for free oil/water mixtures driven merely by gravity. The water permeance of diatomite plates freeze-casted at 5 °C/min reaches 6.9×10^5 Lm^{-2} h^{-1} bar^{-1}, which is one or two order higher than those synthesized by conventional techniques. The intrusion pressure can reach >7.2 kPa of soybean oil due to the stable oil/water interface. High intrusion pressure and high water permeance make diatomite plates capable of treating large amount of oily waste water rapidly, enabling large scale separation. Moreover, diatomite plates can be used for over 30 cycles under difference environmental conditions (1 M HCl solution, sea water, brine) with good mechanical, thermal and chemical stability. The eco-friendly, hierarchically porous diatomite plates fabricated by the facile, non-expensive freeze casting technique can be applied for effective oil/water separation under real environmental conditions at large scale.

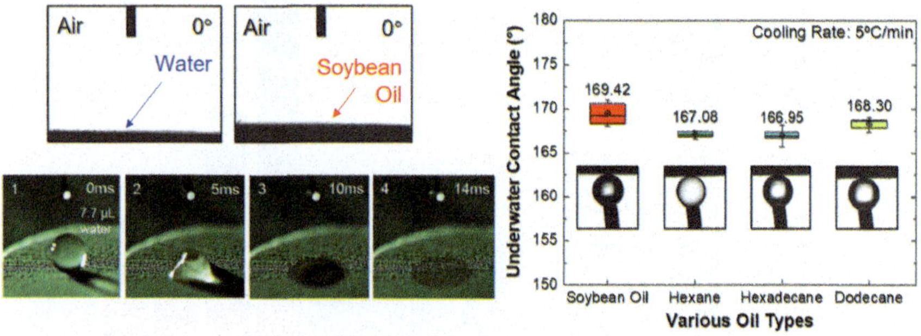

Fig. 9 Contact angle measurements of diatomite plates show superhydrophilicity and superoleophilicity in air and superoleophobicity against various oils underwater [8]

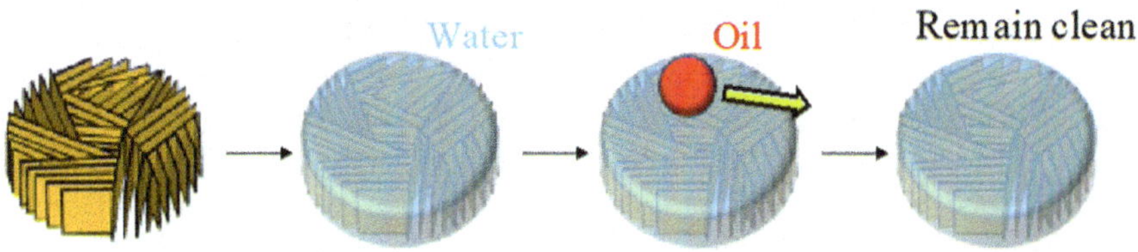

Fig. 10 Schematic illustrations show the oil–water separation process of freeze-casted diatomite plates

3 Fish Scale-Derived Hydroxyapatite Scaffolds

3.1 Introduction

Hydroxyapatite ($Ca_{10}(PO_4)_6(OH)_2$) is the major mineral constituents in bones, teeth, osteoderms, antlers, fish scales, and other mineralized tissues. The hydroxyapatite crystals in natural materials are non-stoichiometric with 4–6% of the phosphate replaced by carbonate groups and typically in the form of platelets, 40–60 nm in length, 20–30 nm in width, and 1.5–4 nm in thickness. Hydroxyapatite is considered as one of the important bio-ceramics and has been widely applied in biomedical fields, such as bone grafting, dental materials, tissue engineering, and coatings on implants. Hydroxyapatite (HA) has also been verified to have excellent heavy ion adsorption ability and can be used to remove heavy metal ions from industrial wastewater. The source of hydroxyapatite can be synthesized by artificial processes or obtained from natural mineralized materials. Artificial production of HA can achieve powders with well controlled sizes and quality yet is more expensive and time-consuming. We utilize fish scales which are considered as fishery waste as the raw materials and extract eco-friendly, low cost HA powder. Fish scale-derived hydroxyapatite scaffolds and hydroxyapatite/chitosan composite scaffolds were fabricated by freeze casting technique and applied in heavy metal ion removal [9, 10] and potentially biomedical fields [7, 11, 12].

3.2 Fabrication Methods

Figure 11 shows the experimental flow chart. Tilapia fish (*Oreochromis mossambicus*) scales were provided by the Kouhu Fisheries (Yunlin, Taiwan). The processing of natural resourced hydroxyapatite from fish scales followed the procedure reported by Mondal et al. [13]. Raw fish scales were ground, ball-milled, deproteinized, washed and finally calcinated in an open-air box furnace (Lindberg/Blue M™ BF51314C, Thermal Product Solutions, America) at 1000 °C for 2 h. Hydroxyapatite-based slurries with various solid loadings (10, 15, 20, 25, 30, 40 vol%) were mixed with DI water, PVA, PEG and dispersant and poured into PTFE mold in the freeze casting system. Different cooling rates (0.5, 1, 2, 5, 8, 10 °C/min) were applied to fabricate scaffolds with varying microstructures. After freeze casting, freeze drying was conducted at low pressure (200mTorr) and temperature (−80 °C) in a freeze dryer (Fisrtek FD4.5/−80, Taiwan) for 48 h to completely sublimate ice dendrites. The green bodies were then sintered at 1300 °C for 2 h in the box furnace to fabricate hydroxyapatite-based scaffolds.

Hydroxyapatie(HA)/chitosan(CS) composite scaffolds were fabricated without sintering process. Fish scale-derived hydroxyapatite powder was mixed with 2 wt% chitosan solution obtained from dissolving commercial 75–85% deacetylated chitosan powder (Sigma-Aldrich, Saint Louis, USA) in 1 wt% acetic acid. The HA/CS slurry was frozen at frozen at 2 °C/min and 5 °C/min cooling rates and sublimated in the freeze dryer following the same procedure. The sublimated HA/CS scaffolds were cross-linked by 1 wt% glutaraldehyde solution for 2 h and rinsed with DI water to preventing constriction. Afterwards, samples were dried at 60 °C for 12 h to remove remaining water content. Finally, freeze-casted and cross-linked HA/CS composites scaffolds were synthesized.

3.3 Structural Characterization

Photographs of tilapia fish, fish scales, calcined HA powder and freeze-casted HA scaffold are shown in Fig. 11. The X-ray diffraction patterns of raw fish scale powder, powder calcinated at 1000 °C, and powder sintered at 1300 °C indicate the intensity

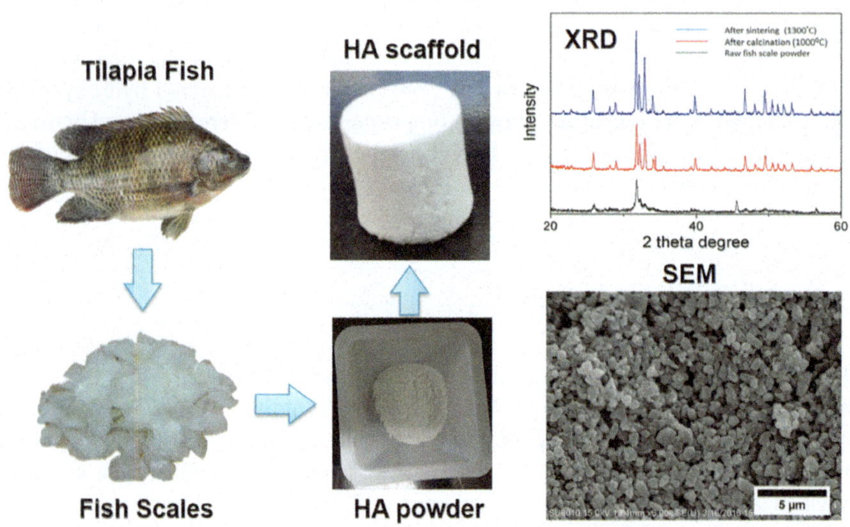

Fig. 11 Photographs of tilapia fish, fish scales, hydroxyapatite powder and freeze-casted scaffold. X-ray diffraction patterns and SEM of HA particles

and crystallinity are enhanced with increasing heat treatment temperatures. After cleaning, calcination and sintering, the characteristic peaks of XRD patterns can be well identified as standard hydroxyapatite (JCPD, 9-432). Fish scale-extracted HA particles after ball milling and calcination were observed under SEM and the particle size ranged from 500 nm to 1.5 μm.

Figure 12 are a series of SEM images of HA scaffolds freeze-casted at various cooling rates, (a) 0.5 °C/min (b) 1 °C/min (c) 2 °C/min (d) 5 °C/min (e) 8 °C/min (f) 10 °C/min, at the same magnification. The aligned lamellae and channels of HA scaffolds can be observed. The channel width or distance between adjacent lamellae

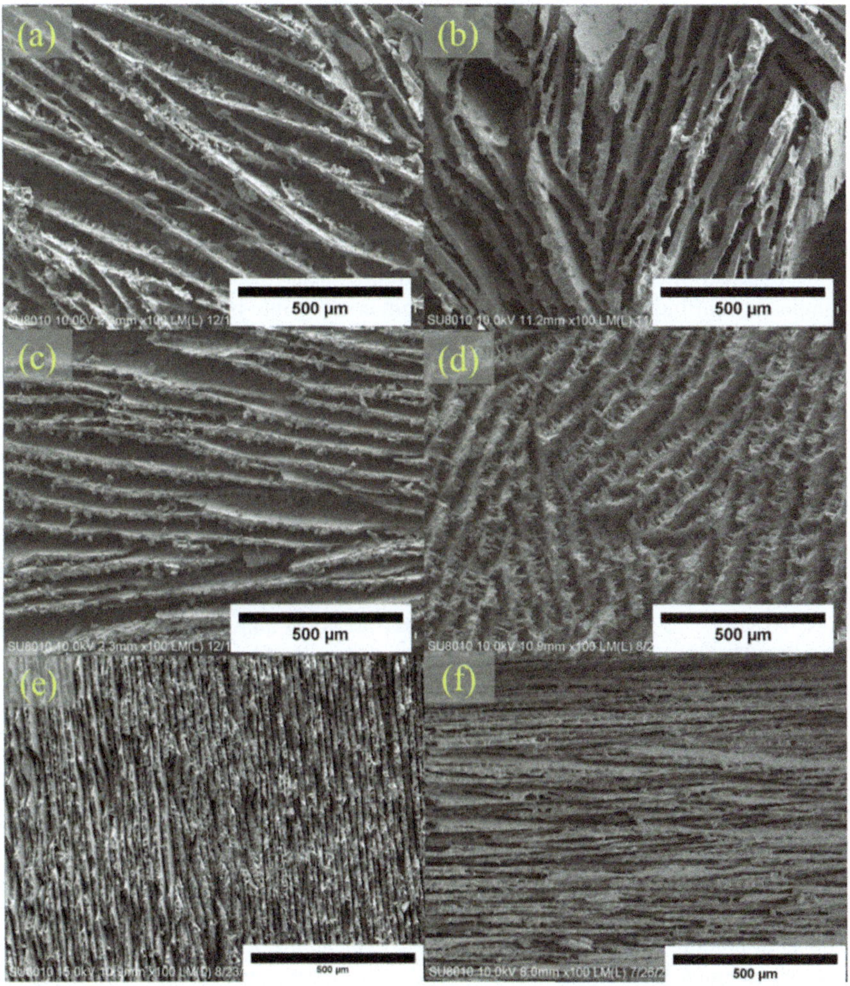

Fig. 12 SEM images of lamellar microstructure of HA scaffolds synthesized at varying cooling rates: **a** 0.5 °C/min, **b** 1 °C/min, **c** 2 °C/min, **d** 5 °C/min, **e** 8 °C/min, **f** 10 °C/min

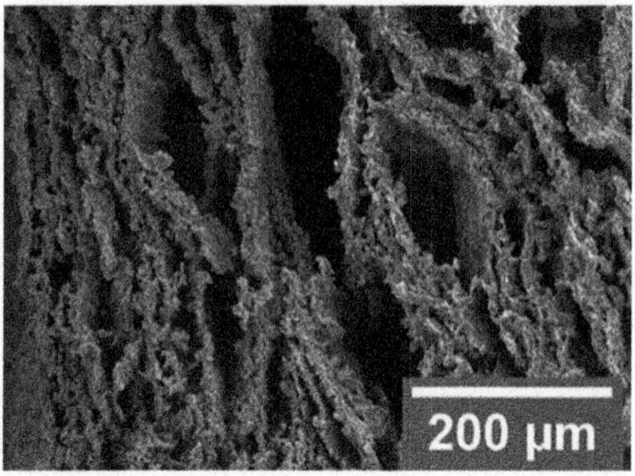

Fig. 13 SEM image of HA/CS composite scaffold freeze-casted at 2 °C/min cooling rate [10]

decreased with increasing cooling rate, from 66.3 ± 14.8 μm, 49.6 ± 21.5 μm, 29 ± 4.5 μm, 15.7 ± 2 μm, 9.1 ± 0.9 μm, to 8.3 ± 0.9 μm, as cooling rate increased from 0.5 °C/min to 10 °C/min. The influence of cooling rate on microstructural features of scaffolds is in agreement with other freeze casting studies and can be applied to design scaffolds with controllable micro-channels. SEM image of the HA/CS composite scaffold freeze-casted at 2 °C/min cooling rate is shown in Fig. 13. The channel widths are non-uniform which may due to different degree of crosslinking.

3.4 Mechanical Properties

The mechanical performance of freeze-casted HA scaffolds with different solid loadings was evaluated by quasi-static compression tests. Representative compressive stress–strain cures of scaffolds freeze-casted at 5 °C/min with varying solid loadings, 10 vol%, 15 vol%, 20 vol%, 25 vol%, 30 vol% and 40 vol%, are shown in Fig. 14a. The average compressive strengths of 10 vol%,15 vol%, 20 vol%, 25 vol%, 30 vol% and 40 vol% samples are 0.5 MPa, 1.3 MPa, 4.3 MPa, 8.8 MPa, 10.5 MPa, 23 MPa, respectively. The average elastic moduli are 45.1 MPa, 51 MPa, 149.1 MPa, 199.3 MPa, 263.4 MPa and 269.4 MPa, correspondingly. The mechanical properties of scaffolds of low solid loadings (10 vol% and 15 vol%) are quite poor due to their high porosity. Scaffolds with solid loadings higher than 20 vol% have proper structural integrity and mechanical stability. The effect of cooling rates on mechanical properties was also investigated. Figure 14b shows representative compressive stress–strain curves of HA scaffolds freeze-casted at 2 °C/min and 10 °C/min cooling. The solid loading of scaffolds was kept as 20 vol.%. For 2 °C/min cooling rate, the average compressive strength is 2.0 ± 0.7 MPa and the average elastic modulus is 84.7 ± 26. MPa, while for 10 °C/min cooling rate, the average compressive strength is 4.3 ± 1.1 MPa and the average elastic modulus is 149.1 ± 37.6 MPa. Both compressive strength and elastic modulus of HA scaffolds synthesized with high cooling rate are

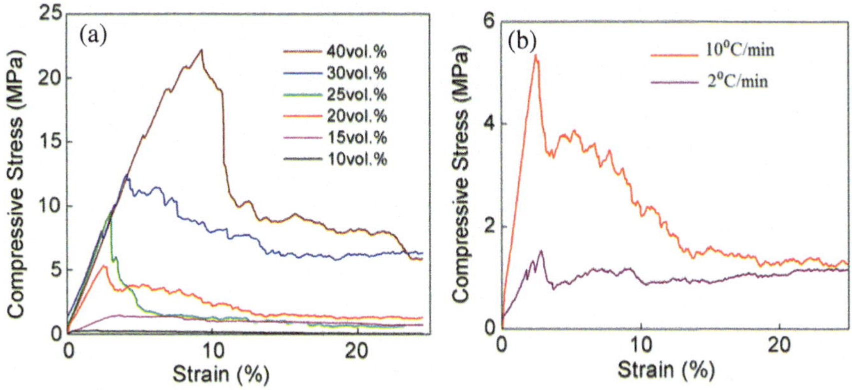

Fig. 14 Representative compressive stress–strain cures of scaffolds made of different amounts of solid loadings and cooling rates

higher than those fabricated with low cooling rate. The results indicate that scaffolds synthesized at lower cooling rates tend to possess poorer mechanical properties due to relatively larger channel space between adjacent lamellae.

3.5 *Adsorption Properties*

The heavy metal ion adsorption capability and mechanisms of HA/CS composite scaffolds were evaluated by batch method and fixed-bed process with different Pb ion initial concentrations (100 and 1000 mg/L) at pH = 2. [10] Typical adsorption mechanisms of hydroxyapatite include ion exchange, surface complexation, precipitation and co-precipitation of heavy metal ion phases. Two types of HA/CS composite scaffolds (2 °C/min and 5 °C/min cooling rates) are fabricated and utilized for adsorption tests. Figure 15 are SEM images of precipitation on the surface of scaffolds after different durations during batch process. The original surface of HA/CS scaffolds is shown in Fig. 15a. After few minutes, small precipitate in the early stage was formed (Fig. 15b). Hexagonal rods hundreds of nanometers in length was developed (Fig. 15c) and further grew to large rods ~20 μm (Fig. 15d). The precipitate was confirmed to be pyromorphite ($(Pb_{10}(PO_4)_6(OH)_2)$), also known as Pb-HA, by XRD analysis. For HA/CS composite scaffolds, the ion exchange mechanism may dominate at early stage and both ion exchanging and precipitation contribute heavy metal ion adsorption at the final stage. The adsorption kinetic of HA/CS composite scaffolds could be fitted by the pseudo second-order model. In the batch process, the maximum adsorption amount of HA/CS scaffold reached 570 mg/g after 15 days for initial Pb ion concentration of 1000 mg/L. In the fixed-bed process, the adsorption amount was 94 mg/g for initial Pb ion concentration of 100 mg/L. Scaffolds with wider channels (2 °C/min cooling rate) possessed higher flow rate, suitable for

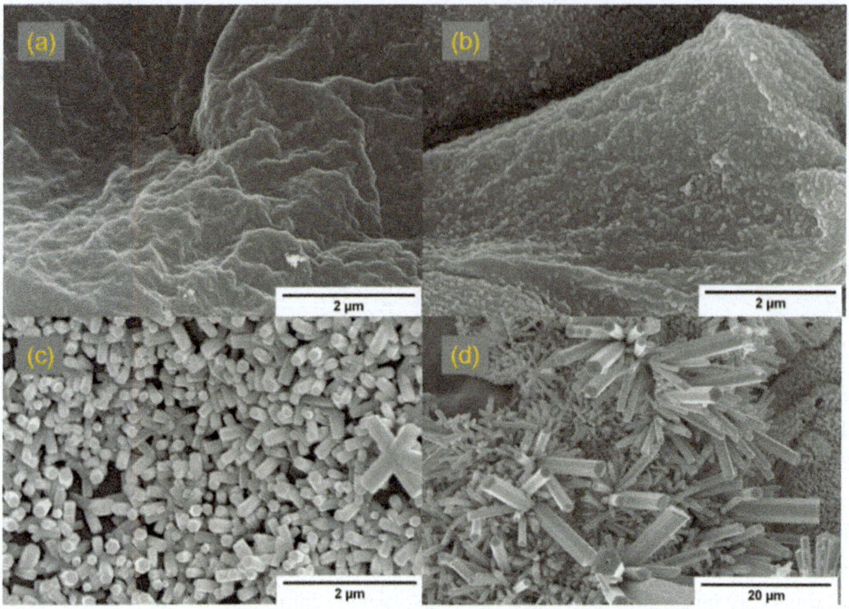

Fig. 15 SEM images show the growth of precipitation at different stages: **a** the original HA/CS scaffold surface, **b** few minutes, **c** few hours **d** few days after absorption [10]

fixed-bed process for wastewater with low metal ion concentration while those with smaller channels (5 °C/min cooling rate) exhibited high removal ability and stability for wastewater with high metal ion concentration. In summary, fish scaled-extracted HA/CS composite scaffolds with tunable, interconnected channels can be designed to adapt varying conditions and potentially applied to industrious wastewater treatment.

3.6 *Biomaterials*

Hydroxyapatite is a natural bio-ceramic commonly found in mineralized tissues and is expected to be non-toxic, biocompatible and osteoconductive. The cytotoxicity of fish scale-derived HA scaffolds was evaluated by the MTS cytotoxicity assay. The results of MTS assay are shown in Fig. 16. The optical density can be considered as the reference corresponding to the viability of osteoblast cells. The HA scaffolds synthesized with 10 °C/min and 2 °C/min cooling rates were investigated. The optical density of control group which cell culturing in a well without scaffold is 0.85 ± 0.16 after 10 days. Both 10 °C/min and 2 °C/min scaffolds showed comparable and slightly higher optical densities than the control group yet the enhancement was not significant.

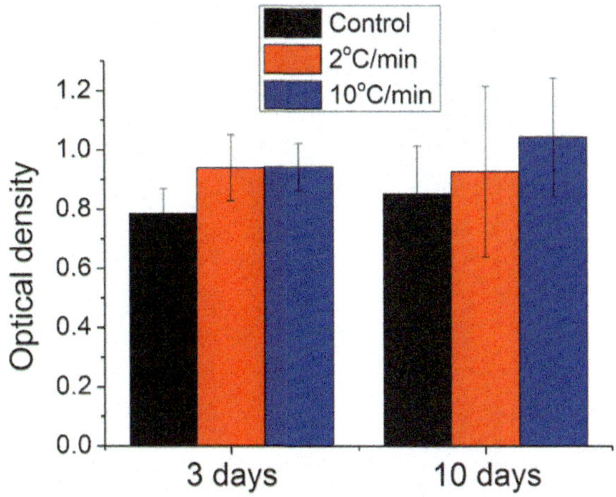

Fig. 16 MTS cytotoxicity results of osteoblast cells cultured on fish scale-derived HA scaffolds fabricated at 10 °C/min and 2 °C/min cooling rates compared to control group

Figure 17a shows the morphology of HA scaffold before cell culturing, and Fig. 17b is the HA scaffold after 10 days of cell culture. It can be observed that most of pores on the scaffold were covered by the extracellular matrix (ECM). At high magnifications (Fig. 17c–d), micro-channels and porous structures in HA scaffolds were covered by the ECM.

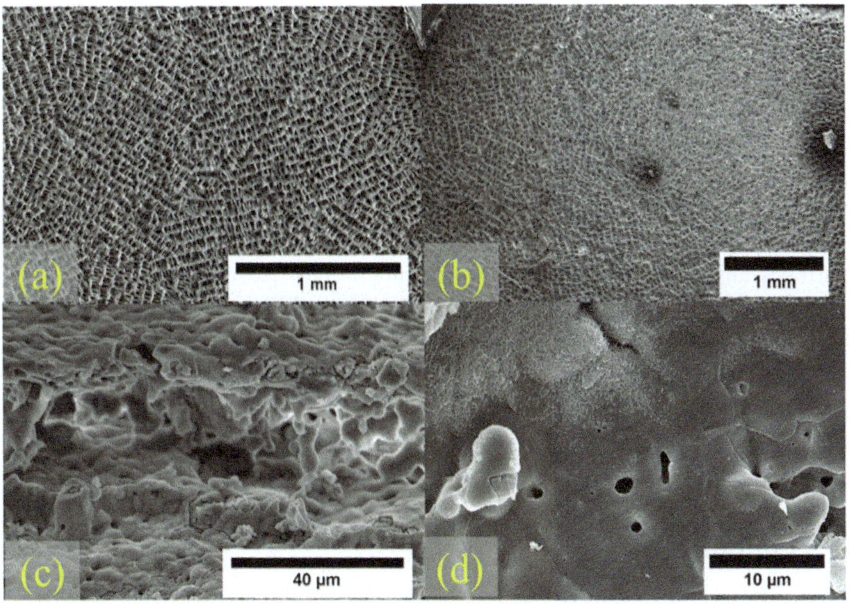

Fig. 17 SEM images of **a** HA scaffold prior to cell culturing, **b** HA scaffold after cell culturing, **c** high magnification observation of channels in scaffold after cell culturing, **d** HA scaffold surface covered by the ECM

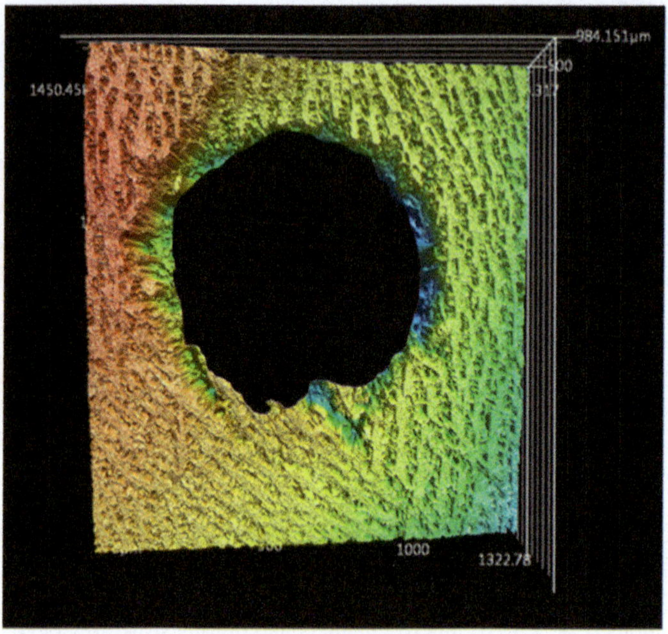

Fig. 18 Laser confocal microscopy image shows the 3D-printing template macro-pore and micro-sized lamellae and channels produced by freeze casting

Jung and McKittrick et al. [12] fabricated hierarchical macro-microporous hydroxyapatite scaffolds by integrating 3D printing templating and freeze casting techniques, mimicking the hierarchical porous structures in natural bones. Polymer-based 3D printed templates with cylindrical diameters of 600, 700, 800 μm were placed in the mold followed by freeze casting of HA slurry. The templates were burnt during the sintering process, resulting sub-millimeter pores and micro-sized channels (Fig. 18). The MG63 cells on macro–micro porous HA scaffolds showed narrowly aligned shapes, whereas those on nonporous HA samples exhibited polygonal shapes with no discernible orientation. Micro-CT analysis indicted that the cells were well distributed in the interior pore spaces via the 3D interpenetrating macro–micro porous networks. The hierarchical macro-microporous HA scaffolds exhibit good biocompatibility and osteo-conductivity and are suitable for biomedical applications.

4 Summary

In this chapter, the solidification-based freeze casting technique is introduced. Scaffolds and composites with controllable microstructures can be fabricated by tuning the experimental parameters (e.g. solid fraction, cooling rate, sintering temperature, post treatments). Two types of natural ceramic sources, diatomites and fish scale-extracted hydroxyapatite, were utilized to fabricate scaffolds and composites. Hierarchically micro-/nano-porous diatomite-based scaffolds are ultra-lightweight and possess superior water absorption/retention, thermal insulating, superhydrophilicity, and oil–water separation efficiency. Fish scale-extracted HA scaffolds and HA/chitosan composite scaffolds have demonstrated good heavy metal ion removal capability. Biocompatible, osteoconductive HA scaffolds are suitable to be applied as biomaterials. The microstructures, mechanical properties and functionalities of scaffolds and composites can be optimized by freeze casting and post treatment processes. The facile, cost-effective, eco-friendly, flexible and scalable freeze casting technique demonstrates capability to manufacture novel porous materials and composites and shows great potential in academic research and industrial applications.

References

1. Lottermoser, A.: Über das Ausfrieren von Hydrosolen. Ber. Dtsch. Chem. Ges. **41**(3), 3976–3979 (1908)
2. Maxwell, W., Gurnick, R., Francisco, A.: Preliminary Investigation of the 'Freeze-Casting' Method for Forming Refractory Powders. NACA Research Memorandum, Lewis Flight Propulsion Laboratory (1954)
3. Deville, S., Meille, S., Seuba, J.: A meta-analysis of the mechanical properties of ice-templated ceramics and metals. Sci. Technol. Adv. Mater. (2016)
4. Deville, S.: Freeze-casting of porous ceramics: a review of current achievements and issues. Adv. Eng. Mater. **10**(3), 155–169 (2008)
5. Scotti, K.L., Dunand, D.C.: Freeze casting—a review of processing, microstructure and properties via the open data repository, FreezeCasting.net. Progr. Mater. Sci. **94**, 243–305 (2018)
6. Zhang, H., Hussain, I., Brust, M., Butler, M.F., Rannard, S.P., Cooper, A.I.: Aligned two- and three-dimensional structures by directional freezing of polymers and nanoparticles. Nat. Mater. **4**(10), 787–793 (2005)
7. Wegst, U.G., Schecter, M., Donius, A.E., Hunger, P.M.: Biomaterials by freeze casting. Philos. Trans. A Math. Phys. Eng. Sci. **368**(1917), 2099–2121 (2010)
8. Lo, Y.H., Yang, C.Y., Chang, H.K., Hung, W.C., Chen, P.Y.: Bioinspired diatomite membrane with selective superwettability for oil/water separation. Sci. Rep. **7**(1), 1426 (2017)
9. Liu, W.-K., Liaw, B.-S., Chang, H.-K., Wang, Y.-F., Chen, P.-Y.: From waste to health: synthesis of hydroxyapatite scaffolds from fish scales for lead ion removal. JOM **69**(4), 713–718 (2017). https://doi.org/10.1007/s11837-017-2270-5
10. Liaw, B.S., Chang, T.T., Chang, H.K., Liu, W.K., Chen, P.Y.: Fish scale-extracted hydroxyapatite/chitosan composite scaffolds fabricated by freeze casting—an innovative strategy for water treatment. J. Hazard Mater. **382**, 121082 (2020). https://doi.org/10.1016/j.jhazmat.2019.121082
11. Deville, S., Saiz, E., Tomsia, A.P.: Freeze casting of hydroxyapatite scaffolds for bone tissue engineering. Biomaterials **27**(32), 5480–5489 (2006)
12. Jung, J.-Y., et al.: 3D printed templating of extrinsic freeze-casting for macro-microporous biomaterials. ACS Biomater. Sci. Eng. **5**(5), 2122–2133 (2019). https://doi.org/10.1021/acsbiomaterials.8b01308
13. Mondal, S., Mahata, S., Kundu, S., Mondal, B.: Processing of natural resourced hydroxyapatite ceramics from fish scale. Adv. Appl. Ceram. **109**, 234–239 (2010)

Preparation and Analysis Methods of Bone Ceramic Substitutes

Said Alkildani, Ole Jung, and Mike Barbeck

Abstract Human bone has an incredible capacity to heal itself, however, in cases of extreme damage, the tissue is unable to do so. Therefore, bone grafts are used to enhance the physiological regeneration. The current gold standard is an autograft but due to the subsequent donor site morbidity and their limited availability, alternative types of grafts are being applied. Aside to allografts and xenografts, alloplastic grafts (synthetic grafts) have been developed and are still under investigation for their potential in the field of bone regeneration for both load-bearing and non-load-bearing defect sites. This chapter covers the most common fabrication techniques for ceramic bone substitute materials in consideration of certain material properties that are matching with the process of bone regeneration. In this context, a focus in the further development of ceramic bone substitutes is to create biomimicking materials. Therefore, characterization is an essential step in the development of a novel bone substitute. This chapter also sheds a light on structural, physical, and chemical characterization methods.

Keyword Bone substitutes · Bone grafts · Bioceramics · Bioactive glass · Injectable bone substitutes · Fabrication · Processing · Imaging techniques · Mechanical characterization · Arheological characterization

S. Alkildani · M. Barbeck (✉)
BerlinAnalytix GmbH, Ullsteinstrasse 108, 12109 Berlin, Germany
e-mail: mike.barbeck@icloud.com

O. Jung · M. Barbeck
Clinic and Policlinic for Dermatology and Venereology, Rostock University Medical Center, 18057 Rostock, Germany

S. Najman et al. (eds.), *Bioceramics, Biomimetic and Other Compatible Materials Features for Medical Applications*, Engineering Materials,
https://doi.org/10.1007/978-3-031-17269-4_10

1 Introduction

1.1 Fundamentals of Bone Substitutes

Bone defects remain a serious problem as the associated critical bone loss dramatically affects the patient's quality of life, causing atrophy of the adjacent bone and soft tissue. The concept of bone tissue regeneration has a long history aiming to restore diseased or damaged tissue by means of so-called bone substitute materials. A wide variety of bone substitutes have been developed and analyzed over the past 50 years.

Thereby, the term bone substitute describes the heterogeneous group of biomaterials that can be of natural or synthetic and also of inorganic or biologically organic origin for the treatment of a bone defect instead of autologous bone grafts [1]. They are broadly categorized into bone grafts (allograft and xenograft), ceramics (e.g. hydroxyapatite (HA), beta-tricalcium phosphate (β-TCP), calcium sulphate etc.), polymers, and different composites [2].

The ideal bone substitute material should fulfill a variety of prerequisites. Mainly, it should be biocompatible and not evoke any adverse inflammatory response [3, 4]. The graft should be durable and be able to maintain its structural properties to be osteoconductive and ideally osteoinductive [5, 6]. In this context, the ideal bone substitutes should resorb in a matching rate with the rate of bone regrowth, following the concept of "creeping substitution" [5]. However, the duration, of which an implant must maintain its structural support, largely depends upon the surgical indication. For instance, spinal fusion requires a material to be degraded within 9 months or longer while in maxillofacial surgery or dentistry the required time period is around 3–6 months [7]. Additionally, an ideal bone substitute material should be thermally nonconducting, sterilizable (without inducing structural/chemical changes and/or cytotoxicity), highly available, and affordable [8].

On a global scale, around 2.2 million bone grafting procedures are performed annually from different resources, including autogenic, allogenic, xenogeneic, or synthetic [9]. This results from the fact that these both material types are believed to optimally occupy the aforementioned properties due to their "natural" characters. However, xenogeneic and synthetic bone grafts are being increasingly applied in the recent years as they are advantageous over autografts/autografts in terms of the following: (i) No need for a second harvesting surgery that can cause chronic donor site morbidity, in case of autografts, (ii) Allografts impose an immunogenic threat, as well as an ethical concern, and (iii) Both autogenic and allogenic bone grafts have a restricted availability, while xenografts/synthetic bone grafts are unlimitedly available. Moreover, new technologies such as 3D printing or novel preparation methods in combination with a deeper understanding of the biology of bone tissue regeneration and graft substitution even on the molecular level shift the focus also onto synthetic bone substitute materials. In this context, it is of special interest that the different preparation methods allow to have influence on different processes in the framework of bone regeneration such as the angiogenesis and the resulting implant bed vascularization or the inflammatory cell responses and cellular material degradation [10, 11]. It has been shown that different physicochemical material properties such as the chemical composition of a bone substitute material or physical characteristics such as porosity and finally the combination of all material properties dictate both the cell responses and finally bone regeneration [10, 11]. Even synthetic materials and their different preparation methods allow for synthesis of bone substitutes with different properties making this type of bone grafts particularly interesting. However, a basic understanding of bone formation including processes like osteogenesis, osteoinduction, osteoconduction, as well as associated cascades like angiogenesis or material-related inflammation is a prerequisite for comprehending the biology of bone substitute-related substitution.

As mentioned above, bioceramics and bioactive glass are largely used clinically for bone augmentation in non-load bearing sites [12–14]. That is based on the fact that such materials have the tendency to fracture under mechanical stress, which restricts their application in load-bearing sites [15, 16]. At a closer look, bone substitutes suffer from the so-called brittleness in material sciences. Thus, these bone substitutes cannot adapt to stress via deformation and are susceptible to fracture that can lead to implant failure. However, different strategies have been developed to overcome this issue. In bone physiology and although the weight of bone constitutes of 70% HA, collagen fibers increase the capacity of bone to absorb energy via increasing the toughness of the tissue (i.e., elasticity and ductility) [17, 18]. Thus, a broad variety of composite materials including both natural and synthetic polymers have been developed. Basically, an understanding of the biomechanics of bone can provide scientists with the insight needed to prepare scaffolds that are mechanically compatible for the regeneration of tissue at a load bearing site. A tradeoff between the required mechanical and structural properties is challenging; however, new fabrication techniques like 3D printing allow for feasible and reproducible investigation of this challenge [17, 19].

Figure 1 shows a Stress–Strain curve of two different materials, where material a is stiff yet brittle, and material b is tough and energy-absorbing. The inorganic part of bone (and bone ceramics/bioglass) will have a similar curve as material (a), while a composition of the inorganic and organic parts of bone will behave similarly as material (b).

In this context, the present chapter covers the most common fabrication techniques for ceramic bone substitute materials in consideration of certain material properties that are matching with the process of bone regeneration. Moreover, a focus in the further development of ceramic bone substitutes is to create biomimicking materials. Therefore, characterization is an essential step in the development of a novel bone substitute. Thus, this chapter also sheds a light on structural, physical and chemical characterization methods.

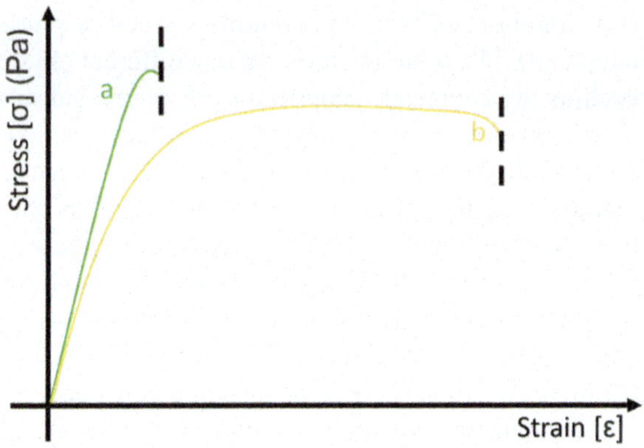

Fig. 1 Stress–Strain curve. Curve a is a behavior of a stiff but brittle material. Curve b is a behavior of a tough and energy-absorbing material. Dotted black lines displays the fracture points of the respective material

1.2 Bioceramics

Bone is a combination of organic (mainly collagen and a variety of associated molecules such as the bone morphogenetic proteins or osteopontin) and inorganic phases (bone minerals). Thus, the so-called bioceramics were developed even based on the mineral part of the extracellular bone matrix few decades ago. Ceramic-based bone substitutes are generally calcium phosphate-based materials and mainly based on hydroxyapatite (HA) and tricalcium phosphate (β-TCP). Even HA is the main component of the bone structure, representing 70% in weight of bone, is an important inorganic compound with the ability to stimulate osteoconduction by promoting the attachment and growth of bone cells [17]. Most often a mixture of both compounds in form of the so-called biphasic calcium phosphate ceramics (BCP) is clinically used. This combination has been developed due to the fact that HA exhibits very high mechanical strength and is a relatively inert substance that has been described to retain within its implantation bed for a prolonged time period, while β-TCP undergoes biodegradation within 6 weeks after its application [9]. To maintain a physiological balance between mechanical and osteoconductive support and bone regeneration up to the condition of a *restitutio ad integrum*, BCP were created by combination of β-TCP (40–60%) and HA (60–40%) [20]. Although they are not used much in clinical practice due to their more or less bad reputation, different studies revealed that synthetic bone substitutes were found to be less painful and relatively less complicated compared to iliac crest grafts [21]. Moreover, comparable regeneration results have been shown for this material type also compared to both allo- and xenografts [22]. Altogether, ceramics are commonly used in many fields for bone regeneration, as they have proven to be biocompatible and successfully promote bone regrowth [17]. However, their mechanical properties are a major drawback. For instance, BCPs have a compressive strength in the range of 10–60 MPa (depending on the TCP:HA ratio) and native cortical bone has a compressive strength of 150–200 MPa (depending on age, gender, and health status) [23]. Thus, their application is most often restricted to non-load-bearing applications such as the treatment of extractions sockets or for sinus lifting in dental surgery. Biphasic bone substitute materials are available in form of blocks, granules, and as injectable materials being the most diverse material class.

1.3 Bioactive Glass

The most common bioactive glass is based on four components: silicon dioxide (SiO_2), sodium oxide (Na_2O), calcium oxide (CaO), and phosphorus pentoxide (P_2O_5). They are known as Bioglass® 45S5 and S53P4, which are available in different forms for clinical use [24, 25]. However, due to their high silica content, these "first generation" bioactive glasses can have manufacturing difficulties, i.e., phase separation, crystallization during melting, and annealing [26]. Therefore, other bioactive glass systems, like the Na_2O-K_2O-MgO-CaO-B_2O_3-P_2O_5-SiO_2 system, have been developed [26].

The chemical mechanism of bioactive glass is the rapid ion exchange within the interface between the bio-glass and bodily fluids [27]. The cellular mechanism of how bioactive glasses work is to induce the recruitment and differentiation of osteoblasts, and promote the fusion of macrophages into pro-inflammatory/anti-inflammatory multinucleated-giant cells (MNGCs) that are essential for wound healing and bone regrowth [28]. In vivo, bioactive glass exhibits high osteoinductivity and osteogenesis [27]. Like bioceramics, bioactive glass is still limited to non-load bearing applications [29].

2 Processing of Ceramic Bone Substitutes

2.1 Ceramic Scaffolds

2.1.1 Primary Fabrication Techniques

Foaming and Foam Replication Ceramics in the form of powders are added to an aqueous solution to create slurries. To these slurries, a foaming agent is added to create a foam. The agents (e.g., hydrogen peroxide, carbonate salt, or baking soda) react with the slurries similarly to how chalk reacts with acid [30]. The foam then is subjected to polymerization and sintering. While this technique produces scaffolds with great mechanical properties, their structure can be compromised (i.e.: low interconnectivity and non-uniform porosity) [30]. Figure 2 shows a simplified flowchart of the foaming process to create ceramic scaffolds. Common foaming techniques are the incorporation of an external gas phase via mechanical mixing and in situ gas evolution which incorporates a foaming agent that decomposes with temperature/chemical stimulation (creating bubbles). Further information regarding foaming and ceramic foams is found in *Processing of Ceramic Foams* [31]. Protein foaming is another foaming method that utilizes proteins (such as albumin, bovine serum albumin, whey proteins or fish collagens) where foaming agents and binders are incorporated to produce a ceramic slurry [32–36]. To this slurry, proteins are added, the protein then adsorbs on the water–air interfaces and stabilizes air bubbles that create a foam [37]. This foam is then exposed to heat, where the polypeptide chains are modified via the formation of new hydrogen bonds. This, in turn, coagulates the protein and creates a porous structure [37]. Advantages of this method are the yielding mechanical strength that is relatively high, the controllability over pore size/porosity [38, 39], and its environmentally friendly process [38–40].

Another process that is similar in naming (but not interchangeable) is foam replication. This process, adopted by numerous groups [41–43], involves the immersion of a polymeric foam (or sponge) in the ceramic slurry followed removal of the polymer through sintering. The polymeric sponges act in this case as positive molds. Thus, this method yields in an opposite replica of the polymeric foam from the ceramic slurry. Such process can produce high porosity (>70%) with roundly shaped pores. Varying the characteristics of the polymeric foams can produce different microstructures, which provides the controllability over the pore size/porosity [43]. Another advantage of this method is structural reproducibility [43]. Cunningham et al. have synthesized ceramic bone scaffolds utilizing marine sponges for replication [44]. A less viscous hydroxyapatite slurry was developed and infiltrated on sponges. After sintering a scaffold structure was obtained that replicated the pore structure and interconnectivity of the natural precursor sponge. The synthesized HA scaffolds demonstrated an overall porosity of 56–61% with an average pore size of 349 μm and an interconnectivity of 99.92% [44].

Particulate Leaching Although the salt-leaching or particulate leaching method has been rarely adopted up-to-now, it offers some relevant advantages. First, the salt-leaching method is conceptually easy as it creates the "voids" by simply washing out the salt. Moreover, it is cost effective, and it does not require specific (and expensive) equipment. The salt-leaching approach is appealing also because it does not imply any dangerous contamination such as polymer residues. Thereby, chemicals such as sodium chloride (NaCl) and sodium bicarbonate ($NaHCO_3$), which are harmless porogens and soluble in water, can be used to create the pores [45]. A disadvantage, however, can be that the number of particles used is limited because of the possible particle entrapment. This limitation can lead to low interconnectivity [46]. For example, Canillo et al. have synthesized highly porous composite scaffolds, since an optimized microstructure is a basic pre-requisite for any advanced application, especially in the biomedical context [47]. Figure 2 shows a flowchart of the particulate leaching process to create ceramic scaffolds.

Gel Casting Fabrication process that depends on casting the ceramic slurry mixed with organic binders on a non-porous mold. Followed by gelation (polymerization), unmolding and burnout of the binder to create a porous structure [48, 49]. Figure 2 depicts a simplified chart of a conventional gel casting process. This technique yields in increased mechanical strength and is cost-effective and highly reproducible [48].

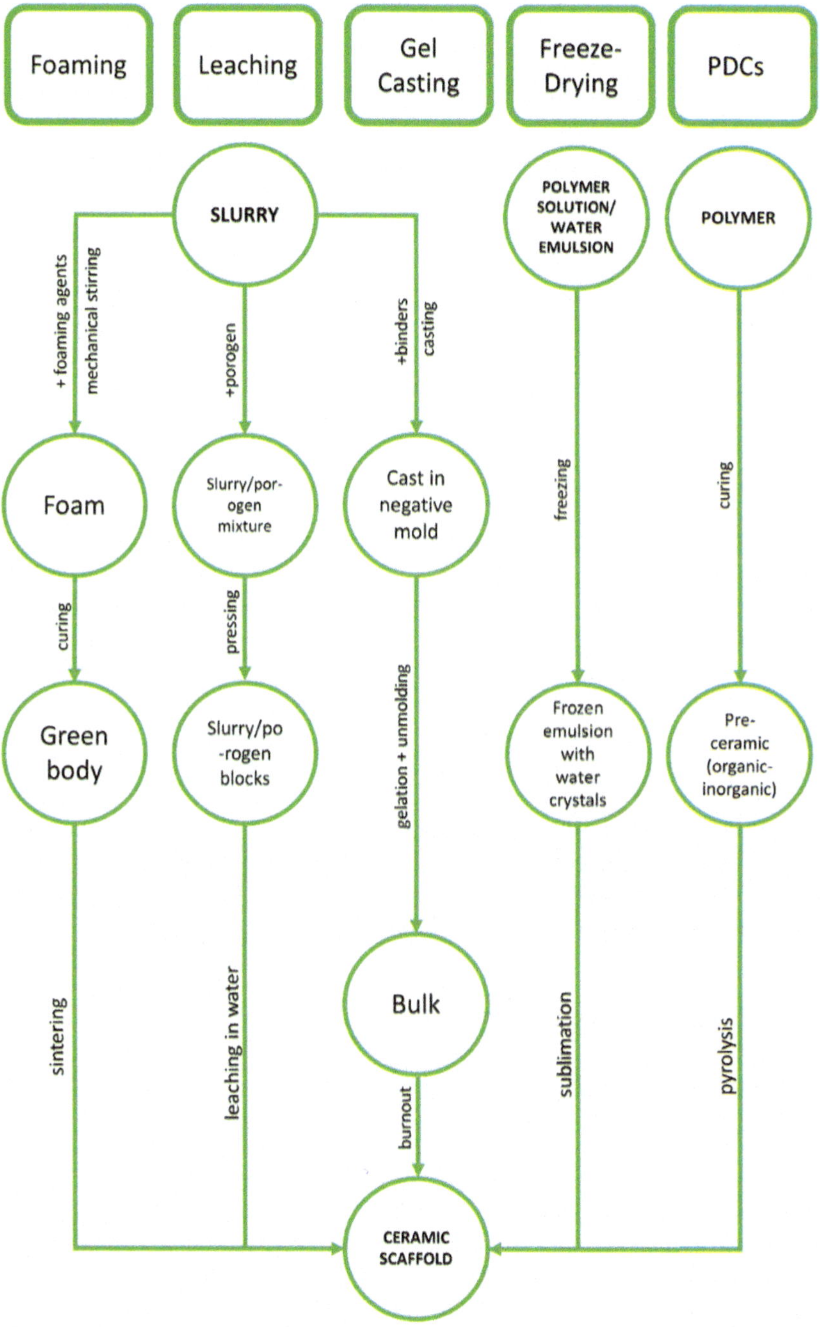

Fig. 2 Schematic flowchart of the different conventional fabrication techniques of ceramic scaffolds

However, burnout time can last up to days and the chemical additives to the slurry are of environmental/safety concerns.

Freeze-Drying Also known as lyophilization, where an emulsion of polymer solution and water is created. This technique is mainly a two-step process [17], seen in Fig. 2. At first, the emulsion is subjected to below-freezing temperatures. The water molecules expand and crystalize within the polymer solution. Subsequently, the frozen emulsion is then dry vacuumed to evaporate the water and solvent via sublimation. The water leaves micropores, creating a porous and interconnected structure.

The advantage of freeze drying is that an extra consolidation agent is unnecessary [50]. However, solvent residuals are a concern, and the porosity/pore size are irregular [17]. The rate of freezing is important here, as rapid freezing can yield in small and finer crystals (decreased pore size), while slower freezing rate will yield in larger crystals (increased pore size). Another parameter of freeze-drying is the freezing time, which must be optimized so that the core of the sample is not left with water molecules that are not frozen.

Polymer Derived Ceramics (PDCs) Polymer-derived ceramics (PDCs) are ceramics derived from preceramic polymers via a pyrolysis process, which makes them much different from materials produced via traditional sintering techniques [51]. Pyrolysis is defined as the decomposition of a material in an inert atmosphere. In the case of PDCs, the organic composition of the polymer is decomposed, leaving the inorganic part [52]. This inorganic part is the yielding amorphous ceramic. Figure 2 depicts a simple flowchart of this process. PDCs arouse a growing interest in ceramic science due to their good suitability in the following points: (a) availability in different forms (fibers, films, porous ceramics, etc.), (b) possibility of micro- and nanoscale porosity, (c) controlling the compositions, and (d) having a heat-stable production process [51]. In PDCs, complex microstructures and functional characteristics are highly tailorable through molecular design and polymer sciences [51]. To some extent, their functionality is rooted in the polymers.

2.1.2 Secondary Fabrication Techniques

Sintering Sintering is an unavoidable step in the processing of advanced ceramic materials that significantly influences the microstructure of products, and thus their mechanical, optical, biological, electrical, or magnetic properties [53]. It is therefore important to optimize the sintering process, i.e., the choice of input powder material, shaping/sintering techniques, heating profile/sintering atmosphere, and so on [53]. In sintering, the pre-shaped and consolidated particles of powder are called the green body. When this green body is subjected to heat, the particles do not melt but they fuse together in a process called densification [54]. Although the sintering process has been known for thousands of years and systematically studied by physicists, chemists, and material engineers since the 1940s, a unified theory of sintering kinetics and its influence on final microstructure still does not exist, even in the case of pressure-less sintering [55]. The reason for that is the complicated nature of mass transport in polycrystalline materials.

Fiber Mesh/Fiber-bonding Although bone bioceramics have been extensively used clinically (in maxillofacial surgeries, spine fusion surgeries and craniofacial therapy—all of which are non-load bearing sites), their utilization in load bearing defects is still restricted. That is due to their compromised mechanical properties (i.e., their brittleness) [17]. Therefore, many have investigated different techniques to improve on the mechanical aspect of bone ceramics [56–58]. One process of interest is fiber reinforcement. The fibers of collagen in bone tissue increase the toughness of the bone (i.e., elasticity and capacity to absorb energy) [59]. Therefore, not only this technique can increase the mechanical properties of bone ceramics, but it is also a step closer to biomimicry. Fiber reinforced calcium phosphate cements (also abbreviated as FRCPC) bear the potential to facilitate the use of degradable bone substitutes in load bearing applications [15].

Powder Milling Milling is a common process to break down structures into particles in micro- and nanoscales. Most common technique is the ball milling, where a mixture of precursor material, milling balls and additives (e.g., surfactants) are rotated inside a cylindrical vessel for a certain period of time [60]. The milling balls collide with each other but with the precursor material entrapped in between, causing it to crush. This technique can be done using a dry or wet media, with the latter yielding in better results. The key factors of this technique are milling ball size, vessel size and rotational speed in rpm [60]. The rotational speed is important to decide the motion of the milling balls inside the vessel. In Fig. 3, the three different motions are depicted (cascading, cataracting and rolling). A critical speed that results in a cataracting motion is optimal as it increases the collision rate of the milling balls; hence, the efficiency of the milling [60].

Granulation/Compaction and Redispersion Due to the high specific area and high surface-to-volume ratio, it is hard to maintain nanoparticles in the nanoscale as these particles tend to agglomerate to each other upon proximity [61]. Intentionally, and sometimes unintentionally, these particles are agglomerated in a granulation/granulation step for purposes of storage and transport [62]. Spray freeze

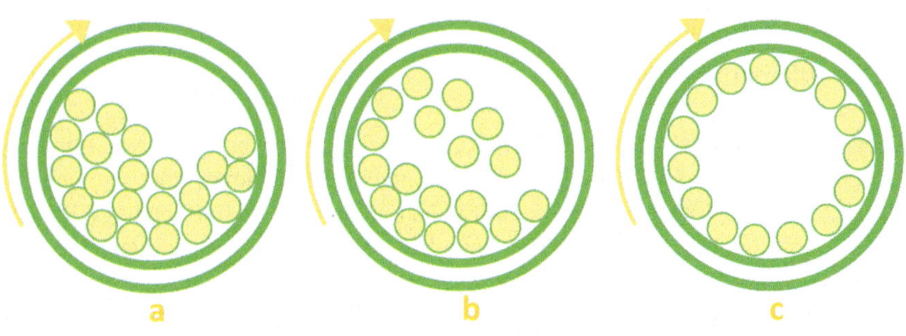

Fig. 3 An adaptation from Burmeister et al. of the three different ball motions during ball milling [60]. **a** cascading, **b** cataracting, and **c** rolling

drying is a novel granulation process, which combines the advantages of a conventional granulation by spray drying and a sublimation drying process [63]. Moritz and Nagy investigated the granulation of different suspensions of nanosized oxide powders via this technique [64]. The yielding granulates were spheric with very low strength, improved flowability and increased bulk density. Improving on the granule properties that result from other conventional granulation techniques (die pressing, roller compaction, high shear mixing, and fluid bed granulation). However, the granules must be completely scaled down through milling or redispersion; otherwise, the advantages of nanoparticles in comparison to conventional powders will not be realized.

2.2 *Composite Materials*

Scaffolds All the aforementioned processes fall under the umbrella of conventional fabrication. These techniques share a disadvantage of compromised tailorability and reproducibility. In additive manufacturing (AM)—also known as rapid prototyping or 3D printing, materials in the form of solutions, melts, powders, slurries, or hydrogels are processed into specific geometries and micro-architectures utilizing patient- and application-specific computer-aided designs (CADs). This gives room to unprecedented optimization of biomaterials. However, the application of AM clinically is still under investigation and not as commercially available as conventionally fabricated biomaterials. The most common 3D printing techniques used up to date are stereolithography, extrusion, inkjet and selective laser sinter. Perić Kačarević et al. comprehensively reviewed 3D printing and their applications in different fields in regenerative medicine, including bone tissue engineering [17]. A subcategory of 3D printing is bioprinting, that is the printing of cell-laden structures [65, 66]. Some studies investigated this technique for bone tissue regeneration, specifically the 3D printing of endothelial cells-osteoblasts co-cultures for enhanced vascularization that in turn supports the regeneration [67, 68]. Figure 4 depicts a simplified flowchart for 3D printing.

2.2.1 Fillers/Injectables

Ceramic Injectables As mentioned before, bioceramics are brittle materials that can hinder their application for load-bearing implants. The brittleness can also compromise the manageability of the material by the clinician. Therefore, bone graft pastes or injectable bone substitutes (IBS) have been adapted by many. Injectables also provide optimal filling capabilities in case of fracture cavities and interspaces that cannot be filled with conventional and granular bone grafts [69, 70]. IBS can also be part biodegradable, which allows for the regrowth of bone in a creeping substitution fashion. BCP granules are combined with various biological or synthetic polymers [70, 71]. To date, different types of injectable/moldable bone substitutes have

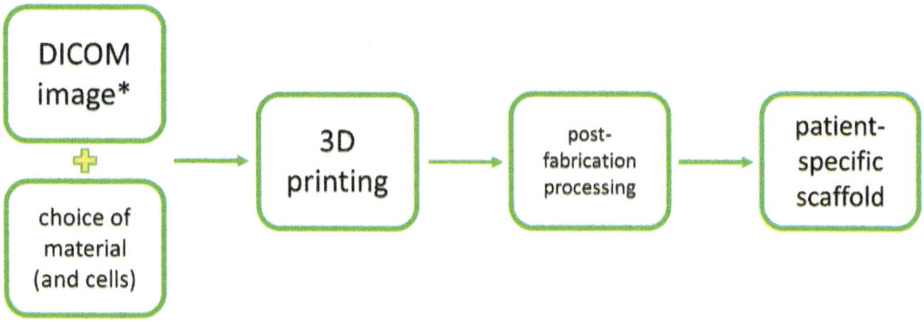

Fig. 4 Flowchart of the 3D printing process for the fabrication of patient-specific scaffolds. *A processing step on the DICOM files is necessary in order to insert the designed 3D structure into a 3D slicing software

been developed such as maxresorb® inject, which is a four-phasic bone graft paste combining a water-based gel containing HA nanoparticles (size 15–50 nm) mixed together with BCP granules (60% HA and 40% β-TCP) [72, 73]. Preclinical in vivo results showed that the application of this material class is associated with a special tissue integration behavior that, unlike conventional bone graft granules, hinders the soft tissue influx into the central regions of the implantation beds [73, 74]. This directed integration behavior has shown to be in accordance with the concept of Guided Bone Regeneration (GBR). In another study, Segredo-Morales et al. prepared injectable thermo-responsive hydrogels for regeneration of osteoporotic bone defects [75]. Natural-synthetic composite hydrogels were loaded with an estrogen hormone and with Bone Morphogenic Proteins (BMPs). The hydrogel allowed for two-phase resorption in vivo in osteoporotic rats. The effect of the loaded biomolecules was described as synergic where the BMPs enhanced the activity of the estrogen, which induced higher bone growth.

Polymer-based Injectable Bone Graft Substitutes Polymer-based bone grafts possess different mechanical, chemical, and physical properties as bioceramics and bioactive glass. Thereby, polymers as bone grafts can be divided into natural and synthetic, and then further divided into degradable and permanent. Kačarević et al. reviewed the most commonly used polymers in bone tissue engineering [17].

One of the most important natural polymers in bone is collagen (type I) being a major component of the natural extracellular bone matrix being the basis molecule for the natural calcification process [76]. The guiding principle for the development of bone substitute materials combining collagen and ceramics is to mimic natural mineralized collagen. Collagen is bioabsorbable and osteoconductive and can promote bone regeneration [77, 78]. Many methods were developed to prepare so-called "mineralized collagen" that consisted of collagen and different natural or synthetic bone substitute materials [79, 80]. Most often, xenogeneic collagen isolated from different sources and tissues is added to bone graft particles to form a composite spongelike implant. Some of the products have been commercialized as medical devices and used to repair bone defects.

Moreover, different composite materials including synthetic polymers have also been introduced. Degradable synthetic polymers should also be resorbed by the body such as natural polymers providing the benefit that they enhance healing without remaining as foreign bodies. For example, Cortoss® resin-based biomaterial that is used for load-bearing applications. The synthetic polymer (difunctional methacrylate) is reinforced with BCP granules. These granules are radiopaque, allowing in vivo visualization via X-ray imaging techniques. Indications for this biomaterial include osteoporotic and metastatic vertebral compression fractures that require vertebroplasty [69]. Other degradable synthetic polymers are polylactic acid (PLA) and poly(lactic-co-glycolic acid) (PLGA), degradability of PLGA can be easily controlled via changing the concentrations ratios of the co-polymers [66].

Curing/Consolidation/Solidification Behavior Consolidation is aimed to harden a composition to provide a suitable material that will have adequate mechanical and rheological behaviors. It also maintains uniform distribution of particles. Consolidation of bioceramics can be done through many methods: starch consolidation (removes water via swelling and acts as a binding agent) [30], combination of bioceramics with biocompatible polymers [81], or cross-linking (natural or chemical) [32, 38].

3 Characterization Techniques of Ceramic Bone Substitutes

3.1 Structure and Composition

Electron Microscopy An analysis of the morphology of ceramic bone substitutes is normally determined by scanning electron microscopy (SEM), Fig. 5. SEM allows for imaging of the material surface via scanning with electron beams. Thereby, the electrons interact with the material atoms producing signals that contain information about the sample's surface topography [82]. Moreover, SEM can provide vivid images of a sample surface via detection of secondary electrons (secondary electron image, SEI) with superior resolution about 1–5 nm [83]. Additionally, SEM imaging can be combined with an Energy Dispersive X-ray Analyzer (EDX) that provides elemental identification and quantitative compositional information [84, 85]. Thereby, analysis via EDX mapping can be used to analyze the chemical composition/conversion of a bone substitute in situ and after in vivo implantation [84], as seen in Fig. 7.

Non-destructive Imaging Techniques Different non-destructive imaging techniques such as X-ray imaging, micro-computed tomography (μCT), high-resolution magnetic resonance imaging (MRI), or synchrotron X-ray microtomography allow for (three-dimensional) imaging of ceramic bone substitutes [86]. Interestingly, these techniques can be used for the analysis of the morphology of bone substitute materials both in vivo and ex vivo [87–90]. Data obtained from these measurement procedures

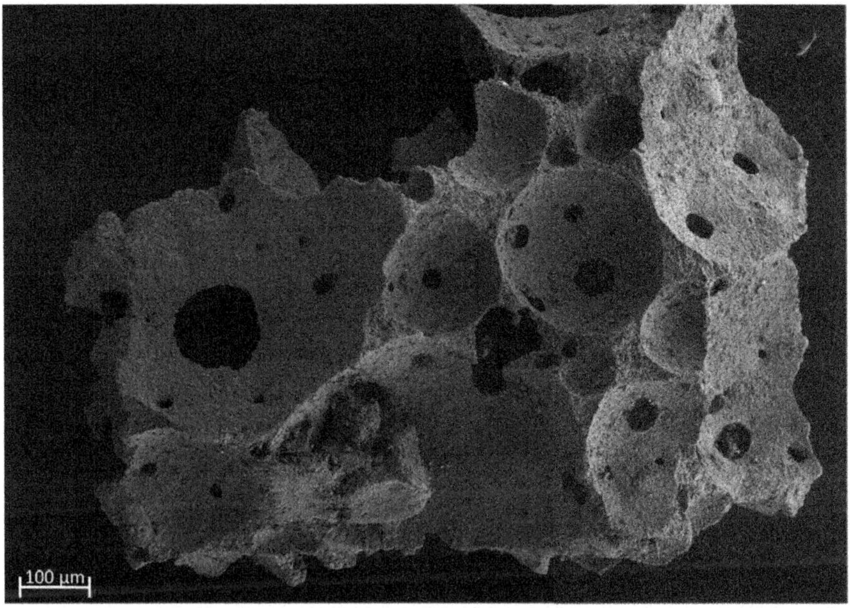

Fig. 5 Scanning electron microscopy image of a synthetic bone substitute (maxresorb®, biphasic calcium phosphate composed from 60% HA and 40% ß-TCP)

result in a set of projections, which can be used for reconstructing a complete 3D-image but can also be used for the measurement of material characteristics such as the pore size distribution [86]. X-ray imaging is a technique that quickly allows for imaging of ceramic bone substitutes but; moreover, X-ray spectrometry investigates important characteristics such as the elemental composition/arrangement, structural arrangement (e.g., crystallinity, pore size, interconnectivity), and compound composition of these biomaterials [91, 92]. Additionally, X-ray fluorescence (XRF) and X-ray diffraction (XRD) are expansions techniques that address these questions further in depth. Thereby, XRF has been applied as an analysis tool for the exact purpose of analyzing the elemental composition of (bone) biomaterils and their arrangement, due to its good sensitivity to the parts per million (ppm) level, wide elemental analysis range, and simple sample preparation techniques. In terms of XRD, it is a tool to detect the chemical compounds of these biomaterials, as well as their degree of crystallinity and amorphous content. Which in turn can provide insight on the in vivo integration and degradation behaviors of these biomaterials. Altogether, XRF and XRD answer different questions, but nowadays devices can carry out both techniques to analyze materials comprehensively.

μCT scanning is also an important tool in ceramic research. It allows for analysis of the material morphology and enables to create three dimensional images of these materials, as seen in Fig. 7. Moreover, different other related measurements like a permeability analysis of porous materials can be done using this technology. In

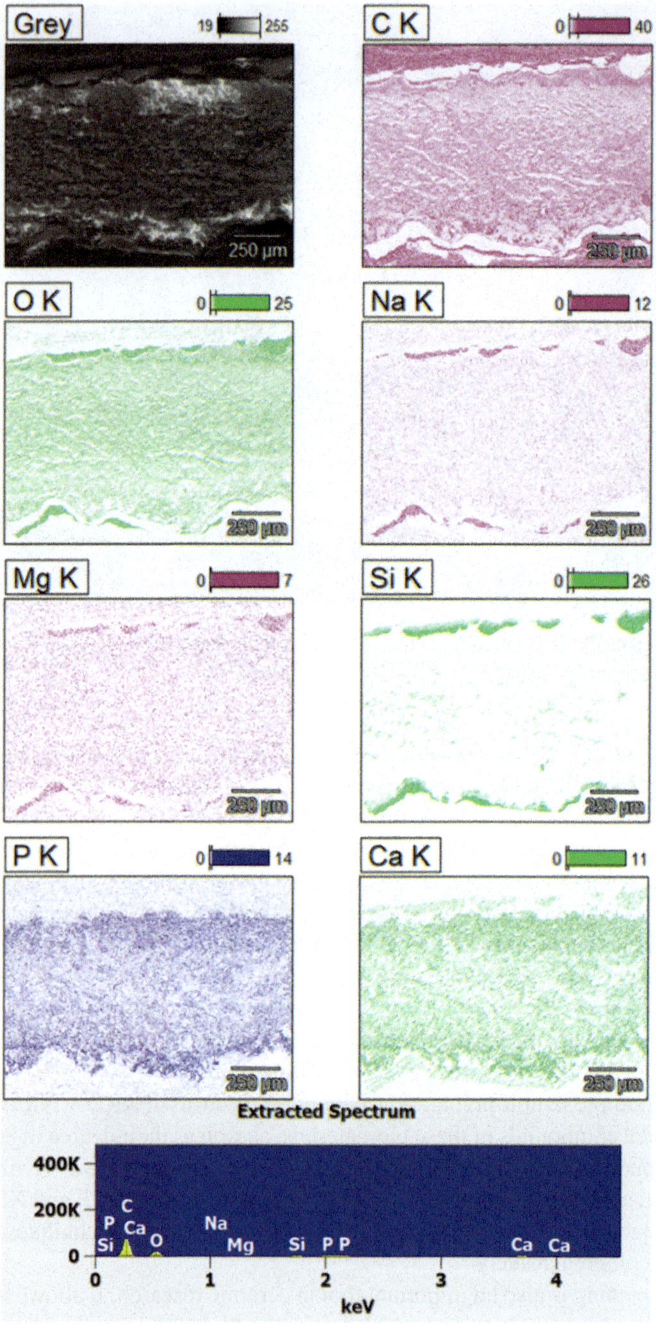

Fig. 6 Elemental analysis via EDX mapping of a vaterite-loaded hydrogel after its subcutaneous implantation in a rat model at day 30 *post implantationem*

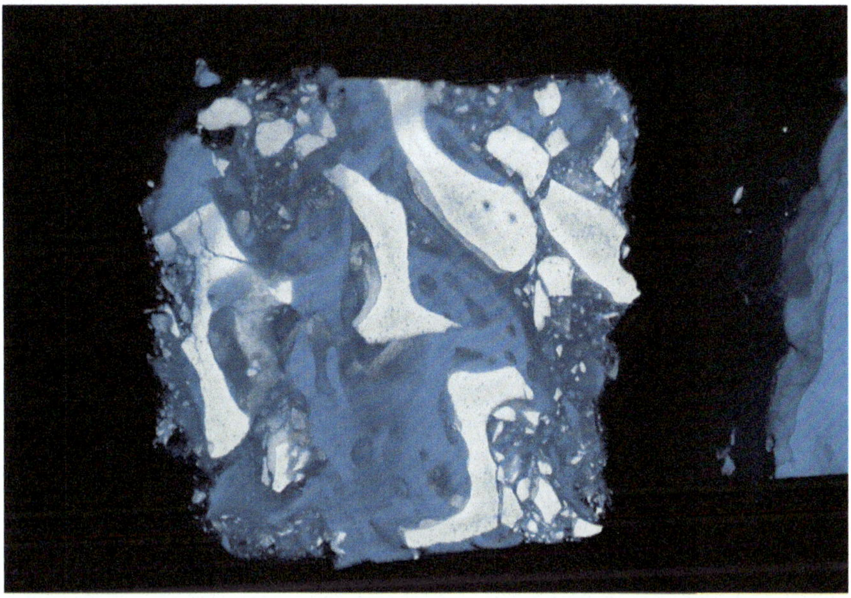

Fig. 7 μCT image of a human biopsy of a sinus augmentation case using a xenogeneic bone substitute after 6 months. White areas represent the bone substitute and darker blue represents the newly formed bone

this context, it should be noted that a significant amount of work has been done in pore characterization and modelling in the last few decades, specifically in the area of X-ray based 3D image analysis [86, 93]. Interestingly, this technique also allows for analysis of bone substitute degradation both in vitro and in vivo [93]. Different protocols for μCT enable to visualize the nature of the bone structure and to quantitatively analyze numerous bone structural parameters with a high degree of accuracy.

Table compares the different characterization processes using imaging techniques (Table 1).

3.2 *Mechanical Properties*

As mentioned before, the unique organic/inorganic composition of human bone allows for a tough and energy-absorbing tissue that can endure the different mechanical stresses subjected to it (i.e., compression, tensile, torsion and shearing) [59]. Bone is subjected to these stresses differently depending on its site. For example, the femoral bone is subjected mainly to compressive loading and torsion while alveolar bone can be subjected to shearing [96]. An understanding of the biomechanics of human bone is essential for developing scaffolds with mechanical adequacy [19].

Table 1 Imaging techniques available for the post fabrication, in vivo and ex vivo (biopsies) characterization of bone substitutes

Imaging	Technique	Sample destruction	Application	Characterization/assessment
SEM [82, 85]	X-ray	Yes	• Post fabrication • Ex vivo (EDX mapping)	• Structural • Chemical (EDX mapping)
μ-CT [93, 94]	X-ray	No	• Post fabrication • In vivo	• Structural • Degradability
XRF [91]	Secondary X-ray	No	• Ex vivo	• Elemental
XRD [92]	Interference between X-ray and crystalline samples	No	• Ex vivo	• Chemical compound • Structural (crystallinity)
Ultrasound [90]	Sound waves	No	• Post fabrication • Ex vivo	• Structural • Biological (real-time) • Mechanical
High-resolution MRI [87, 95]	Magnetic resonance	No	• Post fabrication • In vivo	• Structural • Biological (real-time)

For instance, a bone tissue engineering scaffold should have equivalent mechanical properties to the host bone. Human cancellous bone extracted from the mandible has a compressive strength of 3.9 2.7 MPa, a scaffold should have similar strength [97]. It is important to mention, that a biodegradable implant will lose its mechanical integrity in vivo, which that is of concern and requires investigation. Therefore, the following characterization techniques are commonly carried out post fabrication of the scaffolds.

Tensile Strength Both tensile and compressive tests are carried out using a universal testing machine (UTM). The key factors in each testing are the shape of the specimen (dumb-bell, cylindrical, or rectangular), the loading rate, and the angle of loading [98, 99]. One type of tensile testing is the Brazilian disc test [100]. It is done on short cross-sections of cylindrical samples and can be practical with bioceramics that are brittle. The sample is placed so that its curvature is touching the loading plates. A compressive force is applied until the sample cracks vertically. Even though this technique applies compressive forces, the measured strength is tensile. An advantage of this technique is its independence from surface properties [99]. The tensile strength is then calculated as shown:

$$\sigma = 2P/\pi Dt \quad (1)$$

Equation 1: Calculating tensile strength, where F is the applied load, D is the specimen diameter and t its thickness.

Compressive Strength To calculate the ability of a material to endure compression, compressive strength is measured similarly to tensile. However, Awaji et al. found that dumb-bell shaped specimens are best suitable for compressive testing of ceramics [101]. It has been found that there is a negative linear relationship between compressive strength and the specimen's porosity with a coefficient of determination R2 between 0.8 and 0.99 [102, 103]. It was also found that the scaffolds are more likely to structurally fail at porosities between 89 and 92% due to the buckling phenomenon that causes the microarchitecture to collapse.

Indentation To measure the resistance of a material to indentation, hardness test is carried out. A force is applied to the surface of the material using an indenter, the indented surface is then measured via a microscope [104]. There are many types of hardness tests, all depend on the shape of the indenter (e.g., steel ball or pyramid diamond) [105]. To measure microhardness, Knoop and Vickers tests are most suitable. For nanoindentation, the Berkovich test is the most used [105]. Hardness is not to be confused with stiffness; it is more of a surface characteristic. The hardness test is easy, fast, and used to relate to other properties such as tensile strength.

3.3 Rheology of Injectable Bone Grafts

Fluid characteristics of injectable bone substitutes are important as they the slurries require to be injectable with low resistance and no phase separation during application, which highly depends on the rheological properties of the bone injectables [106]. Rheological properties include the characterization of the fluid into Newtonian or non-Newtonian (Fig. 8), as well as time-dependent viscoelastic properties including rheopectic (apparent viscosity increases with duration of stress) and thixotropic (apparent viscosity decreases with duration of stress) behaviors. In short, Newtonian fluid is one whose viscosity is independent from the applied shear stress (Fig. 8a). In contrast, non-Newtonian fluids have viscosities that are affected by the applied shear stress. Non-Newtonian fluids are either dilatant (shear-thickening) (Fig. 8b), pseudoplastic (shear-thinning) (Fig. 8c), Bingham plastic (flows at higher stresses) (Fig. 8d), or Bingham pseudoplastic (shear-thinning at higher stresses) (Fig. 8e).

When preparing slurries and hydrogels, not only viscosity is studied but also powder content and particle size. In a study, injectability of ß-TCP slurry was enhanced via the decrease of powder/liquid ratio, decrease of particle size, and increasing viscosity via using a thickener [107]. Another important aspect is the sedimentation/setting of slurries as their rheology might differ before and after. For instance, in a study where a calcium phosphate cement was investigated, the slurry exhibited increased thixotropic behavior which, in turn, can have a major impact on its flowability [106]. Vicat needle test is used to measure the setting time of the slurry, which then gives insights to how sedimentation can affect some time-dependent behaviors of the slurry. Furthermore, viscosity can be decreased by ionic

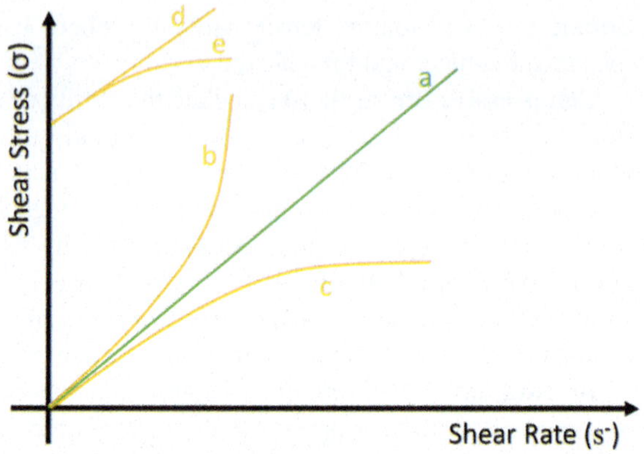

Fig. 8 Classification of Newtonian (green) and non-Newtonian (yellow) fluids where (a) Newtonian fluid, (b) dilatant, (c) pseudoplastic, (d) Bingham plastic, and (e) Bingham pseudoplastic

modification [108, 109] or addition of inert filler particles [110]. Particle size can also modify the viscosity of the injectable; however, can also have impacts on mechanical properties and tendencies of agglomeration [111]. When increasing particle size, particle–particle bonds are strengthened due to proximity which increases viscosity. In contrast, decreasing the particle size enhances hydration or water uptake, which decreases the viscosity of the slurry.

4 Conclusion

In summary, this chapter sheds a light on the fabrication and processing techniques of ceramic bone substitutes, as well as their characterization techniques. A closer look is given at each fabrication technique, from conventional ones to more novel technologies. Characterization techniques covered are used for structural, chemical, and physical assessments. Although bone ceramics are currently being used clinically as alternatives to auto- and allografts, their optimization is still under investigation. Specifically, the improvement of the mechanical properties of bone ceramics for load bearing sites such as femoral augmentation and some cases of spine fusion. The requirements of bone substitutes can differ from one to another depending on their application and the implant site as they need to match the mechanical profile of the host bone.

References

1. Schlickewei, W., Schlickewei, C.: The use of bone substitutes in the treatment of bone defects—the clinical view and history. Macromol. Symp. **253**, 10–23 (2007). https://doi.org/10.1002/masy.200750702

2. Arner, J.W., Santrock, R.D.: A historical review of common bone graft materials in foot and ankle surgery. Foot Ankle Spec. **7**, 143–151 (2014)
3. Yi, H., Ur Rehman, F., Zhao, C., Liu, B., He, N.: Recent advances in nano scaffolds for bone repair. Bone Res. **4**, 16050 (2016). https://doi.org/10.1038/boneres.2016.50
4. Habibovic, P., de Groot, K.: Osteoinductive biomaterials—properties and relevance in bone repair. J. Tissue Eng. Regen. Med. **1**, 25–32 (2007). https://doi.org/10.1002/term.5
5. Ranjan Dahiya, U., Mishra, S., Bano, S.: Application of bone substitutes and its future prospective in regenerative medicine. In: Biomaterial-supported Tissue Reconstruction or Regeneration. IntechOpen (2019)
6. Miron, R.J., Zhang, Y.F.: Osteoinduction: a review of old concepts with new standards. J. Dent Res. **91**, 736–744 (2012)
7. Gupta, A., Kukkar, N., Sharif, K., Main, B.J., Albers, C.E., El-Amin, S.F.: Bone graft substitutes for spine fusion: a brief review. World J. Orthop. **6**, 449–456 (2015). https://doi.org/10.5312/wjo.v6.i6.449
8. Pryor, L.S., Gage, E., Langevin, C.-J.J., Herrera, F., Breithaupt, A.D., Gordon, C.R., Afifi, A.M., Zins, J.E., Meltzer, H., Gosman, A., Cohen, S.R., Holmes, R.: Review of bone substitutes. Craniomaxillofac. Trauma Reconstr. **2**, 151–160 (2009).https://doi.org/10.1055/s-0029-1224777
9. Wang, W., Yeung, K.W.K.: Bone grafts and biomaterials substitutes for bone defect repair: a review. Bioact. Mater. **2**, 224–247 (2017)
10. Ghanaati, S., Barbeck, M., Detsch, R., Deisinger, U., Hilbig, U., Rausch, V., Sader, R., Unger, R.E., Ziegler, G., Kirkpatrick, C.J.: The chemical composition of synthetic bone substitutes influences tissue reactions in vivo: histological and histomorphometrical analysis of the cellular inflammatory response to hydroxyapatite, beta-tricalcium phosphate and biphasic calcium phosphate cer. Biomed. Mater. **7**, 15005 (2012). https://doi.org/10.1088/1748-6041/7/1/015005
11. Ghanaati, S., Barbeck, M., Orth, C., Willershausen, I., Thimm, B.W., Hoffmann, C., Rasic, A., Sader, R.A., Unger, R.E., Peters, F., Kirkpatrick, C.J.: Influence of β-tricalcium phosphate granule size and morphology on tissue reaction in vivo. Acta Biomater. **6**, 4476–87 (2010). PMID: 20624495. https://doi.org/10.1016/j.actbio.2010.07.006
12. Bauer, T.W., Muschler, G.F.: Bone graft materials. An overview of the basic science. Clin. Orthop. Relat. Res. 10–27 (2000)
13. Diez-Escudero, A., Espanol, M., Ginebra, M.P.: Synthetic Bone Graft Substitutes: Calcium-Based Biomaterials. Elsevier Ltd. (2019)
14. Roberts, T.T., Rosenbaum, A.J., Roberts, T.T., Rosenbaum, A.J., Roberts, T.T., Rosenbaum, A.J.: Bone grafts, bone substitutes and orthobiologics. **6278** (2012). https://doi.org/10.4161/org.23306
15. Krüger, R., Groll, J.: Fiber reinforced calcium phosphate cements—on the way to degradable load bearing bone substitutes? Biomaterials **33**, 5887–5900 (2012)
16. Llambés, F., Silvestre, F.-J., Caffesse, R.: Vertical guided bone regeneration with bioabsorbable barriers. J. Periodontol. **78**, 2036–2042 (2007). PMID: 18062126. https://doi.org/10.1902/jop.2007.070017
17. Perić Kačarević, Ž., Rider, P., Alkildani, S., Retnasingh, S., Pejakić, M., Schnettler, R., Gosau, M., Smeets, R., Jung, O., Barbeck, M.: An introduction to bone tissue engineering. Int. J. Artif. Organs. **43**, 69–86 (2020). PMID: 31544576. https://doi.org/10.1177/0391398819876286
18. Tzaphlidou, M.: Bone architecture: collagen structure and calcium/phosphorus maps. J. Biol. Phys. **34**, 39–49 (2008). PMID: 19669491. https://doi.org/10.1007/s10867-008-9115-y
19. Rider, P., Kačarević, Ž.P., Alkildani, S., Retnasingh, S., Schnettler, R., Barbeck, M.: Additive manufacturing for guided bone regeneration: a perspective for alveolar ridge augmentation (2018)
20. Boyan, B., McMillan, J., Lohmann, C.H., Ranly, D.M., Schwartz, Z, Surgeons AA of O and International A: Bone Graft Substitutes: Basic Information for Successful Clinical Use with Special Focus on Synthetic Graft Substitutes, pp. 231–259. ASTM International, West Conshohocken, Pa (2003)

21. Lerner, T., Bullmann, V., Schulte, T.L,. Schneider, M., Liljenqvist, U.: A level-1 pilot study to evaluate of ultraporous β-tricalcium phosphate as a graft extender in the posterior correction of adolescent idiopathic scoliosis. Eur. Spine J. **18**, 170–179 (2009). PMID: 19082847. https://doi.org/10.1007/s00586-008-0844-1
22. Trajkovski, B., Jaunich, M., Müller, W.-D., Beuer, F., Zafiropoulos, G.-G., Houshmand, A.: Hydrophilicity, viscoelastic, and physicochemical properties variations in dental bone grafting substitutes. Materials (Basel) **11**, 215 (2018). https://doi.org/10.3390/ma11020215
23. Campana, V., Milano, G., Pagano, E., Barba, M., Cicione, C., Salonna, G., Lattanzi, W., Logroscino, G.: Bone substitutes in orthopaedic surgery: from basic science to clinical practice. J. Mater. Sci. Mater. Med. **25**, 2445–2461 (2014). PMID: 24865980. https://doi.org/10.1007/s10856-014-5240-2
24. Salinas, A.J., Vallet-Regí, M.: Bioactive ceramics: from bone grafts to tissue engineering. RSC Adv. **3**, 11116–11131 (2013). https://doi.org/10.1039/c3ra00166k
25. Hulsen, D.J., van Gestel, N.A., Geurts, J.A.P., Arts, J.J.: S53P4 bioactive glass. In: Management of Periprosthetic Joint Infections (PJIs), pp. 69–80. Elsevier Inc (2017)
26. Brink, M., Turunen, T., Happonen, R.P., Yli-Urpo, A.: Compositional dependence of bioactivity of glasses in the system Na_2O-K_2O-MgO-Cao-B_2O_3-P_2O_5-SiO_2. J. Biomed. Mater. Res. **37**, 114–121 (1997). PMID: 9335356. https://doi.org/10.1002/(SICI)1097-4636(199710)37:1<114::AID-JBM14>3.0.CO;2-G
27. Välimäki, V.V., Aro, H.T.: Molecular basis for action of bioactive glasses as bone graft substitute. Scand. J. Surg. **95**, 95–102 (2006)
28. Xynos, I.D., Hukkanen, M.V.J., Batten, J.J., Buttery, L.D., Hench, L.L., Polak, J.M.: Bioglass ®45S5 stimulates osteoblast turnover and enhances bone formation in vitro: implications and applications for bone tissue engineering. Calcif. Tissue Int. **67**, 321–329 (2000). PMID: 11000347. https://doi.org/10.1007/s002230001134
29. Yang, J.: Progress of bioceramic and bioglass bone scaffolds for load-bearing applications. In: Orthopedic Biomaterials: Progress in Biology, Manufacturing, and Industry Perspectives, pp. 1–496 (2018)
30. Sopyan, I., Mel, M., Ramesh, S., Khalid, K.A.: Porous hydroxyapatite for artificial bone applications. Sci. Technol. Adv. Mater. **8**, 116–123 (2007). https://doi.org/10.1016/j.stam.2006.11.017
31. Mao, X.: Processing of ceramic foams. In: Recent Advances in Porous Ceramics. InTech (2018)
32. Garrn, I., Reetz, C., Brandes, N., Kroh, L.W., Schubert, H.: Clot-forming: the use of proteins as binders for producing ceramic foams. J. Eur. Ceram. Soc. **24**, 579–587 (2004). https://doi.org/10.1016/S0955-2219(03)00259-0
33. Dhara, S., Pradhan, M., Ghosh, D., Bhargava, P.: Nature inspired novel processing routes for ceramic foams. Adv. Appl. Ceram. **104**, 9–21 (2005). https://doi.org/10.1179/174367605225011007
34. He, X., Su, B.O., Zhou, X., Yang, J., Wang, X., Yang, G., Tang, Z., Qiu, H.: Gelcasting of alumina ceramics using an egg white protein binder system (2011)
35. Berthold, A., Schubert, H., Brandes, N., Kroh, L., Miller, R.: Behaviour of BSA and of BSA-derivatives at the air/water interface. Colloids Surfaces A Physicochem. Eng. Asp. **301**, 16–22 (2007). https://doi.org/10.1016/j.colsurfa.2006.11.054
36. Mazorra-Manzano, M.A., Pacheco-Aguilar, R., Ramírez-Suárez, J.C., Garcia-Sanchez, G., Lugo-Sánchez, M.E.: Endogenous proteases in pacific whiting (*Merluccius productus*) muscle as A processing aid in functional fish protein hydrolysate production. Food Bioprocess Technol. **5**, 130–137 (2012). https://doi.org/10.1007/s11947-010-0374-9
37. Lyckfeldt, O., Brandt, J., Lesca, S.: Protein forming—a novel shaping technique for ceramics. J. Eur. Ceram. Soc. **20**, 2551–2559 (2000). https://doi.org/10.1016/S0955-2219(00)00136-9
38. Yin, L., Peng, H.X., Dhara, S., Yang, L., Su, B.: Natural additives in protein coagulation casting process for improved microstructural controllability of cellular ceramics. Compos. Part B Eng. **40**, 638–644 (2009). https://doi.org/10.1016/j.compositesb.2009.04.016

39. He, X., Zhou, X., Su, B.: 3D interconnective porous alumina ceramics via direct protein foaming. Mater. Lett. **63**, 830–832 (2009). https://doi.org/10.1016/j.matlet.2008.12.021
40. Yin, L.Y., Zhou, X.G., Yu, J.S., Wang, H.L., Zhao, S., Luo, Z., Yang, B.: Preparation of Si_3N_4 ceramic foams by simultaneously using egg white protein and fish collagen. Ceram. Int. **39**, 445–448 (2013). https://doi.org/10.1016/j.ceramint.2012.06.046
41. Muhamad Nor, M.A.A., Hong, L.C., Arifin Ahmad, Z., Md Akil, H.: Preparation and characterization of ceramic foam produced via polymeric foam replication method. J. Mater. Process Technol. **207**, 235–239 (2008). https://doi.org/10.1016/j.jmatprotec.2007.12.099
42. Kim, H.W., Knowles, J.C., Kim, H.E.: Hydroxyapatite/poly(ε-caprolactone) composite coatings on hydroxyapatite porous bone scaffold for drug delivery. Biomaterials **25**, 1279–1287 (2004). PMID: 14643602. https://doi.org/10.1016/j.biomaterials.2003.07.003
43. Ramay, H.R., Zhang, M.: Preparation of porous hydroxyapatite scaffolds by combination of the gel-casting and polymer sponge methods. Biomaterials **24**, 3293–3302 (2003). PMID: 12763457. https://doi.org/10.1016/S0142-9612(03)00171-6
44. Cunningham, E., Dunne, N., Walker, G., Maggs, C., Wilcox, R., Buchanan, F.: Hydroxyapatite bone substitutes developed via replication of natural marine sponges. J. Mater. Sci. Mater. Med. **21**, 2255–2261 (2010). PMID: 20012771. https://doi.org/10.1007/s10856-009-3961-4
45. Chia, O.C., Suhaimin, I.S., Kassim, S.A., Zubir, S.A., Abdullah, T.K.: Effect of modified solvent casting/particulate leaching (SCPL) technique on the properties of bioactive glass reinforced polyurethan. J. Phys. Sci. **30**, 115–126 (2019). https://doi.org/10.21315/JPS2019.30.S2.10
46. Rezwan, K., Chen, Q.Z., Blaker, J.J., Boccaccini, A.R.: Biodegradable and bioactive porous polymer/inorganic composite scaffolds for bone tissue engineering. Biomaterials **27**, 3413–3431 (2006)
47. Cannillo, V., Sola, A., Fabbri, P.: Fabrication of 45S5 bioactive glass-polycaprolactone composite scaffolds. Res. Gate (2009)
48. Yüzbasi, N.S., Graule, T.: Colloid casting processes: slip casting, centrifugal casting, and gel casting. In: Reference Module in Materials Science and Materials Engineering. Elsevier (2020)
49. Pollinger, J.P., Khalfalla, Y.E., Benyounis, K.Y.: Gel casting. In: Reference Module in Materials Science and Materials Engineering. Elsevier (2016)
50. Deville, S.: Freeze-casting of porous biomaterials: structure, properties and opportunities. **3**, 1913–1927 (2010). https://doi.org/10.3390/ma3031913
51. Colombo, P.: Polymer Derived Ceramics: From Nano-structure to Applications. DEStech Publications (2010)
52. Weinmann, M., Ionescu, E., Riedel, R., Aldinger, F.: Polymer derived ceramics. In: Handbood of Advanced Ceramics (2013)
53. Handwerker, C.A., Blendell, J.E., Coble, R.L.: Sintering of ceramics. In: Science of Sintering, pp. 3–37. Springer US, Boston, MA (1989)
54. Rahaman, M.N.: Sintering of Ceramics (2007)
55. German, R.M.: History of sintering: empirical phase. Powder Metall. **56**, 117–123 (2013)
56. Wang, Y., Wang, M., Chen, F., Feng, C., Chen, X., Li, X., Xiao, Y., Zhang, X.: Enhancing mechanical and biological properties of biphasic calcium phosphate ceramics by adding calcium oxide. J. Am. Ceram. Soc. **104**, 548–563 (2021). https://doi.org/10.1111/jace.17450
57. Zhao, J., Xiao, S., Lu, X., Wang, J., Weng, J.: A study on improving mechanical properties of porous HA tissue engineering scaffolds by hot isostatic pressing. Biomed. Mater. **1**, 188–192 (2006). PMID: 18458404. https://doi.org/10.1088/1748-6041/1/4/002
58. Perrotti, V., Iaculli, F., Aragones, Á., Aur, M.: Physical and mechanical properties of composite scaffolds with or without collagen impregnation. Appl. Sci. (2019). https://doi.org/10.3390/app9204296
59. Viguet-Carrin, S., Garnero, P., Delmas, P.D.D.: The role of collagen in bone strength. Osteoporos **17**, 319–336 (2006). PMID: 16341622. https://doi.org/10.1007/s00198-005-2035-9

60. Burmeister, C.F., Kwade, A.: Process engineering with planetary ball millss. Chem. Soc. Rev. **42**, 7660–7667 (2013). PMID: 23389051. https://doi.org/10.1039/c3cs35455e
61. Ashraf, M.A., Peng, W., Zare, Y., Rhee, K.Y.: Effects of size and aggregation/agglomeration of nanoparticles on the interfacial/interphase properties and tensile strength of polymer nanocomposites. Nanoscale Res. Lett. **13** (2018). https://doi.org/10.1186/s11671-018-2624-0
62. Parikh, D.M.: Granulation. In: How to Optimize Fluid Bed Processing Technology, pp. 37–53 (2017)
63. Raghupathy, B.P.C., Binner, J.G.P.: Spray freeze drying of YSZ nanopowder. J. Nanoparticle Res. **14** (2012). https://doi.org/10.1007/s11051-012-0921-6
64. Moritz, T., Nagy, A.: Preparation of super soft granules from nanosized ceramic powders by spray freezing. J. Nanoparticle Res. **4**, 439–448 (2002). https://doi.org/10.1023/A:1021650415563
65. Kačarević, Ž.P., Rider, P.M., Alkildani, S., Retnasingh, S., Smeets, R., Jung, O., Ivanišević, Z., Barbeck, M.: An introduction to 3D bioprinting: possibilities, challenges and future aspects. Materials (Basel) **11** (2018). PMID: 30404222. https://doi.org/10.3390/ma11112199
66. Rider, P., Perić Kačarević, Ž., Retnasingh, S., Alkildani, S., Jung, O., Barbeck, M.: Bioprinting. In: Biomaterial-supported Tissue Reconstruction or Regeneration (2019).https://doi.org/10.5772/intechopen.81135
67. Smeets, R., Alkildani, S., Rider, P., Kačarević, ŽP., Kuhnel, L., Junge, O., Wolff, J., Barbeck, M., Retnasingh, S.: Aktuelle Methoden der additiven Fertigung und des Bioprintings in der Zahnmedizin sowie der MKG-Chirurgie. Quintessenz **69**, 1070–1076 (2018)
68. Rider, P., Kačarević, Ž.P., Alkildani, S., Retnasingh, S., Barbeck, M.: Bioprinting of tissue engineering scaffolds. J. Tissue Eng. **9** (2018). https://doi.org/10.1177/2041731418802090
69. Lorenz, J., Barbeck, M., Kirkpatrick, C.J., Sader, R., Lerner, H., Ghanaati, S.: Injectable bone substitute material on the basis of beta-TCP and hyaluronan achieves complete bone regeneration while undergoing nearly complete degradation. Int. J. Oral. Maxillofac. Implant. **33**, 636–644 (2018). PMID: 29543928. https://doi.org/10.11607/jomi.6026
70. Ryabenkova, Y., Pinnock, A., Quadros, P.A., Goodchild, R.L., Möbus, G., Crawford, A., Hatton, P.V., Miller, C.A.: The relationship between particle morphology and rheological properties in injectable nano-hydroxyapatite bone graft substitutes. Mater. Sci. Eng. C **75**, 1083–1090 (2017). PMID: 28415393. https://doi.org/10.1016/j.msec.2017.02.170
71. Liu, M., Zeng, X., Ma, C., Yi, H., Ali, Z., Mou, X., Li, S., Deng, Y., He, N.: Injectable hydrogels for cartilage and bone tissue engineering. Bone Res. **5** (2017). PMID: 28584674. https://doi.org/10.1038/boneres.2017.14
72. Jelusic, D., Zirk, M.L., Fienitz, T., Plancak, D., Puhar, I., Rothamel, D.: Monophasic ß-TCP vs. biphasic HA/ß-TCP in two-stage sinus floor augmentation procedures—a prospective randomized clinical trial. Clin. Oral. Implants Res. **28**, e175–e183 (2017). PMID: 27683073. https://doi.org/10.1111/clr.12983
73. Barbeck, M., Jung, O., Smeets, R., Gosau, M., Schnettler, R., Rider, P., Houshmand, A., Korzinskas, T.: Implantation of an injectable bone substitute material enables integration following the principles of guided bone regeneration. In Vivo (Brooklyn) **34**, 557–568 (2020). PMID: 32111754. https://doi.org/10.21873/invivo.11808
74. Ahmed, A.G., Awartani, F.A., Niazy, A.A., Jansen, J.A., Alghamdi, H.S.: A combination of biphasic calcium phosphate (Maxresorb®) and hyaluronic acid gel (Hyadent®) for repairing osseous defects in a rat model. Appl. Sci. **10**, 1651 (2020). https://doi.org/10.3390/app10051651
75. Segredo-Morales, E., García-García, P., Reyes, R., Pérez-Herrero, E., Delgado, A., Évora, C.: Bone regeneration in osteoporosis by delivery BMP-2 and PRGF from tetronic–alginate composite thermogel. Int. J. Pharm. **543**, 160–168 (2018). PMID: 29567197. https://doi.org/10.1016/j.ijpharm.2018.03.034
76. Remedios, A.: Bone and bone healing. Vet. Clin. North. Am. Small Anim. Pr. **29**, 1029–44 (1999). https://doi.org/10.1016/s0195-5616(99)50101-0
77. Kleinman, H.K., Klebe, R.J., Martin, G.R.: Role of collagenous matrices in the adhesion and growth of cells. J. Cell Biol. **88**, 473–485 (1981). PMID: 7012158. https://doi.org/10.1083/jcb.88.3.473

78. Ricard-blum, S.: The collagen family. Cold Spring Harb. Perspect. Biol. 1–19 (2011). PMID: 21421911. https://doi.org/10.1101/cshperspect.a004978
79. Yu, X., Xu, L., Cui, F.Z., Qu, Y., Lian, X.J., Wang, X.M., Wang, Y.: Clinical evaluation of mineralized collagen as a bone graft substitute for anterior cervical intersomatic fusion. J. Biomater. Tissue Eng. **2**, 170–176 (2012). https://doi.org/10.1166/jbt.2012.1041
80. Wang, X.-M., Qiu, Z.-Y., Cui, H. (eds.): Mineralized Collagen Bone Graft Substitutes (2019)
81. Delabarde, C., Plummer, C.J.G., Bourban, P.E., Månson, J.A.E.: Solidification behavior of PLLA/nHA nanocomposites. Compos. Sci. Technol. **70**, 1813–1819 (2010). https://doi.org/10.1016/j.compscitech.2010.04.024
82. McMullan, D.: Scanning electron microscopy 1928–1965. Scanning **17**, 175–185 (2006). https://doi.org/10.1002/sca.4950170309
83. Yastrubchak, O., Łusakowska, E., Morawski, A., Demchuk, O., Wosiński, T.: Revealing of threading and misfit dislocations in partially relaxed InGaAs/GaAs heterostructures. Phys. Status Solidi C Conf. **1**, 401–404 (2004). https://doi.org/10.1002/pssc.200303954
84. Maruyama, K., Henmi, A., Okata, H., Sasano, Y.: Analysis of calcium, phosphorus, and carbon concentrations during developmental calcification of dentin and enamel in rat incisors using scanning electron microscopy with energy dispersive X-ray spectroscopy (SEM-EDX). J. Oral. Biosci. **58**, 173–179 (2016). https://doi.org/10.1016/j.job.2016.08.003
85. Abifarin, J.K., Obada, D.O., Dauda, E.T., Dodoo-Arhin, D.: Experimental data on the characterization of hydroxyapatite synthesized from biowastes. Data Br. **26**, 104485 (2019). https://doi.org/10.1016/j.dib.2019.104485
86. Curtis, R.V., Watson, T.F.: Dental Biomaterials: Imaging, Testing and Modelling (2008)
87. Hoehn, M., Küstermann, E., Blunk, J., Wiedermann, D., Trapp, T., Wecker, S., Föcking, M., Arnold, H., Hescheler, J., Fleischmann. B.K., Schwindt, W., Bührle, C.: Monitoring of implanted stem cell migration in vivo: a highly resolved in vivo magnetic resonance imaging investigation of experimental stroke in rat. Proc. Natl. Acad. Sci. USA **99**, 16267–16272 (2002). PMID: 12444255. https://doi.org/10.1073/pnas.242435499
88. Farrar, M.J., Bernstein, I.M., Schlafer, D.H., Cleland, T.A., Fetcho, J.R., Schaffer, C.B.: Chronic in vivo imaging in the mouse spinal cord using an implanted chamber. Nat. Methods **9**, 297–302 (2012). PMID: 22266542. https://doi.org/10.1038/nmeth.1856
89. Osorio, M., Cañas, A., Puerta, J., Díaz, L., Naranjo, T., Ortiz, I., Castro, C.: Ex vivo and in vivo biocompatibility assessment (blood and tissue) of three-dimensional bacterial nanocellulose biomaterials for soft tissue implants. Sci Rep. **9**, 1–14 (2019). PMID: 31332259. https://doi.org/10.1038/s41598-019-46918-x
90. Dalecki, D., Mercado, K.P., Hocking, D.C.: Quantitative ultrasound for nondestructive characterization of engineered tissues and biomaterials. Ann. Biomed. Eng. **44**, 636–648 (2016). PMID: 26581347. https://doi.org/10.1007/s10439-015-1515-0
91. Beckhoff, B., Kanngießer, B., Langhoff, N., Wedell, R., Wolff, H.: Handbook of Practical X-ray Fluorescence Analysis (2006)
92. Birkholz, M.: Principles of X-ray Diffraction (2014)
93. Neldam, C.A., Pinholt, E.M.: Synchrotron μcT imaging of bone, titanium implants and bone substitutes—a systematic review of the literature. J. Cranio-Maxillofacial Surg. **42**, 801–805 (2014). PMID: 24389092. https://doi.org/10.1016/j.jcms.2013.11.015
94. Bae, E.B., Kim, H.J., Ahn, J.J., Bae, H.Y., Kim, H.J., Huh, J.B.: Comparison of bone regeneration between porcine-derived and bovine-derived xenografts in rat calvarial defects: a non-inferiority study. Materials (Basel) **12** (2019). https://doi.org/10.3390/ma12203412
95. Buschmann, J., Welti, M., Hemmi, S., Neuenschwander, P., Baltes, C., Giovanoli, P., Rudin, M., Calcagni, M.: Three-dimensional co-cultures of osteoblasts and endothelial cells in degrapol foam: histological and high-field magnetic resonance imaging analyses of pre-engineered capillary networks in bone grafts. Tissue Eng. Part A **17**, 291–299 (2011). PMID: 20799888. https://doi.org/10.1089/ten.tea.2010.0278
96. Prasadh, S., Wong, R.C.W.: Unraveling the mechanical strength of biomaterials used as a bone scaffold in oral and maxillofacial defects. Oral. Sci. Int. **15**, 48–55 (2018)

97. Misch, C.E., Qu, Z., Bidez, M.W.: Mechanical properties of trabecular bone in the human mandible: implications for dental implant treatment planning and surgical placement. J. Oral. Maxillofac. Surg. **57**, 700–706 (1999). PMID: 10368096. https://doi.org/10.1016/S0278-2391(99)90437-8
98. Mahato, K.K., Biswal, M., Rathore, D.K., Prusty, R.K., Dutta, K., Ray, B.C.: Effect of loading rate on tensile properties and failure behavior of glass fibre/epoxy composite. IOP Conf. Ser. Mater. Sci. Eng. **115** (2016). https://doi.org/10.1088/1757-899X/115/1/012017
99. Downling, N.E.: Mechanical Behavior of Materials: Engineering Methods for Deformation, Fracture, and Fatigue (2012)
100. Fell, J.T., Newton, J.M.: Determination of tablet strength by the diametral-compression test. J. Pharm. Sci. **59**, 688–691 (1970). PMID: 5446428. https://doi.org/10.1002/jps.2600590523
101. Awaji, H., Watanabe, T., Nagano, Y.: Compressive testing of ceramics. Ceram. Int. **20**, 159–167 (1994). https://doi.org/10.1016/0272-8842(94)90034-5
102. Vitale-Brovarone, C., Baino, F., Verné, E.: High strength bioactive glass-ceramic scaffolds for bone regeneration. J. Mater. Sci. Mater. Med. **20**, 643–653 (2009). PMID: 18941868. https://doi.org/10.1007/s10856-008-3605-0
103. Baino, F., Verné, E., Vitale-Brovarone, C.: 3-D high-strength glass-ceramic scaffolds containing fluoroapatite for load-bearing bone portions replacement. Mater. Sci. Eng. C **29**, 2055–2062 (2009). https://doi.org/10.1016/j.msec.2009.04.002
104. Fundamentals of materials science. In: Craig's Restorative Dental Materials, pp. 33–81. Elsevier (2012)
105. Pawelec, K.M., White, A.A., Best, S.M.: Properties and Characterization of Bone Repair Materials, 2nd ed. Elsevier Ltd (2019)
106. Liu, C., Shao, H., Chen, F., Zheng, H.: Rheological properties of concentrated aqueous injectable calcium phosphate cement slurry. Biomaterials **27**, 5003–5013
107. Bohner, M., Baroud, G.: Injectability of calcium phosphate pastes. Biomaterials **26**, 1553–1563 (2005). PMID: 15522757. https://doi.org/10.1016/j.biomaterials.2004.05.010
108. Gbureck, U., Barralet, J.E., Spatz, K., Grover, L.M., Thull, R.: Ionic modification of calcium phosphate cement viscosity. Part I: Hypodermic injection and strength improvement of apatite cement. Biomaterials **25**, 2187–2195 (2004). PMID: 14741634. https://doi.org/10.1016/j.biomaterials.2003.08.066
109. Barralet, J.E., Grover, L.M., Gbureck, U.: Ionic modification of calcium phosphate cement viscosity. Part II: Hypodermic injection and strength improvement of brushite cement. Biomaterials **25**, 2197–2203 (2004). PMID: 14741635. https://doi.org/10.1016/j.biomaterials.2003.09.085
110. Gbureck, U., Spatz, K., Thull, R., Barralet, J.E.: Rheological enhancement of mechanically activated α-tricalcium phosphate cements. J. Biomed. Mater. Res. Part B Appl. Biomater. **73**, 1–6 (2005). PMID: 15627245. https://doi.org/10.1002/jbm.b.30148
111. Liu, C., Shao, H., Chen, F., Zheng, H.: Effects of the granularity of raw materials on the hydration and hardening process of calcium phosphate cement. Biomaterials **24**, 4103–4113 (2003). PMID: 12853240. https://doi.org/10.1016/S0142-9612(03)00238-2

Comparison of Numerical Model with Experimental Measurements for the Purpose of Testing Partially and Fully Biodegradable Stents

Nenad Filipović

Abstract Atherosclerosis is a progressive disease characterized by the accumulation of lipids and fibrous elements in the arterial wall. This accumulation produces plaque in the arteries. Percutaneous transluminal coronary angioplasty (PTCA) is a minimally invasive procedure that opens narrowed coronary arteries because of the plaque growth. A medical device that can hold an artery open in the area of narrowing is called a stent and it usually resembles a mesh tube. Mechanical stent tests are standard preclinical procedure used to simulate stent behavior for different physiological conditions. In this research, a mechanical test called three-point bending test was performed on a partially and fully bioresorbable vascular scaffold (BVS) manufactured by Boston Scientific Limited [1]. Poly-L-lactic acid (PLLA) material model was implemented for the numerical model inside in-house PAK [2] software. Measurements obtained by mechanical testing were compared with the numerical results. There is a strong correlation between the numerical simulation and real experiments with a coefficient of determination (R^2) > 0.99 and a correlation coefficient (R) > 0.99. It can be concluded that in silico mechanical tests can partially or fully replace in vitro stent tests, which can open a new avenue for regulatory submission and change regulatory ISO standard procedures.

Keywords Partially biodegradable stent · Fully biodegradable stent · Numerical model · Mechanical testing · Three-point bending test

1 Introduction

Cardiovascular diseases are one of the leading causes of death globally. Coronary artery disease (CAD), the most common type of heart disease, is caused by the narrowing of the coronary arteries as a result of atherosclerosis.

N. Filipović (✉)
Faculty of Engineering, University of Kragujevac, Kragujevac, Serbia
e-mail: fica@kg.ac.rs

Biomedical Research and Development Center, BioIRC, Kragujevac, Serbia

S. Najman et al. (eds.), *Bioceramics, Biomimetic and Other Compatible Materials Features for Medical Applications*, Engineering Materials,
https://doi.org/10.1007/978-3-031-17269-4_11

Atherosclerosis is characterized by endothelial dysfunction, vasculitis and accumulation of lipid, cholesterol and cell elements inside blood vessels' walls. Cholesterol deposition inside the wall is called plaque and it is the main contributing factor to the process of stenosis.

Percutaneous transluminal coronary angioplasty (PTCA) is a minimally invasive therapy in which a catheter balloon is inflated to a nominal pressure, compressing the atherosclerotic plaque inside the arterial wall and deploying the stent. It directly opens the artery and enables normal blood flow to other organs.

It is has been shown that PCTA has a very good success rate; however, in some patients, plaque can build again 6–12 months after the procedure. This process is called restenosis and it is the principal limitation of PCTA procedure [3].

It is quite demanding to experimentally measure the performance of a stent deployed in a coronary artery. Numerical simulations can be regarded as a good alternative and facilitate all procedures for stent design and performance assessment.

Finite element method is a well-known methodology used in solid and fluid mechanics. There are many biomechanics studies which have shown benefits of using this methodology in the investigation of structural properties of a stent during deployment phase [4–8].

Due to the rapid growth of computing power in recent years, the possibilities of finite element method application have significantly increased.

During stent deployment procedure, corresponding boundary conditions are applied. Expansion of the balloon is modeled with pressure boundary condition, while the nonlinear model of the balloon and arterial wall is taken into consideration. Stent model is also nonlinear with specific material characteristics. There are different unknown values which need to be calculated when using the finite element methodology such as displacement, stress, strain, shear stress, pressure etc.

In standard structural analysis, two different methodologies are applied: static and explicit. Obviously, in non-linear static structural analysis, dynamics effects are not considered. Nonlinearity also demands small time steps for calculation of large deformations. In order to solve these high nonlinear equations, iterative solver Newton–Raphson [9] is implemented.

Different stent designs have been investigated which include geometry and material properties [9–11]. Dumoulin and Cochelin [10] were among the first scientists who investigated the Palmaz-Schatz stent during deployment. They used a simple numerical model based on the repeated unit cellapproach. As a boundary condition, a constant pressure load was applied. Additionally, buckling and fatigue life cycle were simulated. Calculated data were validated using manufacturer's data. Good matching between the results was achieved.

Etave et al. [11] investigated coil and tubular stents' deployment characteristics. A displacement-driven loading condition was applied on the stent nodes during stent expansion.

Migliavacca et al. [12] examined the effect of geometrical parameters of the Palmaz-Schatz stent on its deployment characteristics. Numerical results were compared to the Carbostent and Multi-Link Tetra stent [13]. The results showed that geometrical parameters have a significant impact on the deployment characteristics.

Several studies examined stent performance using the expansion model [14–17]. Other authors considered idealized arterial geometry [13, 18–21].

Karanasiou et al. [22] made a three-dimensional reconstruction of the coronary artery based on IVUS and angiography of a real patient.

Biodegradable stents should keep an artery open and support it mechanically for a period of time that is necessary for the artery to heal. This is not a trivial task. It is very demanding to create and design such a stent under complex material, geometry and loading conditions.

Normal vasomotion and arterial function can be restored with permanent metal drug-eluting stents. The same can be achieved using a biodegradable stent but they can also make a reservoir for larger drug doses and improve drug delivery design [23]. After some time, the biodegradable stent degrades making the artery clean for further treatment, if necessary, which is not the case for metallic stent.

Some authors investigated material properties that include the effects of mechanical deformation in conditions of accelerating biodegradation [24–26].

It is a simple model where material is characterized with a neo-Hookean, purely elastic model. The energy density function for neo-Hookean material is dependent on shear modulus and the first principal invariant of the right Cauchy-Green deformation tensor.

Shear modulus is typically a material constant estimated from load-deformation experiments. However, in the case of biodegradable material, this material property changes over time as material degrades. For fully degraded material, it has value 1, while for undegraded material it has value 0 [25].

Usually, polymers are used for manufacturing biodegradable stents. This material exhibits complex nonlinear stress versus strain responses. Simple material models based on the Taylor expansion in strain invariant space such as neo-Hookean or Mooney-Rivlin models are not suitable to fully describe their behavior. Vieira et al. [27] defined the observed responses from experimental research with the neo-Hookean, Mooney-Rivlin and reduced 2nd order hyperelastic models.

Vieira et al. [28] considered a Bergstrom-Boyce microstructurally inspired hyperelastic material model [29]. This material is able to record the strain softening behavior of blends of PLA and PCL under multiple uniaxial loading–unloading cycles of different magnitude.

In this study, a partially BVS stent (SYNERGY™ BP (Bioabsorbable Polymer) Everolimus-Eluting Platinum Chromium Coronary Stent—Boston Scientific Limited) and a fully BVS stent (prototype polymeric bioresorbable stent made from PLLA—Boston Scientific Limited) were investigated experimentally and using a finite element model.

PLLA experimental curves with three different strain rates: 0.001, 0.01 and 0.1 s^{-1} were used to define the material model. Three-point bending test is presented in the Results section. A comparison of the results obtained from the simulation and real experiments is provided with the coefficient of determination and correlation coefficient.

2 Method

The SYNERGY™ BP stent is made of a platinum-chromium alloy (Pt-Cr) which exhibits bi-linear elastoplastic behaviour. Material properties such as material density, Young's modulus, Poisson's ratio and yield stress were taken from [30].

Geometrical model of the polymeric prototype of a bioresorbable stent has a length of 16 mm and an internal diameter of 3 mm, the same as the tube used for laser cutting of the stent, with a strut width of 184 μm and a strut thickness of 115 μm.

The stent is made from PLLA and the geometrical model is presented in Fig. 1. The length of the stent is 16 mm with the internal diameter of 3 mm, with a strut width of 184 μm and a strut thickness of 115 μm.

There are 49,464 hexahedral elements in the model which are presented in Fig. 2.

PLLA stent is elasto-visco-plastic polymer which has non-trivial mechanical behaviour dependent on the strain rate and operating temperature.

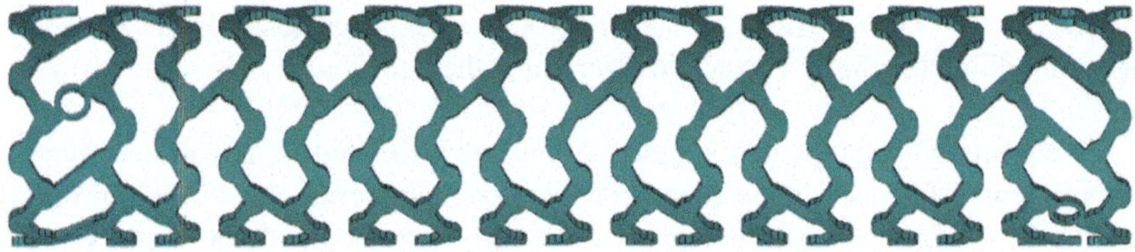

Fig. 1 Geometrical model of the bioresorbable stent prototype

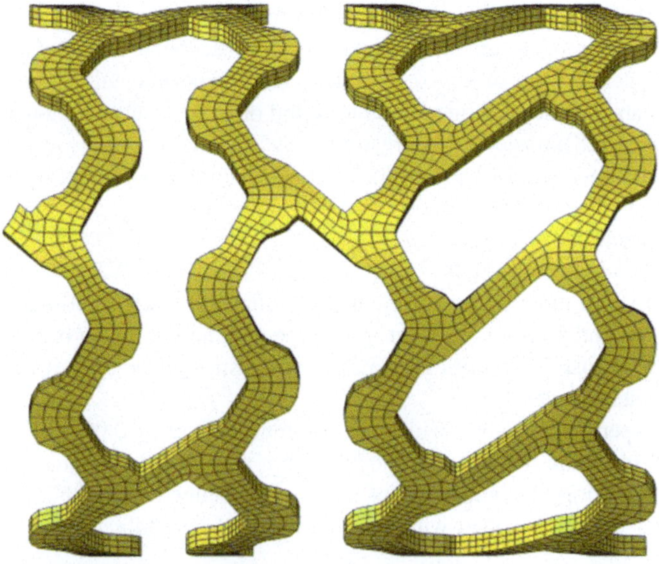

Fig. 2 Details of meshed bioresorbable stent prototype

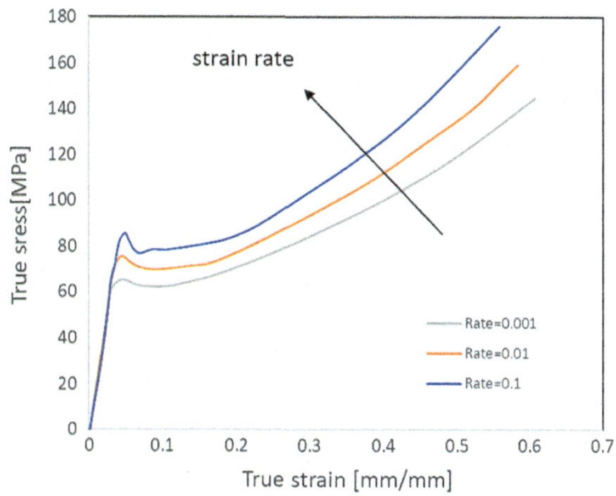

Fig. 3 Average tensile test results provided by BSL and strain rates

Experimental curves presented in Fig. 3 were used for the model implemented in PAK solver [2].

Uniaxial tensile tests are performed on a number of dog-bone samples at three different temperatures—25, 37 and 48 °C. There are also three different strain rates for each temperature: 0.001, 0.01 and 0.1 s^{-1}. It can be seen that the three curves show a common initial elastic response, a strain rate dependent yield point and plastic behavior ending with a strong hardening.

Standard equilibrium equations [4, 31, 32] are used for the finite element method:

$$\frac{\partial \sigma_{ik}}{\partial x_k} + f_i^V = 0, \quad i, j = 1, 2, 3 \tag{1}$$

including inertial and dissipative forces and satisfying loading and displacement boundary conditions [33]. Solid dynamics is defined in the discrete form:

$$\boldsymbol{M}\ddot{u} + \boldsymbol{B}\dot{u} + \boldsymbol{K}u = \boldsymbol{F} \tag{2}$$

where:

$\boldsymbol{M} = \int_V \rho N^T N \mathrm{d}V$—mass matrix,
$\boldsymbol{B} = \int_V b N^T N \mathrm{d}V$—damping matrix,
$\boldsymbol{K} = \int_V B^T C B \mathrm{d}V$—stiffness matrix,
$\boldsymbol{F}$—vector of external forces.

Interactions between the two bodies [34–36] are shown in Fig. 4.

Contact interaction between the bodies comes and disappears as an elastic support in the contact points. It is applied to both bodies since outer nodes of the first body can come in contact with surfaces of the second body and vice versa.

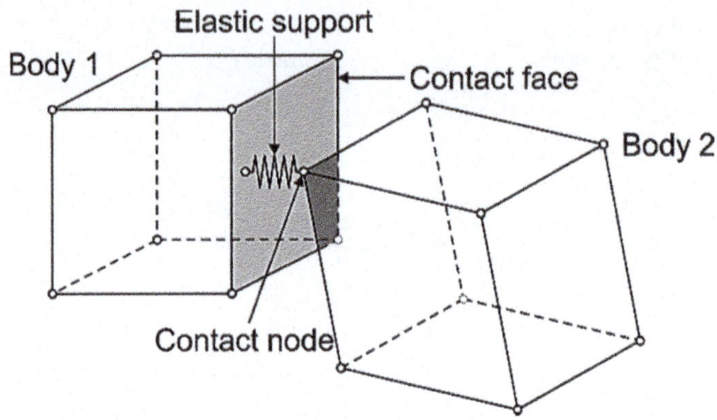

Fig. 4 Interaction between two solid bodies

3 Results for Three-Point Bending Test

Stent flexibility is defined with the three-point bending test. The stent is positioned so that the central stent axis is collinear with the Z-axis. Three rigid body cylinders are positioned in such a way that their central axis is collinear with the X-axis. Axial force is applied on the top cylinder, and bottom cylinders are fixed. The corresponding boundary conditions for this test are shown in Fig. 5 (right).

The stress distribution from applied numerical model is shown in Fig. 6. In Fig. 7, there is a comparison of the displacement-force curve results between the numerical model and real experimental measurements. There are two representative diameter-pressure curves from actual test articles. Data from all n = 4 curves were used in the numerical simulation (Table 2).

The results from mechanical testing are presented in the form of force—displacement curves in Fig. 9.

The stress distribution from the three-point bending numerical model is presented in Fig. 8. Force–displacement (dash) curve is shown in Fig. 9.

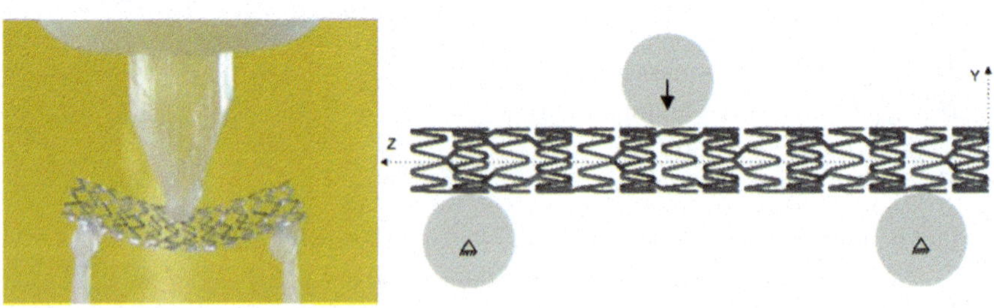

Fig. 5 Real mechanical test setup for three-point bend test (left); three-point bend test simulation (right)

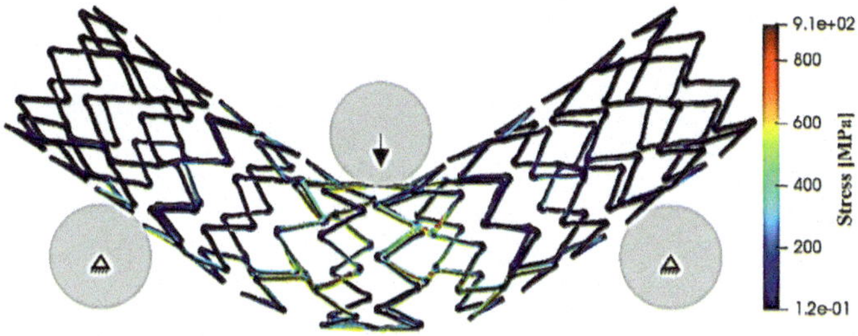

Fig. 6 Stress distribution—three-point bending test for partially BVS stent

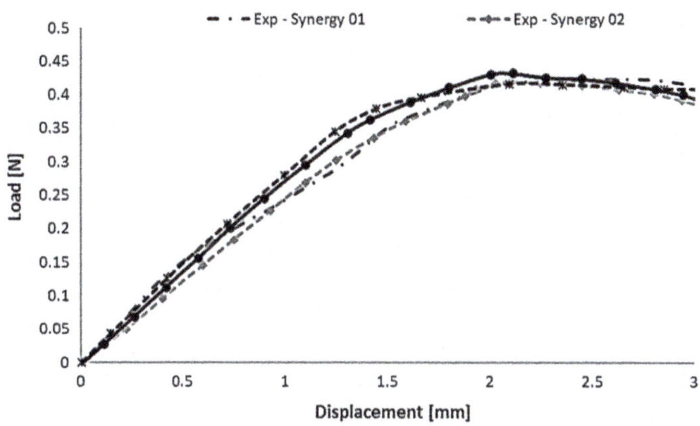

Fig. 7 Comparison of displacement-load curves, PAK versus experiment for stent device, three-point bending test for partially BVS stent

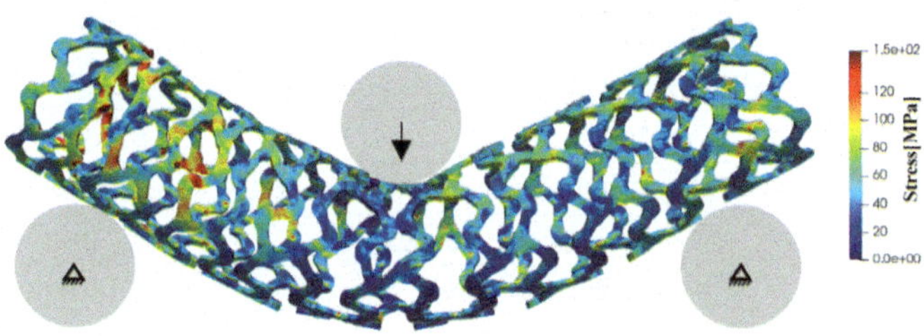

Fig. 8 Stress distribution—three-point bending model for fully BVS stent

4 Discussion

It can be seen from Fig. 7 that results for the displacement-force in the three-point test numerical model are very close to the experimental measurements. This comparison was validated and quantified by the coefficient of determination (R^2) and correlation

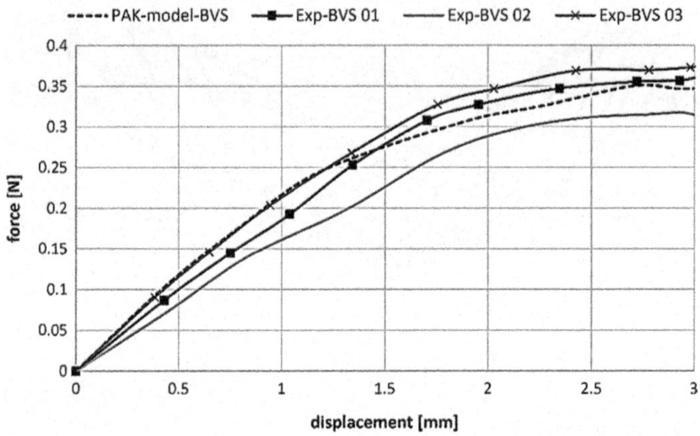

Fig. 9 Comparison of displacement-force curves, PAK versus experiment three-point bending test for fully BVS stent

coefficient (R) calculated between the simulation curve and all points from all experimental curves (Table 1). Bland–Altman plots for the graphs (Fig. 7) are presented in Fig. 10. Quantification showed a strong correlation between the numerical model and experiments with $R^2 = 0.99$ and $R = 0.995$. Bland–Altman plot with data points located within mean ±1.96 standard deviations is shown in Fig. 10.

It can be seen from Fig. 9 that the three-point test numerical model in the case of BVS stent devices is in good agreement with the experimental test. The precision of the numerical model is quantified by the coefficient of determination (R^2) and correlation coefficient (R) calculated between the numerical model curve and all experimental curves (Table 2) as well as with the Bland–Altman plot presented in Fig. 11.

Table 1 Statistical analysis of results—three-point bending

Model	Synergy N = 4
Coefficient of determination R^2	0.9900
Correlation coefficient R	0.995
Significance level	$P < 0.0001$

Table 2 Coefficient of determination (R^2)—longitudinal tensile test, fast protocol

Model	BVS prototype devices N = 4
Coefficient of determination R^2	0.9954
Correlation coefficient R	0.996
Significance level	$P < 0.0001$

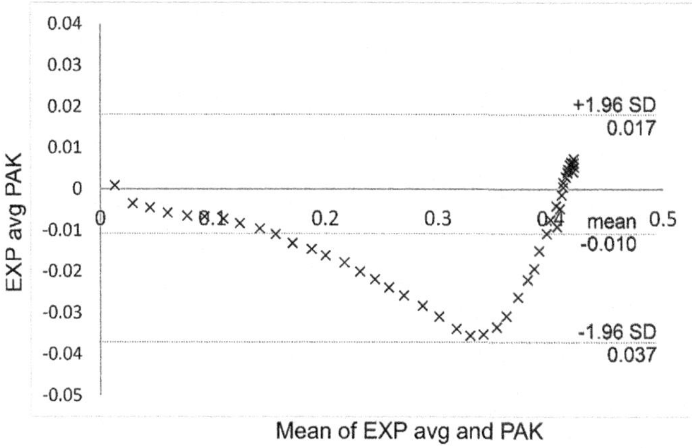

Fig. 10 Bland–Altman plot for center position of partially BVS stent device—three-point bending

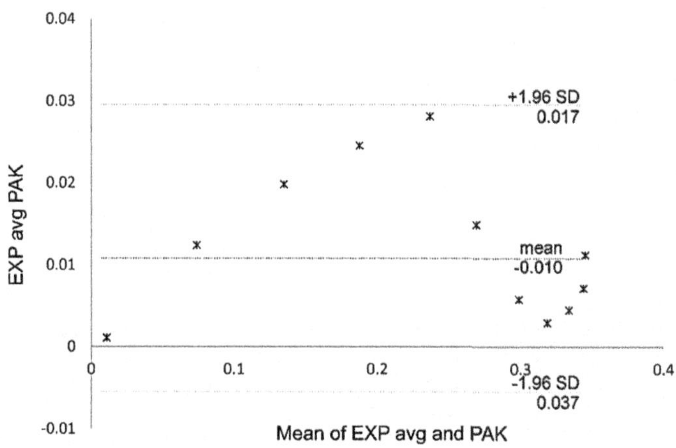

Fig. 11 Bland–Altman plot for fully BVS prototype stent device—three-point bending test

5 Conclusion

Experimental and numerical mechanical tests with two different types of stents were presented. The first stent is a partially BVS device and Boston Scientific Limited is a fully BVS device. The curves for experimental measurement and numerical modeling have been shown for comparison. It can be observed that diameter—load curves or pressure—diameter curves show a high correlation with results from the real mechanical tests. A strong correlation exists between the numerical model and experimental test for the coefficient of determination ($R^2 > 0.99$) and correlation coefficient ($R > 0.99$).

It can be concluded that numerical modeling and in silico tests have demonstrated to be capable of partially or fully replacing in vitro mechanical tests, which can open a new avenue for regulatory submission for stent as a medical device.

Acknowledgements This study was funded by the European Project H2020 InSilc [grant number 777119] and Serbian Ministry of Education, Science, and Technological Development [451-03-68/2020-14/200107 (Faculty of Engineering, University of Kragujevac). This chapter reflects only the author's view. The Commission is not responsible for any use that may be made of the information it contains.

References

1. Jovicic, G., Vukicevic, A., Filipovic, N.: Computational assessment of stent durability using fatigue to fracture approach. J Med Dev **8**(4), 041002 (2014). https://doi.org/10.1115/1.4027687
2. Kojic M, Filipovic N et al (2022). http://www.bioirc.ac.rs/index.php/software/5-pak. Last visited: 29 September 2022
3. Martin, D., Boyle, F.J.: Computational structural modelling of coronary stent deployment: a review. Comput Methods Biomech Biomed Eng **14**(4), 331–348 (2011). https://doi.org/10.1080/10255841003766845
4. Balossino, R., Gervaso, F., Migliavacca, F., Dubini, G.: Effects of different stent designs on local hemodynamics in stented arteries. J Biomech **41**(5), 1053–1061 (2008). https://doi.org/10.1016/j.jbiomech.2007.12.005
5. LaDisa, J., Hettrick, D., Olson, L., Guler, I., Gross, E., Kress, T., Kersten, J., Warltier, D., Pagel, P.: Stent implantation alters coronary artery hemodynamics and wall shear stress during maximal vasodilation. J Appl Physiol **93**(6), 1939–1946 (2002). https://doi.org/10.1152/japplphysiol.00544.2002
6. LaDisa, J., Olson, L., Guler, I., Hettrick, D., Audi, S., Kersten, J., Warltier, D., Pagel, P.: Stent design properties and deployment ratio influence indexes of wall shear stress: a three-dimensional computational fluid dynamics investigation within a normal artery. J Appl Physiol **97**(1), 424–430 (2004). https://doi.org/10.1152/japplphysiol.01329.2003
7. Pontrelli G, de Monte F (2007) Modelling of mass convection diffusion in stent-based drug-delivery. Paper presented at: XXV Congresso Nazionale UIT sulla Trasmssione del Calore, 18–20 May 2007, Trieste
8. Zunino, P., D'Angelo, C., Petrini, L., Vergara, C., Capelli, C., Migliavacca, F.: Numerical simulation of drug eluting coronary stents: mechanics, fluid dynamics and drug release. Comput Methods Appl Mech Eng **198**, 3633–3644 (2009). https://doi.org/10.1016/j.cma.2008.07.019
9. Mac Donald BJ (2007) Practical stress analysis with finite elements. Glasnevin Publishing, Dublin
10. Dumoulin, C., Cochelin, B.: Mechanical behaviour modelling of balloon-expandable stents. J Biomech **33**, 1461–1470 (2000). https://doi.org/10.1016/S0021-9290(00)00098-1
11. Etave, F., Finet, G., Boivin, M., Boyer, J.C., Rioufol, G., Thollet, G.: Mechanical properties of coronary stents determined by using finite element analysis. J Biomech **34**(8), 1065–1075 (2001). https://doi.org/10.1016/s0021-9290(01)00026-4
12. Migliavacca, F., Petrini, L., Montanari, V., Quagliana, I., Auricchio, F., Dubini, G.: A predictive study of the mechanical behaviour of coronary stents by computer modelling. Med Eng Phys **27**(1), 13–18 (2005). https://doi.org/10.1016/j.medengphy.2004.08.012
13. Chua, D., MacDonald, B., Hashmi, M.: Finite element simulation of slotted tube (stent) with the presence of plaque and artery by balloon expansion. J Mater Process Technol **155–156**, 1772–1779 (2004). https://doi.org/10.1016/j.jmatprotec.2004.04.396

14. Chua, D., MacDonald, B., Hashmi, M.: Effects of varying slotted tube (stent) geometry on its expansion behaviour using finite element method. J Mater Process Technol **155–156**, 1764–1771 (2004). https://doi.org/10.1016/j.jmatprotec.2004.04.395
15. Bathe, K.J.: Finite element procedures. Prentice-Hall, Englewood Cliffs, NJ (1996)
16. De Beule, M., Mortier, P., Carlier, S.G., Verhegghe, B., Van Impe, R., Verdonck, P.: Realistic finite element-based stent design: the impact of balloon folding. J Biomech **41**(2), 383–389 (2008). https://doi.org/10.1016/j.jbiomech.2007.08.014
17. Petrini, L., Migliavacca, F., Auricchio, F., Dubini, G.: Numerical investigation of the intravascular coronary stent flexibility. J Biomech **37**, 495–501 (2004). https://doi.org/10.1016/j.jbiomech.2003.09.002
18. Auricchio, F., Di Loreto, M., Sacco, E.: Finite element analysis of a stenotic artery revascularisation through a stent insertion. Comput Methods Biomech Biomed Eng **4**, 249–263 (2001). https://doi.org/10.1080/10255840108908007
19. Capelli, C., Gervaso, F., Petrini, L., Dubini, G., Migliavacca, F.: Assessment of tissue prolapse after balloon-expandable stenting: influence of stent cell geometry. Med Eng Phys **31**(4), 441–447 (2009). https://doi.org/10.1016/j.medengphy.2008.11.002
20. Holzapfel, G.A., Stadler, M., Gasser, T.C.: Changes in the mechanical environment of stenotic arteries during interaction with stents: computational assessment of parametric stent designs. J Biomech Eng **127**(1), 166–180 (2005). https://doi.org/10.1115/1.1835362
21. Lally, C., Dolan, F., Prendergast, P.J.: Cardiovascular stent design and vessel stresses: a finite element analysis. J Biomech **38**(8), 1574–1581 (2005). https://doi.org/10.1016/j.jbiomech.2004.07.022
22. Karanasiou GS et al (2018) In Silico analysis of stent deployment-effect of stent design. In: 40th annual international conference of the IEEE engineering in medicine and biology society (EMBC), Honolulu, HI, pp 4567–4570. https://doi.org/10.1109/EMBC.2018.8513205
23. Soares JS, Moore JE (2015) Biomechanical challenges to polymeric biodegradable stents. Ann Biomed Eng 44:560–579. https://doi.org/10.1007/s10439-015-1477-2
24. Soares JS, Moore Jr JE, Rajagopal KR (2007) Modeling of biological materials. Mollica F, Preziosi L, Rajagopal KR (eds). Birkhauser Basel, pp 125–177
25. Soares JS, Moore Jr JE, Rajagopal KR (2008) Constitutive framework for biodegradable polymers with applications to biodegradable stents. ASAIO J 54(3):295–301. https://doi.org/10.1097/MAT.0b013e31816ba55a
26. Soares JS, Rajagopal KR, Moore Jr JE (2010) Deformation-induced hydrolysis of a degradable polymeric cylindrical annulus. Biomech Model Mechanobiol 9:177–186.https://doi.org/10.1007/s10237-009-0168-z
27. Vieira, A.C., Vieira, J.C., Ferra, J.M., Magalhaes, F.D., Guedes, R.M., Marques, A.T.: Mechanical study of PLA–PCL fibers during in vitro degradation. J Mech Behav Biomed Mater **4**, 451–460 (2011). https://doi.org/10.1016/j.jmbbm.2010.12.006
28. Vieira, A.C., Guedes, R.M., Tita, V.: Constitutive modeling of biodegradable polymers: hydrolytic degradation and time-dependent behavior. Int J Solids Struct **51**, 1164–1174 (2014). https://doi.org/10.1016/j.ijsolstr.2013.12.010
29. Bergstrom, J.S., Boyce, M.C.: Constitutive modeling of the large strain time-dependent behavior of elastomers. J Mech Phys Solids **46**, 931–954 (1998). https://doi.org/10.1016/S0022-5096(97)00075-6
30. O'Brien, B.J., Stinson, J.S., Larsen, S.R., Eppihimer, M.J., Carroll, W.M.: A platinum-chromium steel for cardiovascular stents. Biomaterials **31**(14), 3755–3761 (2010). https://doi.org/10.1016/j.biomaterials.2010.01.146
31. Kojic, M., Bathe, K.J.: Inelastic analysis of solids and structures. Springer, Berlin-Heidelberg-New York (2005)
32. Kojic M, Filipovic N, Stojanovic B, Kojic N (2008) Computer modeling in bioengineering—theoretical background, examples and software. Wiley, England. 978-0-470-06035-3
33. Isailovic, V., Kojic, M., Milosevic, M., Filipovic, N., Kojic, N., Ziemys, A., Ferrari, M.: A computational study of trajectories of micro- and nano-particles with different shapes in flow through small channels. J Serbian Soc Comput Mech **8**(2), 14–28 (2014). https://doi.org/10.5937/jsscm1402014I

34. Djukic, T., Saveljic, I., Pelosi, G., Parodi, O., Filipovic, N.: Numerical simulation of stent deployment within patient-specific artery and its validation against clinical data. Comput Methods Prog Biomed **175**, 121–127 (2019). https://doi.org/10.1016/j.cmpb.2019.04.005
35. Krsmanovic D, Filipovic N, Koncar I, Petrovic D, Milasinovic D, Davidovic L (2014) Computer modelling of maximal displacement forces in endoluminal thoracic aortic stent graft. Comput Methods Biomech Biomed Eng 17(9):1012–1020. https://doi.org/10.1080/10255842.2012.735661
36. Vukicevic, A.M., Stepanovic, N.M., Jovicic, G.R., Apostolovic, S.R., Filipovic, N.D.: Computer methods for follow-up study of hemodynamic and disease progression in the stented coronary artery by fusing IVUS and X-ray angiography. Med Biol Eng Comput **52**(6), 539–556 (2014). https://doi.org/10.1007/s11517-014-1155-9

Structural and Morphological Characterization of Strontium Ferrite-Ethylcellulose Nanocomposite for Application in Membrane Technology

Aleksandar Stajčić and Ivana Radović

Abstract Among many possible fields of application, membrane technology is very valuable for biological and medical purposes. As a young field with high potential for further expansion, it is of great interest for researches. This chapter presents preparation and characterization of magnetic nanocomposite membranes. Ethylcellulose-strontium ferrite (EC-$SrFe_{12}O_{19}$) nanocomposites were prepared via solvent casting method with applied low magnetic field. In order to identify morphological and topological changes induced by membrane processing, scanning electron microscopy (FESEM) and atomic force microscopy (AFM) were performed. Orientation of nanoparticles and formation of two-phase structure caused by the influence of magnetic field were observed. Infrared spectroscopy with Fourier transformation (FTIR) was used to prove the stability of starting components during processing of nanocomposite membrane. Nanoparticles' high reinforcing potential was proved by micro Vickers method and tensile test. Modulus of elasticity in EC-$SrFe_{12}O_{19}$ samples has increased up to 135%, compared to pure EC. The permeability of magnetic nanocomposite membranes was tested by monitoring the output pressure change of the nitrogen/oxygen mixtures, as well as pure nitrogen, using custom-made laboratory device. This technique also enabled investigation of membranes' mechanical performance by following changes in permeability with the pressure for each sample. Orientation of magnetic $SrFe_{12}O_{19}$ nanoparticles led to a formation of highly reinforced membranes that have potential application in membrane technology.

Keyword Membranes · Ethylcellulose · Air separation · Mechanical properties · Polymer nanocomposites

---

A. Stajčić (✉)
Center of Microelectronic Technologies, Institute of Chemistry, Technology and Metallurgy—National Institute of the Republic of Serbia, University of Belgrade, Belgrade, Serbia
e-mail: stajcic@nanosys.ihtm.bg.ac.rs

I. Radović
Department of Physical Chemistry-050, "VINČA" Institute of Nuclear Sciences—National Institute of the Republic of Serbia, University of Belgrade, Belgrade, Serbia
e-mail: ivana_r@vinca.rs

S. Najman et al. (eds.), *Bioceramics, Biomimetic and Other Compatible Materials Features for Medical Applications*, Engineering Materials,
https://doi.org/10.1007/978-3-031-17269-4_12

1 Introduction

Membrane technology is a relatively new and a fast growing multidisciplinary field emerging from the increased environmental concerns. This field includes mostly water and gas treatment, i.e. removal of potentially dangerous elements from water and the enrichment of gas mixtures with certain components, depending on the application demands [1–3]. Rising industrial need for membrane gas separation leads to diversity in their use, from nitrogen production, over purification of hydrogen and natural gas, to air enrichment by oxygen. So far, air enrichment industry has mostly been relying on old and energy consumptive cryogenic methods that further require high production costs. Polymer membranes are becoming attractive, due to their low cost production, good mechanical and chemical properties, as well as their diversity in composition and structure. They have a wide range of applications in industry and medicine, from different types of filtration, to gas separation [4–10]. The choice of polymer is based on specific properties, such as thermal, chemical and mechanical, which depend on structural factors [11]. In general, all polymers can be used as membrane materials, but the chemical and physical properties are so different that only a certain number of polymers are used in practice [12, 13]. Polymer membranes can be porous or non-porous [14]. In porous membranes, the process of membrane preparation, chemical and thermal stability, influences the choice of material, while in non-porous membranes the composition of the membrane has a significant influence. The most important properties of membranes, such as selectivity and permeability, depend on various factors in porous and non-porous polymer-based membranes. The selectivity of porous membranes is mostly determined by the pore dimensions, while in non-porous ones the influencing factor is the possibility of the membrane interacting with the permeate. The choice of material also affects adsorption and chemical stability, which means that the polymeric material is chosen not only on the basis of the required flow and selectivity, but also the chemical and thermal properties of the material [15, 16]. The major drawback of non-porous membranes represents a low selectivity/permeability ratio, as well as instability during processing (swelling, plasticization) [17–19]. The most commonly used polymers for membrane preparation are polyetarsulfone, cellulose esters and ethers, polyimide, polyamides, poly (vinylidene fluoride), polyetharetarketone [20]. Cellulose belongs to polysaccharides that can easily be converted to esters (cellulose acetate or nitrate) or to ethers (ethylcellulose). Since cellulose-based membranes have low adsorption characteristics, they are very useful for biopharmaceutical processes, where proteins cause rapid membrane contamination [21–23]. Ethyl ether of cellulose is nearly insoluble in water, glycerol and propane-1,2-diol, but it is soluble in certain organic solvents, depending on the ethoxyl fraction. Ethylcellulose (EC) is a non-toxic, inert and hydrophobic polymer, widely used for the preparation of pharmaceutical dosage forms. Figure 1 shows the structural formula of EC used as the matrix membrane material in this research.

Ethylcellulose has already been employed as a membrane for separation, dominantly in medical devices [24]. It is a biocompatible and widely used polymer, but with poor selectivity for separation of gas mixtures, especially O_2/N_2, where

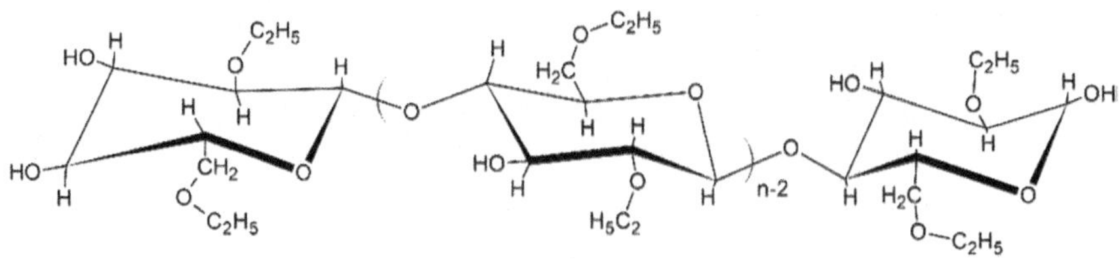

Fig. 1 Chemical structure of ethylcellulose (EC)

the elements have quite similar properties and it is hard to control the flow of the components separately.

Composite materials are multicomponent materials composed of two or more phases separated by an interfacial boundary [25–27]. The physical–mechanical properties of composites differ significantly from the properties of the initial constituents [28, 29]. The idea of combining several different materials into a composite stems from the need to modify existing materials. With the development of civilization and the need to use new materials, there was an expansion of production and improvement of composite materials at the industrial level. The formation of composites improves the structural, thermal, chemical and other properties of the starting components. As a result of the synergy of properties of different starting materials, composites have some of the following properties: high strength and stiffness, low density and mass, resistance to corrosion and high temperatures, chemical inertness, ability to process and shape into various shapes, and durability [30]. The development of modern composites is based on the possibility of designing their structure and properties by different methods of synthesis and processing. The resulting set of properties of the composite material can be achieved by combining the starting components at the macro-; micro- and nanoscopic scale [31–36]. As the need for new, more advanced materials is constantly growing, continuous research is being conducted into the possibilities of different basic materials classes' combinations: metals, ceramics and polymers. By targeted selection of constituents and the production process, it is possible to process composites of different properties and purposes—from materials intended for everyday life, through materials for construction, military, automotive, aerospace, medicine and electronics, to special purpose materials such as space industry [37–39]. Membrane technology belongs to the young branches of industry in which in recent years research has also turned to composites, with the aim of improving the separation and mechanical properties of existing materials.

In the initial development of composite membranes, the first approach was surface polycondensation, with the aim of forming a thin polymer layer on a substrate [40–42]. The contribution of this approach, known as surface polymerization (SP), was of paramount importance to membrane science and technology and is considered a quantum leap toward processing high-flow membranes at low pressures, with good salt removal ability. It is generally known that by using the SP technique, the properties of the upper and lower part of the film can be cut separately, with the aim of obtaining the desired rate of water permeation and solution separation.

Polymer-inorganic nanocomposite membranes could improve the permeability and selectivity of polymer membranes because they have the properties of polymer and inorganic membranes—high permeability and selectivity, mechanical strength and thermal/chemical stability [43]. Although there has been a huge progress in the polymers structure modification, with the aim of improving their separation properties, inorganic materials are still superior in this area. Major drawback in the use of inorganic membranes lies in the lack of technology for the formation of continuous membranes without damage, the cost of membrane production, as well as handling problems (brittleness). Therefore, a new approach of processing composite membranes could provide an alternative membrane with separation properties well above the upper limit between permeability and selectivity [44, 45].

1.1 Oxygen Enrichment

In addition to the separation of polluting elements from water using polymer membranes, the separation of gas mixtures is also an important industrial problem, with the aim of enriching gases with oxygen. Today, obtaining cheap high-purity gases or enriched gas mixtures (especially air) is a great challenge in industry and medicine, as well as in everyday life [46–48]. Oxygen separation is used in many applications, among which are medical devices [49, 50]. The three branches of technology for extracting oxygen from the air that currently exist include distillation, adsorption, and membranes [51, 52]. Membrane technology is the youngest of these three technologies and includes polymer and high-temperature ion transport membranes [53]. With an induced pressure difference, a selective O_2/N_2 polymer membrane, if it has properties that allow oxygen molecules to pass through the membrane more easily than nitrogen molecules, can partially extract oxygen from the air. However, the use of such membranes does not allow the complete separation of oxygen from the air; it can only be used to increase the oxygen concentration, while some nitrogen molecules will also pass through the membrane. This process is called *oxygen enrichment.* Some advantages offered by polymer membranes are: continuity of separation, low costs, energy efficiency, and regeneration is not required [54].

In general, membrane gas separation performance can be described by a dissolution/diffusion mechanism, which regulates permeability and selectivity. Permeability describes the ability of a membrane to allow gas to flow as a result of the difference in membrane pressure. It can be calculated using the following equation [55]:

$$P_A = \frac{N_A l}{(p_2 - p_1)}$$

where P_A stands for the membrane permeability, N_A represents the flux of the permeate gas, p_1 is the pressure at the front, and p_2 is the pressure at the back side.

When polymer membranes are used, the challenge in air separation is to create conditions for differences (other than sorption and diffusion properties) in mass transport between oxygen and nitrogen due to their similarity in properties and size. However, oxygen and nitrogen have completely different magnetic properties, the former is a paramagnetic element, while the latter is diamagnetic, which led to the idea for the processing of the so-called *magnetic membranes* [56–58].

By inserting magnetic nanoparticles into the polymer matrix, it is possible to obtain a nanocomposite of satisfactory separation properties, with a significant improvement in the mechanical properties of the polymer matrix itself. Ethylcellulose (EC) nanocomposite membranes will be presented in this chapter, where nanoparticles of strontium hexa-ferrite ($SrFe_{12}O_{19}$) magnetic powders were used as functional and mechanical reinforcement. Through the results and discussion, an insight will be given into the magnetic properties of nanoparticles, as well as their behavior in the polymer.

2 Ethylcellulose-Based Magnetic Nanocomposite Thin Films

Polymer solution casting method was used for the preparation of ethyl cellulose (EC) flat films (thickness 77–100 μm) and magnetic EC-$SrFe_{12}O_{19}$ (thickness 80–109 μm, depending on the filler content). The solution of EC in 40:60 ethanol/toluene mixture was left to dry at room temperature for 24 h exposed to a magnetic field of 30 mT using magnetic stripes. Prepared nanocomposite membranes had 10, 20 and 30 wt% of $SrFe_{12}O_{19}$, denoted EC-SrFe10, EC-SrFe20 and EC-SrFe30, respectively. Influence of the magnetic field on the nanocomposite membranes' morphology was investigated by Field Emission Scanning Electron Microscope (TESCAN MIRA 3). Software analysis of FESEM images was performed in *Image-Pro Plus*. Composition of particle-rich and polymer-rich zones was investigated using Fourier transform infrared spectroscopy- FTIR (Hartmann and Braun, MB-series). Spectra were recorded in transmission mode from 4000 to 400 cm^{-1}, with resolution of 4 cm^{-1}. Tensile test was performed on Autograph AG–X plus Universal Testing Machine (Shimadzu, Japan), at room temperature, in accordance with the ASTM D3039 standard. Tested samples had dimensions 60 $mm^2 \times 10$ mm^2. Each mechanical property is presented as the average value of the three measurements. Vickers microhardness tester "Leitz, Kleinharteprufer DURIMET I" (load at 4.9 N) was used for the investigation of nanoparticles' influence on microhardness. [59–61]. Atomic force microscopy (AFM) was performed using AutoProbe CP-Research SPM (TM Microscopes-Veeco) with Veeco Phosphorous (n)—sensor probe, model MPP-31123-10. Measurements were conducted in noncontact mode; scan surface was from 1×1 to 80×80 μm^2, with resolution of 256×256 dpi. Average roughness values (Ra) were calculated using software Veeco SPMLab NT Ver.6.0.2 on 2D images (0.8 $\mu m^2 \times 0.8$ μm^2).

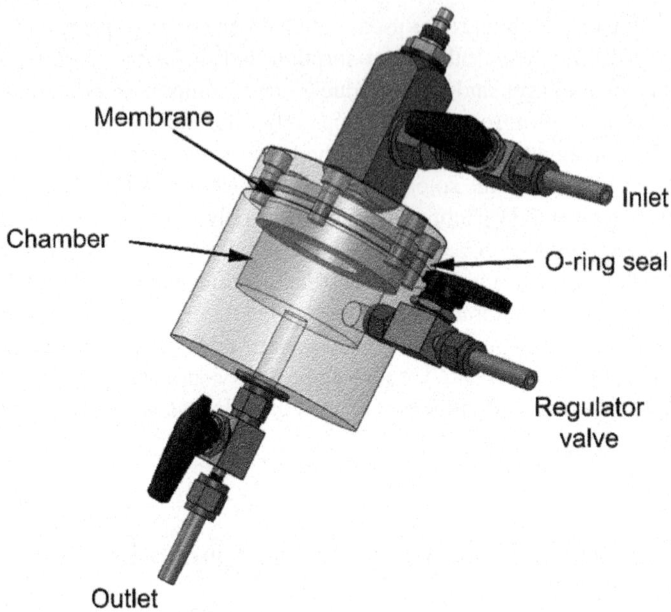

Fig. 2 3D model of diffusion chamber

Diffusion chamber used for permeability measurements was made at the Center of Microelectronic Technologies, ICTM, Belgrade. The three-dimensional model made in Solid Works, used in the design of the device, is shown in Fig. 2.

Pressurized gas has been introduced into the chamber, and the pressure was kept constant during each measurement. The inlet gas pressure ranged from 2 to 9 bar. The change in the output pressure was monitored on a device connected to the computer. The mixture used for the permeability test consisted of nitrogen and oxygen in a 95:5% ratio. Based on the measured changes in the values of the outlet pressures over time, the permeability for the gas mixture P (O_2/N_2) was calculated, as well as for pure nitrogen, P (N_2).

2.1 SQUID Analysis of $SrFe_{12}O_{19}$ Nanoparticles

Figure 3 shows the hysteresis loop of the $SrFe_{12}O_{19}$ nanoparticle, formed as a result of the SQUID analysis. The resulting hysteresis loop is typical for this type of material [62]. Considering that this is a magnetic ferrite, it is to be expected that the powder has higher coercivity. This can also be seen from the shown hysteresis, where the coercivity value was Hc = 363 kA/m = 4651 Oe.

Considering that the maximum strength of the applied magnetic field of 50 kOe is more than enough to achieve saturation magnetization (the proof is seen from the

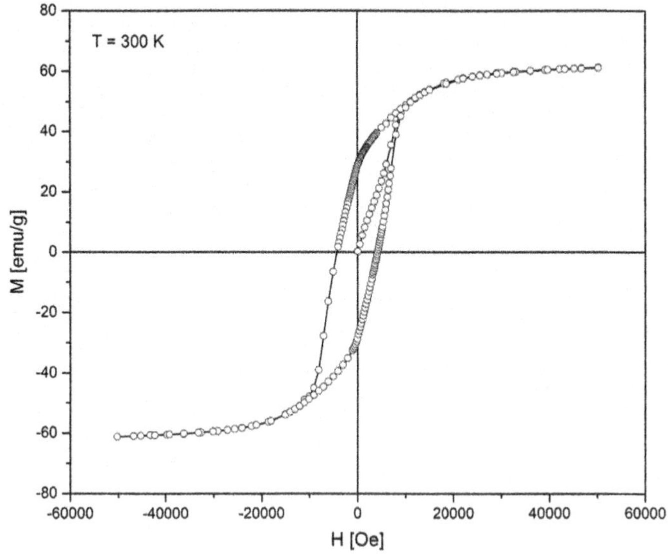

Fig. 3 Hysteresis loop for nanoparticles $SrFe_{12}O_{19}$

figure because the curves are both in the negative and the positive region practically parallel to the x axis), it can be concluded that the values for Ms and Mr read from the obtained hysteresis represent the real values of these parameters.

2.2 *FESEM Analysis of the EC-SrFe Nanocomposite Membrane Thin Films*

Images of EC-SrFe10 and EC-SrFe20 obtained by FESEM analysis are shown in Figs. 4, 5, 6 and 7. The magnetization of samples during processing was expected to induce orientation of nanoparticles, which could further lead to improved mechanical properties. As shown in Fig. 4, FESEM micrograph revealed a clear separation between $SrFe_{12}O_{19}$-rich (bright areas) and EC-rich (dark areas) areas. Obviously, exposure of the sample to a magnetic field during processing led to the phase separation, that is, a controlled formation of agglomerates. The orientation of nanoparticles in polymer-rich areas is obvious with a 50× magnification (Fig. 4 left).

The magnification of 500× showed the formation of branched nanoparticle structures (light areas) in the polymer-rich phase, along with formed clusters (Fig. 4 right).

The particles were oriented by the magnetic field lines in such a way that there is an almost continuous path filled with them in the polymer-rich phase, which indicates the potential for oxygen separation.

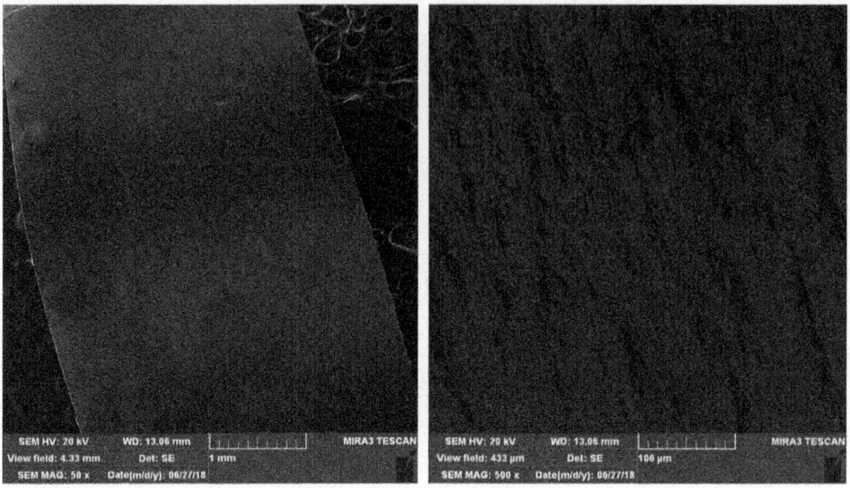

Fig. 4 FESEM of the nanocomposite EC-SrFe20

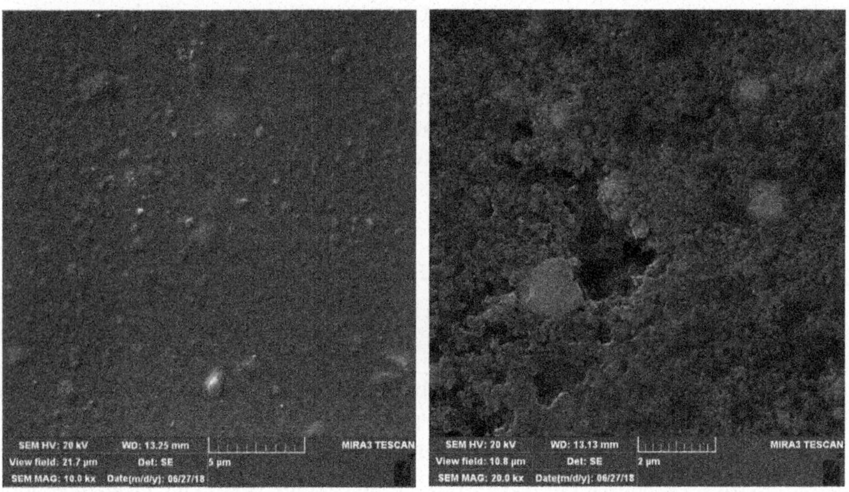

Fig. 5 Areas rich in EC (left) and nanoparticles $SrFe_{12}O_{19}$ (right) in EC-SrFe10

Figures 5 and 6 show the difference between polymer-rich and nanoparticles-rich areas for the membranes with 10 and 20% of $SrFe_{12}O_{19}$. For the purpose of software image analysis, FESEM images obtained with 50 and 100 kx magnification were used.

For illustration purposes, Fig. 7 (left) shows $SrFe_{12}O_{19}$ nanoparticles and their agglomerates in the nanoparticles-rich area. A mask made in image analysis software (*Image Pro Plus*) based on which the particle size is determined is also shown in Fig. 7

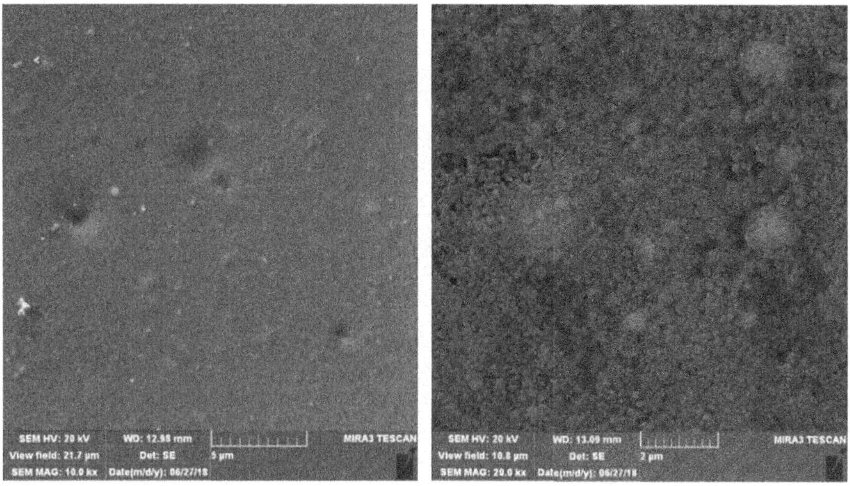

Fig. 6 Areas rich in EC (left) and nanoparticles $SrFe_{12}O_{19}$ (right) in EC-SrFe20

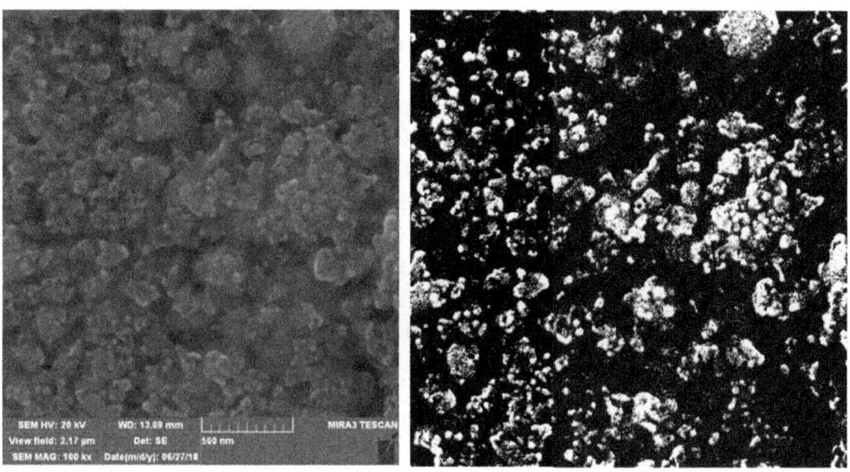

Fig. 7 Enlarged nanoparticles $SrFe_{12}O_{19}$ in EC-SrFe20

(right). Software analysis is done by identifying individual objects and agglomerates based on contrasting zones. The particle size distribution is shown in Fig. 8.

As can be seen, the particle diameter ranges from 10 nm to near 100 nm, which is in accordance with the data obtained by the manufacturer. Over 90% of the particles had a diameter below 50 nm.

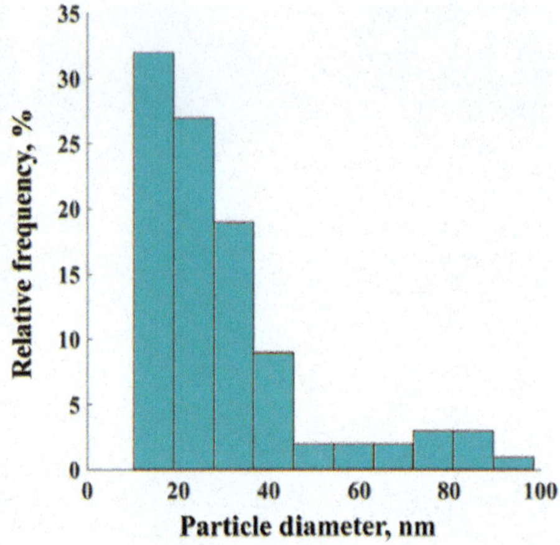

Fig. 8 Distribution of nanoparticle $SrFe_{12}O_{19}$ diameters

2.3 AFM Analysis of Thin Films

Changes in Nanocomposite Morphology The magnetic nanoparticles' influence on nanocomposite topology surface and morphological changes were studied by atomic force microscopy (AFM). Figure 9 shows phase and three-dimensional images of sample surfaces of pure EC, EC-SrFe10 and EC-SrFe30, respectively, with scanning surfaces of 40 $\mu m^2 \times 40 \mu m^2$ and 10 $\mu m^2 \times 10 \mu m^2$. It has been observed that EC-$SrFe_{12}O_{19}$ samples had two-phase topology, composed of hard and soft domains. As with FESEM microscopy, the darker regions are polymeric, a softer phase, while the lighter region was filled with strontium hexa ferrite particles, i.e. hard segment domains. Phase images showed a heterogeneous character, which is a result of segregation between hard and soft segments within the polymer matrix. EC and EC-SrFe samples with a higher content of nanoparticles show a more heterogeneous character, due to the higher amount of magnetic particles that cover a part of the examined surface. Phase images of EC-SrFe30 show more pronounced differences between soft and hard domains than EC-SrFe10.

Nanocomposite Membrane Roughness By measuring and comparing different areas of membrane ultrastructure, it was observed that the roughness increased with the content of magnetic nanoparticles. Figure 10 presents histogram of peak heights and it shows that nanoparticles addition significantly contributes to a height increase. Actually, detected peak to valley roughness (Rp-v), root-mean-square roughness (Rq), average roughness (Ra) and mean height (mean Ht) of the nanocomposite membrane surface all increased with $SrFe_{12}O_{19}$ concentration.

The R_q values ranged from 25.7 to 201.8 nm and generally increased with increasing content of hard segments in the samples (Fig. 11). From the three-dimensional image of the sample surface and the data from Fig. 11, it can be concluded that the increase in the nanoparticle content leads to a significant increase

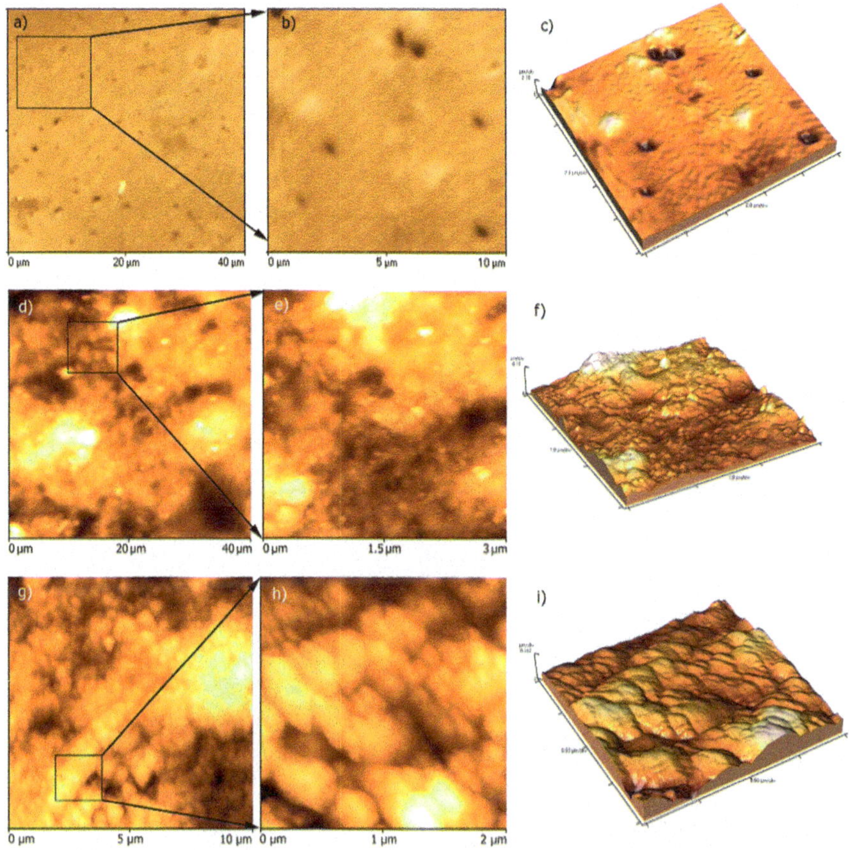

Fig. 9 Changes in morphology detected by AFM in membranes: **a–c** EC; **d–f** EC-SrFe10 and **g–i** EC-SrFe30

in the thickness of the nanocomposite membranes, which is a consequence of the nanoparticle grouping due to a magnetic field exposure during processing.

2.4 *FTIR Analysis of Thin Films EC and EC-SrFe*

Figure 12 shows the infrared spectra of pure EC and EC-SrFe nanocomposite membrane. Both spectra of ethylcellulose and EC-SrFe show a clear peak at 3477 cm^{-1}, which originates from the –OH groups present in the cellulose.

Peaks occurring in both spectra around 2978 and 2867 cm^{-1} originate from $-CH_2$ stretching [35, 63]. The $-CH_3$ bending can be seen at 1378 cm^{-1}, while the $-CH_2$ bending occurs at 1456 cm^{-1}. The peak at 1111 cm^{-1} comes from C–O–C stretching in cyclic ether. Strontium ferrite was identified with two characteristic bands, at 547

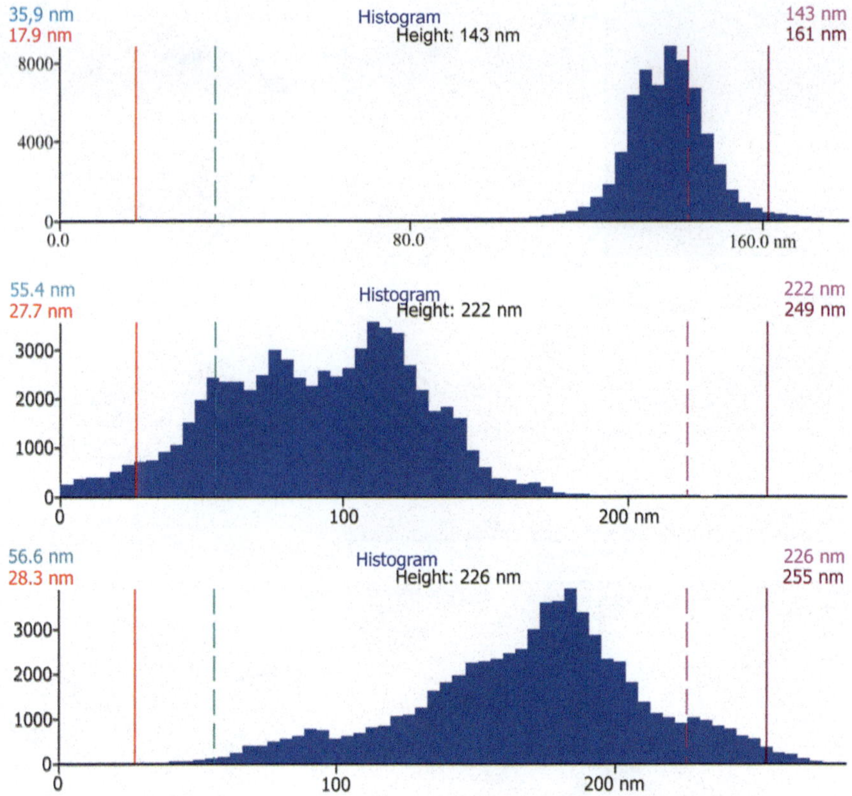

Fig. 10 Peak height histogram

Fig. 11 Membrane roughness parameters depending on the nanoparticle content

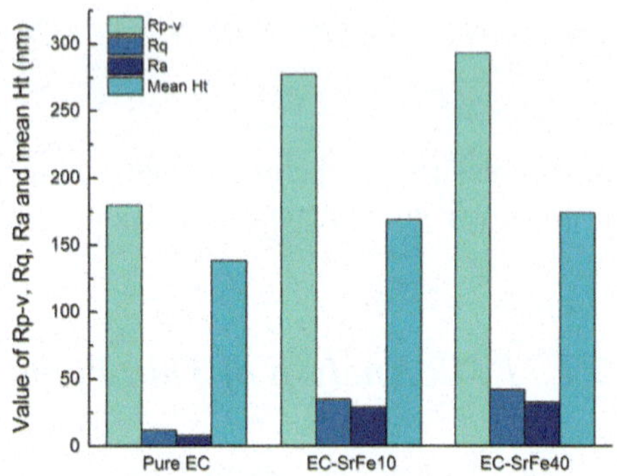

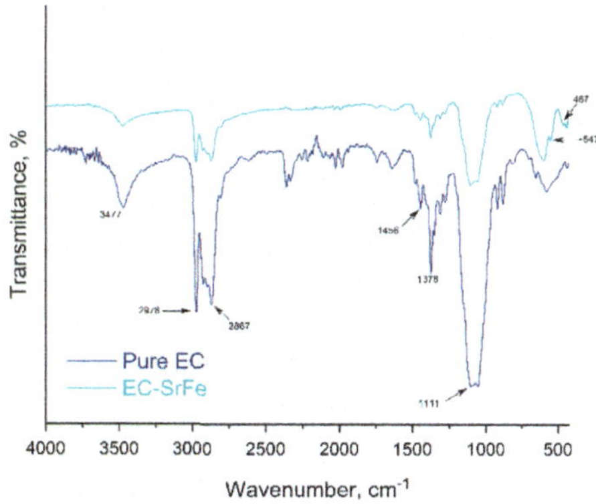

Fig. 12 FTIR spectra of pure EC and nanocomposite membranes EC-SrFe

and 467 cm^{-1}, which come from stretching vibrations of metal oxygen bond (Fe ↔ O, Sr ↔ O) on the tetrahedral and octahedral positions, respectively. These vibrations confirm the presence of hexa ferrite $SrFe_{12}O_{19}$ in EC [64]. Taking into account that there are only subtle differences between the obtained EC and EC-SrFe spectra, it can be assumed that the nanoparticles remain stable during processing in the polymer.

2.5 *Vickers Microhardness Test*

Figure 13 shows the impression formed during the indentation of the micro-Vikers diamond pyramid in the nanoparticles-rich area. Films of pure EC had a microhardness value of 21 MPa, while the addition of 10 wt% nanopowder led to an increase of 10%. A sample with 20 wt% of $SrFe_{12}O_{19}$ nanoparticles showed a significant increase in microhardness of 13% compared to pure EC, which suggested that film casting is a suitable method for treating thin nanocomposite thin films based on the EC.

By increasing the fraction of nanoparticles, the hardness values continued to rise, and with 30 wt% of $SrFe_{12}O_{19}$, the value was over 14% higher. These results showed that the increase in the content of nanopowders magnetized during processing results in an improvement of the nanocomposite mechanical properties. The indicated microhardness values are the average values from the measurement in three different places. Given that polymer-rich and nanoparticles-rich areas are separated, it is necessary to show the difference in the microhardness value for each measurement. This difference is shown in Fig. 14.

For each measurement there is a value that is significantly lower than the others, indicating that the region is rich in polymer. Considering that the lowest concentration of nanoparticles was in the first sample, it is expected that there is a larger area rich in polymer, and therefore two lower values of microhardness are measured. These results indicate how much nanoparticle-rich area is harder than pure ethylcellulose, and that the average hardness values cannot be taken into account alone because

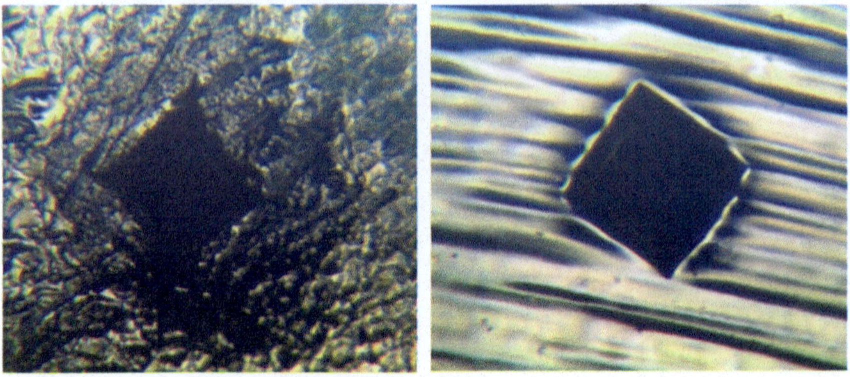

Fig. 13 Imprints in areas rich in nanoparticles (left) and polymer (right)

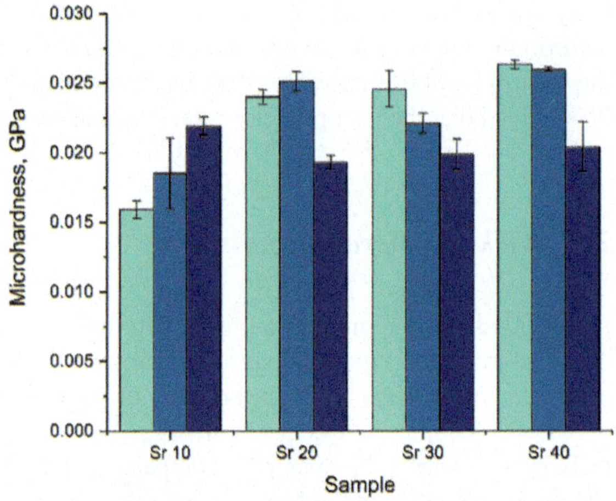

Fig. 14 Microhardness dependence on nanoparticle fraction in the nanocomposite

they do not provide an overall picture of the matrix reinforcement by the magnetic nanoparticles of strontium ferrite.

2.6 *Tensile Test*

Figures 15 and 16 show the results obtained by the tensile test. Deformation, or elongation at break, can be presented depending on the concentration of $SrFe_{12}O_{19}$ in tested nanocomposites (Fig. 15). With the addition of 10 wt% of nanoparticles in the EC, elongation decreased from 6.35 to 3.16%. By increasing the concentration of magnetic nanoparticles, the elongation decreases to 1.85% for the sample with 30 wt% of $SrFe_{12}O_{19}$. An abrupt decrease in elongation suggests that the effect of nanoparticles' clustering under the influence of the magnetic field is evident already

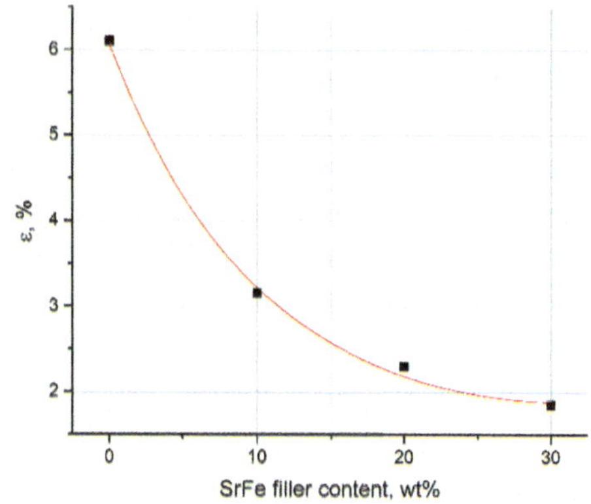

Fig. 15 Elongation at brake dependence on nanoparticle fraction in composite

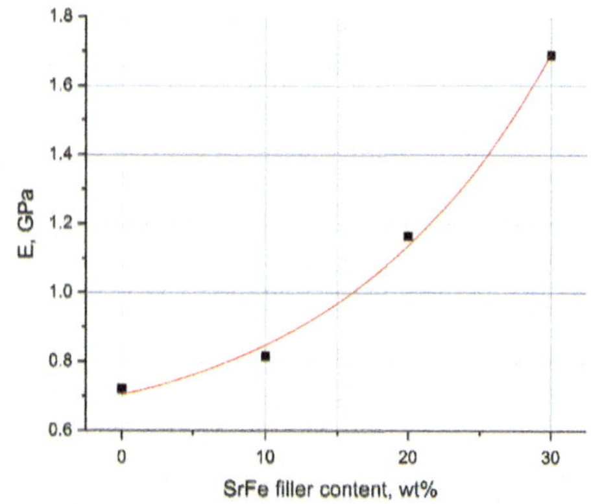

Fig. 16 Modulus of elasticity dependence on nanoparticle fraction in composite

with 10 wt% of their content. Brittle segments rich in $SrFe_{12}O_{19}$ lead to a reduction in the elongation at break.

The change of the elastic modulus with $SrFe_{12}O_{19}$ is shown in Fig. 16. The sample EC-SrFe10 showed 13% increase in modulus, compared to pure EC. At 20 wt% fraction of nanoparticles, the value of the module increased as much as 62%, while for 30 wt%, the value increased by 135%.

These results show that, at the same load, nanocomposite membrane EC-SrFe30 exhibits approximately 2.5 times less deformation than the pure EC. Obviously, the formation of polymer-rich and nanoparticles-rich areas has a significant reinforcing effect on EC, and could widen the use of this material.

2.7 *Permeability Test of Nanocomposite Membranes EC-$SrFe_{12}O_{19}$*

The permeability test of EC-SrFe nanocomposite membranes was performed with the aim of determining the efficiency of magnetic nanoparticles in the separation of similar gases mixture, such as N_2/O_2. It should be noted that the membranes withstood the work at high pressures, which further confirms the results of mechanical analysis that indicated a significant strengthening of the EC matrix by inserting magnetic nanoparticles $SrFe_{12}O_{19}$. Based on the pressure difference at the inlet and outlet of the membrane, the values of membrane permeability were calculated using Eq. (1).

Figure 17 shows the change in the value of the outlet pressure of the N_2/O_2 mixture (95%:5%), as well as the change in the value of the outlet pressure of pure N_2 with increasing inlet pressure when testing a representative nanocomposite membrane with 30 wt% $SrFe_{12}O_{19}$ of nanoparticles. As can be seen, an increase in inlet pressure leads to an increase in outlet pressure in a mixture of oxygen and nitrogen, as well as in pure nitrogen.

Permeability values ranged from about 250 Barrer to 2100 Barrer and classify nanocomposite membranes as highly efficient membranes [65]. In a series of membranes with 10 wt% $SrFe_{12}O_{19}$, there was an increase in permeability with increasing inlet pressure, which may indicate that membranes with a lower content of nanoparticles are not designed to work at higher pressure. Figure 18 shows the change in permeability with inlet pressure for EC-SrFe10 membrane.

Comparing the permeability values for a mixture of N_2/O_2 and pure N_2, a significant difference is observed for membranes of the same nanoparticle concentrations. The permeability of all membranes is higher for the H_2/O_2 mixture, which indicates that the membranes perform separation. Given that the initial N_2:O_2 ratio was

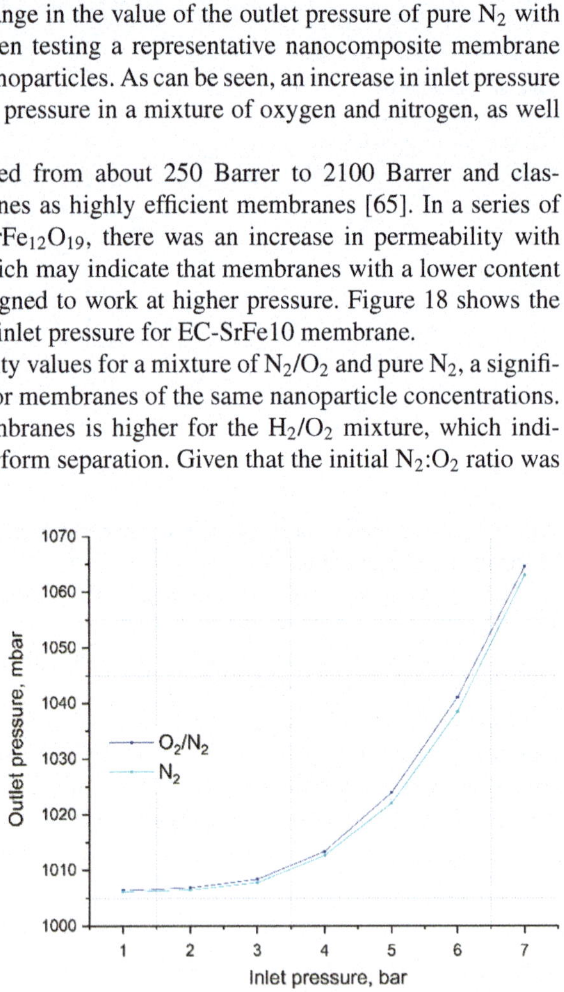

Fig. 17 Change of outlet pressure with inlet pressure for N_2/O_2 mixture

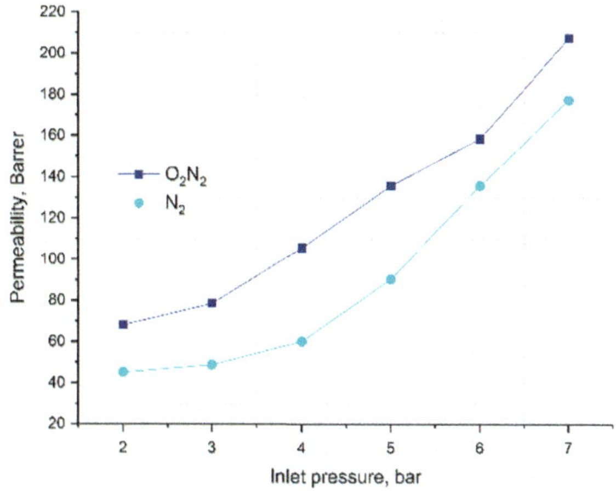

Fig. 18 Change of permeability with inlet pressure for EC-SrFe10 membrane

95%:5%, and the permeability ratios for the mixture and pure nitrogen deviate from the initial ratio, it is assumed that the output mixture is enriched with oxygen.

For a better insight into the difference between the permeability for the N_2/O_2 mixture and for pure N_2, Fig. 19 shows the change in permeability with the concentration of nanoparticles for the mixture and pure nitrogen. A significant difference is observed for each concentration of magnetic nanoparticles.

The results obtained by the permeability analysis indicate that the processing of nanocomposite magnetic membranes by simple solution casting, results in obtaining membranes of high separation possibilities. From these findings, it can be concluded that the processed nanocomposite EC-SrFe membranes show a high potential for use in the separation of the N_2/O_2 mixture, because in addition to separation, they also show good mechanical properties, which will allow their use at high pressure.

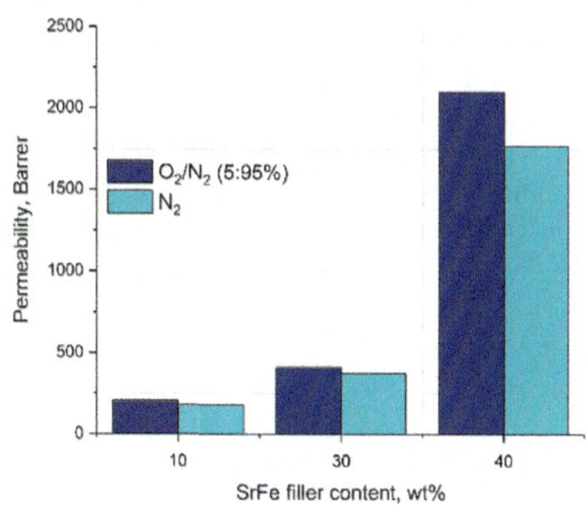

Fig. 19 Permeability change for N_2/O_2 and pure N_2 mixture with $SrFe_{12}O_{19}$ nanoparticle content in the nanocomposite

3 Conclusion

Nanocomposites with ethylcellulose matrix were processed with the aim of improving poor mechanical properties of the polymer, introducing novel technique for the processing of nanocomposites with magnetic nanoparticles of $SrFe_{12}O_{19}$. Using magnetic stripes, low magnetic field was applied on the samples during drying of nanocomposite films, inducing orientation of $SrFe_{12}O_{19}$, which led to a formation of two-phase structure. Composites were consisted of alternating polymer-rich and nanoparticle-rich areas. In order to investigate the influence of the nanoparticles content, their concentrations were in the range from 10 to 30 wt%. FESEM confirmed phase separation; observed branch-like orientation of the particles proved that applied magnetic field had influence on nanocomposite morphology, showing potential of a new approach for incorporation of magnetic particles in polymers. AFM also recognized two-phase structure, identifying larger area of 'hard' segments (nanopariticles-rich) for the samples with 30 wt% of nanopowder, along with an increased thickness of the nanocomposite. Micro-Vickers test was used to investigate the overall influence of the reinforcement, as well as to emphasize the difference in local microhardness values, depending on whether the indented area was polymer-rich or nanoparticle-rich. As expected, average microhardness obtained from three indentations increased with the particles' content, while each indentation showed that the lowest values were for the polymer-rich segment. Young's modulus of elasticity increased from 13% for the sample with 10 wt%, up to 135% for composite with 30 wt% of $SrFe_{12}O_{19}$, compared to pure ethylcellulose. The diffusion chamber showed pressure increase of the N_2/O_2 gas mixture after passing through magnetic nanocomposite membranes. Membrane permeability increased with an increase in nanoparticle content, from 120 Barrer with 10 wt%, up to 2100 Barrer with 30 wt%. Based on all of these findings, it can be concluded that the presented technique is promising for the processing of nanocomposites with magnetic particles, leading to significant reinforcement of polymer matrix. Easy processing, the possibility of inserting a high content of magnetic nanoparticles with continuous improvement of mechanical properties encourage further research for their potential application in the field of membrane technology.

Funding The research was funded by the Ministry of Education, Science and Technological Development of the Republic of Serbia (Grant No. 451-03-68/2020-14/200026 and 451-03-68/2020-14/200017).

References

1. Stajčić, A., Nastasović, A., Stajić-Trošić, J., Marković, J., Onjia, A., Radovanović, F.: Novel membrane-supported hydrogel for removal of heavy metals. J. Environ. Chem. Eng. **3**, 453–461 (2015)

2. Stajčić, A., Nedeljković, D., Panić, V., Radović, I., Grujić, A., Stajić-Trošić, J., Jančić-Heinemann, R.: Adsorption kinetics of polyethersulfone membrane-supported hydrogels. Desalin. Water. Treat. **131**, 43–49 (2018)
3. Nedeljković, D.M., Stevanović, M.P., Stijepović, M.Z., Stajčić, A.P., Grujić, A.S., Stajić-Trošić, J.T., Stevanović, J.S.: The possibility of application of zeolyte powders for the construction of membranes for carbon dioxide separation. Chem. Ind. Chem. Eng. Q **21**, 277–284 (2015)
4. Sanders, D.E., Smith, Z.P., Guo, R.L., Robeson, L.M., McGrath, J.E., Paul, D.R., Freeman, B.D.: Polymer **54**, 4729–4761 (2013)
5. Lau, C.H., Li, P., Li, F., Chung, T.S., Paul, D.R.: Prog. Polym. Sci. **38**, 740–766 (2013)
6. Budd, P.M., McKeown, N.B.: Polym. Chem. **1**, 63–68 (2010)
7. Yampolskii, Y.: Macromolecule **45**, 3298–3311 (2012)
8. Geens, J., Peeters, K., Van der Bruggen, B., Vandecasteele, C.J.: J. Membr. Sci. **255**, 255–264 (2005)
9. Natara, S.K., Hosamani, K.M., Aminabhavi, T.M.: Desalination **249**, 12–17 (2009)
10. Rahimpour, A., Jahanshahi, M., Mortazavian, N., Madaeni, S.S., Mansourpanah, Y.: Appl. Surf. Sci. **256**, 1657–1663 (2010)
11. Mulder, M.H.V.: Basic Principles of Membrane Technology. Kluwer Academic, Dordrecht, the Netherlands (1996)
12. Cabasso, I.: Encyclopedia of Polymer Science and Engineering, pp. 598–605. Wiley, New York (1990)
13. Mulder, M.H.V.: Membranes in Bioprocessing: Theory and Applications, pp. 13–54. Chapman & Hall, London (1993)
14. Van der Bruggen, B., Vandecasteele, C., Van Gestel, T., Doyen, W., Leysen, R.: Environ. Prog. **22**, 46–56 (2003)
15. Strathmann, H., Giorno, L., Drioli, E.: An Introduction to Membrane Science and Technology. CNR Publisher, Roma (2006)
16. Strathmann, H., Giorno, L., Drioli, E.: Basic aspects in polymeric membrane preparation. In: Comprehensive Membrane Science and Engineering, pp. 91–111. Elsevier BV (2010)
17. Pereira Nunes, S., Peinemann, K.V.: Membrane Technology in the Chemical Industry. Wiley-VCH Verlag GmbH, Weinheim, Germany (2001)
18. Pandey, P., Chauhan, R.S.: Prog. Polym. Sci. **26**, 853–893 (2001)
19. Ismail, A.F., Lorna, W.: Sep. Purif. Technol. **27**, 173–194 (2002)
20. Warsinger, D.M., Chakraborty, S., Tow, E.W., Plumlee, M.H., Bellona, C., Loutatidou, S., et al.: Prog. Polym. Sci. **81**, 209–237 (2018)
21. Gomes, M., Azevedo, H., Malafaya, P., Silva, S., Oliveira, J., Silva, G., Sousa, R., Mano, J., Reis, R.: Handbook of Biopolymers and Biodegradable Plastics, pp. 385–425. Elsevier Inc. (2013)
22. Ghadi, R., Jain, A., Khan, W., Domb, A.J.: Wound Healing Biomaterials, pp. 203–225. Elsevier Inc. (2016)
23. Trombino, S., Poerio, T., Ferrarelli, T., Mauro, M.V., Giraldi, C., Giorno, L., Cassano, R.: Polym. Int. **64**, 344–351 (2015)
24. Rajabi-Siahboomi, A.R., Mehta, R.Y., Ambudkar, V., Dias, V., Tiwari, S.: Ethylcellulose applications in multiparticulate systems. In: Multiparticulate Drug Delivery, pp. 267–299 (2017)
25. Kaw, A.K.: Mechanics of Composite Materials. CRC Press, Boca Raton (2005)
26. Chung, D.D.L.: Composite Materials: Science and Applications, pp. 1–34. Springer, London (2010)
27. Reddy, J.N.: Mechanics of Laminated Composite Plates and Shells: Theory and Analysis. CRC Press, Boca Raton (2003)
28. Aleksić, R., Živković, I., Uskoković, P.: Kompozitni materijali. TMF Beograd (2015)
29. Radojević, V., Aleksić, R.: Mehanička svojstva materijala. TMF Beograd (2015)
30. Shi, C., Mo, Y.L.: Engineering Materials for Technological Needs, vol. 1, World Scientific Publishing Co. Pte. Ltd, Singapore (2004)

31. Radovic, I., Stajcic, A., Radisavljevic, A., Veljkovic, F., Cebela, M., Mitic, V.V., Radojevic, V.: Solvent effects on structural changes in self-healing epoxy composites. Mater. Chem. Phys. **256**, 123761 (2020)
32. Radovic, I.M., Stojanovic, D.B., Kojovic, A., Petrovic, M., Uskokovic, P.S., Radojevic, V.J., Aleksic, R.R.: Healing efficiency of polystyrene electrospun nanofibers with Grubbs' catalyst in thermosetting composite. J. Compos. Mater. **51**, 3003–3016 (2017)
33. Grujić, A., Stajić-Trošić, J., Stijepović, M., Putić, S., Nedeljković, D., Stajčić, A., Aleksić, R.: Dynamic mechanical behaviour of polymer bonded Nd-Fe-B composite materials. Mater. Trans. **53**, 395–400 (2012)
34. Stajčić, A.P., Stajić-Trošić, J.T., Grujić, A.S., Stijepović, M.Z., Lazić, N.L., Žák, T., Aleksić, R.R.: Hybrid Nd-Fe-B/barium ferrite magnetic materials with epoxy matrix. Hem. Ind. **66**, 301–308 (2012)
35. Stajcic, A., Radovic, I., Cosovic, V., Grujic, A., Stajic-Trosic, J., Jancic-Heinemann, R.: The influence of barium ferrite nanoparticles on morphological and mechanical properties of ethyl cellulose based nanocomposites. Sci. Sinter. **51**, 277–283 (2019)
36. Nedeljković, D.M., Stajčić, A.P., Grujić, A.S., Stajić-Trošić, J.T., Zrilić, M.M., Stevanović, J.S., Drmanić, S.Z.: The application of zeolite nanopowder for the construction of the dense composite polymer membranes for carbon dioxide separation. Dig. J. Nanomater. Bios. **7**, 269–782 (2012)
37. Dukali, R.M., Radovic, I., Stojanovic, D.B., Uskokovic, P.S., Romcevic, N., Radojevic, V., Aleksic, R.: Preparation, characterization and mechanical properties of $Bi_{12}SiO_{20}$-PMMA composite films. J. Alloy. Comp. **583**, 376–381 (2014)
38. Elmadani, A.A., Radović, I., Tomić, N.Z., Petrović, M., Stojanović, D.B., Jancic-Heinemann, R., Radojevic, V.: Hybrid denture acrylic composites with nanozirconia and electrospun polystyrene fibers. PLoS ONE **14**, e0226528 (2019)
39. Yerro, O., Radojević, V., Radović, I., Kojović, A., Uskoković, P.S., Stojanović, D.B., Aleksić, R.: Enhanced thermo-mechanical properties of acrylic resin reinforced with silanized alumina whiskers. Ceram. Int. **42**, 10779–10786 (2016)
40. Morgan, P.W.: Polymer Reviews, vol. 10, pp. 19–64. Wiley, New York (1965)
41. Lau, W.J., Ismail, A.F., Misdan, N., Kassim, M.A.: Desalination **287**, 190–199 (2012)
42. Prakash Rao, A., Desai, N.V., Rangarajan, R.: Membr. Sci. **124**, 263–272 (1997)
43. Chung, T.S., Jiang, L.Y., Kulprathipanja, S.: Prog. Polym. Sci. **32**, 483–507 (2007)
44. Scholes, C.A., Stevens, G.W., Kentish, S.E.: Fuel **96**, 15–28 (2012)
45. Funk, C.V., Lloyd, D.R.E.: J. Membr. Sci. **313**, 224–231 (2008)
46. Bodzek, M.: Pol. J. Environm. Stud. **9**, 1 (2000)
47. Freeman, B., Yampolskii, Y., Pinnau, I.: Materials Science of Membranes for Gas and Vapor Separation. Wiley, Chichester, UK (2006)
48. Vansant, E.F., Dewolfs, R.: Gas Separation Technology. Elsevier, Antwerp, Belgium (1990)
49. Zaidaoui, H., Boushaki, T., Sautet, J.C., Chauveau, C., Sarh, B., Gökalp, I.: Combust. Sci. Technol. **189**, 784–802 (2017)
50. Favre, E., Bounaceur, R., Roizard, D.: Separ. Purif. Technol. **68**, 30–36 (2009)
51. Koros, W.J., Mahajan, R.: J. Membr. Sci. **175**, 181–196 (2000)
52. Gaffney, T.R.: Curr. Op. Solid State Mater. Sci. **1**, 69 (1996)
53. Smith, A.R., Klosek, J.: Fuel Process. Technol. **70**, 115–134 (2001)
54. Strzelewicz, A., Grzywna, Z.J.: J. Membr. Sci. **60**, 294 (2007)
55. Rao, H.-X., Liu, F.-N., Zhang, Z.-Y.: J. Membr. Sci. **296**, 15–20 (2007)
56. Rybak, A., Grzywna, Z.J., Kaszuwara, W.: J. Membr. Sci. **79**, 336 (2009)
57. Rybak, A., Krasowska, M., Strzelewicz, A., Grzywna, Z.J.: Acta Phys. Pol. B **40**, 1001 (2009)
58. Lazouzia, G., Vuksanović, M.M., Tomić, N.Z., Mitrić, M., Petrović, M., Radojević, V., Jančić Hainemann, R.: Optimized preparation of alumina based fillers for tuning composite properties. Ceram. Int. **44**, 7442–7449 (2018)
59. Iost, A., Bigot, R.: Hardness of coatings. Surf. Coatings Technol. **80**, 117–120 (1996)
60. ASTM E384-16, Standard Test Method for Microindentation Hardness of Materials. ASTM International, West Conshohocken, PA (2016). www.astm.org

61. Song, F., Shen, X., Xiang, J., Song, H.: Mater. Chem. Phys. **120**, 213–216 (2010)
62. Desai, J., Alexander, K., Riga, A.: Int. J. Pharm. **308**, 115–123 (2006)
63. Mali, A., Ataie, A.: Scripta Mater. **53**, 1065–1070 (2005)
64. Meng, Y.Y., He, M.H., Zeng, Q., Jiao, D.L., Shukla, S., Ramanujan, R.V., Liu, Z.W.: J. Alloys. Compd. **583**, 220–225 (2014)
65. Rybak, A., Rybak, A., Kaszuwara, W., Awietjan, S., Jaroszewicz, J.: Mater. Lett. **183**, 170–174 (2016)

Unusual Chemical Reactivity at Low Temperatures of Buckminsterfullerene C_{60}

Jih Ru Hwu, Shuey-Fang Shu, Tsong-Ming Chang, Tung-Ying Kuo, Wen-Chieh Huang, Shwu-Chen Tsay, and Vojislav Mitić

Abstract Unusual properties of buckminsterfullerene C_{60} were explored, which reacted more efficiently with primary and secondary amines at low temperatures than at elevated temperatures in a solvent, such as benzene, toluene, and xylene. Low temperatures favor the formation of a charge-transfer complex, which can be detected by UV spectrometry. Furthermore, a series of electron spin resonance experiments were performed at various low temperatures to detect the formation of $C_{60}^{\bullet-}$. The "low-temperature" acceleration effect on the amination of fullerene C_{60} is closely related to solvent and temperatures. The new findings provide an avenue to functionalize buckminsterfullerene C_{60} so that the resultant adducts may have controllable solubility in various media. The outcome may offer a solution to enhance its biological and medicinal applicability.

Keyword Buckminsterfullerene C_{60} · Amination · Low temperature · Electron spin resonance (ESR)

J. R. Hwu (✉) · S.-F. Shu · T.-M. Chang · W.-C. Huang · S.-C. Tsay
Department of Chemistry, National Tsing Hua University, Hsinchu 300, Taiwan
e-mail: jrhwu@mx.nthu.edu.tw

J. R. Hwu · W.-C. Huang · S.-C. Tsay
Frontier Research Center on Fundamental and Applied Sciences of Matters, National Tsing Hua University, Hsinchu 300, Taiwan

J. R. Hwu · S.-F. Shu · T.-M. Chang
Academia Sinica, Nankang, Taipei 11529, Taiwan

T.-Y. Kuo
Industrial Technology Research Institute, Hsinchu 310, Taiwan

V. Mitić (Deceased)
Institute of Technical Sciences of the Serbian Academy of Science and Arts, Knez Mihailova 35/IV, 11000 Belgrade, Serbia

Faculty of Electronic Engineering, University of Niš, Niš, Serbia

S. Najman et al. (eds.), *Bioceramics, Biomimetic and Other Compatible Materials Features for Medical Applications*, Engineering Materials,
https://doi.org/10.1007/978-3-031-17269-4_13

1 Introduction

Chemical reactivity of molecules usually increases along with temperatures [1]. Compounds of few types undergo chemical reactions more efficiently at low temperatures than at high temperatures; yet a sequel to low temperature chemistry is essential to material science. Buckminsterfullerene C_{60} possesses a unique framework and electronic configuration [2, 3]. Many scientists pay attention to its physical and chemical properties at low temperatures [4]. We report herein an unusual property of C_{60}, which reacted with amines more efficiently at low than at high temperatures.

Electron transfer is among a few types of chemical reactions that can proceed at low temperatures [5]. Wudl et al. [6] first reported the reaction of C_{60} with amines to give adducts at room temperature or higher. These reactions involve electron transfer mechanism. To the best of our knowledge, performance of reactions of this type at low temperatures has never been reported [7].

Since the discovery in 1985, buckminsterfullerene C_{60} has become an appealing subject in biological science and medicinal chemistry. For example, upon irradiation with UV light, fullerene can produce singlet oxygen and then cleaves DNA [8]. It can function as a radical scavenger [9] and antioxidant [10] in biological systems and has been used for serum protein profiling for biomarker development [11]. Fullerene also fits inside the hydrophobic cavity of HIV proteases to inhibit the substrates from getting into the catalytic site of enzymes [12]. Moreover, fullerene has been modified by chemical methods as a carrier for drug and gene delivery [13].

Although applications of buckminsterfullerene C_{60} attract much attention, the low solubility due to its carbon sphere is problematic in physiological media. One way to overcome this obstacle is to functionalize its spherical surface. Therefore, we considered to develop an efficient way to aminate fullerenes. Amination is one of the early studied reactions in fullerene chemistry [14]. Owing to the nucleophilicity of primary and secondary amines, they could react with the electron deficient C_{60} to generate different adducts depending on the structures of amines and reaction conditions [15]. The solubility could be improved and the resultant aminofullerenes would have potential applications in biological and medicinal fields [16].

2 Results and Discussion

We first added an amine **1** to a benzene solution of C_{60} at room temperature. The amines included $MeNH_2$, $EtNH_2$, *n*-$PrNH_2$, *n*-$BuNH_2$, Me_2NH, pyrrolidine, and piperidine. Solidification of the solution at various low temperatures between –21 and –196 °C caused a color change from purple to dark blue. After the reaction mixture returned to room temperature, we obtained the adducts of C_{60} with up to four amine molecules (i.e., **2**) as brown solids (Scheme 1). The fast atom bombardment mass spectrometry (FABMS) was applied to determine their molecular formulas. The yields of the adducts are listed in Table 1. The lower temperature we applied,

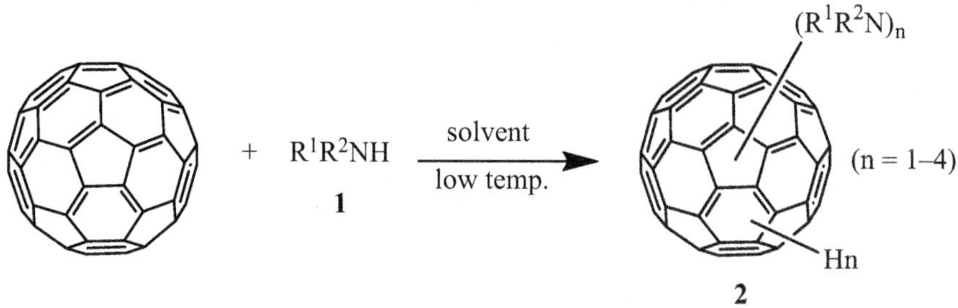

1 and 2	$R^1 =$	$R^2 =$		$R^1 + R^2 =$
a.	H	Me	**f.**	$(CH_2)_4$
b.	H	Et	**g.**	$(CH_2)_5$
c.	H	*n*-Pr		
d.	H	*n*-Bu		
e.	Me	Me		

Scheme 1 Addition of various amines to C_{60} generating C_{60}–amine adducts at low temperatures

the higher yields were obtained. Direct addition of a benzene solution containing C_{60} and an amine to liquid nitrogen at its boiling temperature (–196 °C) produced the corresponding adducts in high yields (83–95%). Their structures were further characterized by means of ^{1}H NMR and IR spectroscopy.

Performance of these addition reactions at various low temperatures gave the adducts in lower yields by replacement of benzene with toluene or in neat amines. Furthermore, the addition reaction did not proceed to a significant extent either at 25 °C for 3.0 h or by replacement of amines with alcohols or sulfides.

We carried out a series of electron spin resonance (ESR) experiments by detecting the signals of $C_{60}^{\bullet -}$ ($g = 2.0007$) [17, 18] in a solution containing C_{60} and *n*-propylamine at 25, 5, 0, –21, –32, –64, –78, –96, –110, –131, and –196 °C. No signals showed up during cooling from 25 to –196 °C. While we warmed up the frozen matrices starting at any temperature below the critical temperature (Tcritical) as indicated in Table 2, a strong signal always started appearing at the temperature called Tsignal and then it gradually decayed at 25 °C (see Fig. 1). The media included benzene, toluene, as well as *o*-, *m*-, and *p*-xylenes, among which benzene solution generated the strongest signals.

A charge transfer (CT) complex with absorption at 450–650 nm [19–22] can be generated from buckminsterfullerene C_{60} and an amine. We found that the frozen matrices of C_{60} and *n*-propylamine in benzene, *o*-, or *p*-xylene showed ESR signals at the melting points of the solvents; yet a big gap existed between Tsignal and the melting points of toluene and *m*-xylene. Thus the reaction of C_{60} with *n*-propylamine in toluene between –32 and –95 °C provided us a window to detect the CT complex by UV spectrometry. Accordingly, we obtained the UV spectra as shown in Fig. 2. Because its ESR signal started showing up at –32 °C (see Table 2), the two curves

Table 1 Percentage yields of adducts from reactions of buckminsterfullerene C_{60} with various amines in benzene (PhH) or toluene (PhMe) at various temperature for 10 min

Temp (°C)	$MeNH_2$		$EtNH_2$		n-$PrNH_2$		n-$BuNH_2$		Me_2NH		Pyrrolidine		Piperidine	
	PhH	PhMe	PhH	PhMe	PhH	PhMe	PhH	PhMe	PhH	PhMe	PhH	PhMe	PhH	PhMe
– 21	50	20	49	25	50	27	53	28	58	25	54	29	60	31
– 32	53	24	73	27	68	29	54	32	60	28	65	32	74	40
– 64	58	33	75	35	69	35	55	35	61	35	67	37	75	43
– 78	61	47	76	53	75	49	70	46	63	48	68	47	76	62
– 96	62	59	78	63	76	57	73	58	65	54	71	68	77	65
– 110	73	70	79	70	78	60	75	71	66	64	76	70	78	70
– 131	75	72	81	71	81	68	79	72	74	65	79	71	79	71
– 196	79	74	85	75	82	70	88	74	73	67	93	86	87	81
– 196[a]	83	30	89	32	93	35	92	39	85	40	95	52	95	50

[a] A benzene solution containing C_{60} and an amine was cooled down by liquid nitrogen.

Table 2 Parameters on temperatures related to ESR experiments involving the reactions of C_{60} with *n*-propylamine in various aromatic solvents

Solvent	Tcritical[a] (°C)	Tsignal[b] (°C)	mp (°C)	ε
p-xylene	0	12	12	2.27
Benzene	– 21	5	5	2.28
o-xylene	– 32	– 23	– 23	2.57
m-xylene	– 78	– 21	– 48	2.37
Toluene	– 78	– 32	– 95	2.38

[a] Tcritical: the highest temperature allowed to start showing up ESR signals in the process of decreasing solution temperatures and then followed by raising temperatures from –196 to 25 °C; [b] Tsignal: the temperature at which an ESR signal of $C_{60}{}^{\cdot -}$ showing up in the process of raising temperatures from –196 to 25 °C.

measured at –20 and –30 °C (i.e., curves D and E) belonged to the mixture containing $C_{60}{}^{\bullet -}$. These three curves having different absorption patterns at –50, –70, and –80 °C (i.e., curves A–C) indicate the formation of CT complexes of C_{60} and *n*-propylamine [23, 24]; this dark blue solution exhibited a stronger absorption between 750–900 nm than that of C_{60} itself (i.e., curve F).

Color of the toluene solution containing C_{60} and an amine changed along with the temperatures. The solution was purple during cooling from 25 to –95 °C; the frozen matrix kept dark blue between –95 and –196 °C. While it was gradually warmed up, the dark blue color resulting from the CT complex remained unchanged up to –32 °C. Once the radical ions were formed around at this temperature, the color changed to brown.

We rationalize the unusual phenomenon of low temperature acceleration on addition of amines to C_{60} as shown in Scheme 2. The C_{60} is an electron sink [25] and the amines can act as electron donors. When C_{60} is mixed with amines, an exothermic process [26] leads to the CT complexes **3** favorably at low temperature as indicated in Fig. 3. Subsequently, the radical ion pairs **4** containing $C_{60}{}^{\bullet -}$ and amines$^{\bullet +}$ are generated from the CT complexes **3** when the reaction temperature is raised. Finally, combination of these two ionic radicals gives the adducts **2**.

Application of low temperatures favors the formation of CT complexes, which were detected by UV spectrometry. Furthermore, a series of ESR experiments were performed at various low temperatures to detect $C_{60}{}^{\bullet -}$. These results demonstrate an unusual way to accelerate a reaction by "low temperature effect."

3 Conclusion

We established an efficient method for obtaining the adducts of buckminsterfullerene C_{60} and amines by decreasing, instead of increasing, the reaction temperatures. The

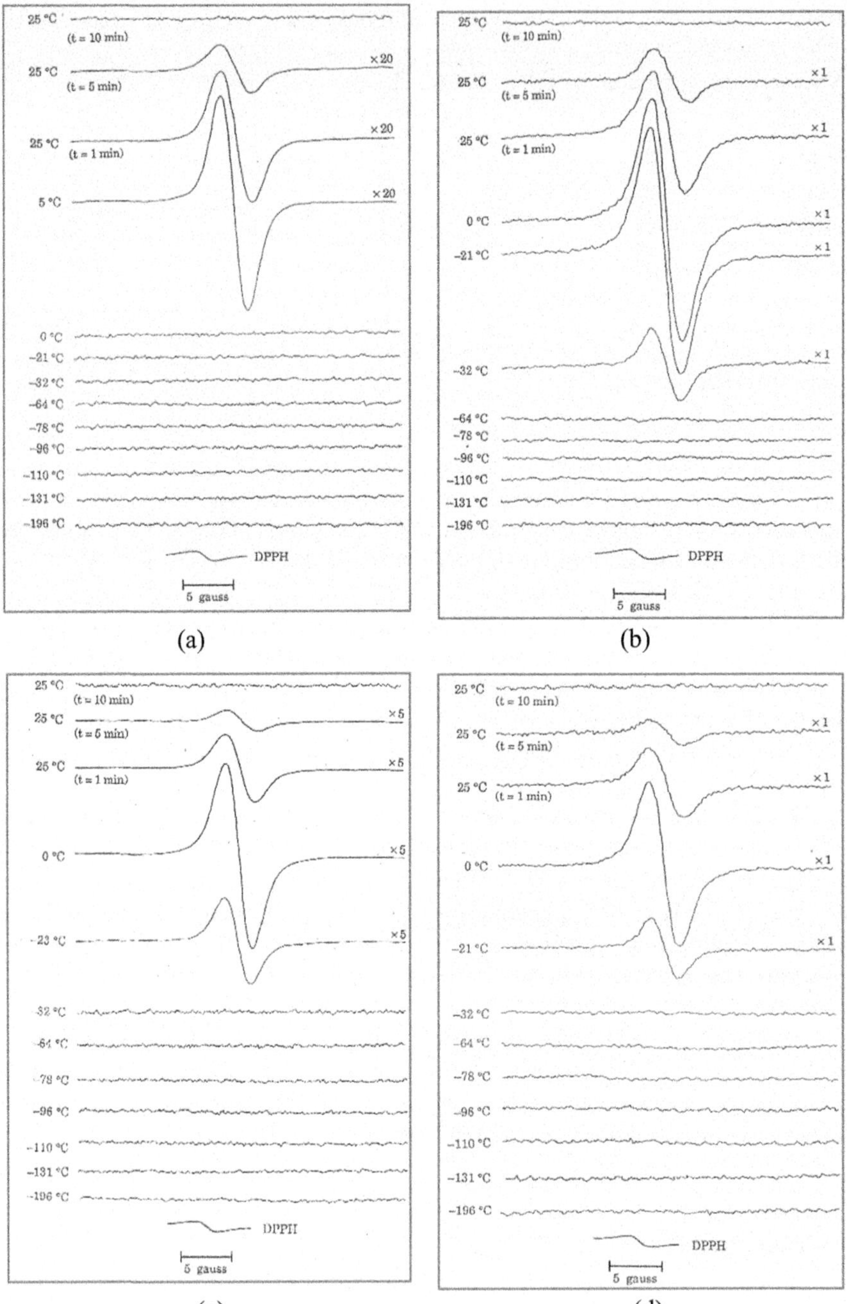

Fig. 1 A series of ESR spectra of an organic solvent containing C_{60} (1.39×10^{-4} M) and *n*-propylamine (1.39×10^{-2} M) recorded at the temperatures from −196 to 25 °C. The solvents were benzene (**a**), toluene (**b**), *o*-xylene (**c**), *m*-xylene (**d**), and *p*-xylene (**e**)

Fig. 1 (continued)

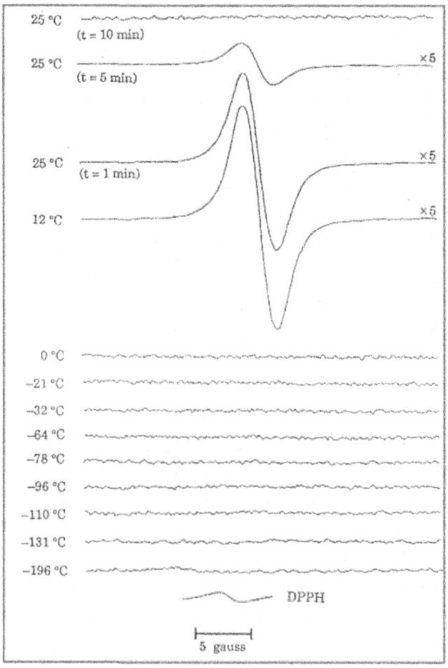

(e)

new method provides an easy and efficient way to generate aminofullerenes for their biological and biomedical utilization.

4 Experimental Procedures

General and Standard Procedures were the same as those reported before [27], which included the preparations of C_{60}–methylamine (**2a**), C_{60}–*n*-propylamine (**2c**), and C_{60}–dimethylamine (**2e**) adducts. The following methods were used for the preparation of low temperature baths, which involved addition of dry ice (CO_2) or liquid nitrogen (LN) to a solvent followed by stirring until a slush was formed. Temperature and composition of the bath are −196 °C (LN), −131 °C (*n*-pentane/LN), −110 °C (ethanol/LN), −95 °C (hexanes/LN), −78 °C (acetone/CO_2), −63 °C (chloroform/CO_2), −32 °C (iodobenzene/LN), and −21 °C (carbon tetrachloride/CO_2).

C_{60}–Ethylamine Adducts (**2b**) The standard procedure was followed by use of C_{60} (12.2 mg, 0.0169 mmol), ethylamine (**1b**, 75.3 mg, 1.67 mmol), and benzene (10.0 mL). The desired C_{60}–ethylamine adducts were obtained in 85% yield as brown solids: ^{1}H NMR (C_6D_6, 300 MHz) δ 1.35–2.28 (br, 4 H, $NCCH_3$ + CH), 2.66–3.43 (br, 3 H, NCH_2 + NH); IR (KBr) 3409 (s, N–H), 2913 (m, C–H), 1631 (m), 1449 (m),

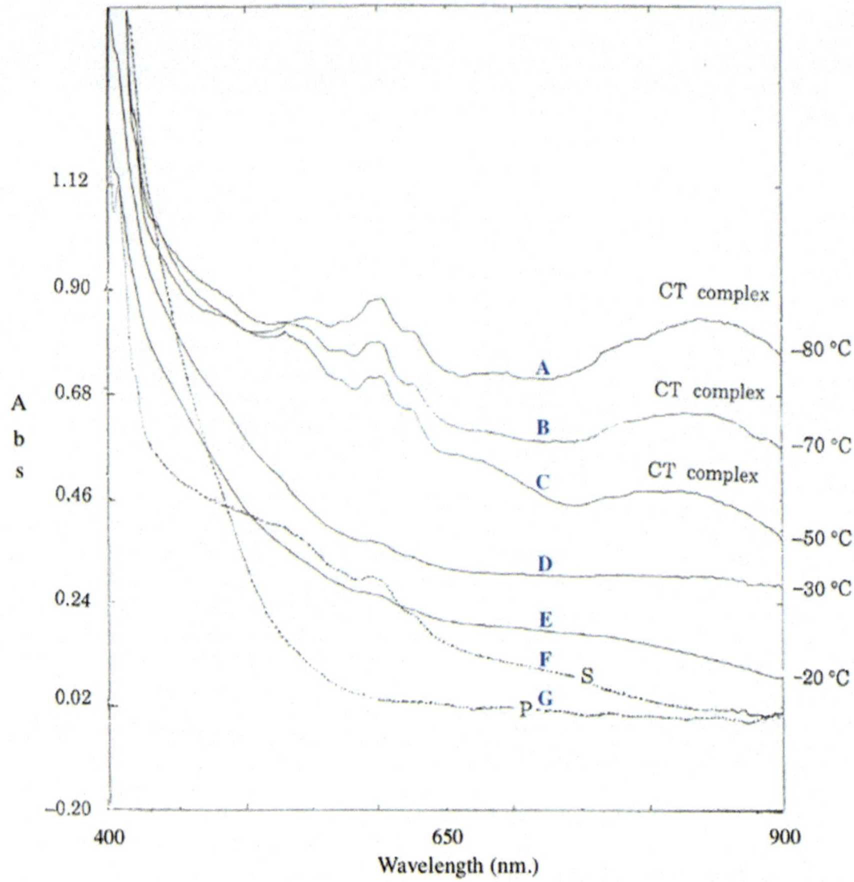

Fig. 2 A–E: UV–vis spectra of a toluene solution containing C_{60} (1.39×10^{-4} M) and *n*-propylamine (1.39×10^{-2} M) recorded by increment of temperatures from –196 to –20 °C. F: Spectrum of a toluene solution containing C_{60} (1.39×10^{-4} M) recorded at –80 °C. G: Spectrum of a toluene solution containing adducts of C_{60} and *n*-propylamine (1.39×10^{-4} M) recorded at –80 °C

1096 (m, C_{60}–N), 539 (m) cm^{-1}; FABMS: clusters of peaks at 900 ($C_{60}(EtNH_2)_4$), 855 ($C_{60}(EtNH_2)_3$), 810 ($C_{60}(EtNH_2)_2$), 765 ($C_{60}(EtNH_2)$), and 720 (C_{60}) amu.

C_{60}–*n*-Butylamine Adducts (2d) The standard procedure was followed by use of C_{60} (10.7 mg, 0.0148 mmol), *n*-butylamine (**1d**, 108.5 mg, 1.486 mmol), and benzene (10.0 mL). The desired C_{60}–*n*-butylamine adducts were obtained in 88% yield as brown solids: ^1H NMR (C_6D_6, 300 MHz) δ 0.83–1.34 (br, 3 H, CH_3), 1.32–2.00 (br, 5 H, $NCCH_2CH_2$ + CH), 2.72–3.64 (br, 3 H, NH + NCH_2); IR (KBr) 3389 (s, N–H), 2958 (m, C–H), 1639 (m), 1456 (m), 1086 (m, C_{60}–N), 528 (m) cm^{-1}; FABMS: clusters of peaks at 1012 ($C_{60}(n\text{-}BuNH_2)_4$), 939 ($C_{60}(n\text{-}BuNH_2)_3$), 866 ($C_{60}(n\text{-}BuNH_2)_2$), 793 ($C_{60}(n\text{-}BuNH_2)$), and 720 ($C_{60}$) amu.

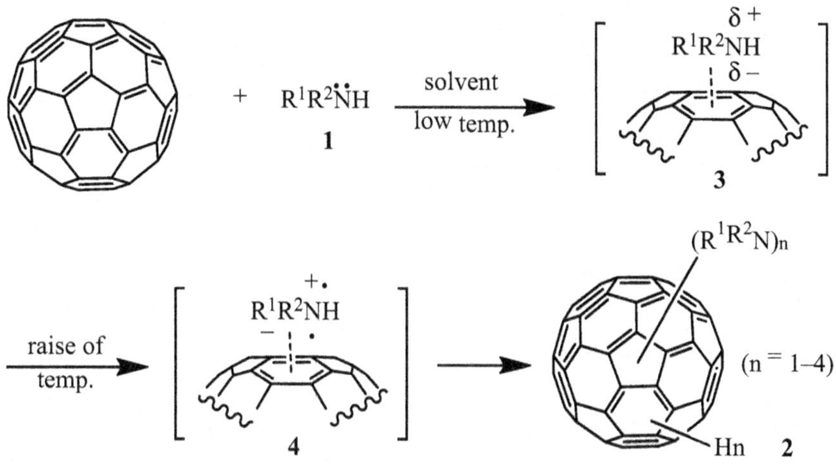

Scheme 2 Mechanism of amination of C_{60}

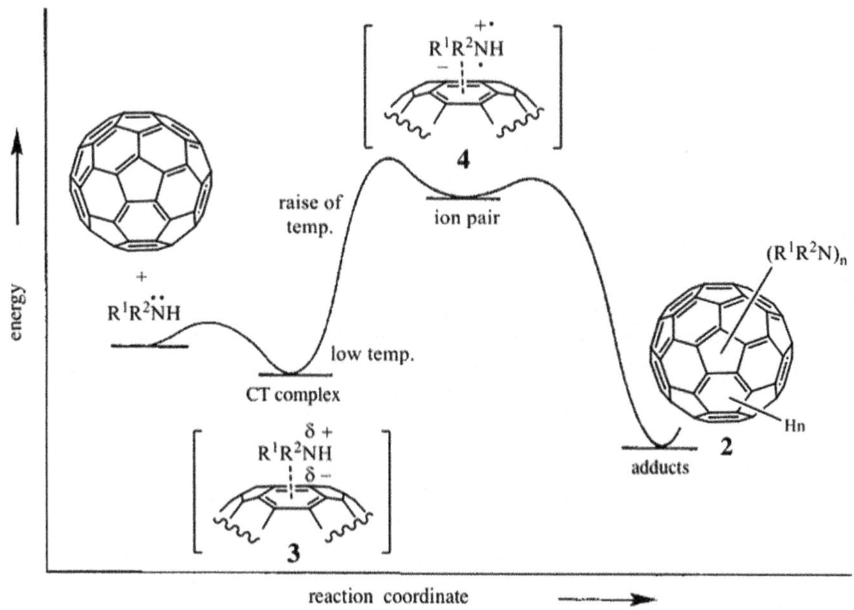

Fig. 3 Schematic energy diagram of the relationship between starting materials C_{60} and amines **1**, intermediates CT complexes **3** and ion pairs **4**, as well as the final adducts **2**

C_{60}–Pyrrolidine Adducts (2f) The standard procedure was followed by use of C_{60} (12.8 mg, 0.0178 mmol), pyrrolidine (**1f**, 126.2 mg, 1.777 mmol), and benzene (10.0 mL). The desired C_{60}–pyrrolidine adducts were obtained in 93% yield as brown solids: ^{1}H NMR (C_6D_6, 300 MHz) δ 1.65–2.07 (br, 5 H, 2 × $NCCH_2$ + CH), 3.04–3.40 (br, 4 H, 2 × NCH_2); IR (KBr) 2909 (m, C–H), 1635 (m), 1426 (m), 1128 (s, C_{60}–N), 853 (w), 533 (w) cm^{-1}; FABMS: clusters of peaks at 1004 (C_{60}(pyrrolidine)$_4$), 933 (C_{60}(pyrrolidine)$_3$), 862 (C_{60}(pyrrolidine)$_2$), 791 (C_{60}(pyrrolidine)), and 720 (C_{60}) amu.

C_{60}–Piperidine Adducts (2 g) The standard procedure was followed by use of C_{60} (8.70 mg, 0.012 mmol), piperidine (**1 g**, 101.8 mg, 1.198 mmol), and benzene (10.0 mL). The desired C_{60}–piperidine adducts were obtained in 87% yield as brown solids: ^{1}H NMR (C_6D_6, 300 MHz) δ 1.06–1.52 (br, 2 H, $NCCCH_2$), 1.61–2.10 (br, 5 H, 2 × $NCCH_2$ + CH), 3.11–3.38 (br, 4 H, 2 × NCH_2); IR (KBr) 2900 (m, C–H), 1642 (m), 1429 (m), 1089 (m, C_{60}–N), 996 (w), 525 (m) cm^{-1}; FABMS: clusters of peaks at 1060 (C_{60}(piperidine)$_4$), 975 (C_{60}(piperidine)$_3$), 890 (C_{60}(piperidine)$_2$), 805 (C_{60}(piperidine)), and 720 (C_{60}) amu.

Addition of Different Amines to Fullerene C_{60} at Various Low Temperatures Reaction between various amines with C_{60} were performed at different low temperatures as described in the standard procedure to give the same C_{60}–amine adducts. The amines included methylamine, ethylamine, *n*-propylamine, *n*-butylamine, dimethylamine, pyrrolidine, and piperidine; the temperatures included –21, –32, –64, –78, –96, –110, –131, and –196 °C. The yields are summarized in Table 1.

Yields of Fullerene C_{60}–Amine Adducts Yields of C_{60}–amine adducts were obtained by the total weight of isolated products. Nevertheless, some of the adducts had very low solubility in most organic solvents. Accordingly, the yields of C_{60}–amine adducts were further confirmed by measurement of the amount of recovered C_{60}. When the system was warmed up to room temperature, acenaphthylene (1.0 equiv) was added to the mixture in one portion. Condensation of the solution under reduced pressure formed the solids, which were dried over P_2O_5 (s) under vacuum for 24 h. Infrared spectrum of the solid was taken, from which the peak height of C_{60} (525 cm^{-1}) and acenaphthylene (730 cm^{-1}) was measured for analysis. For Table 1, the amount of recovered C_{60} was determined by use of IR instrument and acenaphthylene as the internal standard.

Detection of $C_{60}{}^{\cdot -}$ by ESR Spectrometer Samples for the ESR studies were taken from a freshly prepared solution containing C_{60}, solvent, and an amine. The solvent included benzene, toluene, *m*-, *o*-, and *p*-xylenes. This mixture was transferred into an ESR tube, which was capped and sealed by use of Teflon tape and a regular tube cap. The tube was then placed in a pre-cooled ESR probe at low temperatures for 3 min. Studies by ESR were performed at X-band on a Bruker ER 200D 10/20 spectrometer equipped with a variable temperature apparatus. The *g* values were measured versus (DPPH; $g = 2.0037$), which was used as the external reference. Whilst the temperature of the solution was increased, the ESR signals were detected as the results shown in Fig. 1.

Detection of Charge–Transfer Complex by UV–vis Spectrometer Samples for the UV–vis studies were taken from a freshly prepared solution containing C_{60} (1.39

$\times$ 10^{-4} M), toluene, and *n*-propylamine (1.39 $\times$ 10^{-2} M). The mixture was stirred vigorously at room temperature for 30 s, cooled down in a bath at −196 °C and kept for 10 min, then warmed up gradually to −95 °C (melting point of toluene). Then it was quickly transferred to the UV cell, which was pre-cooled at −80 °C. While the temperature of the UV cell was increased, the absorption spectra were detected as the results shown in Fig. 2. The CT complex has an absorption band at 700–800 nm, which is directly different from C_{60} and (C_{60} + amines) at low temperatures.

Acknowledgements For financial support, we thank Ministry of Science and Technology (Grant Nos. 110-2113-M-007-011 and 110-2634-F-007-023) and Ministry of Education (Grant Nos. 109QR001I5 and 110QR001I5) of R.O.C. We also thank the MOST in Taiwan for supporting The Featured Areas Research Center Program within the Framework of the Higher Education Sprout Project through the Frontier Research Center on Fundamental and Applied Sciences of Matters.

References

1. Anslyn, E.V., Dougherty, D.A.: Modern Physical Organic Chemistry. University Science, Mill Valley (2005)
2. Kroto, H.W.: The story of C_{60} buckminsterfullerene. In: Bawa, R., Audette, G.F., Rubinstein. I. (eds.) Handbook of Clinical Nanomedicine: Nanoparticles, Imaging, Therapy, and Clinical Applications, pp. 409–434. Jenny Stanford, Centennial Tower, Singapore (2016)
3. Evstigneev, M.P., Buchelnikov, A.S., Voronin, D.P., Rubin, Y.V., Belous, L.F., Prylutskyy, Y.I., Ritter, U.: Complexation of C_{60} fullerene with aromatic drugs. ChemPhysChem **14**(3), 568–578 (2013)
4. For examples, see (a) Suzuki, H., Nakano, M., Hashikawa, Y., Murata, Y.: Rotational motion and nuclear spin interconversion of H_2O encapsulated in C_{60} appearing in the low-temperature heat capacity. J. Phys. Chem. Lett. **10**(6), 1306–1311 (2019); (b) Lin, J., Zhong, Z., Li, Q., Tan, Z., Lin, T., Quan, Y., Zhang, D.: Facile low-temperature synthesis of cellulose nanocrystals carrying buckminsterfullerene and its radical scavenging property in vitro. Biomacromolecules **18**(12), 4034–4040 (2017); (c) Michinobu, T., Okoshi, K., Murakami, Y., Shigehara, K., Ariga, K., Nakanishi, T.: Structural requirements for producing solvent-free room temperature liquid fullerenes. Langmuir **29**(17), 5337–5344 (2013)
5. Carey, F.A., Sundberg, R.J.: Advanced Organic Chemistry, 5th edn. Springer, New York (2007)
6. Hirsch, A., Li, Q., Wudl, F.: Globe-trotting hydrogens on the surface of the fullerene compound $C_{60}H_6(N(CH_2CH_2)_2O)_6$. Angew. Chem. Int. Ed. Engl. **30**(10), 1309–1310 (1991)
7. For related works, see (a) Wu, S.-L., Gao, X.: Copper-catalyzed aerobic oxidative reaction of C_{60} with aliphatic primary amines and CS_2. J. Org. Chem. **83**(4), 2125–2130 (2018); (b) Lim, S.H., Jeong, H.C., Sohn, Y., Kim, Y.-I., Cho, D.W., Woo, H.-J., Shin, I.-S., Yoon, U.C., Mariano, P.S.: Single electron transfer-promoted photochemical reactions of secondary *N*-trimethylsilylmethyl-*n*-benzylamines leading to aminomethylation of fullerene C_{60}. J. Org. Chem. **81**(6), 2460–2473 (2016)
8. Hashimoto, A., Takamura-Enya, T., Oda, Y.: Synthesis and in vitro biological evaluation of psoralen-linked fullerenes. Photochem. Photobiol. **95**(6), 1403–1411 (2019)
9. Ma, H., Zhao, J., Meng, H., Hu, D., Zhou, Y., Zhang, X., Wang, C., Li, J., Yuan, J., Wei, Y.: Carnosine-modified fullerene as a highly enhanced ROS scavenger for mitigating acute oxidative stress. ACS Appl. Mater. Interfaces **12**(14), 16104–16113 (2020)
10. Gudkov, S.V., Guryev, E.L., Gapeyev, A.B., Sharapov, M.G., Bunkin, N.F., Shkirin, A.V., Zabelina, T.S., Glinushkin, A.P., Sevost'yanov, M.A., Belosludtsev, K.N., Chernikov, A.V., Bruskov, V.I., Zvyagin, A.V.: Unmodified hydrated C_{60} fullerene molecules exhibit antioxidant

properties, prevent damage to DNA and proteins induced by reactive oxygen species and protect mice against injuries caused by radiation-induced oxidative stress. Nanomed. Nanotechnol. Biol. Med. **15**(1), 37–46 (2019)
11. Dellinger, A.L., Zhou, Z., MacFarland, D., Sandros, M.G., Sawafta, A., Kepley, C.L.: Molecular interactions of fullerene derivatives in human serum and inflammatory cells. Insci. J. **1**(3), 102–114 (2011)
12. Acton, O., Grant, T., Nicastro, G., Ball, N.J., Goldstone, D.C., Robertson, L.E., Sader, K., Nans, A., Ramos, A., Stoye, J.P., Taylor, I.A., Rosenthal, P.B.: Structural basis for fullerene geometry in a human endogenous retrovirus capsid. Nat. Commun. **10**, 5822 (2019). https://doi.org/10.1038/s41467-019-13786-y
13. Kazemzadeh, H., Mozafari, M.: Fullerene-based delivery systems. Drug Discov. Today **24**(3), 898–905 (2019)
14. Hirsch, A., Brettreich, M.: Fullerenes: Chemistry and Reactions. Wiley-VCH, Weinheim (2005)
15. Rašović, I.: Water-soluble fullerenes for medical applications. Mater. Sci. Technol. **33**(7), 777–794 (2016)
16. Castro, E., Garcia, A.H., Zavala, G., Echegoyen, L.: Fullerenes in biology and medicine. J. Mater. Chem. B **5**(32), 6523–6535 (2017)
17. Wudl, F., Hirsch, A., Khemani, K.C., Suzuki, T., Allemand, P.-M., Koch, A., Srdanov, G., Webb, H.M.: Survey of chemical reactivity of C_{60}, electrophile and dieno—polarophile par excellence. ACS Symp. Ser. **481**, 161–175 (1992)
18. Moriyama, H., Kobayashi, H., Kobayashi, A., Watanabe, T.: Electrocrystallization and ESR spectra of the single crystal $[N(P(C_6H_5)_3)_2]{\cdot}C_{60}$. J. Am. Chem. Soc. **115**(3), 1185–1187 (1993)
19. Wang, Y., Cheng, L.-T.: Nonlinear optical properties of fullerenes and charge-transfer complexes of fullerenes. J. Phys. Chem. **96**(4), 1530–1532 (1992)
20. Ghosh, H.N., Pal, H., Sapre, A.V., Mittal, J.P.: Charge recombination reactions in photoexcited fullerene C_{60}-amine complexes studied by picosecond pump probe spectroscopy. J. Am. Chem. Soc. **115**(25), 11722–11727 (1993)
21. Sun, Y.-P., Bunker, C.E., Ma, B.: Quantitative studies of ground and excited state charge transfer complexes of fullerenes with *N, N*-dimethylaniline and *N, N*-diethylaniline. J. Am. Chem. Soc. **116**(21), 9692–9699 (1994)
22. Li, J., Feng, J., Sun, C.: Calculations on the electronic structure and nonlinear second-order optical susceptibility of the C_{60}/aniline charge-transfer complex. J. Phys. Chem. **98**(35), 8636–8640 (1994)
23. Konarev, D.V., Troyanov, S.I., Otsuka, A., Yamochi, H., Saito, G., Lyubovskaya, R.N.: Charge transfer complexes of fullerenes containing $C_{60}{}^{\cdot-}$ and $C_{70}{}^{\cdot-}$ radical anions with paramagnetic $Co^{II}(dppe)_2Cl^+$ cations (dppe: 1,2-bis(diphenylphosphino)ethane). Dalton Trans. **45**(15), 6548–6554 (2016)
24. Seshadri, R., Rao, C.N.R., Pal, H., Mukherjee, T., Mittal, J.P.: Interaction of C_{60} and C_{70} with aromatic amines in the ground and excited states. evidence for fullerene—benzene interaction in the ground state. Chem. Phys. Lett. **205**(4–5), 395–398 (1993)
25. Zhou, Z., Xu, S., Song, J., Jin, Y., Yue, Q., Qian, Y., Liu, F., Zhang, F., Zhu, X.: High-efficiency small-molecule ternary solar cells with a hierarchical morphology enabled by synergizing fullerene and non-fullerene acceptors. Nat. Energy **3**, 952–959 (2018)
26. Song, H., Lee, K., Choi, M.-G., Park, J.T.: [60]Fullerene as a versatile four-electron donor ligand. Organometallics **21**(9), 1756–1758 (2002)
27. Hwu, J.R., Kuo, T.-Y., Chang, T.M., Patel, H.V., Yong, K.-T.: Amination of buckminsterfullerene C_{60} at low temperature: application in polyamide synthesis. Fullerene Sci. Technol. **4**(3), 407–422 (1996)

The Nanomaterials Fractal Characterization and Bioforensic Science

Ana Radosavljević-Mihajlović, Vojislav V. Mitić, Bojana Marković, and Dragan Simeunović

Abstract Nanotechnology and nanomaterials are beginning to have an impact on the bioforensic science, regarding handling of evidence at crime scenes, its analysis in the laboratory and its presentation in the courtroom. Many different nanomaterials are used for processing of the samples, as DNA, gun powder residues, body fluids etc. Nevertheless, nanopowders, especially luminescent, are the most important for the fingerprinting method. The application of each nanomaterial in the forensic examination depends on its structure and properties, which can successfully be determined by applying fractal nature analysis, as an excellent method for micro and nanomaterials characterization. In our research we successfully synthesized photoluminescent Bi, Y and Ag zeolite$_{LTA}$ topology nanopowders, which could be used for taking fingerprints from different materials, and therefore, they should be well characterized by fractal analysis. This article aims to highlight some of the major advances in forensic science brought about by nanomaterials fractal characterization, but is not exhaustive of the subject matter.

Keyword Forensic science · Nanobiotechnology · Nanomaterials · Fractals · Luminescent nanopowders

---

A. Radosavljević-Mihajlović (✉)
Institute for Technology Nuclear and Other Raw Materials, Franse d'Epere Blvd. 86, 11000 Belgrade, Serbia
e-mail: a.radosavljevic@itnms.ac.rs

V. V. Mitić (Deceased) · B. Marković
Faculty of Electronic Engineering, University of Niš, Aleksandra Medvedeva 14, 18000 Niš, Serbia

V. V. Mitić (Deceased)
Institute of Technical Sciences of the Serbian Academy of Science and Arts, Knez Mihailova 35/IV, 11000 Belgrade, Serbia

D. Simeunović
Faculty of Political Science, University of Belgrade, 11000 Belgrade, Serbia

National Security Academy, 11000, Belgrade, Serbia

S. Najman et al. (eds.), *Bioceramics, Biomimetic and Other Compatible Materials Features for Medical Applications*, Engineering Materials,
https://doi.org/10.1007/978-3-031-17269-4_14

1 Introduction

Nanobioforensic science is a new forensic discipline related to various nanotechnological methods for crime scene investigation, especially in the case of explosive gases detection, and biological and chemical reagents during terroristic activities [1].

Nanotechnology, as a science, studies physical, chemical and biological properties of nanoparticles, and as a technology, applies research from different materials consolidation engineering fields, and special characteristic functional systems, as well. Despite the fact that nanotechnology is one of the most exploited topics today, there is no consensus about its definition and nano-domain scope, thus from different angles, nanotechnology is defined as a technology dealing with structural units up to 100 nm, submicron elements or particles on atom and molecular level.

Nanomaterials are solid materials with nanodimensions from 1 to 100 nm, including 3D nanoparticles, 2D thin films and 1D thin wires [2]. Features of 1 to 250 nm particles size materials are somewhere in between atoms and molecules quantum effects, and voluminous samples macroscopic characteristics [2]. It is just in this "no man's land", that the majority of physical properties is controlled by the critical nanoscale boundary phenomena. Nowadays, nanomaterials are more and more present in our everyday life, as components of pharmaceutical and medical products and water purifying filters, in soil remediation process, in chemical and biological sensors production, in military industry, in controlled and improved chemical and biological features materials synthesis processes [1], etc. The application of nanomaterials in characterization and identification processes of different materials from the crime scene, has given outstanding results.

Fractal application in the field of nanomaterials used in forensic science is a new and perspective idea. By applying fractal nature analysis on nanomaterials we can determine and predict its structure and properties, which is very important for its adequate implementation. Also, this method can help us design the nanomaterial with desired characteristics that can fulfill certain forensic demands.

1.1 Nanomaterials

In the crime scene forensic investigation, the domain of nanotechnology involved in application of nanomaterials in the sample (like fingerprints, DNA, body fluids, etc.) processing and analyzing, has a huge significance (Fig. 1).

Nanopowders There are three groups of nanopowders standard, metal and luminescent.

Standard nanopowders consist of resin based polymer for pasting and contrast generating colorant, often with Fe_2O_3, TiO_2, MnO_2, $PbCO_3$, or pigments, like rosin, lamp black. Minerals, like hematite, rutile and cerussite, are also used as pigments due to their structural properties. Hematite, an intensively red mineral, consists of iron oxide, clay, mica and accessory minerals, whilst rutile, an intensively white mineral,

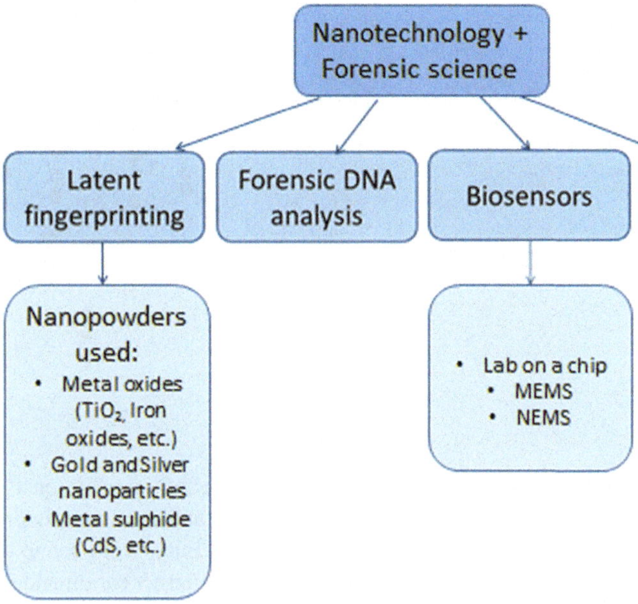

Fig. 1 Shematic diagram of nanotechnology analysis

light, acid and atmosferic conditions resistant, with uniformly shaped crystal grains which gives colour the smoothness and shine, is used as a mixed pigment with $BaSO_4$, ZnO i $CaCO_3$.

Metal nanopowders often contain Ag, Pb or Au metal nano-net, which provides large specific surfaces and great porosity.

Luminescent nanopowders, based on lanthanides with luminescent properties characteristic for rare-earth elements, contain sensitive organic complexes, like 1,10-phenanthroline [3, 4]. Nanopowders synthesized on the ZnO, TiO_2, EuO, FeO_2, CdS and CdSe basis, necessarily contain luminescent substances [5, 6]. By using this way synthesized nanopowders, spectra are formed, from UV to red, which provides a great choice flexibility and possibility in this field of forensic science.

Red nanopowder Lumicyano, a mixture of 99% cyanoacrylate ($C_5H_5NO_2$) and 1% fluorescent chemical compound fluorophore, synthetized by French scientists [7], has shown exceptional features, as well as phosphorus nanopowders doped with $Y_2Zr_2O_7$ nanoparticles imprinted in silicon matrix (Fig. 2), which can successfully be applied for fingerprints detection on different surfaces [7].

To enhence desired effects of nanopowders, various dopants are used, such as rare earth elements and Bi, Ag, Pd, Cu, Fe, Co, Ni, Zn, which have an important role in photoluminescence and luminescence, because these processes depend on the doped cation position. As precursors for this kind of nanomaterials, synthetic zeolites, structures with (Si, Al) O_4 tetrahedral scaffold and vacancies with big motile cations and water molecules, which enables cation exchange and rehydration, are used [8].

Fig. 2 $Y_2Zr_2O_7$ structure

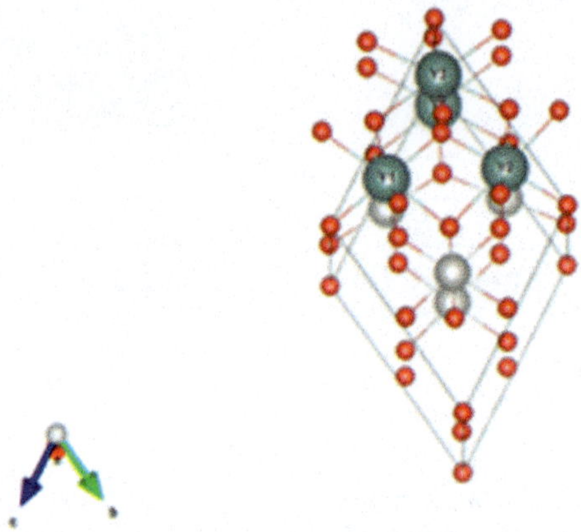

Low density, great empty space volume in cages after dehydration, intensive cation exchange, significant presence of various sized channels and vacancies, intensive absorbing capacity, catalitic properties, high ion conductivity, wide scope of Si-Al ratio in tetrahedral positions, as well as the presence of outernet cation and its coordination with aluminosilicate net oxygen, make zeolites very interesting precursors for different extraquality nanomaterials synthesis [9–11]. During the thermal treatment zeolites pass into structures with greater net density and directly produce another cristal or amorphous phase, which present new materials.

$Zeolite_{LTA}$ and $zeolite_{FAU}$ topology, as the most often used due to their great ion exchange features and low density aluminosilicate net [12–14], are presented in Fig. 3.

In Fig. 4 synthetic $zeolite_{LTA}$ topology, after processes of ion exchange and thermal treatment, are presented.

1.2 Fingerprinting Method

One of the most important analyses for person identification is a fingerprinting method. The first sistematization and fingerprints data base, enabling suspects identification, was established in New York Civile Service New Scotland Yard/Metropolitan Police in 1902 [15, 16], whilst the first application of fingerprinting method at the crime scene was done by the French police in the case of Henri-Leone Scheffer murder the same year [16, 17]. At the beginning, ink and mixture of tannins water solution and iron salts, were used for taking fingerprints, and later, mixture of acrylic colours with glycerin and alcohol was introduced. Today, there are various techniques, like combination of different optical methods (absorption, diffuse reflection, luminescence, UV absorption) [5, 18, 19], physical methods (nanopowders, nanoparticles as reagents) [20], physico-chemical methods [21] and various chemical methods [22]. The basic physico-chemical method for crime scene

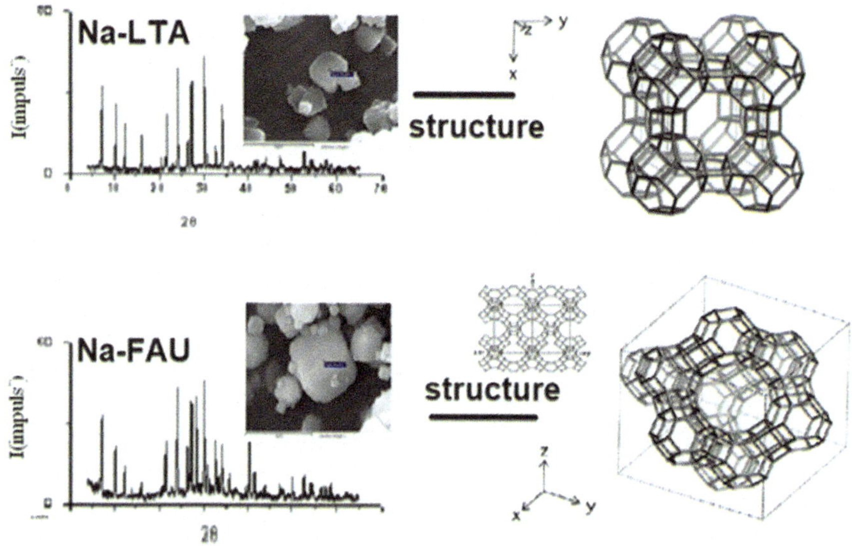

Fig. 3 The X-ray diagrams and structure of zeolite$_{LTA}$ and zeolite$_{FAU}$ topology nanopowders

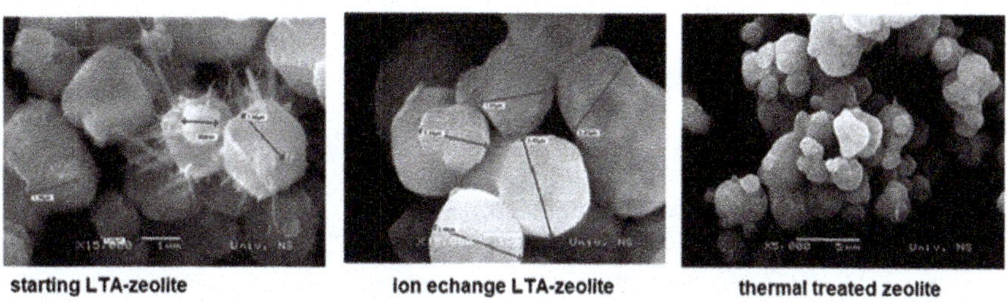

Fig. 4 SEM micrographs of zeolite$_{LTA}$ topology (starting, ion exchange and thermal treated)

fingerprints identification is the application of nanopowders on the investigating surface.

1.3 Short Intro to Fractals

Fractals are irregular geometric objects, that can be found everywhere in nature. They are named after the Latin adjective *fractus*, which means broken, fractured, due to their fragmented, ragged and shattered form. Fractal patterns exist at all scale sizes in nature, from nano and microstructures up to the huge objects, thus snowflakes, seashells, tree branching, vegetables, like Romanesco broccoli, crystals, coral reefs, coastlines, clouds, etc., express fractal nature. Fractals are not only morphological phenomena—they can be observed in various processes, like heart sounds, Brownian motion, lightning, stock market fluctuation, and many more.

The main characteristic of fractals is selfsimilarity, which means that every part of the fractal resembles the whole, displaying repeating similarities. Mathematical fractals, like Cantor set, Koch curve, Sierpinski triangle, etc. are selfsimilar ideal fractals. Physical fractals, like aforementioned snowflakes, trees, clouds, etc. are still closer to mathematical fractals than to Euclidean geometry objects, even though they do not possess ideal selfsimilarity characteristics. Because of their irregular and complex features, fractals cannot be adequately and sufficiently defined by Euclidean geometry, therefore they are the subjects of the fractal geometry. Mathematical studies of fractals began in the seventeenth century and continued to develope throughout the next few centuries, until Benoit Mandelbrot in the 1980s [23] systematized all previous research, introducing a modern approach, and the term "fractal ".

One of the most commonly used parameters for characterizing fractals is fractal (Hausdorff) dimension (FD), a non-integer which describes the shape, structure and related properties of a fractal object. Unlike FD, classical geometry topological dimension (TD) is an integer, and the mathematical relation between these paremeters is FD-TD = FD-2 > 0 [24, 25]. The value of an object's fractal dimension is always greater than its topological dimension.

2 Experimental Part

The first part of the experiment implied the consolidation of the ionically modified zeolite, as a precursor for further synthesis process.

2.1 Photoluminescent Bi-Sillenite Nanopowder Synthesis and Characterization

The synthesis procedure involves mixing of zeolite (Na-LTA) water solution with native bismuth in autoclave at 170 °C for 7 days. The new synthesized materials (Bi + $zeolite_{LTA}$ topology) is annealed up to 350 °C for 1 h and its structural transformation to sillenite phase occured. The results of chemical, AAS and EDAX analyses are presented in Fig. 5.

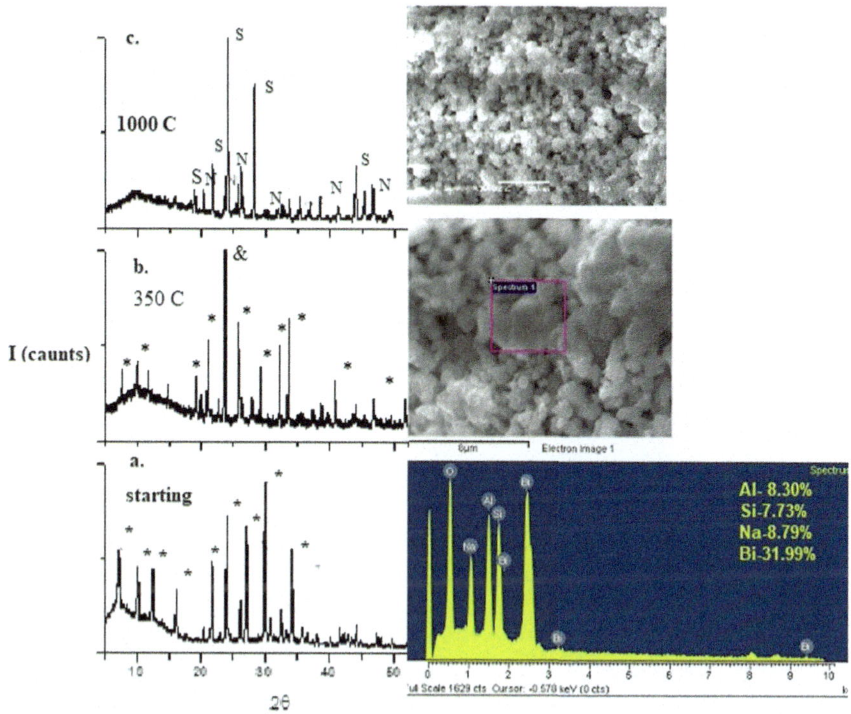

Fig. 5 SEM microphotographs and X-ray diffraction pattern of zeolite LTA topology doped with Bi cation. **a** Starting doped LTA zeolite whit Bi cation. **b** Thermal treated Bi doped LTA zeolite at 350 °C/1 h. **c** Bi-LTA sample annealed at 1000 °C/1 h

2.2 *Photoluminescent Y and Ag Doped Nanopowders Synthesis and Characterization*

Ion exchange of precursor LTA zeolite outernet Na^+ cation with Y and Ag was performed. At the beginning of the procedure, Y and Ag content in $YCl_2 \cdot 2H_2O$ and AgCl solutions was measured, and the solution molarity was 0.21 M. Next, 15 g of the Na-LTA zeolite sample was put in contact with 300 ml 0.21 M $YCl_2 \cdot 2H_2O$ and 300 ml 0.21 M AgCl, in order to ion exchange occurrence. Results of SEM/EDAX analysis are presented in Figs. 6 and 7.

2.3 *Preparation for the Fractal Analysis*

To characterize microstructure and properties of photoluminescent Bi, Y and Ag doped zeolite nanopowders, fractal nature analysis should be applied and that is the aim of our future research. At this point, we will show application on the clay sample,

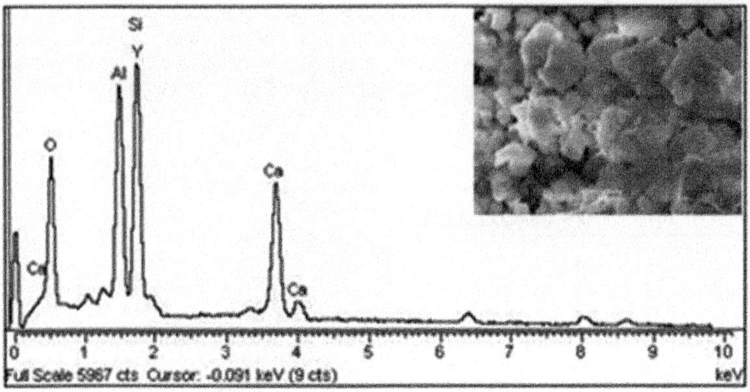

Fig. 6 SEM/EDAX analysis of Y cation doped LTA zeolite

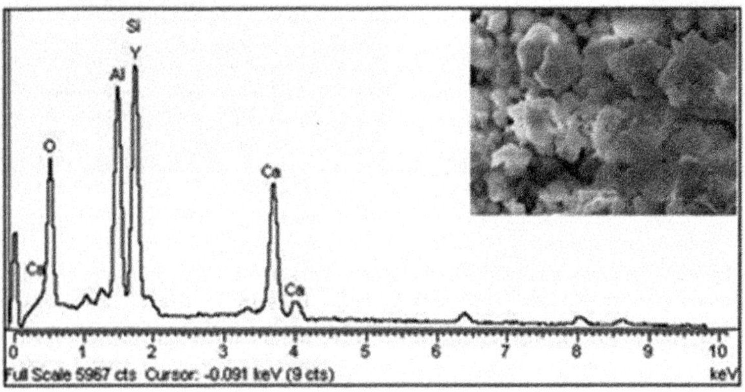

Fig. 7 SEM/EDAX analysis of Ag cation doped LTA zeolite

as an example of a nanomaterial (can constitute any material as long as it's within the particle size range of $< 2\ \mu m$).

In order to apply fractal analysis on the clay sample, we prepared a couple of SEM images of the samples under different magnification. Next, we selected one SEM image, the most suitable for the fractal characterization that follows (Fig. 8).

SEM images of the same part of the sample were taken under four different magnifications, and presented in Fig. 9.

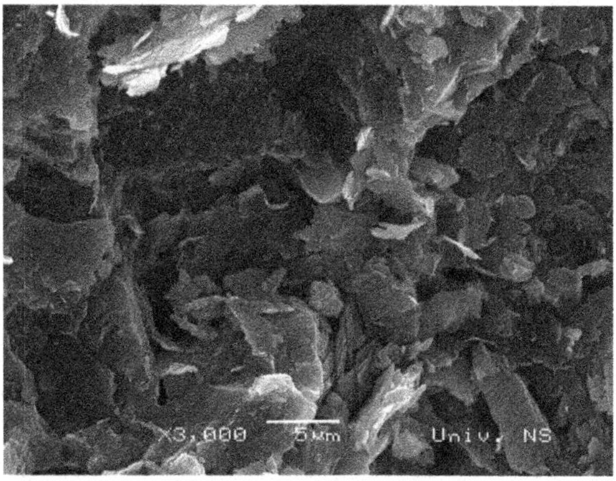

Fig. 8 SEM image of the clay sample prepared for the fractal characterization

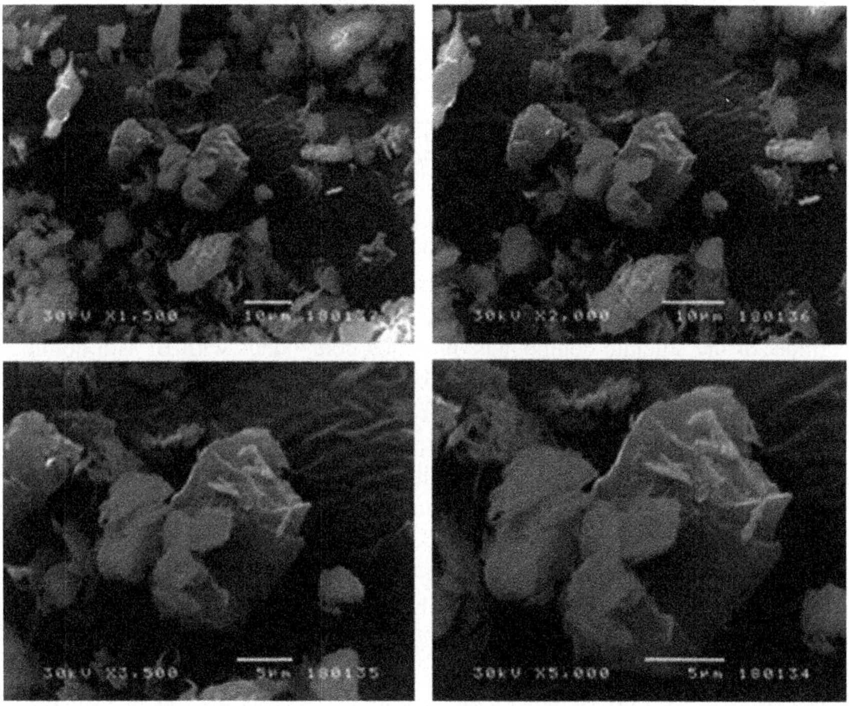

Fig. 9 SEM images of the selected part of the sample under different magnifications (1500, 2000, 3500 and 5000)

3 Results and Discussion

3.1 *The Application of Nanopowders in Forensic Science*

Nanopowders are widely used in forensic science, but their most significant application is for the fingerprinting method. All three groups of nanopowders, standard, metal and luminescent, have their advantages in cases of taking fingerprints from the crime scene, nevertheless luminescent nanopowders show the greatest potential. That is the reason we focused on the luminescent nanopowders synthesis and characterization.

3.2 *Nanomaterials Based on Doped Bi, Y and Ag Cations*

The work deals with a possibility of using zeolite LTA topology doped with different cations Bi, Y and Ag, as precursors for obtaining new nanophase. In all three cases nanopowders with luminescent properties are obtained. Bi doped nanopowder displays yellow-green, Ag doped paleyellow, and Y doped light orange luminescent colour.

Bi Doped Nanopowder Structural Characteristics We presented the data regarding the photoluminescent Bi-sillenite nanopowder in this research paper, which could be applied in the forensic science for fingerprints detection.

In the ion exchange process with Bi cations sillenite was obtained. The general formula of the sillenite compounds, in which compounds with Bi as a dominant cation belong, is $Bi_{12}MO_{20}$, with the cation M = Ge, Si, Ti or the cation in the form of isomorphic mixtures M = (Bi, Ga), (Bi, V), (Bi, Zn), (Bi, Fe), (Fe, P) [26, 27]. It is known that the intensive orange-red photoluminescence in Bi-doped materials, comes from Bi^{2+} ions. The center responsible for this phenomenon is paired electrons system with integer total spin, or Bi^{2+} ions and oxygen vacancies system. Based on the occupation factors Bi (0.93451) Si (0.15907), and oxygen positions O_2 (0.333) and O_3 (0.333), cation oxygen vacancies are observed.

The X-ray powder diffraction profiles for thermal treated LTA + Bi zeolite shows the increase in zeolite component cristalinity and crisps aggregates morphology, with sillenite and nephelin phase (Fig. 10). The sillenite phase was refined in the cubic space group *I23*, for different distrbutions of Si and Bi over the cation sites [28].

The interest in this Bi-based materials is a consequence of the wide-range near-infrared photoluminescence discovery [29, 30].

Y Doped Nanopowder Structural Characteristics In the ion exchange process with Y cations, anorthite, unknown in nature, was obtained. Y doped LTA zeolite was thermaly treated at the temperature of 800 °C when the cristal structure starts to amorphize, whilst at 1000 °C cristalization of a new anorthite phase occurs. SEM images of initial and thermal treated Y-LTA zeolite are shown in Fig. 11. Anorthite structure with Y cations has not been described in available literature yet, so it will

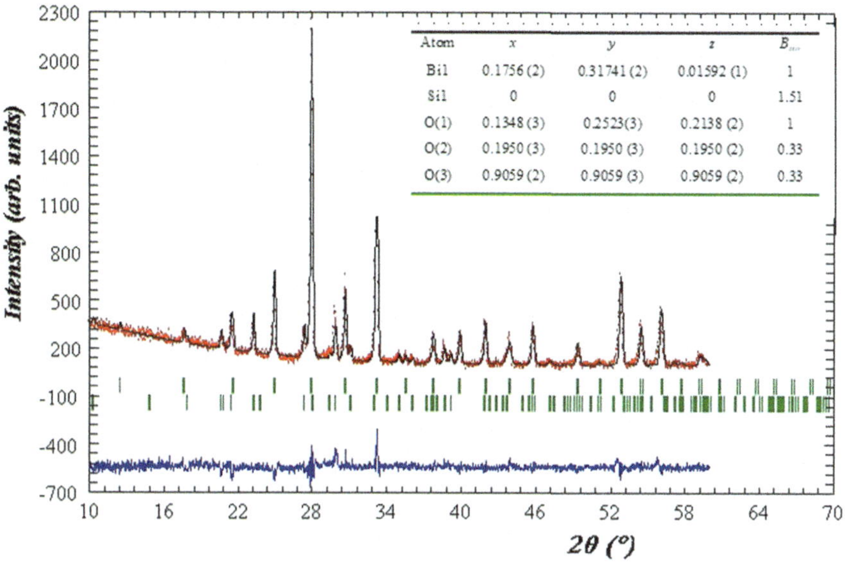

Atom	x	y	z	B_{iso}
Bi1	0.1756 (2)	0.31741 (2)	0.01592 (1)	1
Si1	0	0	0	1.51
O(1)	0.1348 (3)	0.2523(3)	0.2138 (2)	1
O(2)	0.1950 (3)	0.1950 (3)	0.1950 (2)	0.33
O(3)	0.9059 (2)	0.9059 (3)	0.9059 (2)	0.33

Fig. 10 The observed (circles), calculated (continuous line) and difference powder diffraction profiles for thermal treated LTA+Bi compuonds. Table presents the final atomic coordinates and occupations factors for sillenite (S.G. I23)

be the subject of our future research regarding fractal nature analysis application on nanopowders used in forensic science.

The results of the X-ray diffraction analysis of zeolite LTA topology doped with Y cations and thermaly treated are presented as diagrams in Fig. 12.

Ag Doped Nanopowder Structural Characteristics Anorthite, unknown in nature, was obtained in the ion exchange process with Ag cations, which was thermaly treated at 800 °C, giving the hexacelsian phase, and at 1000 °C, anorthite mineral. In Fig. 13 the X-ray diffraction diagram of Ag doped LTA zeolit, initial and thermaly treated at 800 °C and 1000 °C is presented. Since the anorthite with Ag as

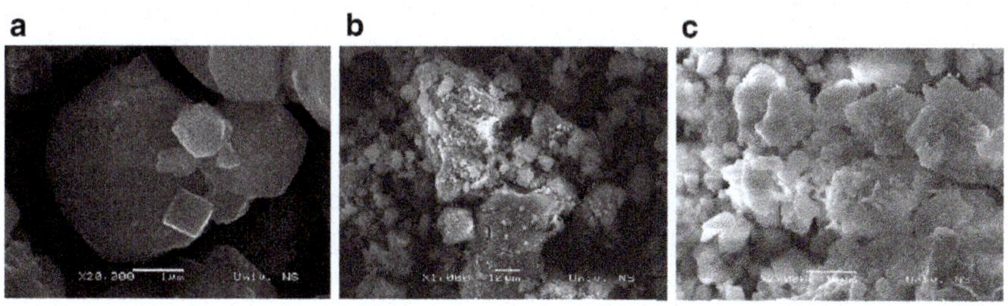

Fig. 11 SEM microphotographs of Y doped zeolite LTA-topology. **a** initial zeolite LTA topology doped with Y cation. **b** Thermal treated Y doped zeolite at temperature 800 °C/1 h. **c** Thermal treated Y doped zeolite at temperature 1000 °C/1 h

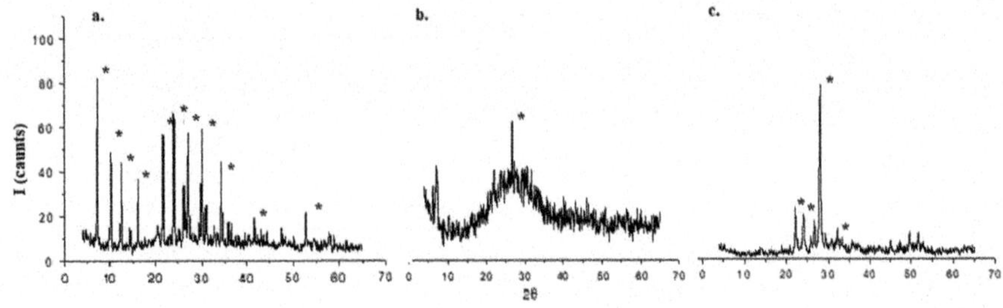

Fig. 12 The X-ray powder diffraction pattern of Y doped LTA zeolite. **a** Starting zeolite LTA topology doped with Y cation (* LTA zeolite); thermal treated Y doped zeolite at temperature thermally treated at 800 °C (* amorphe phase), thermal treated Y doped zeolite at temperature thermally treated at 1000 °C (* Y anorthite)

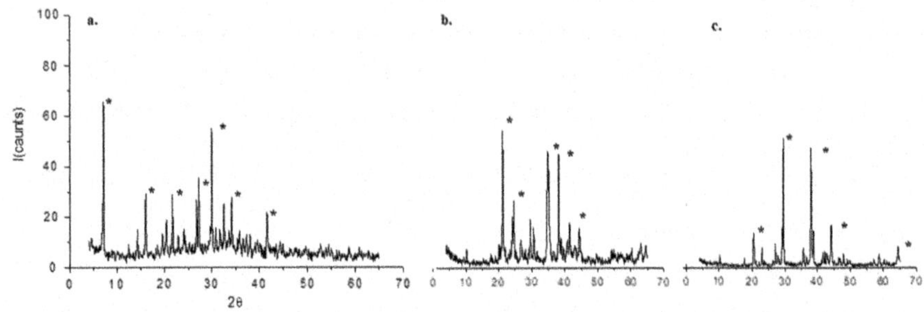

Fig. 13 The X-ray powder diffraction pattern of Ag doped zeolite LTA topology. **a** Starting zeolite Ag-LTA. **b** Thermal teatred Ag-LTA zeolite at temperature 800 °C. **c** Thermal treated zeolite Ag-LTA at temperature 1000 °C

a dominant cation, nor the hexacelsians, has not been studied in details yet, it will be included in our further luminescent nanopowders fractal characterization research.

3.3 The Nanomaterials Fractal Analysis

Depending on the surface on which the fingerprints are found, adequate nanopowders are applied, however, the problem exists when taking fingerprints from inaccessible surfaces. Conventional nanopowders are not often able to develop a fingerprint image, due to the surface and type of a material which they are taken from [31].

Here, fractal characterization of the nanopowder's structure is of a great assistance, considering that the nanostructure highly affects the application on the inaccessible surfaces. Sinthesis of nanomaterials applicable for taking fingerprints from versatile surfaces is a new research direction, where the fractal analysis could be implemented, as a method for nanomaterials structure and properties determination and prediction.

Each nanopowder, as well as zeolite LTA topology doped nanomaterials with different cations Bi, Y and Ag, synthesized in this research, finds its application in different forensic methods and investigations, according to its features, thus, it is very important to examine and designate them. The structure and properties of luminescent Bi, Y and Ag-LTA nanopowders, as potential nanomaterials for application in the fingerprinting method, have to be clearly defined by applying the fractal nature analysis.

Our aim, in this research paper, is to emphasize the importance of fractal nature analysis application in forensic science, as a new approach opening the perspectives for predicting and designing of nanomaterials implemented in various forensic fields. By this efficient and accurate method, based on fractal self-similarities, we can precisely determine morphological microstructure and related properties of a nanomaterial, which is significant for its further application in the forensic investigation.

As an example of fractal nature analysis, based on our previous research results [32], in Fig. 14 fractalization of the natural clay sample is shown.

Boundary of the selected fractal sample is designated in blue colour on the SEM micrography, and transfered into a linear function, whose graph is a straight line,

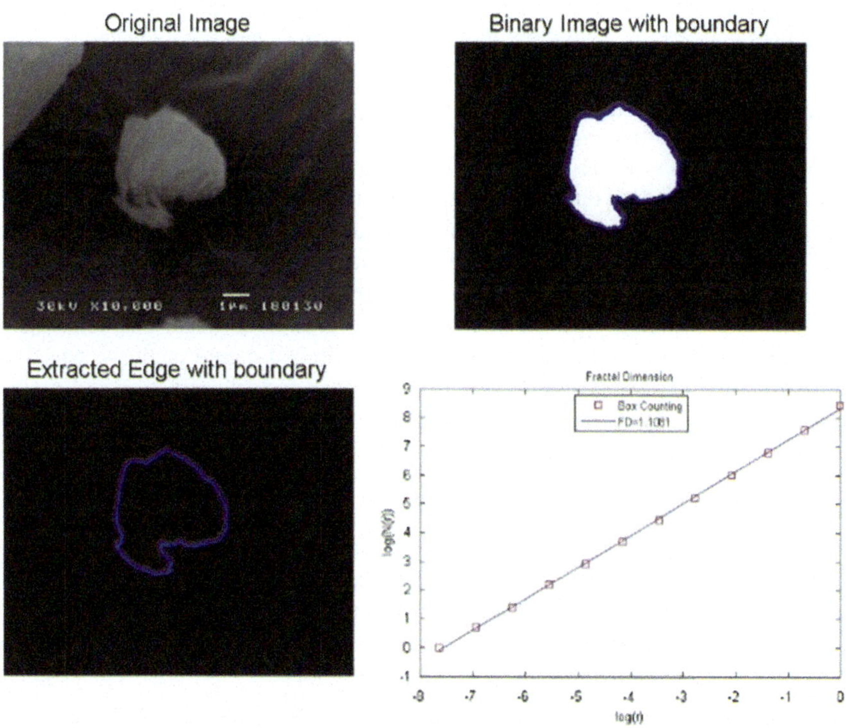

Fig. 14 Fractalization of the ceramic clay sample and obtained fractal dimension [32]

by applying the box-counting method. In this procedure, N is the number of parts (boxes) into which the original object is divided to, and h is the magnification (scaling factor), representing the number how many times the part needs to be magnified in order to be as the whole object. Next, the graph is created, with $\log(h)$ on x-axis, and $\log(N)$ on the y-axis. The purpose of this mathematical technique is to obtain fractal dimension represented as the slope of the graph, $FD = \log N/\log h$, and calculated by the least-squares method. The obtained fractal dimension provides us with very important data about the fractal object of interest, including the fact that the greater fractal dimension means the greater complexity of the object. FD indicates material's morphological characteristics which directly imply its physicochemical properties, and that is why FD is an essential parameter in determination and prediction process of nanomaterials in forensic science synthesis and application.

4 Conclusion

Accuracy and precision of the obtained data is one of the major demands in the forensic investigation, thus the forensic techniques and materials applied have to be characterized in details, due to their big impact on final results regarding the presented evidences in the court. Therefore, the choice of adequate and suitable nanomaterials is of a great importance in the whole process. It is necessary to define and predict microstructure and properties of each nanomaterial used, in order to implement it in the best way possible.

When it comes to the fingerprinting method, various nanopowders are used, according to the surface on which the fingerprints are located, including luminescent nanopowders. In our research we synthesized and characterized photoluminescent Bi, Y and Ag doped zeolite LTA topology nanopowders, potential nanomaterials for taking fingerprints, by applying the X-ray powder diffraction, crystallographic analysis and scanning electron microscopy, nevertheless, fractal characterization would provide some very important new data. Fractal nature analysis, based on self-similarity, is an outstanding scientific approach for determination and prediction of material's properties. It gives us an excellent insight into the microstructure, and accordingly, related properties, which is significant for nanopowders application regarding the investigated surface.

We demonstrated how to fractally characterize a clay sample, as an example of a nanomaterial, and how fractal analysis could be applied on different materials, like luminescent nanopowders. The idea and the aim of this paper is to stress all the advantages of fractal nature analysis application on nanomaterials used in forensic science research, which opens new frontiers for conventional forensic nanomaterials improved implementation, as well as introducing innovative and advanced nanomaterials characterized by fractal self-similarities scientific approach.

Acknowledgements The authors gratefully acknowledge the support of Ministry of Education, Science and Technological Development of the Republic of Serbia (Contract No. 451-03-68/2022-14/200023).

References

1. Nanotechnology and human health:Scientific evidance and risk governance. Report of the WHO expert meeting 10–11 December 2012, Bonn, Germany, Copenhagen, WHO Regional Office for Europe (2013)
2. Matovic, B., Boškovic, S.: Terminologija nanomaterijala i nanotehnologije. Metalurgija **13**, 155–157 (2007)
3. Smith, W.C., Kinney, R.W., De Partee, D.G.: The report of the International Assotiation for Identification. Standardization II Committee. J. Forensic Identification **43**, 563–570 (1993)
4. Seah, L.K., Dinish, U.S., Phang, W.F., Chao, Z.X., Murukeshan, V.M.: Fluorescence optimization and lifetime studies of fingerprints treated with magnetic powders. Forensic Sci. Inter. **152**, 249 (2005)
5. Saferstein, R., Graf, S.L.: Evaluation of a reflected ultraviolet imaging system for fingerprint detection. JFI **51**, 385–393 (2001)
6. Radosavljevic-Mihajlovic, A., Vulic, P., Matovic, B., Devecerski, A.: Synthesis of sillenite-type compounds from zeolite precursors: XRPD and SEM/EDS analyses. J. Optoelcctron. Adv. Mater. **10**, 887–890 (2008)
7. Cosimo, P., Laurent, G., Quenum-Possy-Berry, F.-G., Clemence, A., Th, N., Thomas, C.: Lumicyano: A new fluorescent cyanoacrylate for a one-step luminescent latent fingermark development. Forensic Sci. Int. **233**, 104–112 (2013)
8. Breck, D.W.: Zeolite Molecular Sieves Structure, Chemistry and Use. J. Wiley & Sons, New York (1974)
9. Barrer, R.M.: Zeolites and Clay Minerals as Sorbent and Molecular Sieves. Acedem. Press, New York (1978)
10. Betekhtine, A.G.: Manuel de mineralogie descriptive. Editions MIR, Moscou (1966)
11. Baerlocher, Ch., Meier, W.M., Olson, D.H.: Atlas of zeolite framework types. Structure Commission of International zeolite Association, Elsevier, Amsterdam (2001)
12. Rakic, V.M., Hercigonja, R.V., Dondur, V.T.: CO interaction with zeolites studied by TPD and FTIR: transition-metal ion-exchanged FAU-type zeolites. Microporous Mesoporous Mater. **27**, 27–39 (1999)
13. Dondur, V.T., Rakic, V.M., Damjanovic, L., Hercigonja, R., Auroux, A.: Temperature-programmed desorption of n-hexane from hydrated HZSM-5 and NH4ZSM-5 zeolites. J. Ther. Anal. Calorimet. **84**, 233–238 (2006)
14. Rakic, V.M., Dondur, V.T., Hercigonja, R.V.: Thermal effects of the interactions of carbon monoxide with zeolites. Thermochim. Acta **379**, 77–84 (2001)
15. https://www.ncjrs.gov/pdffiles1/nij/225320.pdf
16. Abraham, J., Champod, C., Lennard, C., Roux, C.: Modern statistical models for forensic fingerprint examinations A critical review. Forensic Sci. Int. **232**, 131–150 (2013)
17. http://www.police-scientifique.com/dossier-scheffer
18. Margot, P., Lennard, C.: Fingerprint Detection Techniques, 6th edn. University of Lausanne, Lausanne, Institut de Police Scientifique et de Criminologie (1994)
19. Lee, H.C., Gaensslen, R.E.: Advances in Fingerprint Technology, 2nd ed., CRC Press (2001)
20. Jones, N., Stoilovic, M., Lennard, C.J., Roux, C.: Vacuum metal deposition: factors affecting normal and reverse development of latent fingerprints on polyethylene substrates. Forensic Sci. Int. **115**, 73–88 (2001)

21. Schnetz, B., Margot, P.: Technical note: latent fingermarks, colloidal gold and multimetal deposition (MMD) optimisation of the method. Forensic Sci. Int. **118**, 21–28 (2001)
22. Pounds, C.A., Grigg, R., Mongkolaussavaratana, T.: The use of 1,8-diazafluoren- 9-one (DFO) for the fluorescent detection of latent fingerprints on paper: a preliminary evaluation. J. Forensic Sci. **35**, 169–175 (1990)
23. Mandelbrot, B.: Fractals and the Geometry of Nature. Freeman, San Francisco (1982)
24. Mitic, V.V., Kocic, L., Paunovic, V., Lazovic, G., Miljkovic, M.: Fractal nature structure reconstruction method in designing microstructure properties. Mater. Res. Bull. **101**, 175–183 (2018). https://doi.org/10.1016/j.materresbull.2018.01.019
25. Mitic, V.V., Kocic, L., Paunovic, V., Bastic, F., Sirmic, D.: The fractal nature materials microstructure influence on electrochemical energy sources. Sci. Sinter. **47**, 195–204 (2015)
26. Radev, S.F., Simonov, V.I.: Structures of sillenites and atomic mechanisms of their isomorphic substitutions. Sov. Phys. Crystallogr. **37**, 484 (1992)
27. Dos Santos, T.O., Carvalho, J.F., Hernandes, A.C.: Synthesis and cristal growth of sillenite phase in the Bi_2O_3-TiO_2-Nb_2O_5 system. Cryst. Res. Technol. **39**, 868–872 (2004)
28. Neov, S., Marinova, V., Reehuis, M., Sonntag, R.: Neutron-diffraction study of Bi2 M O20 single crystals with sillenite structure (M = Si, Si0.995 Mn0.005, Bi0.53 Mn0.47). Appl. Phys. A **74**, 1016–1018 (2002)
29. Murata, K., Fujimoto, Y., Kanabe, T., Fujita, H., Nakatsuka, M.: Bi-doped SiO2 as a new laser material for an intense laser. Fusion Eng. **44**, 437–439 (1999)
30. Fujimoto, Y., Nakatsuka, M.: Infrared luminescence from Bismuth-doped silica glass. Jpn. J. Appl. Phys. **40**, 279–281 (2001)
31. Menzel, E.R., Menzel, L.W., Schwierking, J.R.: Talanta **67**, 383 (2005)
32. Mitic, V.V., Lazovic, G., Radosavljevic-Mihajlovic, A.S., Milosevic, D., Markovic, B., Simeunovic, D., Vlahovic, B.: Forensic science and fractal nature analysis. Mod. Phys. Lett. B **35** (2021). S0217984921504935

Natural Patterns, Theoretical Models and New Insights in Material Characterization

Medical Devices Based on Mimicry in Light-Matter Interaction: "Structured Matter Meets Structured Light"

Djuro Koruga, Lidija Matija, Ivana Stanković, Branislava Jeftić, and Noel Thompson

Abstract Methods and designs of mimicry taken from nature and biology and implemented in photonic science and engineering are presented. Order of geometrical features and process based on the symmetry, and harmony, are given. Symmetry and harmony give rise to beautiful geometrical structures in nature and biology, and engineers have been trying to copy and apply these into various devices. A selection of examples of mimicry are presented based on light-matter interaction and its application in health sciences. Two basic mimetic approaches are identified; the first, "mirror mimicry" (reflection), when photons and electrons have the same energy values and reflected photons (without matter damage) give information about the state of matter. The second "absorbed mimicry" (absorption), when electrons of matter absorb photons and change the state of matter according to the order of photons. The first approach is used for matter characterisation and diagnostics in medicine, while the second one is used for therapy. Brewster mirror effect of light-matter interaction is used for tissues diagnostics, while nano photonic devices based on molecule C_{60} have been used for therapy. This is due to the symmetrical similarity of C_{60} and collagen, microtubules, centrioles and water molecules around biomolecules. In

D. Koruga (✉) · L. Matija · I. Stanković · B. Jeftić
NanoLab, Biomedical Engineering, Faculty of Mechanical Engineering, University of Belgrade, Belgrade, Serbia
e-mail: dkoruga@mas.bg.ac.rs

L. Matija
e-mail: lmatija@mas.bg.ac.rs

I. Stanković
e-mail: imileusnic@mas.bg.ac.rs

B. Jeftić
e-mail: bjeftic@mas.bg.ac.rs

D. Koruga
TFT Nano Center, Belgrade, Serbia

N. Thompson
ZeptoHyperTech, Belgrade, Serbia
e-mail: noel.thompson@zeptohypertech.rs

S. Najman et al. (eds.), *Bioceramics, Biomimetic and Other Compatible Materials Features for Medical Applications*, Engineering Materials,
https://doi.org/10.1007/978-3-031-17269-4_15

order to test both approaches we have made and tested nano photonic devices on skin, scars, burns, cancers, etc. According to our investigation, the symmetries of structure and the harmonies of processes in nature and biology are direct consequences of process optimization; mass-energy, energy-information and information-control. The same principles of symmetry and harmonisation should be implemented, via mimicry, into future process and machine development since this will lead to greater system optimization.

Keywords Mimicry · Symmetry · Harmony · Nano photonics · Reflection · Absorption · Skin · Cervix · Colon · Cancer

1 Introduction

In everyday life, from time-to-time, we ask ourselves from time to time why something looks as it does? When the outside form of some object fascinates us we are usually trying to understand its inner composition. Answering this question becomes even more difficult when one looks at complex, animate objects such as insects, birds and humans. However, the magic word that explains the connection between the geometry (shape of the object), kinematics (elements of the object) and dynamics (regulation of the relationship between parts—whole—environment) is optimization: mass, energy, information, organisation and control [1, 2]. Optimization is a consequence of three pairs; two internal opposites and one external object-environment opposite. The first pair of internal opposites is symmetry/asymmetry, and the second pair is harmony/chaos, while the object-environment opposite is classical-quantum information pairing in time. Quantum information processing is billions of times faster than classical, and it sets up concurrent possible events that could become reality, depending on its matching with a classical counterpart. This classical counterpart is established through evolution ("arrow of time"). To summarise, the final reality is the code entity of pairing quantum and classical information processing [3].

From a scientific point of view, it is very important to understand how internal structure relates to the final external form. Sunflower geometry is an example of system optimisation in nature, biology and in engineering, as human mimicry. The crux of understanding sunflower geometry is its icosahedral symmetry, which is a part of the general point symmetry group [4].

Since the essence of the photon and electron existence is unknown, we are unaware of the essence of our own existence, i.e., of the life phenomenon. However, we do know many characteristics of the photon and electron, and regarding life, we know that, according to Leibniz, health is the most important issue after peace of mind. This monograph originated from the need to contribute to the maintenance of good health as efficiently as possible in a natural way, using light. To achieve this, it is necessary to be well acquainted with the structural, energetic, and informational foundations of biomolecules, that is, with the organisation and regulation mechanisms of the human organism. After we have understood the laws governing the main rules of biomolecules, which are essential as life itself, the next step is to design a device capable of inducing structural organisation in photons according to the same laws that govern biomolecular organisation; that is, in the way biochemical/physical processes are realised based on Gibbs free energy. Biomolecules are, by their structure and energy, via entropy, related to information. Thus the newly created light can influence the molecules' information states, and therefore act on their structural-energy-information processes as well. Structuring photons, according to some biomolecular features, should follow the tally principle—the ancient method of recognition, pairing, i.e. identification of ownership. For example, it was historically used by millers; a farmer would bring a sack of wheat, take a stick upon which notches would be made. The stick would then be split longitudinally so that on both halves the notches would be visible; one half would be kept by the miller, and the other by the farmer, and when the farmer came to claim the flour the notches on the two sticks would be compared and, if they aligned, the farmer would receive his flour. In this Chapter we will explain how a light polarization phenomenon was applied to achieve harmonisation and interaction between light and biomolecules, directly affecting the behaviour of the organism [4].

2 Mimicry from Nature and Biosystems

Contemporary science considers that biological life on Earth originated in water, under the influence of light (Sun and atmospheric discharges) and Earth's microwave radiation. Other preconditions were also satisfied such as gravity, appropriate temperature, atmosphere, etc. The importance of initial conditions for the origin of life is significant. It is compared, within the science of deterministic chaos, to the "butterfly effect" [5].

Clathrin is found in many human tissues as a carrier of substances such as neurotransmitters. It also clears the cell debris into extracellular space. Clathrin naturally forms a triskelion, and these triskelia form pentagons and hexagons so the clathrins in the CNS (composed of 36 triskelia) form 12 pentagons and 20 hexagons, whilst in other tissues they are made of 12 pentagons and a varying number of hexagons. Clathrin within the CNS is considered, alongside the dodecahedron, the most perfect symmetrical structure that can exist in nature (based on the law of point symmetry) [6].

Microtubules did not attract attention until 1974 when the New York Academy of Sciences organized the first scientific meeting on the subject, with emphasis on the structural and biochemical aspects of microtubules. Since this topic aroused the interest of researchers all over the world, the same Academy organized another scientific conference in 1986 on the dynamic aspects of microtubules [7]. It was demonstrated that microtubules have an important role in biology, in intracellular transport, cell shape definition, and as the main compound of the cell mitotic spindle. Microtubules also create more complex structures such as cilia, flagella, and centrioles [8].

3 Mimetic in Light-Matter Interaction

Light—water interaction was crucial to start building biological life as we know it. But what is a photon? Science still does not have the exact answer to this question, but many photon characteristics are known and, based on this insight, many devices have been constructed for diagnostic and therapy or used by man in day-to-day life, starting with the simple light bulb and radio, up to the high-powered laser.

Especially significant is the use of light in medicine (both in diagnostics and therapy). Beside ordinary, diffuse daylight, polarized light (linear, circular, elliptical) is also used for technical and medical purposes. It is known that the photon exhibits wave-particle duality i.e. under certain conditions it behaves like a wave, and under others like a particle. However, recent experimental findings demonstrate that the photon exhibits wave-particle duality simultaneously [9], enabling better understanding of the light-matter interaction. The concept of wavelike light has been dominant until 1905, when Einstein explained the photoelectric experiment and demonstrated that the moving photon also has a particular nature. The Nobel Prize was awarded to him for this discovery in 1921. Asked once what a photon is, he replied that, despite the fact that he devoted most of his time to the study of light, he does not know what a photon is, and added: "it would also be nice to know what an electron is" [10].

We should ask ourselves what is an electron. Most people would assume that this question has been satisfactorily resolved, because it seems that the electron is an simpler object than the photon. However, contemporary science still does not have the answer to this question. As in the case of the photon, whilst many of its characteristics have been established the essential answer is still lacking. Whilst light was the subject of human curiosity and investigation since the beginning of time, the electron was first discovered in 1897 by the British scientist Joseph John Thomson. It was initially represented as a cloud filling the majority of atomic volume, then later as a particle orbiting the nucleus at a given distance. The electron has corresponding energy depending on its distance from the nucleus. As Einstein established that the photon exhibits wave-particle duality, Luis de Broglie demonstrated in 1924 that the electron similarly exhibits wave-particle duality (he was awarded the Nobel Prize for this discovery in 1929). A short history of the development of the electron model (in the hydrogen atom) is presented in Table 1. Today, many devices have been constructed based on the wave-particle duality of the electron, such as the scanning tunnelling microscope (STM), which records molecules at the atomic scale [11].

In light–matter interaction, photons of various energies interact with valence electrons. In the case of visible light, photons interact exclusively with electrons from the external orbital, leaving the essential electron organisation unchanged.

Table 1 The short history of electron model development in hydrogen atom [4]

Electron in the hydrogen atom	Description
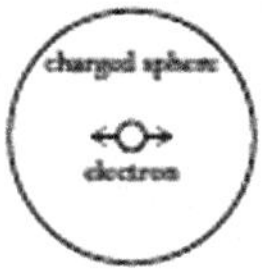	**1897 J.J. Thomson:** Electron is subatomic corpuscle filling a sphere with uniform positive charge. Atoms of order number Z are positively charged bonding the electron with electric forces
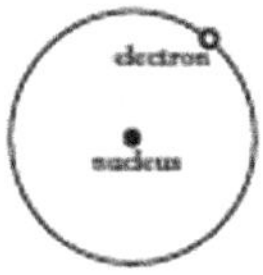	**1911 E. Rutherford:** Electron is a three-dimensional corpuscular, negatively charged particle in the nuclear atom model. In the proposed planetary model, the electrons rotate at a great distance from the positively charged nucleus on exactly defined circular paths. The overall negative electron charge is equal to the positive nucleus charge
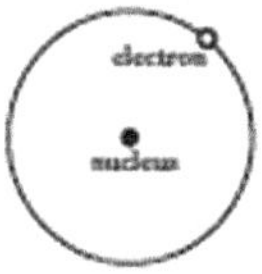	**1913 N. Bohr:** Electron is a point-lite three-dimensional charged particle on a circular path, Each orbit has a different energetic Level. Electrons do not emit energy while moving, on stationary paths. When the electron transits from a path, of a higher energy level to a path of a lover energy level it radiates electromagnetic radiation ($h\nu$) equal to the difference of energies of these two energy levels
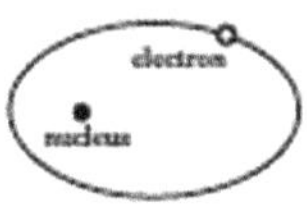	**1916 A. Sommerfeld:** Electron orbits a quantized elliptical orbital the electron position is defined by the radius of the orbital and the azimuth angle. Electron mass depends on its velocity along quantized orbitals
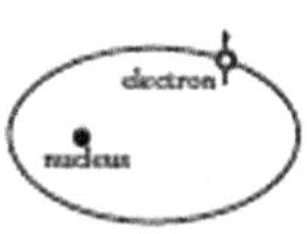	**1925 S, Goudsmit:** Besides moving along elliptical orbitals, electron rotates about its own axis (spin). As the electron is negatively charged. it has a proper magnetic held. Electron has its own momentum and a proper magnetic moment, which explains the splitting of atomic levels
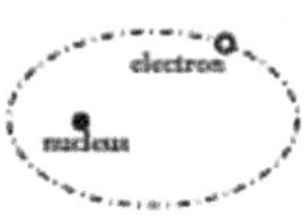	**1925 W. K. Heisenberg:** Electron is not considered from the aspect of the classical formalism (Poisson notation); the concept of uncertainty is introduced according to which the product of two related quantities cannot exceed the Planck constant (electron's position and its velocity cannot be determined at the same time)
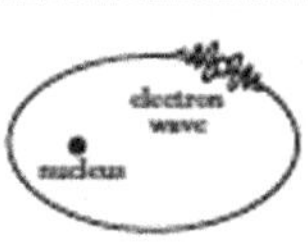	**1926 E. Schrödinger:** Electron is considered from the aspect of wave mechanics (De Broglie. 1923), according to which paths of particular electrons within the atom are not described classically spatially and temporally, but are determined based on probability. Therefore, particular electron energy levels within the atom are given only as average values of the distribution of the electron charge cloud with respect to the nucleus. The solution of the Schrödinger's equation gives the electric charge distribution around the nucleus

(continued)

Table 1 (continued)

Electron in the hydrogen atom	Description
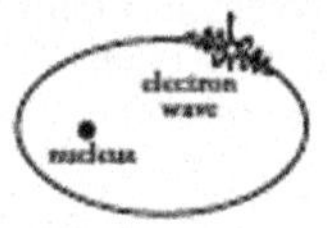	**1928 P. Dirac:** The electron is a quantum–mechanical object whose motion can be described relativistically. This approach forecast the existence of the *positron,* a particle having the same mass and spin as the electron, but opposite charge. Using relativistic theory for electron motion, the best conformity to spectral lines for the hydrogen atom was demonstrated
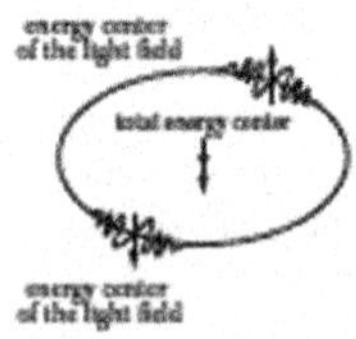	**1978 H. Salhofer:** The electron is at the same time a quantum–mechanical (microscopic) and an electrodynamic (macroscopic) entity (Maxwell-Dirac isomorphism—MDI). There are two electromagnetic fields with energy centers symmetrically distributed on "Keplerian" electron orbitals (antipodal action)

However, high-energy photons interact with valence electrons and eject them from their orbitals, thus causing matter ionization. X-rays penetrate yet deeper into atoms, reaching electrons in internal shells, resulting in the reorganisation of electrons within the atom; atoms transit into higher energy orbitals—that is, into an excited state [12]. This paper discusses the interactions of matter with visible and infrared light of wavelengths 380–780 nm. In order to fully understand the interaction of VIS–NIR light with tissue, it is necessary to be well acquainted with characteristics of biomolecules, tissues and the organism itself. Biomolecules, such as proteins, lipids, fat, etc., constitute about 15% of the organism's total mass. Until now, the absorption characteristic of biomolecules was dominant in selecting the type of light for diagnostics and therapy—a necessary, although not sufficient condition for the optimal interaction between light and biomolecules. Beside classical vibration complexes (C–O, C = C, O–H, N–H, etc.) it is necessary to understand vibration modes of the molecule (structure) as a whole.

In order to grasp this, we have to know the symmetry group to which a molecule or structure belongs to as a whole. Therefore, this Chapter will place special emphasis on the investigation of the symmetry features of particular biomolecules, such as clathrin, microtubules, collagen, actin, cilia, centrioles, etc. These characteristics will define how light acts on biomolecules in order to preserve their organisation, or improve their impaired structure and functionality. Both light and matter structures should have the same type of symmetry and organisation, so that, during their interaction, mutual recognition of structural "patterns", occurs, resulting in resonant interaction [13]. Epithelial tissues are the first biological structure that light interacts with, whether in diagnostics or in therapy. Skin is one of the best examples of this interaction because it is exposed to the effects of daylight (diffuse light) on a daily basis. Owing to the presence of water in the skin (approximately 70%), blue light penetrates the tissue very slightly, only 5–10 μm, green light penetrates the skin slightly deeper up to the basement membrane (100–150 μm), whilst red light penetrates deep into the dermis (800–1600 μm), and infrared light (of wavelength greater than $\lambda \geq 800$ nm) up to 0.5–3 cm. Water's absorption spectrum is 100–1000 times greater for red and infrared light than for blue light; since, in the Sun's spectrum, the percentage of red and infrared light is small compared to blue, green and yellow lights, the origin and sustenance of life on Earth is possible. A high proportion of red and infrared light would result in body temperatures in excess of 65 °C, preventing the synthesis of nucleic and amino acids into DNA and protein chains. Even in the instance of DNA and protein chain formation under specific local conditions, such structures would rapidly denature under high red/infrared conditions. Collagen is the protein most prevalent in the human organism (40% of all proteins), and plays an important role in extracellular space, especially in the basement membrane.

Embryogenesis is, after the evolution of the Universe, probably one of the most complex and miraculous processes we know. The anatomical-physiological stages in the development of the fetus, from the fertilized ovum to childbirth, are mostly known. They can be divided into three main phases: from the zygote to the formation of the three-layered germ (embryonal period of development), the forming of ectoderm, endoderm and mesoderm until the end of the second lunar month (embryonal period), and from the third month until childbirth (fetus period). Based on perfect numbers and Fibonacci numbers, a light model of embryogenesis is developed, i.e., it is demonstrated that the embryogenesis can be represented using the RGB system (colour system starting with black, them moving successively through blue, green, and red, ending in white). This light model improves understanding of the interconnectedness of parts of the human organism developed over the course of embryogenesis [14]. Further, embryogenesis is one of the key processes for the understanding of the formation of extra-bioactive body loci and channels of hydrogen bonds body network presenting the flow network of electromagnetic signals (of light), and quantum gravity signals (biological "black hole" effect of 4D space–time, as -1_4), Yin (gravity) and Yang (light). Taking all this into account, it seems that Einstein was right when he said:"One thing I have learned in a long life: that all our science, measured against reality, is primitive and childlike, and yet it is the most precious thing we have" [15].

The quantum-electronic Bloch sphere was defined in 1946 for fermions and spin-1/2 particles (such as electrons). Equations defining this sphere follow from the time-dependent Schrödinger's equation for a system of two levels, i.e., two states. Using the Hamiltonian, the Bloch sphere can be defined using smaller modifications such that Pauli's matrix is included as part of the Bloch vector defining the sphere. If we compare Fig. 1, which represents Poincare sphere, and Fig. 2, which representing the Bloch sphere, we can see that there is a one-to-one correspondence between term for light and for the electron. In the Bloch sphere, "north" and "south" pole are defined by the characteristic that electron has two orientations "↑" (up, "north") and "↓" (down, "south"). However, since this is the consequence of the fourth quantum number, this determination defines the quantum bit (qubit) denoted by $|0\rangle$ and $|1\rangle$.

Comparative analysis of Poincaré and Bloch spheres yields the following relations: [0, 0, 1]—the right-hand circular polarization is equivalent to ["↑"]—that is $|0\rangle$, [0, 0, −1]—left-hand circular polarization is equivalent to ["↓"]—that is $|1\rangle$. [−1, 0, 0]—the vertical linearly polarized light corresponds the superposed

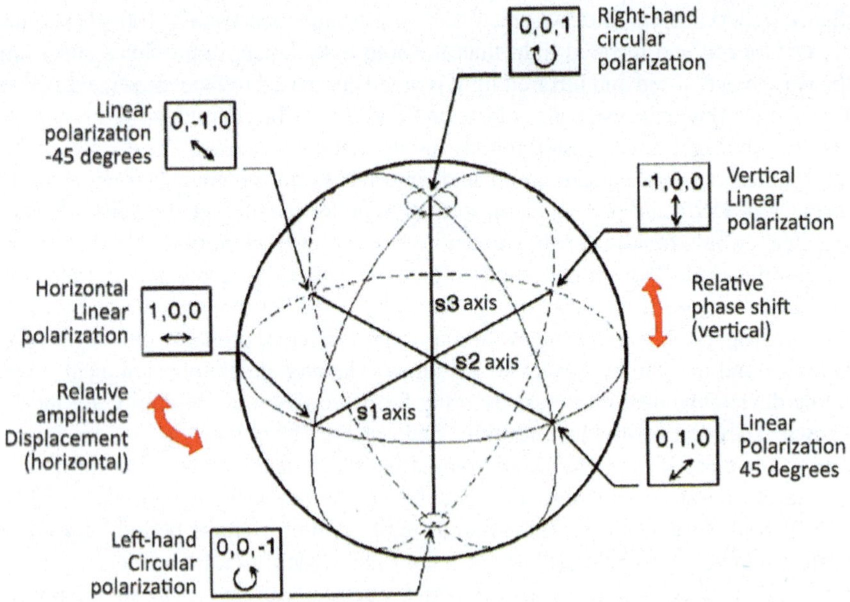

Fig. 1 Poincare sphere with layout and interdependence of basic linear and circular polarizations. *Source* Koruga [4], p. 91

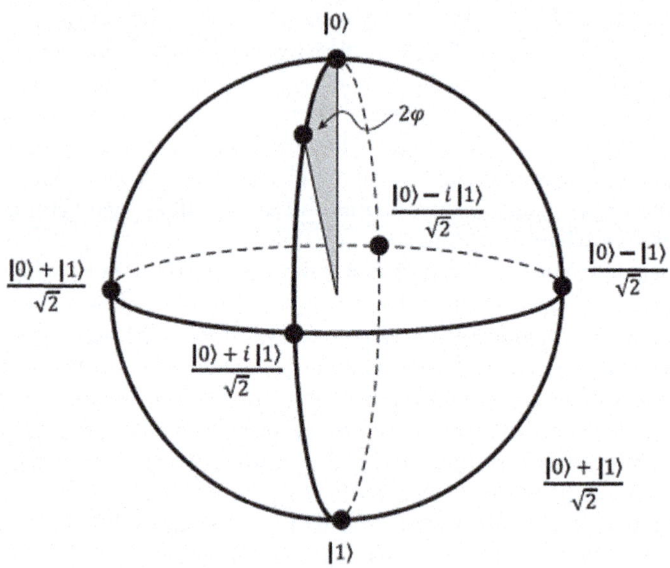

Fig. 2 Bloch sphere with two basic $|0\rangle$ and $|1\rangle$, and four superposed states. *Source* Koruga [4], p. 97

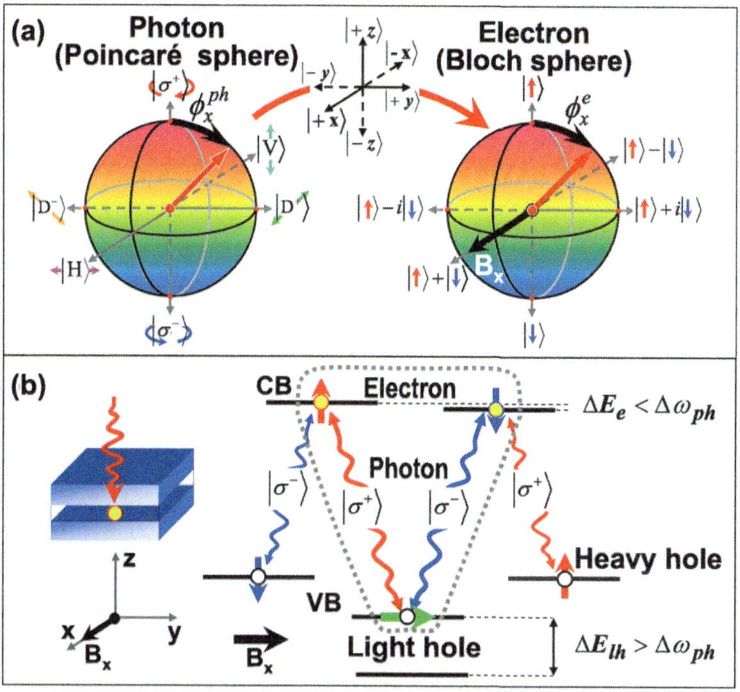

Fig. 3 **a** Schematic representation of photon-to-electron quantum information transfer and correspondence between photon (Poincare sphere) and electron (Bloch sphere), **b** photon-electron interaction with heavy hole and light hole. *Source* Kosaka [16]

state $(1/\sqrt{2})[|0\rangle — i|1\rangle]$, and [1, 0, 0]—the horizontal linear light polarization corresponds the superposed state $(1/\sqrt{2})[|0\rangle + i\,|1\rangle]$. The transfer and correspondence of quantum information between photon (Poincare sphere) and electron (Bloch sphere) is presented in Fig. 3.

3.1 *Mirror Mimetic in Light-Matter Interaction*

The basis of mirror mimetic light-matter is the interaction between diffuse visible lights; one is perpendicular to the sample and the other, under the Brewster angle, is based on the equivalence of valence electrons and incoming light energy. This novel technique identifies the average energy states of valence electrons and hydrogen bonds within the sample material. Calculations based on the valence electron velocity of matter give the ratio between the magnetic force (FM) and electrical force (FE) of the matter FM/FE = 10^{-4}. Since force (F) is directly related to action (A = F × d × t, where F is force in range 0,01–1.0 nN, d is displacement in range 0, 1–1.0 nm, and t is time in range 10^{-8}–10^{-10} s), it can be concluded (based on Planck constant/action

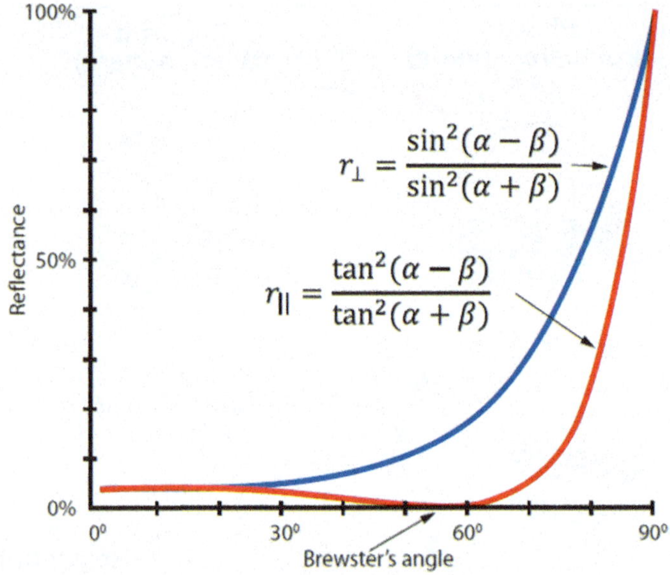

Fig. 4 Reflectance percentage from sample depending of incident light angle. For Brewster's angle the magnetic component is zero, while for angle of 90° reflectance is maximum for both electrical and magnetic component of light. *Source* Koruga [4], p. 95

of 6.626 9 10^{-34} Js), that the magnetic force is four orders of magnitude closer to its quantum state of matter than the electrical force. This opens an opportunity to detect conformational states and changes in the matter at the nanoscale using opto-magnetic imaging spectroscopy (OMIS) via light-matter interaction [17, 18]. The light, as an electromagnetic phenomenon, consists of electric and magnetic waves. When a sample is illuminated at a specific angle (Brewster's angle) the reflected light is perfectly polarized (Fig. 4). The value of Brewster's angle varies from material to material [4]. Reflected polarized light, which travels to the sensor (camera) from a sample contains dominantly (or, ideally, solely) the electrical component of the sample's light-matter interaction. By subtracting the reflected polarized light (electrical properties) from the reflected white diffuse light (electromagnetic properties), the result provides information about the magnetic properties of the sample based on light-matter interaction (Fig. 5).

3.2 Capture Mimetic in Light-Matter Interaction

The capture mimetic is based on the absorption phenomena when structured light meets structured matter [13]. Light and matter recognise each other by symmetries of structure, electronic states and vibration–rotation energy (with quantum energy states of photons based on angular momentum). The most important property is the spin

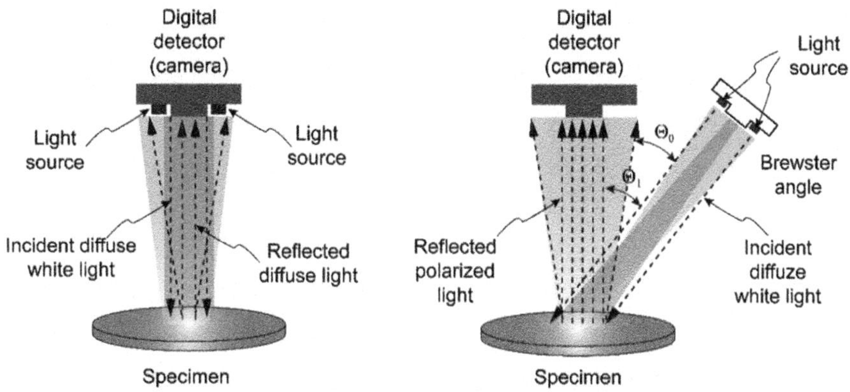

Fig. 5 Schematic arrangement of the positions of diffuse incident light and reflected diffuse white light (left), and incident diffuse light which under Brewster angle become white polarized and reflected polarized light (right). Total polarization efficiency is 95.4%, while angular diffusion of the light source (six white LEDs arranged in a circle) is ± 1:6° (the difference between the angles θ and θ1) [17]

of both photons and electrons, as they play an important role in energy-state pattern recognition, as well as in information storage. For spin-based quantum information technology, preparation and read-out of the electron spin state must be spin-coherent. However, both the traditional preparations and read-outs of spin states are projective to up/down spin states, which do not exhibit spin coherence. Interestingly, it was recently demonstrated that the polarization coherence of light can be transferred to the spin coherence of electrons in matter [16]; these results have opened up the possibility of making a quantum media converter between flying photon qubits and stationary electron spin qubits in matter.

Biological structures which are good candidates for capturing mimicry on the principle of "structured light meets structured matter" [13] are collagen, microtubules, centrioles, clathrin, etc.

Collagen. Depending on external influences, reversible transitions between collagen states exist (Fig. 6a and b). The collagen fibres organise into a pentagonal structure (a) as an elementary unilayer lattice of fibres. Double-layered organisations of pentagonal fibres and multi-layered forms of collagen fibres have quasi-crystalline properties with characteristics ϕ and Φ. Quantitative energy values of the hydrogen bond N–H…O = C are determined the collagen of type I, which includes polypeptide planes of amino acids glycine and proline. These findings can explain the physical basis of collagen stability, having a very important structural role in connecting tissues. Numerous experiments on collagen were conducted: infrared spectroscopy, quartz piezogravimetry, and differentia scanning calorimetry [4].

Centrioles. The centriole is the central enigma of molecular biology. What are the physical processes behind such a beautiful geometric figure, inciting not only a feeling of beauty but of sublime? This is the question which scientists have tried to

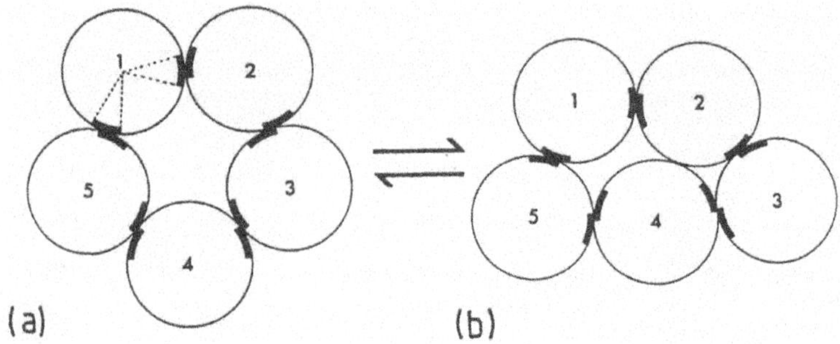

Fig. 6 **a** Organisation of collagen fibres into pentagons, bias-voltage state with the ϕ and Φ characteristic. **b** Collagen shape that endures high pressure strain. *Source* Koruga [4], p. 128

answer in the last 30 years. We discussed this with many biologists, but no satisfactory answer was found; the majority displayed the attitude: it is a structure having a so and so function. Most of them were satisfied with this answer. Why is it so was not of much interest to them from the professional viewpoint (because they were taught so); however some expressed interest to find out. Our model is based on the following mathematical and physical premises: for a random point having coordinates x, y, z, uniformly distributed within a sphere of radius r, the mathematical expectation of the point distance from the centre of the sphere should be determined (Fig. 7). Left and right centriole organisation in each cell is presented in Fig. 8 and a classical magnet model with magnetic lines of force between the north and the south pole, and the distribution of microtubules along magnetic lines of force during cell division, is presented in Fig. 9. Discrete two-dimensional representations of the icosahedral energy eigenvalues T_{1g}, T_{2u}, T_{1g}, and T_{2g}, can be seen, with the three last points representing microtubular protofilaments which form centrioles (Fig. 10) [4].

By observing a biological process—in one case the growth of a rabbit population—Fibonacci arrived at the discovery of a special class of numbers, belonging to the set of natural numbers Φ (1.61803...) and ϕ (0.61803...). Why do we say natural numbers? Because these numbers belong to the mathematica naturalis—they are at the foundation of nature (Greek φυσιζ), i.e., of physical reality, as opposed to mathematica instrumentalist, for which the mind is a sufficient instrument. Fibonacci published this discovery in 1202 in his book Liber Abaci. Here is what his contemporaries said of him: "... Leonardo from Pisa, known as Fibonacci, played an important role in the revival of the ancient mathematics and made a significant contribution by his approach. His Liber Abaci introduced the Hindu-Arabic positional decimal number system and the usage of Arabic numerals into Europe, which incited a renaissance in science" [20]. It is important to note that Roman numerals, previously used in Europe, had enjoyed very limited scientific application.

Fibonacci numbers Φ, −Φ, ϕ, −ϕ are solutions of these two simple quadratic equations:

$$x^2 + x - 1 = 0 \tag{1}$$

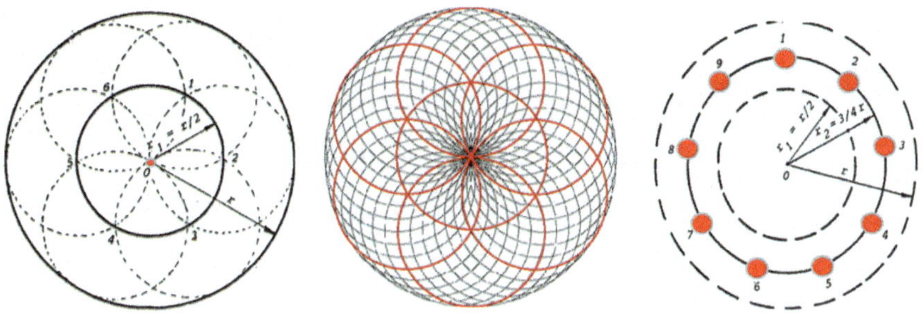

Fig. 7 Cross section of the sphere (S_0) of radius r through its centre, with the cross section of sphere (S_1) of radius $r_1 = 1/2$ r. The circle (k_1) of radius r_1 is divided into 6 equal parts. Each point of the divided circle k_1 circumference becomes the centre of six circles (1, 2… 6) passing through the centre 0 (left). When the structure has icosahedral (or dodecahedral) symmetry as in Table 2, left and right-leading lines of electromagnetic twisted force " are created from the centre (middle). When there is a systemic symbiosis between structure and energy, mass points are organized as enneads (nines), such as the one displayed in the right-hand image. *Source* Koruga [4], p. 123

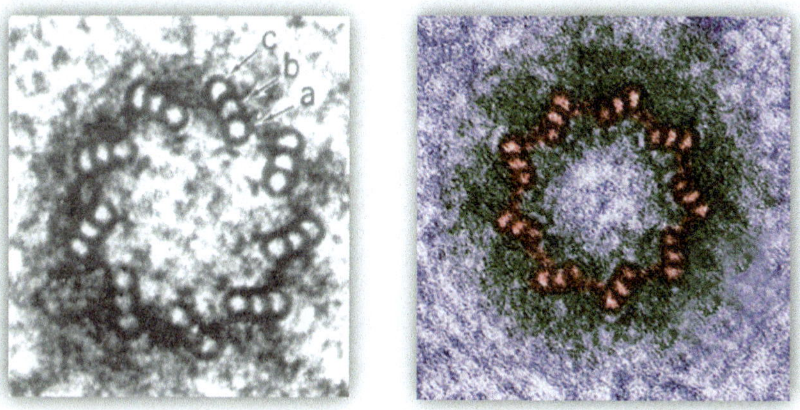

Fig. 8 Left and right centriole organisation: the microtubule "a" has 13 protofilaments, while microtubules "b" and "c" have 10 protofilaments each (left). The angle of angulation of the microtubule triplet is 222.50, that is 3600 × 0.61803 = 222.50. *Source* Dustin [8], p. 184

$$x^2 - x - 1 = 0 \tag{2}$$

which give rise to the logical square of Fibonacci numbers (Fig. 11).

Number Φ and ϕ can be determined in several ways, and here we will demonstrate three methods; the first is by observing the reproduction of rabbits, as Fibonacci did (mathematica naturalis). Let us take the first pair of rabbits (the first "1") that reproduced—during this time there is only one pair (the second "1"). A new pair follows from this pair, so now there are two pairs ("2"). The original pair continues

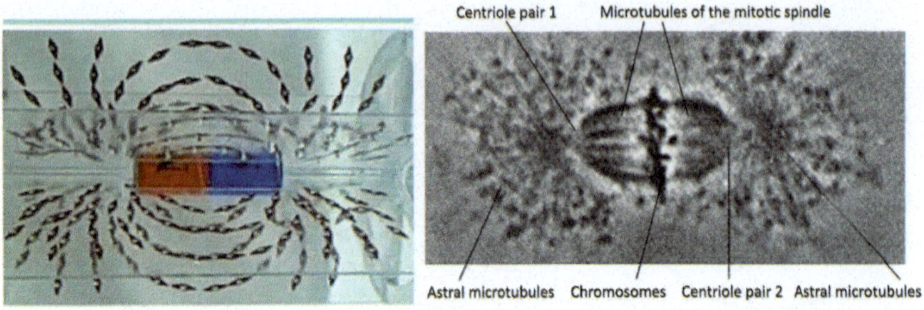

Fig. 9 Classical magnet with magnetic lines of force between the north and the south pole (left) and the distribution of microtubules along magnetic lines of force during cell division. Centrioles have the role of poles, and the "astral" microtubules are present as the result of the law of magnetism [4]

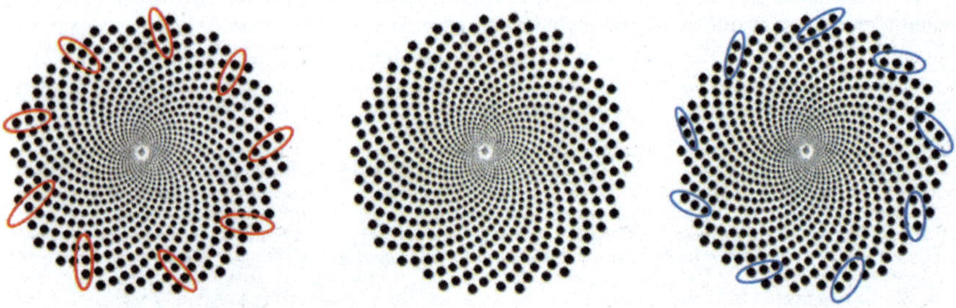

Fig. 10 Discrete two-dimensional representation of the icosahedral energy eigenvalues T_{1g}, T_{2u}, T_{1g}, and T_{2g}, where the peripheral angle (of each point on the circle circumference) is 222.50 (middle). We observe a left and a right orientation, as on Fig. 8, where the three last points represent microtubular protofilaments which are forming centrioles

Table 2 Dependence between symmetry and energy eigenvalues of a structure or process based on icosahedral symmetry

Table of the icosahedral symmetry group

I/I_h	E	$12C_5$	$12C_5^2$	$20C_3$	$15C_2$	i	$12S_{10}$	$12S_{10}^3$	$20S_6$	15σ	III	IV	
A_g	1	1	1	1	1	1	1	1	1	1		$x^2+y^2+z^2$	
T_{1g}	3	$\frac{1}{2}(1+\sqrt{5})$	$\frac{1}{2}(1-\sqrt{5})$	0	−1	3	$\frac{1}{2}(1-\sqrt{5})$	$\frac{1}{2}(1+\sqrt{5})$	0	−1	(R_x, R_y, R_z)		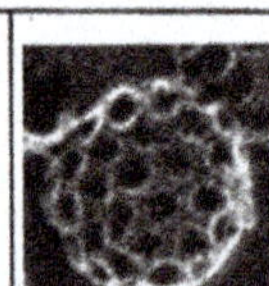
T_{2g}	3	$\frac{1}{2}(1-\sqrt{5})$	$\frac{1}{2}(1+\sqrt{5})$	0	−1	3	$\frac{1}{2}(1+\sqrt{5})$	$\frac{1}{2}(1-\sqrt{5})$	0	−1			
G_g	4	−1	−1	1	0	4	−1	−1	1	0			
H_g	5	0	0	−1	1	5	0	0	−1	1		$(2z^2-x^2-y^2,$ $x^2-y^2,$ $xy, yz, zx)$	
A_u	1	1	1	1	1	−1	−1	−1	−1	−1			
T_{1u}	3	$\frac{1}{2}(1+\sqrt{5})$	$\frac{1}{2}(1-\sqrt{5})$	0	−1	−3	$-\frac{1}{2}(1-\sqrt{5})$	$-\frac{1}{2}(1+\sqrt{5})$	0	1	(x, y, z)		
T_{2u}	3	$\frac{1}{2}(1-\sqrt{5})$	$\frac{1}{2}(1+\sqrt{5})$	0	−1	−3	$-\frac{1}{2}(1+\sqrt{5})$	$-\frac{1}{2}(1-\sqrt{5})$	0	1			(x^3, y^3, z^3)
G_u	4	−1	−1	1	0	−4	1	1	−1	0			$[x(z^2-y^2), y(z^2-x^2),$ $z(x^2-y^2), xyz]$
H_u	5	0	0	−1	1	−5	0	0	1	−1			

Source Koruga et all 1993, p. 81 [19]

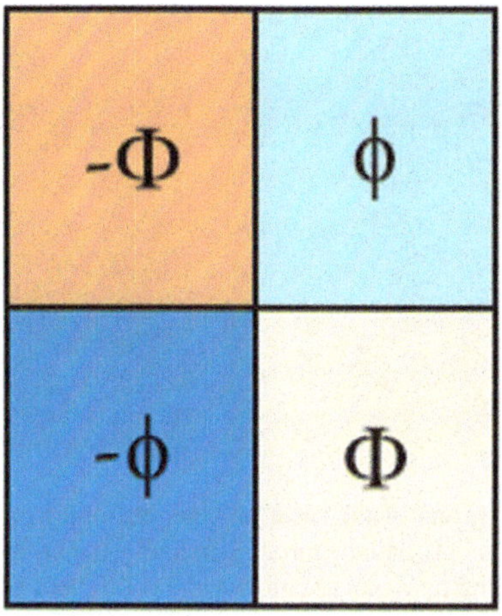

Fig. 11 Logical square of Fibonacci numbers Φ, $-\Phi$, ϕ, $-\phi$, which may generate any number of decade system ($\Phi - \Phi = 0$, $\Phi - \phi = 1$, $\Phi^1 + \phi^2 = 2$, $\Phi^2 + \phi^2 = 3$.......$(\Phi^3 + \phi^3)^2 = 20$......)

to reproduce (while the new pair is coming to the age for reproduction) and produces another pair, so now three pairs exist ("3"). This process continues and the original pair produces yet another new pair, but now the first new pair has come to the reproduction age, so now we have five pairs ("5"), etc. [21].

Another approach is via a series of numbers created in our mind (mathematica instrumentalist): 0, 0!, 1, 2, 3, 5, 8, 13, 21, 34, 55, 89, 144.... These numbers are put into proportion: the smaller number (n) to the next larger number (n + 1), then inversely, the larger number (N) to the preceding smaller number (N − 1). It should be noted that we introduced 0! as a logical transition between 0 and 1, i.e., there is no repetition of 1, as is usually denoted (0, 1, 1, 2, 3 ...) (Fig. 12).

Clathrin. Clathrin is a complex protein spherical structure composed of two main protein chains: the "light" chain (25 000 D) and the "heavy" chain (190 000 D). The overall molecular mass is about 215 000 D (Dalton: 1D ~ weight of atomic hydrogen), the size is 20 – 80 nm. Human chromosomes 17 and 22 respectively are responsible for the synthesis of the "heavy" and "light" chains. These two protein chains form a more complex structure called the triskelion (trimer). It was discovered in 1969 by the Japanese scientists Kanaseki and Kadota using the electron microscope [6], and is found in many human tissues as a carrier of substances such as neurotransmitters. It also clears cell debris into extracellular space. The triskelia naturally form pentagons and hexagons, so the clathrins in the CNS, composed of 36 triskelions, form 12 pentagons and 20 hexagons, whilst in other tissues they are made of 12 pentagons and a varying number of hexagons (Fig. 13). Clathrin of the CNS is considered the most symmetrical structure that can exist in nature based on the law of point symmetry (exhibiting perfect symmetry). This is the icosahedral symmetry group (dual to dodecahedron) whose energy states T_{1g}, T_{2g}, T_{1u} and T_{2u} are determined

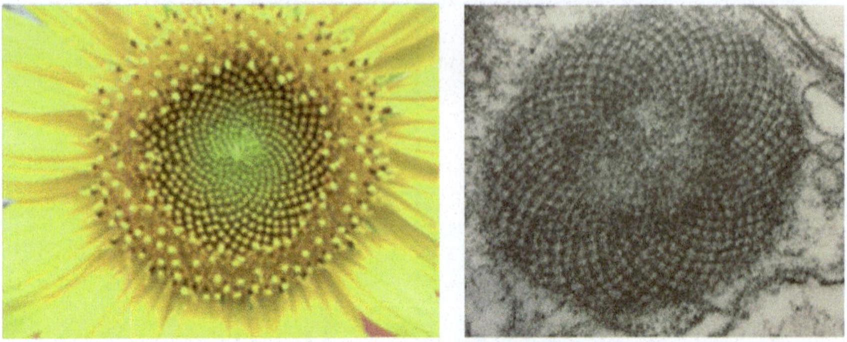

Fig. 12 The sunflower (left), one of the most obvious examples of the realisation of Fibonacci numbers in nature (realised in 2D), and the toroidal organelle (right, realised in 3D) within eye cells for night vision (rods) enabling hyperpolarization of the cell. These two examples demonstrate the realisation of Fibonacci numbers as the mathematica naturalis in nature and in biological systems. *Source* Koruga [4], p. 151

by the ordered quadruple Φ, −Φ, ϕ, −ϕ (1.61803..., −1.61803..., 0.61803..., −0.61803).

When we have a headache, feel sleepy, or have a mental or neurological disorder, the cause in many cases is one of the neurotransmitters: serotonin (5-HT), acetylcholine (ACh), melatonin, catecholamine, GABA etc. For example, serotonin (colloquially known as the hormone of happiness) is formed from the amino acid tryptophan via the oxidation of this amino acid into 5-oxytryptophan, and its subsequent decarbonization. Serotonin has a very important regulatory functions in the body, and is stored in the presynaptic vesicles, in clathrin. When the action potential acts on the presynaptic termination, the depolarized presynaptic membrane interacts with vesicles (clathrin). This opens them and their contents (neurotransmitter) is released into the intersynaptic space to activate the postsynaptic membrane. The catecholamine group includes three compounds: dopamine, noradrenalin and adrenaline, originating from the amino acid tyrosine. They are released at the sympathetic peripheral nerve

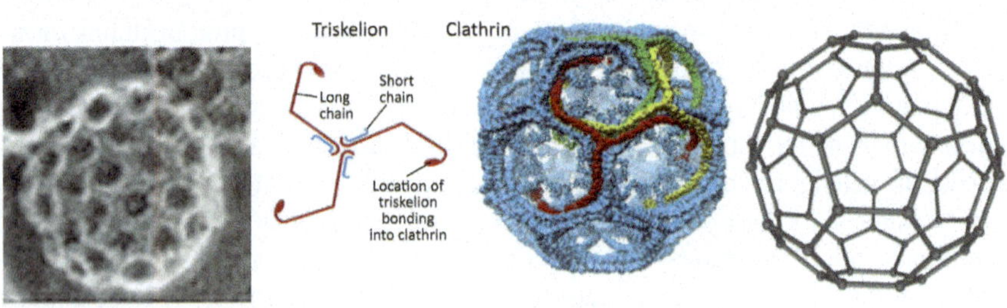

Fig. 13 Microscopic image of clathrin (left), triskelion shape and the network of 36 triskelions forming clathrin with 12 pentagons and 20 hexagons. Schematic structure with pentagons and hexagons (right) is displayed. *Source* Koruga [4], p. 116

terminations, synapses, and various zones of the central nervous system (CNS). Catecholamines are accumulated in secretory vesicles—again in clathrin.

4 Biomimetics Light Devices

4.1 Mirror Mimicry: Opto Magnetic Imaging Spectroscopy (OMIS)

The design of OMIS is based on the concept of unpaired and paired electrons (explained in Sect. 3.1 and Fig. 14), with its technical realisation presented in Fig. 15. Devices may be used in vivo, in vitro and extempore. Results of tissue examinations are obtained in 5 min, important for cancer screening, monitoring and diagnostics where rapid analysis is essential. OMIS can be used in vivo and in vitro characterisations of skin, in vitro characterisation of cervix, colon and oral cavity (Fig. 16). The OMIS method has also been used to characterise the quality of water, determining the concentrations of water solutions, polymers, gels, solid materials as well as viscoelastic materials. In these applications the Brewster angle is the only parameter that differs, ranging from 53° (water) to 76° (metal).

4.2 Capture Mimicry: Hyperpolarized Light

Problem Identification and its Conceptual Solution. The main reasons why biomedical engineering experts are seeking a new light type are:

1. Diffuse, linearly polarized and laser lights are considered "wild" energies, acting strictly energetically without recognizing which stimulants are actually necessary for particular biomolecules, tissues and organs. They do not cover all energy states of biomolecules and tissues, but primarily the electronic energetic states (1.4–3.4 eV) of valence electrons without acting on the basic energy, vibrational and rotational states. It is not easy to cover all energy states of biomolecules, cells and tissues; however, we shall focus on the domain 0.012–1.6 eV from an energy perspective (starting at fundamental vibrations and vibro-rotational energies, all the way to the ground electronic states of biomolecular valence electrons). Present devices, such as BIOPTRON (~40 m W/cm^2) generate linearly polarized light: the new apparatus should generate ~ 28 m W/cm^2, granting enough energy and spatial information to act upon the basic electronic, vibrational and rotational states of biomolecules and tissues (30% of light energy is lost through the ordering of the photons).

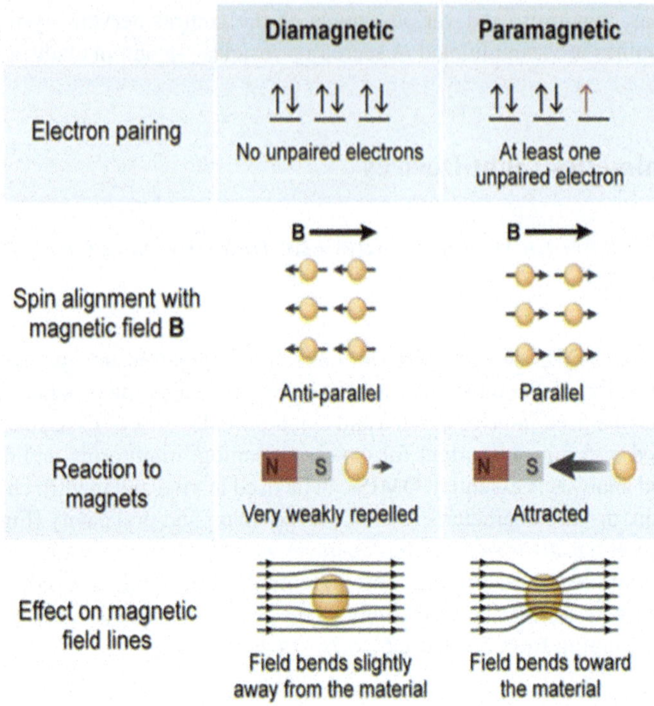

Fig. 14 The paramagnetic and diamagnetic properties of matter depend **on** unpaired and paired electrons. Magnetic quantum number of the electron spin m_s may has two values + ½ and − ½, "up" or "down". If all electrons are paired then material is diamagnetic and external magnetic field near material will slightly decrease. However, if at least one electron is unpaired then material is paramagnetic and external magnetic field near material will increase [22]

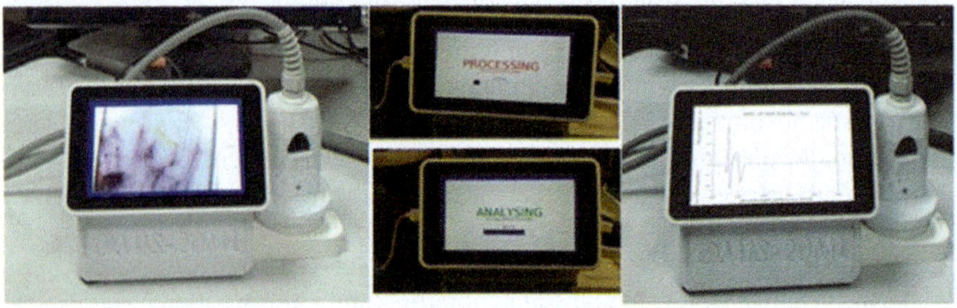

Fig. 15 OMIS device with different images on screen: *(left)* image of stain PAP slide, (*middle*) screen during processing and analysing, and (*right*) result presented as diagram

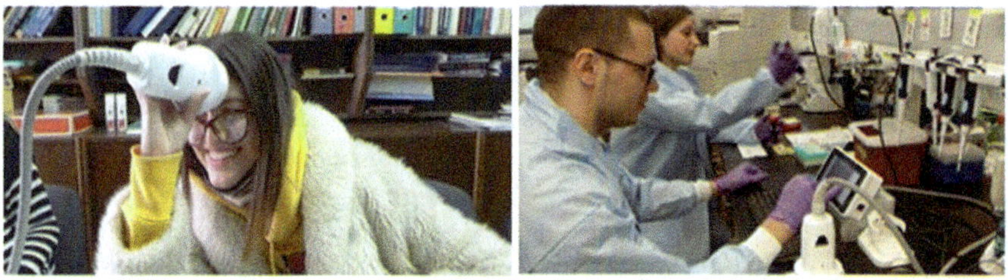

Fig. 16 OMIS as "mirror mimicry" device based on reflection may characterise tissues in vivo (left) and in vitro (right). It can be used in lab, clinic, home, working place, etc. Three main processes are: taking images (PROCESSING), data analysis (ANALYSING) and result presenting (DIAGRAMS or REPORT), presenting on right side of picture

2. All three present light energy types (diffuse, linearly polarized and laser) act primarily locally, although linearly polarized light can act regionally (via organised water) due to its ability to affect the organisation of dipole moments of water molecules.
3. Biomolecules and tissues are based on the union of structure, energy and information, not only on structure and energy.
4. Biological information processes are very important for the maintenance of function and repair of biomolecules, tissues and organs.
5. Biomolecule symmetry defines electronic states (ground and excited) and vibrational–rotational energy, thus defining signal (information) propagation from one end of a cell to another (via the principle of resonant biomolecular recognition at a distance through water).
6. Light (photons) for the conservation and treatment of biological structures must be compatible with biostructures; photonic (spatial–temporal) organisation must correspond to the symmetry of the biological structure, defining its electronic, vibrational, and rotational energy states.
7. Based on the above, the task is to generate light compatible with biomolecules according to the principle:

   SYMMETRY of biomolecules = SYMMETRY of photonic organisation.

   Analogous conclusion is made in the paper by Natalie Litchinitser, 2012 "It can be expected that by synergy of complex materials and complex light a new breakthrough in the science on light and its application will be made" [13]. The paper, however, did not recognize that for biological systems icosahedral and dodecahedral symmetry is the basis for this recognition.
8. By establishing synergy of light and matter based on icosahedral and dodecahedral symmetries, a resonant recognition is established between organisation patterns, including (beside their energy states) the entropy states and, consequently, the information states.
9. We observed that the icosahedral symmetry is found in clathrin, collagen, microtubules, cilia, centrioles and water (in water molecule clusters dodecahedral

symmetry is present as well). Technological solutions will be sought that induce photonic organisation in-line with icosahedral (and dodehaderal) symmetry prior to interaction with tissue.

First of all, it is necessary to determine the type of symmetry dominant in biological structures and processes responsible for signal (information) generation and transfer. On the other hand, it is also necessary to observe the relationship between the electric and the magnetic component in biological structures. The previous part of Chapter emphasized the importance of water for the human organism (70% of the human organism; water is prevalent in all body parts), collagen (40% of all protein, one of the most important extracellular structures), microtubule ("brain of the cell", dominant cytoplasmic protein structure responsible for matter transportation within the cell, determines cell shape, and combined with actin and intramedial protofilaments determines the cell bias voltage state, provides signalization between the cell membrane–nucleus membrane and, through interaction with clathrin and water, generates pre-process activity in the brain in neurons responsible for memory, learning and possibly for the generation of consciousness), cilia (very important for the function of epithelial tissue surfaces), flagella (important in male reproductive cells-spermatozoids), and centrioles (microtubular structure that, together with DNA, represents the central enigma of molecular biology; responsible for cell division, cytoskeleton organisation and regulative functions in the cytoplasm).

In this chapter (Sect. 3.1) we earlier demonstrated that the ratio of the magnetic to the electric component of valence electrons is $F_M/F_E \approx 10^{-4}$, consequently it is necessary to investigate light–matter interaction as action $A_E = F_E \times d \times t$ for the electric component, and $A_M = F_M \times d \times t$ for the magnetic component. The electric force in biomolecules equals 0.01–1.0 nN, displacement 0.01–0.5 nm, and action time is 10^{-8}–10^{-10} s. The average electric action (A_E) is therefore:

$$A_E = 10^{-10} \times 10^{-10} \times 10^{-10} = 10^{-30}\,\text{Js} \quad (3)$$

For the magnetic component, action (A_M) is:

$$A_M = 10^{-30} \times 10^{-4} = 10^{-34}\,\text{Js} \quad (4)$$

which is very close to the quantum action. Consequently it can be stated that the electric component is primarily responsible for classic action and the magnetic component for quantum action ($h = 6.626 \times 10^{-34}$ Js).

As the conformation states of biomolecules are primarily quantum–mechanical phenomena, the correction of biomolecular functionality is established primarily using the conversion of light energy into magnetic energy, at the nano and pico Tesla level, because the magnetic component of biomolecules is by 4 orders of magnitude closer to quantum phenomena than the electric component.

Therefore, the new light type should act on the basic energetic, vibrational and rotational states of biomolecules, tissues and processes in the organism (above all on the generation of Gibbs free energy) and must satisfy the following conditions:

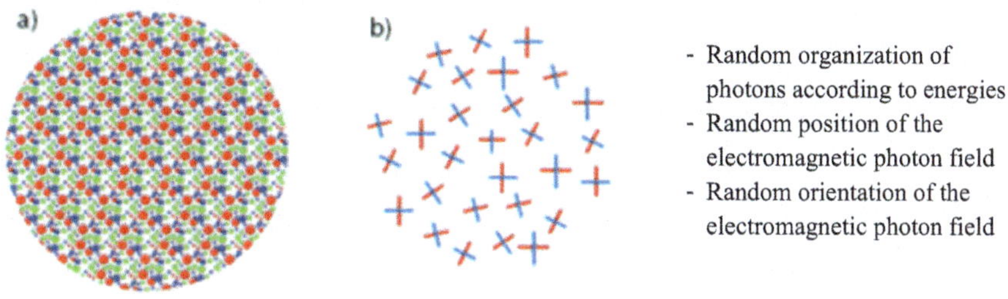

Fig. 17 **a** Polychromatic diffuse light as a random set of photons with respect to energies. **b** Random positions of the electromagnetic photon rotating field (blue—electric photon field, red—magnetic photon field); photons have random orientation along the light propagation direction (rays are not parallel, they can intersect)

1. The energy level should be within the interval 0.012–1.6 eV, meaning that a part of light (approximately 62%) coming from the light source should pass through (0.6–1.6 eV), to act on basic electronic states and processes.
2. The other part (about 38%) should be transformed via the "nanophotonic transformer" into energies 0.012–0.6 eV (to act on vibrational and rotational states of biomolecules and processes).
3. Photons transmitted through the "nanophotonic generator" and the newly transformed electromagnetic energy in the light–nanomatter interaction should be organized according to the icosahedral (and dodecahedral) symmetry ("structured light meets structured matter").

Nanophotonic Generator of Hyperpolarized Light. The nanophotonic generator (NPG) of hyperpolarized light should transform diffuse light or linearly polarized light into a new light form characterized by icosahedral symmetry, harmonized with the organisation of biomolecules or bioprocesses (the Fibonacci law ϕ and Φ, i.e., values in the Table 2 relating symmetry and energy eigenvalues). The first task of the NPG is to generate photon organisation, and the second to generate photon energies through the light–matter interaction. This energy will be based on overall orbital momentums that are not within the electromagnetic spectrum of visible light, but within the far infrared domain.

In diffuse light, the position of the electromagnetic component of each photon is arbitrary in space and variable in time; "crosses" in Fig. 17 rotate randomly.

In linearly polarized light, two main phenomena can occur: vertical polarization and horizontal polarization. Polarization is defined with respect to the electric photon field (Figs. 18 and 19).

4.3 Material for the Fibonacci Light Structure

In order to establish the interaction between Fibonacci light structures and biological Fibonacci material structures we need technical devices to generate the Fibonacci

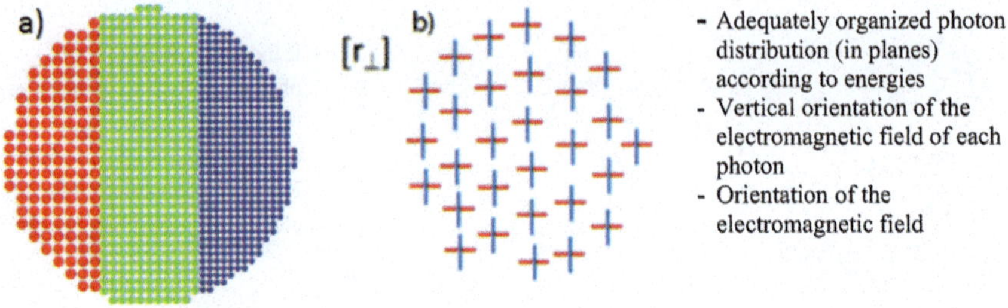

Fig. 18 **a** Polychromatic vertically-polarized light as an ordered set of photons with respect to energies. **b** Fixed position of the electromagnetic photon field (blue—electric photon field, red—magnetic photon field), and complete orientation of the electromagnetic photon field along the light propagation direction (rays are parallel). As the electrical field (blue) is vertical, this type of polarization is called the vertical linearly polarized light

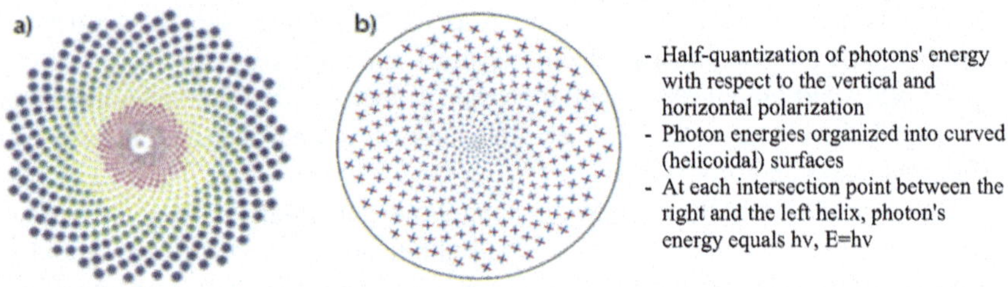

Fig. 19 Hyperpolarized light as an organized photon structure according to the Fibonacci law, with angular structural organisation $\varphi\alpha = 137.4908$. *Source* Koruga [23]

light (photonic) structure. The first technical realisation of a Fibonacci structure, associated with light transportation, was performed by the Italian-Dutch research team headed by Dal Negro [24]. In order to better understand the advantages and problems of using nanomaterials with real icosahedral symmetry (quasi crystals), let us first remember that the C60 molecule is one of the most serious candidates for building nanophotonic devices.

This material was discovered in 1985, and its discovery was awarded the Nobel Prize for chemistry in 1996 [25]. C60 is a molecular crystal of diameter 0.71 nm (at the level of the carbon atom position), i.e., 1.02 nm (on the external position of the π electron ($1.02-0.71 = 0.31$ nm), consequently π is an electronic cloud $\delta\pi = 0.155$ nm thick). The π electrons are located on the internal side of the carbon atom, thus, there is empty space within the C60 (vacuum) of $0.71-0.31 = 0.4$ nm. Therefore atoms can be encapsulated within the C60 icosahedron, such as a water molecule (endohedral fullerenes) [26].

The C60 molecule is a very dynamic vibrational–rotational structure built from sixty carbon atoms. These are arranged in 12 pentagons and 20 hexagons, forming a truncated icosahedron. Its dual structure is the dodecahedron, resulting from Euler's formula on polyhedra. The pentagons are energetically closed, whilst hexagons

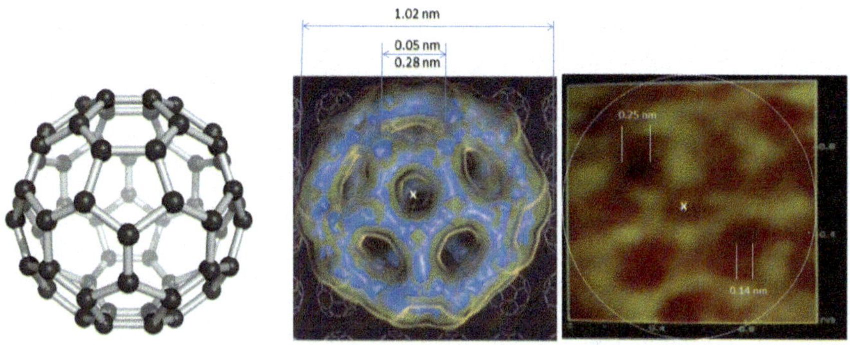

Fig. 20 The 3D view of the C60 molecule (left) [25] and its shape based on quantum–mechanical calculations (published in 1991 on the cover of Science in December, as the molecule of the year) (middle). The STM image of the C60 molecule experimentally confirms the quantum–mechanical calculations, including punctures in hexagons (right) [27]

"breathe"; they can have holes up to 0.28 nm so that in the interior of the shape, under certain conditions, smaller atoms can be encapsulated. However, from the perspective of hyperpolarized light, these punctures in the hexagons are interesting regarding photonic transition (collision between a photon and an electron of C60). We established experimentally the existence of punctures in hexagons using the STM (Fig. 20).

The C60 molecule rotates fast, about $10^{-10}\ s^{-1}$, whilst photons travel much faster, 3×10^8 m/s, and when the size of the C60 molecule is considered, interstitial spaces between C60 molecules and punctures in hexagons combine to make the C60 molecule highly porous to photons. Therefore to successfully establish the interaction between photons and C60 many layers of this molecule are required. Note that its rotation is not oriented in one direction, it is random in all directions (twisting, the "bang-bang" concept).

C60 furthermore represents a quantum pirouette because, according to the laws of classical physics, a particle (body) can spin either to the left or to the right. However, a quantum entity could exist in a superposition of both possibilities. This sounds fantastic, but for C60 and other quantum particles this is an experimentally-confirmed reality [28].

Another interesting feature of the C60 molecule relating to its pentagons and hexagons is that it is one of the rare molecules simultaneously exhibiting paramagnetic (hexagon) and diamagnetic (pentagon) features. Vertical linearly polarized light is sequentially changed into horizontal linearly polarized light according to the Fibonacci order—"sunflower"—firstly its 20 hexagons (paramagnetics) generate the Faraday effect which rotates the plane of polarization of the electromagnetic wave proportionally to the thickness of the material through which the light passes. Meanwhile its 12 pentagons (diamagnetics) are changed by rotation sequentially according to the Fibonacci law. If it was not rotating randomly and if its rotation was directed it would be an ideal nano motor (a selfpropelled vehicle on "four wheels" could be built).

Beside the quantum–mechanical appearance of the C60 molecule recorded using the STM, its surface energy was determined to correspond very well with its vibrational properties (Fig. 20). Although the C60 molecule includes hexagons it does not have symmetry axes of the sixth order (as would seem likely at first sight), the axis is instead of the third order (symmetry element 3:6 = ½). This reminds us of the electron spin ½: it has to perform two revolutions to coincide with itself. The C60 molecule is the closest structure in nature to exhibiting perfect point symmetry (more perfect than diamond, which has 48 symmetry transformations), having 60 symmetry transformations (it could have 120, 60 $\times$ i symmetry transformations: E (inversion centre), 12 C_5, 12 C_5^2, 20 C_3, 15C_2, and, 12S_{10}, 12 S_{10}^3 10,20S_6, 15σ (symmetry planes)). The total number of (energy) eigenvalues is 46 (there is a small discrepancy of 5 to 10% between theoretical and experimental values).

The C60 molecule, as a molecular crystal, has the role of an atom in classical crystallography, thus we have a crystal within a crystal (because of its distribution into the crystal lattice T_h as the fcc lattice). The first crystal structures of the C60 molecule were experimentally detected by Huffman [29].

The topological similarity between a sphere (h = 1 connected) and a torus (h = 3 connected) via the Fibonacci numbers ϕ and Φ is presented in Fig. 21. The dynamics of a system with two independent frequencies f1(Φ) and f2(ϕ) are described as quasiperiodic motion on the torus (Fig. 22). However, when the process is observed in a plane, the "sunflower seed" shape is obtained where frequencies f1(Φ) and f2(ϕ) are coupled. Figure 23 [23] depicts a schematic representation of hyperpolarized light generation from linearly polarized photons coming to interact with electrons through the icosahedral structure, performing the "bang-bang" motion relative to spatial (x, y, z) and temporal (t) dynamics with rotation ("twisting") 10^{10} per second. This generates "deterministic chaos" and provides coupling of the orbital angular momenta of photons and electrons, forming a 2-D (Φ, ϕ) "pattern" which is actually a 3D twisting torus with f1(Φ) and f2(ϕ) group frequencies. Photonic orbital angular momenta with left and right orientation [30] is presented in Fig. 24.

4.4 Thin Films Based on the C_{60} Molecule

Thin C60 films are produced either via the CVD method (chemical deposition of C60 molecules on a scaffold) or by spattering (physical method). Via CVD the C60 molecules are in the form of powder, and in the second case solid monoliths (usually powder pressed into tablets). The energetic HOMO–LUMO gap in the C60 molecule varies depending on how the C60 molecules are distributed in the thin film. When molecular organisation is adequate the powder turns from black to yellow in colour, resulting in a thin film with transparency up to 95%. The thickness of the thin film can vary; thicknesses of 30 nm to 250 nm are usually produced for various usages

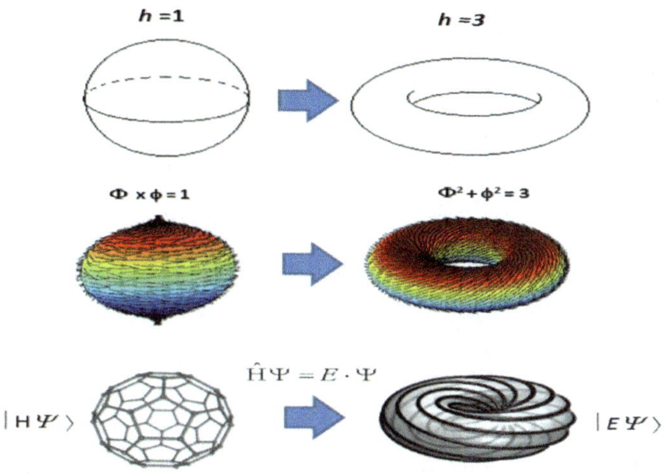

Fig. 21 Topological similarity between the sphere (h = 1 connected) and torus (h = 3 connected) via the Fibonacci numbers φ and Φ. This correspondence enables the photon energy to be coupled with the C60 molecule based on the total angular momentum

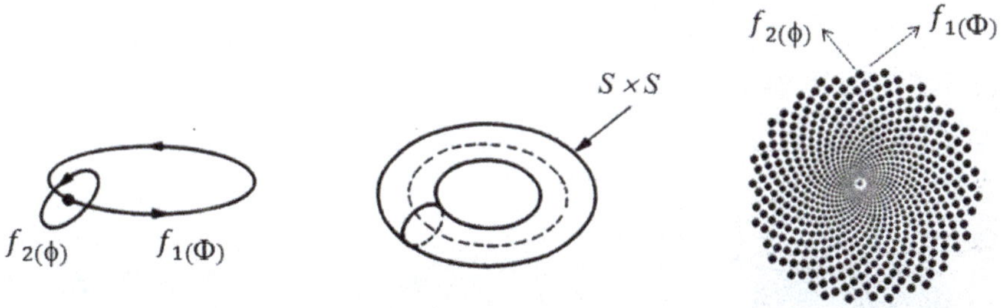

Fig. 22 The dynamics of a system with two independent frequencies f1(Φ) and f2(φ) is described as quasiperiodic motion on the torus. However, when the process is observed in a plane, the "sunflower seed" shape is obtained where frequencies f1(Φ) and f2(ϕ) are coupled. Adapted from: Strogatz [31]

(presently for protection from the UV radiation and for the modification of the EEG signal under the influence of light on the CNS via eyesight).

The physical method for the production of the photonic material based on C60 is by incorporating C60 molecules into a transparent polymer material. Why does the basic material have to be a monomer? The answer is that the base material should enable the C60 molecule to be physically placed between monomers. The material should not bind chemically, thus working temperatures must not exceed 289 °C (as these would severe the double C = C bonds in hexagons, one liberated bond would later bind the C60 molecule to the polymer and thus prevent rotation of the C60 molecule).

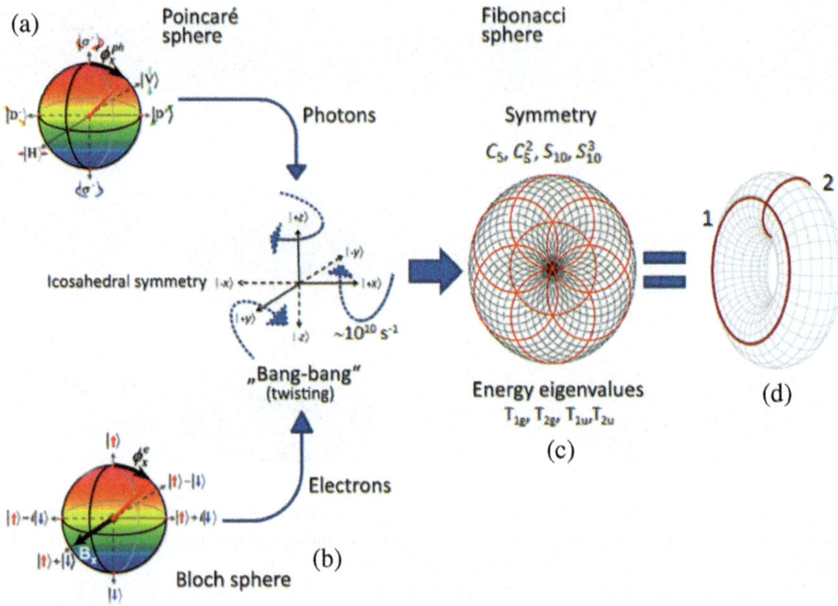

Fig. 23 Schematic representation of hyperpolarized light generation: **a** linearly polarized photons coming to interact with electrons. **b** which belong to the icosahedral structure performing the "bang-bang" motion. **c** spatial (x, y, z) and temporal (t) dynamics with velocity 10^{10} per second. This generates "deterministic chaos" and provides coupling of the orbital angular momenta of photons and electrons, forming a 2-D (Φ, φ) "pattern". **d** which is actually a 3D twisting torus with f1(Φ) and f2(ϕ) group frequencies. *Source* Koruga [23]

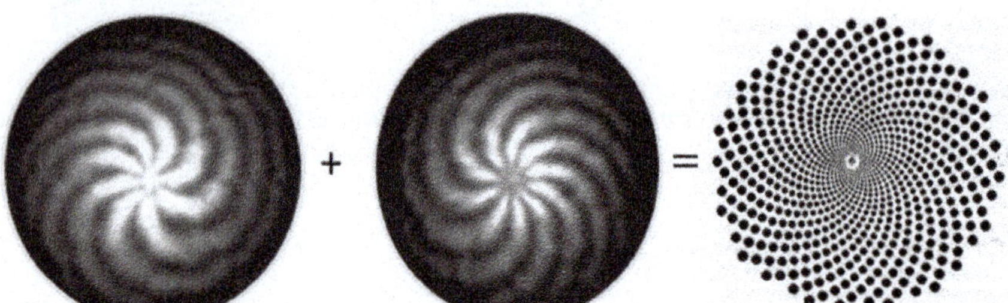

Fig. 24 Photonic orbital angular momenta with left and right orientation [30]. When the first two images are "overlapped", their intersecting points result in a Fibonacci [Φ,ϕ] system (right)

4.5 System for the Generation of Hyperpolarized Light

The system for the generation of hyperpolarized light has three main elements: (1) diffuse light source (2) polarizer transforming diffuse light into the vertical linearly

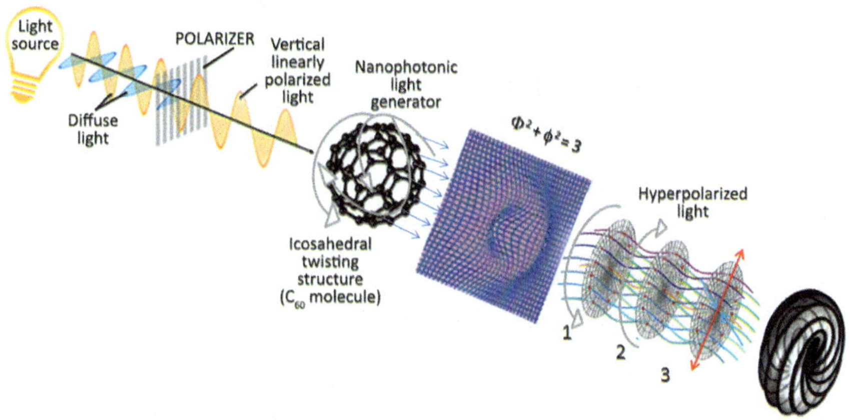

Fig. 25 Schematic representation of the nanophotonic light generation. The key element is the icosahedral twisting structure (C60 molecules incorporated into the polymer material) generating photon distribution by creating a 2D energy membrane [$\Phi^2 + \phi^2 = 3$] which "filters" propagating photons according to the Fibonacci law [Φ, ϕ]. The final output is a Fibonacci twisting torus resulting from the dynamics of three (1, 2, 3) energy forms (left helix ϕ, right helix Φ, and attractive-repulsive interactions determining the value at each intersection of the left and the right helix) [23]

polarized light (3) nanophotonic polarizer transforming vertically polarized light into hyperpolarized light (Fig. 25).

However, we need to clarify the nature of the influence (from the aspect of covalent and noncovalent bonds) of stability, Gibbs free energy, the nature of the reaction (chemical reaction or physical interaction), the influence of the solvent and the establishment of cooperative bonds. An explanation of these effects is displayed in the table of Fig. 26. The same Figure (right) shows the successful primary effects of linearly polarized and hyperpolarized light. Linearly polarized light has a better effect in covalent bonds due to the higher energy photon emission in equilibrium states, where there is a primary effect of enthalpy (ΔH) in chemical reactions, and the effect of cooperative bonds (e.g. interaction with the solvent, water) is secondary. However, in nonequilibrium states, where establishing cooperative bonds is very important and where the solvent (water) plays a primary role and physical (intermolecular) interactions are significant; where entropy (ΔS, associated with information via probability states) is significant, hyperpolarized light exhibits better therapeutic results (Table 3). Hyperpolarized light has, in case of the water–lipid layers system, a better effect on water which is one of the Fibonacci structures with pronounced dependence on entropy and significance of cooperative bonds (non-covalent hydrogen bonds), whilst linearly polarized light has a positive effect, via dipole moments, on lipids (it acts as a "comb").

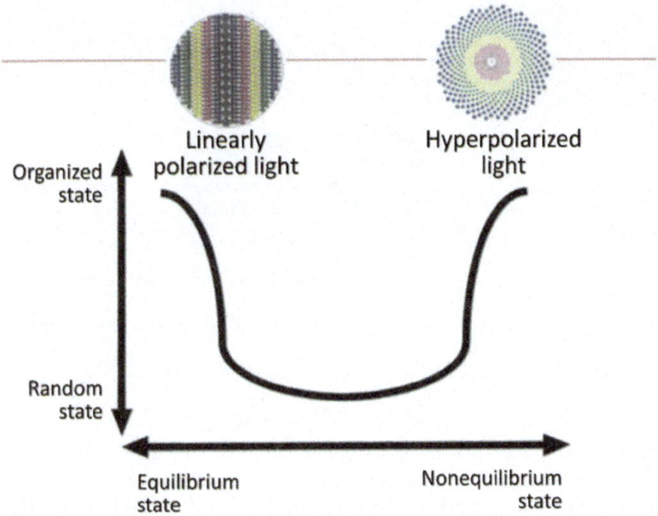

Fig. 26 Table of interaction categories (covalent interactions) needing photons of higher energies (in the visible light spectrum) (left), and categories needing photons of lower energies (non-covalent interactions) (right)

Table 3 Intensity of bonding depends of bond type

Interaction type	Covalent (molecules)	Non-covalent (intermolecular)
Bond type	Chemical	Physical (Van der Waals, hydrogen, ionic, dipole, etc.)
Energy (KJ/mol)	4–60	0.02–4.5
Stability	Stable	Open to change
Contribution to free energy ΔG	Primary ΔH	Both ΔH and ΔS
Nature	Chemical reaction	Physical interaction
Solvent influence	Secondary	Primary
Establishment of cooperative bonds	Little importance	Very important

5 Applications of Biomimetic Light Devices in Medicine

5.1 *OMIS Devices Based on Mirror Mimicry of Matter in Light-Matter Interaction*

The microtubules of the age spindle of the cell follow the magnetic laziness of the forces generated by the cell. In this case, the centrioles represent the poles of the magnet as shown in Fig. 27. During cell division, the symmetry of the process occurs and instead of two magnetic poles, three or more magnetic poles appear. Then there is an uncontrolled division of chromosomes and the cell dies or becomes carcinogenic.

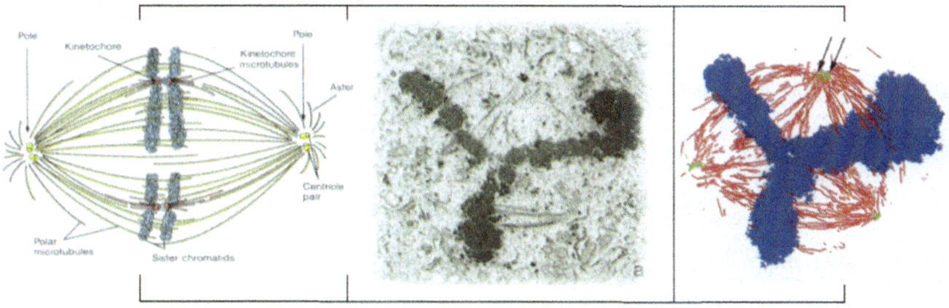

Fig. 27 Chromosome separation during cell differentiation: (*left*) schematic presentation of normal process of cell differentiation with two poles (two pairs of centrioles), (*middle*) microscopic image of chromosome separation with three poles, which leads to cancer, (*right*) schematic presentation of process when cell differentiation has three poles

Cervical Cancer. The Papanicoulaou (PAP) test is a primary screening test for cervical tissue exanimation, and has been considered a significant breakthrough ever since its introduction to the world of public health. However, the PAP test is a subjective test that depends upon the expertise of the technician who prepares the slides and the pathologist who inspects them. Some adjustments to PAP test have been made over the past years, and consequently Liquid Based Cytology (LBC) was developed. LBC improved the process of sample preparation, but studies have shown varying results when it comes to deciding whether LBC has overall better sensitivity and specificity compared to conventional cytology [32, 33]. The fact that almost every cervical cancer is linked to one of the high-risk HPVs enables early detection of cervical cancer, giving molecular tests an advantage over other, more conventional screening tests. However, the issue that has not yet been resolved is that the HPV DNA test alone cannot determine whether the infection is transient or persistent. The approval of an application to use a HPV test as the primary screening test was recommended by FDA Advisory Panel in March 2014. Still, recent studies show that greatest optimization of sensitivity and specificity is achieved when HPV DNA testing is combined with cytology [34]. Finally, early-age HPV vaccination would significantly reduce the incidence of cervical cancer and, thus, the burden of cervical cancer screening [35]. Its implementation would have undeniable impact in developing countries, but the cost of implementation is, at the time of writing, still too high and unaffordable in less-developed countries.

Since current screening tests have not absolutely met requirements to be cost-effective, accurate and efficient, there is still a need for new screening methods for cervical cancer detection. Here we are present a semi-automated method for the detection of abnormal cervical cells based on optomagnetic imaging spectroscopy (OMIS) and its application in the field of cervical cancer detection. Previous studies reported OMIS as a fast and accurate method, and showed it to have real potential to become a new standard screening test for cervical cancer detection. Classification results provided a high degree of accuracy in cervical cancer detection (85.18%) using the OMIS method on stained cervical smears [18, 36]. In this study we present

Table 4 Comparation of performance measures of OMIS data classification using Naïve Bayes classifier [36]

Performance measures for binary classification	Sensitivity (%)	Specificity (%)	Accuracy (%)
II Pa–III Pap	56	84	83
II Pap–IV Pap	82	99	98
II Pap–V Pap	75	91	96
II Pap–(III, IV and V Pap)	73	82	81

results of an algorithm for the detection of abnormal cervical cells in unstained cervical smears using Optomagnetic Imaging Spectroscopy (Table 4). The algorithm takes Optomagnetic spectra of the cervical sample, decides if the sample is healthy or abnormal based on characteristic peaks, wavelength difference shifts, and classifies it using a naïve Bayes classifier.

OMIS, in its current state, is a semi-automated method intended to be used in cervical cytology screening. It scans cervical cell samples taken from endocervix and exocervix and produces Optomagnetic diagrams which reflect the energy state of cervical cells in cytology samples (Fig. 28). Differences in OMIS diagrams obtained for normal cells (II Pap group) abnormal (III Pap group) and cancerous cells (IV and V Pap group) were used as inputs for a classifier which separates samples into four Papanicolaou groups. Compared to stained samples, where classification results achieved with a naïve Bayesian classifier showed a high degree of accuracy in cervical cancer detection using the OMIS method (85,18%), unstained sample classification with naïve Bayesian classifier gave even better results, with an accuracy of 96% achieved for classification into healthy/cancerous group, with a sensitivity of 75% and specificity of 97% (Fig. 29). The advantages of the OMIS method are multiple: results with the OMIS method can be obtained within 10 min (unlike screening tests used in clinical practice today); OMIS can be applied on unstained samples, thus the cost of the screening test implementation is significantly reduced; high specificity, and sensitivity in the range no lower than the range of sensitivity of Papanicolaou test. Further investigations on larger sample sets are needed and will be conducted in future studies in order to choose the efficiency classifiers and show the true potential of Optomagnetic Imaging Spectroscopy as a new screening test.

Colon cancer. It has been predicted that by 2035 the global number of the new cases of colorectal cancer (CRC) will increase to 2.4 million annually [37]. Many diagnostic methods already exist for the detection of colorectal cancer, such as faecal occult blood testing, colonoscopy, virtual colonoscopy, sigmoidoscopy and a combination of barium enema and sigmoidoscopy. Colonoscopy is considered to be a "gold standard" procedure and has a significant advantage because the removal of adenomas or early cancer can be performed during the exploratory or diagnostic procedures. Furthermore, it can be used at long intervals, since the risk of developing CRC after a negative colonoscopy remains decreased for more than 10 years. Due to the development of methods for the removal of large, flat colorectal polyps, i.e. endoscopic mucosal resection along with other minimally invasive transanal techniques (used

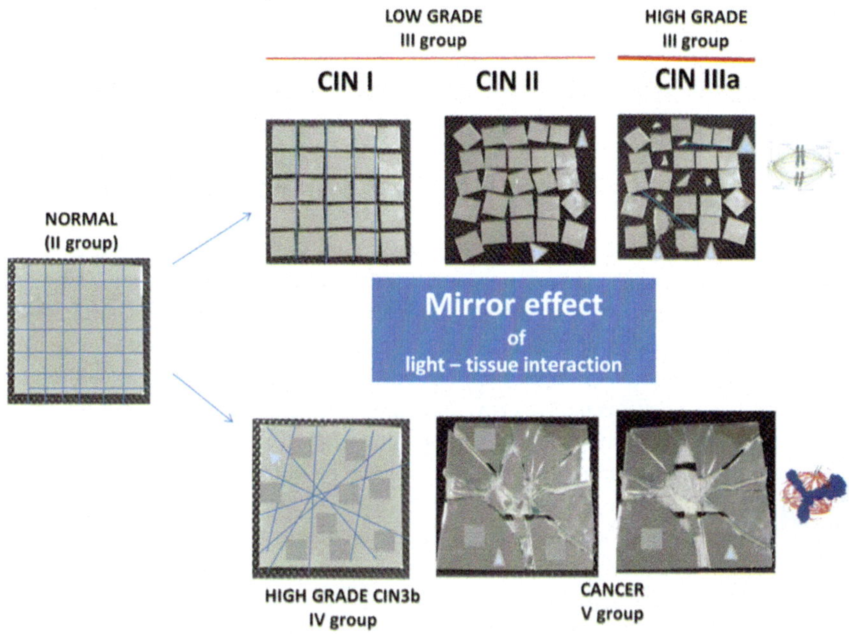

Fig. 28 Mirror effect of light-matter interaction and difference between normal and cancer cells

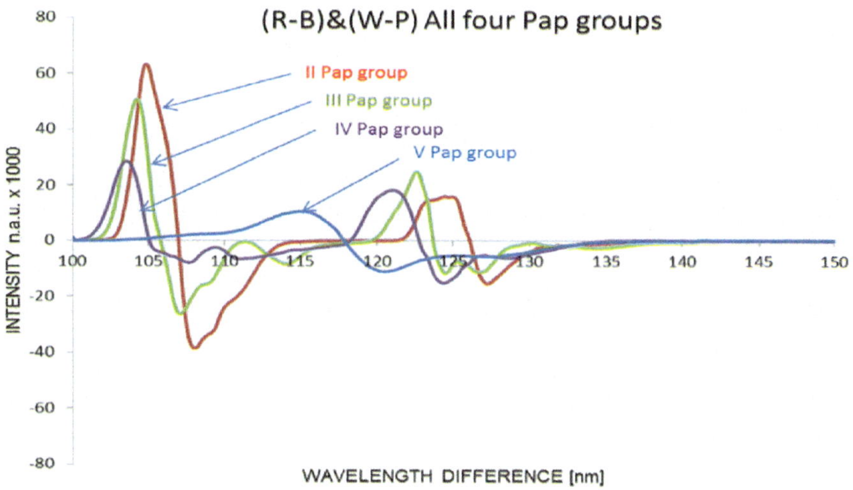

Fig. 29 OMIS diagram obtained for PAP groups [36]

for selected cases of rectal carcinomas), more and more cases are treated with these minimally-invasive techniques. Nevertheless, the incidence of local recurrence after diagnosis is still rather high, in excess of 20% [38]. Furthermore there is always the risk that malignancy already exists in large polyps. In these settings it would be very useful to have a method that would enable inspection of the lesion in detail and visualization of all the layers of the bowel wall before deciding on definitive treatment.

Standard methods used in the definitive verification of CRC are expensive and time consuming. The optical method presented in this paper, as an auxiliary diagnostic method, is less expensive than the standard. However, some other optical methods require special sample preparation, many are not portable and only few can be used for in vivo investigations in addition to in vitro. It is crucial for in vivo methods to be non-invasive. OMIS is non-invasive, efficient, utilising portable equipment which does not require any particular sample preparation (guaranteeing fresh sample state). It shows good results in the detection of colorectal carcinoma based on light-tissue interaction *ex vivo*. The differences in OMIS diagrams obtained for normal and cancerous tissue, with the values of healthy tissue higher than 20 n.a.u. for intensity and tissue activity in the domain of wavelength difference of 110–130 nm. This was compared to carcinoma tissue with intensity less than 10 n.a.u. and a wavelength difference in range of 105 to 170 nm. These were used as inputs to a classifier, which separates samples into two groups. These achieved accuracies of 92,59% (Multilayer perceptron Neural Network) and 89.87% (Naïve-Bayes classifier) in predicted sets for crop size 710 × 710 pixels, indicating OMIS as a possible new method for cancer detection [39]. Results of Naïve-Bayes classifier indicate as well high percentage of accuracy for two different size of crop region, 710 × 710 pixels and 1700 × 1700 pixels (Table 5).

As the existing OMIS method can differentiate healthy tissue and tumour ex vivo, this opens up the possibility of further development for in vivo application. In addition the knowledge gained over the course of this research gave us the opportunity to improve our hardware and software solutions, which will contribute to successful in vivo research. In order to extend the results obtained by the OMIS method, future measurements will be made to measure remanent magnetism of healthy and cancer tissue of colon. This will be done because the OMIS and spinner magnetometer (JR-6A speed spinner magnetometer [40]) are two complementary methods, with the first one measuring the paramagnetic/diamagnetic properties of tissue layers on surface and the second one measuring the permanent magnetism of the whole sample of tissue.

Table 5 Predicted set of two different size of cropped region (1700 × 1700 pixels and 710 × 710 pixels)

Size of cropped region	710 × 710 pixels	1700 × 1700 pixels
Sensitivity	92.11	76.32
Specificity	87.80	73.17
Accuracy	89.87	74.68

Skin Cancer. The skin consists of three main parts: the epithelial tissue (which makes up the upper layer of the skin, the epidermis), the middle layer (dermis), and the deepest layer of the skin, containing fat and connective tissue (hypodermis). The epidermis is keratinized stratified squamous epithelium and is made of keratinocytes (95%), melanocytes, Langerhans cells and Merkel cells. Keratinocytes are the main and most numerous cells that produce keratin and also synthesize the following: specific proteins (that form the inner lining of keratinized cells), products such as cytokines, enzymes, proteins, inflammatory mediators (that are important when it comes to the inflammatory process).

The layers of epidermis are, in ascending order: stratum basale, stratum spinosum, stratum granulosum, stratum lucidum (only in the epidermis on the palm and the sole of the foot) and stratum corneum. The stratum basale (basal layer) is the deepest layer of epidermis, consisting of one line (row) of cylindrical cells. Ultrastructural analysis shows that the basal cells transform into keratinocytes, which means that the basal cell is a stem cell from which multiplication begins. The stratum spinosum (spinous layer) has several layers of large polygonal cells (called desmosomes) which are tightly interconnected with the nexus. In this layer the transformation of the keratinocytes continues. The stratum granulosum (granulosa layer) consists of several flat, polygonal cells. In this layer the transformation of a keratinocyte continues. The stratum corneum (horny corneal layer) consists of 15–20 layers of flat, dead cell, called corneocytes. In this layer the keratinization process is completed. Corneocytes separate from each other and gradually the whole process ends with desquamation (peeling), and the cells of the basal layer replenish the epithelium. It takes about 30 days to restore the stratum corneum. This means that during this time the cells of the basal layer divide, multiply, and go through all the layers of skin to become corneocytes in the stratum corneum. The dermis (loose connective tissue) is just under the epidermis. Components of the dermis provide mechanical support, rigidity and thickness (1–4 mm). The dermis is composed of two layers: papillary and reticular. Loose connective tissue and extracellular matrix consist of collagen fibres (collagen type I and III) and elastin, which form the basis of the papillary layer of the dermis. Irregular, loose, thick connective tissue is the basis of the reticular layer. The dense network of the thick, erratically-positioned collagen bundles, which lies parallel to the surface of the skin in the direction of the force stretching the skin, provides mechanical stability. The hypodermis is the deepest layer of the skin, composed of lobules of adipose tissue separated by connective tissue. It is a thermal insulator, the depot of energetic materials and binds the skin to the muscle and bones, providing its mobility. The boundary between the dermis and the epidermis is the basement membrane, which is important because of its prognostic significance of skin tumours [41, 42].

The optical properties of skin in in vivo conditions were investigated for two different types of skin lesions that exist or occur on the skin due to damage. These changes were divided into two basic categories: benign and malignant pigment changes. Each category was further divided into appropriate subgroups. The device was put directly onto the lesion and pictures were taken with both white diffuse and polarized light. In 97% of cases, the results obtained using OMIS agreed with

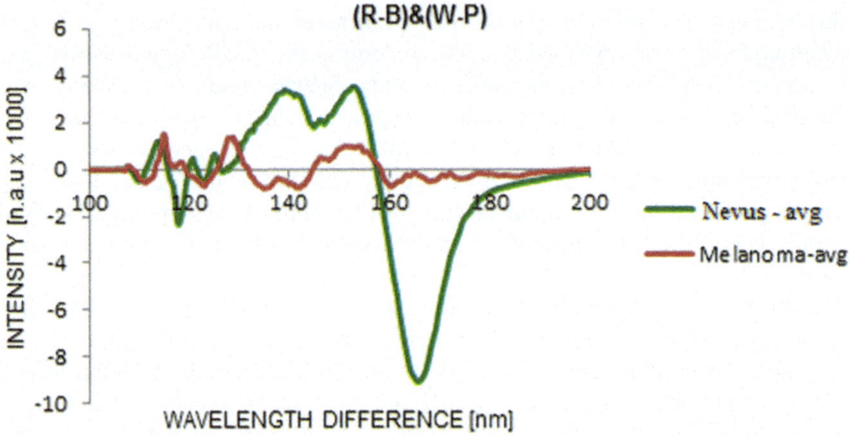

Fig. 30 Comparison of the mean opto-magnetic spectra for the dataset of 48 melanoma cases and the mean optomagnetic spectrum for the dataset of 48 nevus cases [18]

dermoscopy and histopathology findings. Samples were obtained from 96 patients (48 samples belong to the melanoma group and the other 48 to the nevus group) (Fig. 30).

Opto-magnetic Imaging Spectroscopy was applied in vitro and in vivo on cervical, colon, and skin samples. Research included 280 cervical samples, 112 colon samples and 96 skin samples. The optomagnetic spectra exhibited good differentiation between healthy and cancerous samples based on characteristic OMIS spectra intensities and peak positions. They also showed that spectra intensity decreases towards lower values in cases of precancerous and cancerous tissues in all three varieties of epithelial tissue. Classification results provided a high degree of accuracy in cancer detection (skin 91.67%, colon 96.43%, cervix 85.18) using the OMIS method (Table 6). Research efforts are underway and are geared towards expanding the databases of the opto-magnetic spectra of cancer and healthy cases, and also research of an optimal classification method in order to develop a method which would complement the efforts of medical professionals in quick screening and early cancer diagnostics.

5.2 *Biomedical Devices Based on Captured Mimicry in Light-Matter Interaction*

The aim of biomedical photonics is to aid the prevention of cancer and maintenance of the functional status of tissues, organs and the overall human organism. However, when a dysfunction occurs it should be eliminated—i.e. the impaired function of the biomolecule, tissue, organ or the organism should be restored (Fig. 31).

Three basic light types are used today in biology and medicine: diffuse, polarized (linearly or circularly) and laser light. Circularly polarized light is applied mostly for

Table 6 Summary of classification results using Naïve Bayes classifier with kernel density estimation

Type of tissue	Number of samples			Total	Average (%)		
	Serbia	India	UK		Sensitivity	Specificity	Average
Skin (in vivo)	96	–	–	96	97.62	87.04	91.67
Cervix (in vitro) PAP, LBC	600	PAP: 1006 LBC: 641	– LBC: 132	PAP: 1.606 LBC: 773	PAP: 77.18 LBC: 78.20	PAP: 96.50 LBC:97.84	PAP: 87.54 LBC: 88.47
Colon (ex tempura)	112	–	–	112	91.97	96.85	92.59

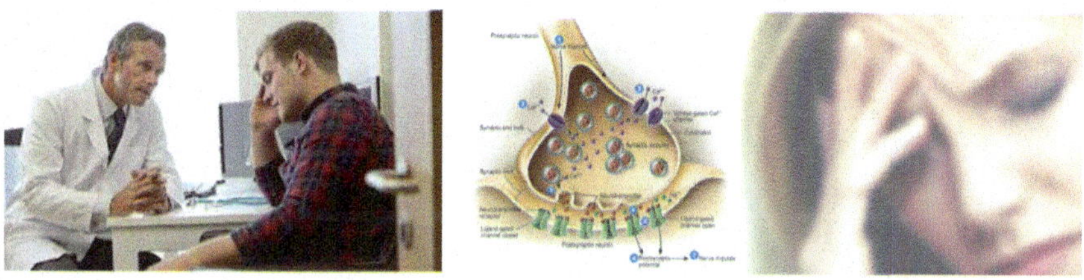

Fig. 31 Most disorders of brain functioning, such as headache (left), depression (right) etc., are caused by inadequate neurotransmitter discharge at the synapses [45, 46]

the determination of optically active chromophores and secondary protein structures (α-helix, β-plate, and R-"random structure") [43].

This section investigates light and its influence on biological systems when diffuse light interacts with C60 molecules in a thin film (C60 can also be incorporated into polymer material or some other material having transparency greater than 92%). We named this kind of light hyperharmonized because the electromagnetic photon fields are organized according to the degree of curvature, and not as "aligned soldiers" (as in the case when linearly polarized light is transformed into hyperpolarized light); they are distributed randomly with respect to energy, but are hyperharmonized as an active (information) pattern [44]. We have already seen how the linearly polarized light affects the "shift" of wavelengths (left and right of 680 nm), this being very significant for the protection of the human eye from intense blue light. This study examined the effect of hyperharmonized light on the human brain, primarily the modification of EEG signals (Figs. 33, 35 and 36).

Similarities and differences between hyperharmonized and hyperpolarized light are displayed in Fig. 32. In diffuse light, the direction and orientation of the electromagnetic photon field (EM) and photon intensity are arbitrary. When photons of different energies (wavelengths/frequencies) interact with the C60 molecule, the orbital angular momenta are oriented according to the Fibonacci laws [ϕ, Φ], however, the energy intensities remain diffusely distributed. Regarding the hyperpolarized light originating in the interaction with the C60 molecule, the orbital angular

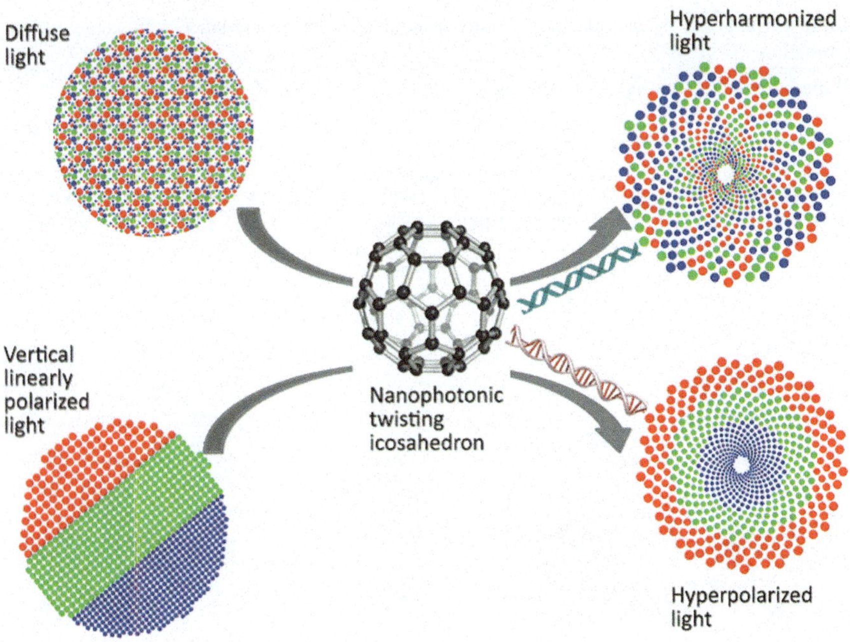

Fig. 32 Similarities and differences between hyperharmonized and hyperpolarized light: the first originates in the interaction between the diffuse light and C60 molecules, twistingly rotating at $\sim 10^{10}$ s − 1, and the HPL is formed in the interaction between the linearly polarized light and C60 molecules [4]

momenta (J = L + S) and energies are organized according to their intensities (in the hyperpolarized light; the organisation of energies according to intensities was "prepared" by the linearly polarized light because photons of the same wavelength are already "packed" in a plane).

The study examined twelve research subjects (volunteers); three subjects were recorded at the Military Medical Academy in Belgrade, and nine research subjects at the Medical Faculty in Belgrade. Recorded data were processed at the "Siniša Stanković" Biological Institute at the Department for Multidisciplinary Research. It is known that the EEG (electrical) and MEG (magnetic) brain signals are modified under the influence of daylight, and that signals are different when the eyes are open versus when they are closed (Fig. 33).

The dynamics of neurotransmitters discharged at synapses is one of the main mechanisms of EEG and MEG signal generation (Fig. 34). The character of the electrical and magnetic dynamics established depends mainly on the carrier of neurotransmitters to the presynaptic part of the neuron. This is the role of the clathrin structure (Fibonacci biomolecular structure). Since the hyperharmonized light is organized according to Fibonacci laws [ϕ/Φ] with respect to the orbital angular momenta (OAM), the study's aim was to determine whether hyperharmonized light via clathrin affects the EEG signals and how.

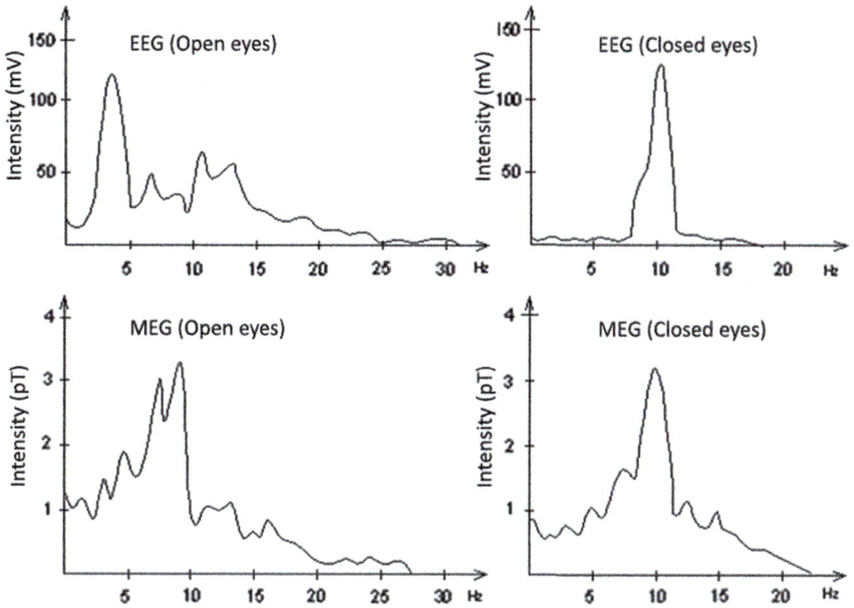

Fig. 33 Light influence on the functioning of the CNS when eyes are open and when eyes are closed. Electrical (EEG) and magnetic (MEG) brain signals operate at approximately the same frequencies when eyelids are closed (the main magnetic peak is at 9 Hz, and the electrical peak is at 10 Hz), and are different when the eyes are open: the main magnetic peak is at 9 Hz, and the electrical peak at 3 Hz). Adapted from: Kato [47]

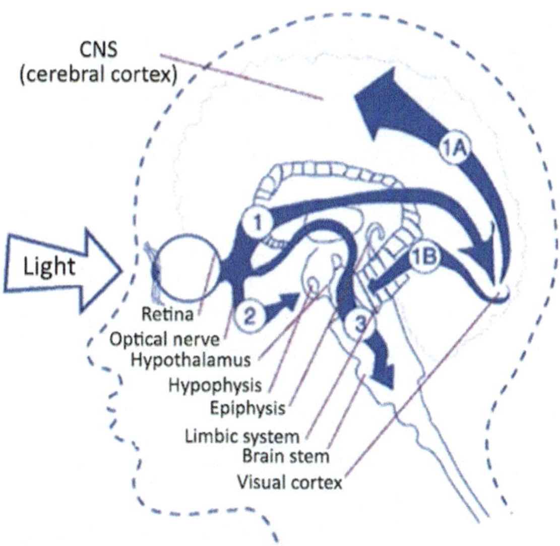

Fig. 34 Light via the eyesight affects the hypothalamus, the visual cortex, the cerebral cortex, and other CNS structures. Since the regulation system is the integral neuro-endocrine-immune system, the influence of light through the CNS on the endocrine and immune system is possible

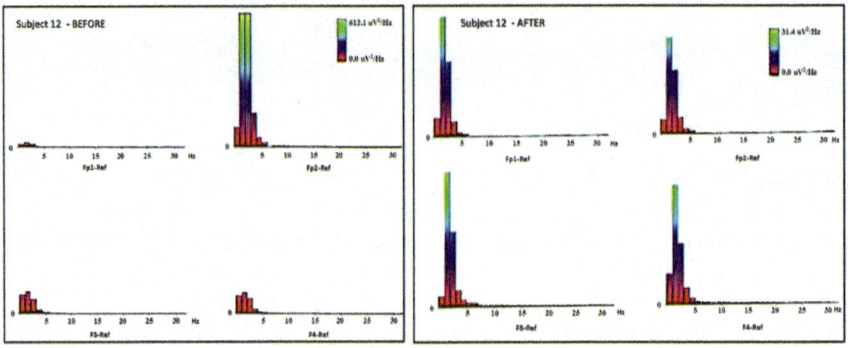

Fig. 35 Example of EEG signals in one of the 9 research subjects when electrodes were positioned at locations Fp1, Fp2, F3, F4 of the "brain cap"; (left) before the treatment; and (right) 10 min after exposure to daylight. The second case is more characteristic: at first, three signals were not adequate (Fp1, F3 and F4). They were improved after the treatment, that is, a more more realistic performance of brain structures was obtained

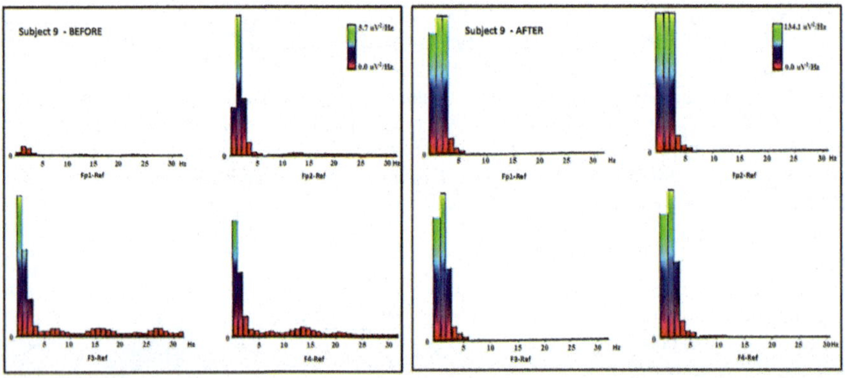

Fig. 36 Example of EEG signals in one of the 9 research subjects when electrodes were positioned at locations Fp1, Fp2, F3, F4 of the "brain cap"; (left) before the treatment, and (right) 10 min after exposure to daylight

EEG signals and Tesla Hyper light glasses. Nanophotonic glasses were constructed for this study by applying a thin film of 100 nm C60 molecules on glass 1.5 mm thick. Above the thin film a 1 mm thick covering glass was mounted, and the edges of these two glass surfaces were connected with adhesive tape so that air could not infiltrate the space where thin film was applied.

Four positions were used (Fp1, Fp2, F3, F4) for the recording of EEG signals, which were connected to the apparatus and the analyser via the EEG headpiece. At these four points the intensity of EEG signals (under good neurological functional conditions) is approximately the same. Before the glasses were put on, the EEG signals were recorded during 10 min, and diagrams determined giving the average value in this period. Under the same ambient conditions, research subjects put on the nanophotonic glasses and the recording of EEG signals was continued during the next 10 min. Average values were calculated based on the recorded data for all four positions during this period.

All research subjects experienced changes in EEG signals. Figures 35 and 36 show two characteristic cases. In the first case signal Fp1 was not of adequate intensity with respect to the other three signals. Ten minutes later, the intensity of the Fp1 signal reached an adequate value. The other three signals were improved as well (Fp2, F3, F4), especially signal Fp2.

The mechanism of the hyperharmonized light action on the modification of EEG signals is explained by the effect, via the visual cortex, of clathrin having the same structural (icosahedral) matrix as the harmonized light.

Research conducted in the USA by leading psychiatrists also points to the conclusion that the entire human brain functions according to the principle of the Fibonacci law Φ [48]. Giulio Tononi is a professor at the University of Wisconsin (USA) and one of the leading researchers in consciousness. He cooperated with Gerald Edelman (Nobel Prize winner for physiology and medicine 1972) in the field of immune system research.

Acquired, preliminary results point strongly to the conclusion that we can influence brain functioning by hyperharmonized light to regulate the normal discharge of neurotransmitters at synapses. Since good results were achieved in the treatment of psoriasis by hyperpolarized light, it would be desirable to organize a study where, via application of hyperpolarized light through the eyes (whilst the eyes were closed) we would act on the brain in tandem with another device treating the region afflicted by psoriasis. This is because psoriasis is cause by psychosomatic factors in addition to being of organic origin. Gerald Edelman believes that not only the brain, but in fact the entire human organism functions according to the "Φ" law. His belief is based primarily on the information transmission viewpoint because information is central to investigations of the consciousness phenomenon.

One more paper points to the conclusion that the brain is functioning according to Fibonacci laws [49]. This paper proposes that the principle of information coding within the brain is based on the Fibonacci law Φ, and that this is the missing link between psychometric intelligence measurement and comprehension. Metrics of brain waves, according to the authors, can always be represented as a superposition of n harmonics multiplied by 2Φ, where half of the basic state is represented precisely by Φ ($= 1.618$) and has the meaning of a resonant point. Such wave series represent bifurcation processes occurring in the brain, and these function as "deterministic chaos" [50] because $2\Phi = 3 + \phi^3$. Bearing in mind that $\Phi^2 + \phi^2 = 3$ (the basis of the twisting torus of C_{60}), neurological function as a system operating in the domain of "deterministic chaos" can be corrected (brought to a functional state by the influence of hyperharmonized and hyperpolarized light: $2\Phi = \Phi^2 + \phi^2 + \phi^3$).

Results of the initial study of the effect of hyperharmonized light (synchronized spatial–temporal effects of diffuse light on the C60 molecule) on the EEG signals, in twelve research subjects, clearly point to the modification of signals. Everything points to the fact that the action mechanism is established through Fibonacci structures: the orbital angular momenta of the photon and of clathrin in the brain have the same symmetry. This is a classical example and realisation of the principle "structured light meets structured matter", which researchers predicted several years ago [13].

Acknowledgements We are grateful to Prof. Dr Nikola Ilanković and his associates at the Medical Faculty in Belgrade and the Military Medical Academy for assistance in the measurement of EEG signals. My gratitude goes extends to the associates of the "Siniša Stanković" Biological Institute for assistance in processing EEG signals. Zepter international provided important support to the studies and also took part in the study. Our special gratitude goes to the volunteers—students of master, specialist, and doctoral studies from the Department of Biomedical Engineering at the Faculty of Mechanical Engineering, University of Belgrade. Željko Ratkaj's contribution to study on nanophotonics is especially valuable and outstanding.

References

1. Koruga, Đ: Neuromolecular computing. Nanobiology **1**, 5–24 (1992)
2. Matija, L.: Nanotechnology: artificial versus natural self-assembly. FME Trans. **32**, 1–14 (2004)
3. Vedral, V.: Decoding Reality: The Universe as Quantum Information. Oxford University Press, Oxford (2010)
4. Koruga, D.: Hyperpolarized Light: Fundamentals of Nanobiomedical Photonics. Zepter Book World, Belgrade (2018)
5. Schuster, H.G., Just, W.: Deterministic Chaos: An Introduction. John Wiley & Sons (2006)
6. Kanaseki, T., Kadota, K.: The "vesicle in a basket". A morphological study of the coated vesicle isolated from the nerve endings of the guinea pig brain, with special reference to the mechanism of membrane movements. J. Cell. Biol. **42**, 202–220 (1969). https://doi.org/10.1083/jcb.42.1.202
7. Koruga, D.L.: Microtubular screw symmetry: packing of spheres as a latent bioinformation code. Ann. N. Y. Acad. Sci. **466**, 953–955 (1986). https://doi.org/10.1111/j.1749-6632.1986.tb38483.x
8. Dustin, P.: Microtubules, 2nd edn. Springer-Verlag, Berlin Heidelberg (1984)
9. Piazza, L., Lummen, T.T.A., Quinonez, E., et al.: Simultaneous observation of the quantization and the interference pattern of a plasmonic near-field. Nat. Commun. **6**, 1–7 (2015)
10. Band, Y.B.: Light and Matter: Electromagnetism, Optics, Spectroscopy and Lasers. Hoboken, NJ, John Wiley, Chichester (2007)
11. Binnig, G., Rohrer, H., Gerber, C., Weibel, E.: Surface studies by scanning tunneling microscopy. Phys. Rev. Lett. **49**, 57 (1982)
12. Weiner, J., Nunes, F.: Light-Matter Interaction: Physics and Engineering at the Nanoscale. Oxford University Press, Oxford (2012)
13. Litchinitser, N.M.: Structured light meets structured matter. Science (80-) **337**, 1054–1055 (2012). https://doi.org/10.1126/science.1226204
14. Carlson, B.M.: Human embryology and developmental biology. Mosby/Elsevier, Philadelphia (2009)
15. Goodreads: Albert Einstein Quotes. https://www.goodreads.com/quotes/3653-one-thing-i-have-learned-in-a-long-life-that
16. Kosaka, H.: Photon-to-electron quantum information transfer. J. Appl. Phys. **109**, 102414 (2011)

17. Koruga, D., Tomic, A.: System and method for analysis of light-matter interaction based on spectral convolution. US Pat. App. No.61/061,852, 2008, PCT/US2009/030347, Publication No: WO/2009/089292 (2009)
18. Matija, L., Jeftic, B., Nikolic, G., et al.: Nanophysical approach to diagnosis of epithelial tissues using Opto-magnetic imaging spectroscopy. In: Seifalian, A. (ed.) Nanomedicine, pp. 156–186. One Central Press Ltd., Manchester (UK) (2014)
19. Koruga, D., Hameroff, S., Withers, J., et al.: Fullerene C60: History, Physics, Nanobiology, Nanotechnology. Elsevier Science Ltd (1993)
20. Devlin, K.: Finding Fibonacci. Princeton University Press (2017)
21. Vajda, S.: Fibonacci and Lucas Numbers, and the Golden Section : Theory and Applications. Ellis Horwood Limited; John Wiley & Sons, Chichester, New York (1989)
22. Coey, J.M.D.: Magnetism and Magnetic Materials. Cambridge University Press, Cambridge (2015)
23. Koruga, D.: Optical filter and method of manufacturing an optical filter. Pat. App. No.16734563.6 EP 3 469 406. B1, International publication No: WO 2017/211420 (2020)
24. Dal Negro, L., Oton, C.J., Gaburro, Z., et al.: Light transport through the band-edge states of Fibonacci quasicrystals. Phys. Rev. Lett. **90**, 55501 (2003)
25. Kroto, H.W., Heath, J.R., O'Brien, S.C., et al.: C 60: buckminsterfullerene. Nature **318**, 162–163 (1985)
26. Matija, L.: Endohedralni fulereni. Zadužbina Andrejević (1999)
27. Koruga, D., Simic-Krstic, J., Trifunovic, M., et al.: Imaging fullerene C60 with atomic resolution using a scanning tunnelling microscope. Fuller. Sci. Technol. **1**, 93–100 (1993). https://doi.org/10.1080/15363839308015518
28. Arndt, M., Nairz, O., Vos-Andreae, J., et al.: Wave–particle duality of C 60 molecules. Nature **401**, 680–682 (1999)
29. Huffman, D.R.: Solid C60. Phys. Today **44**, 22–29 (1991)
30. Wang, J., Yang, J.-Y., Fazal, I.M., et al.: Terabit free-space data transmission employing orbital angular momentum multiplexing. Nat. Photonics **6**, 488–496 (2012). https://doi.org/10.1038/nphoton.2012.138
31. Strogatz, S.H.: Nonlinear Dynamics and Chaos: with Applications to Physics, Biology, Chemistry, and Engineering. Westview, Cambridge (1994)
32. Monsonego, J., Autillo-Touati, A., Bergeron, C., et al.: Liquid-based cytology for primary cervical cancer screening: a multi-centre study. Br. J. Cancer **84**, 360–366 (2001)
33. Ronco, G., Cuzick, J., Pierotti, P., et al.: Accuracy of liquid based versus conventional cytology: overall results of new technologies for cervical cancer screening: randomised controlled trial. BMJ BMJ **335**, 28 (2007)
34. Chevarie-Davis, M., Ramanakumar, A.V., Ferenczy, A., et al.: Assessment of the performance of algorithms for cervical cancer screening: evidence from the Ludwig-McGill cohort study. YGYNO Gynecol. Oncol. **128**, 415–419 (2013)
35. Van Kriekinge, G., Castellsagu, X., Cibula, D., Demarteau, N.: Estimation of the potential overall impact of human papillomavirus vaccination on cervical cancer cases and deaths. JVAC Vaccine **32**, 733–739 (2014)
36. Jeftic, B., Papic-Obradovic, M., Muncan, J., et al.: Optomagnetic imaging spectroscopy application in cervical dysplasia and cancer detection: comparation of stained and unstained papanicolaou smears. J. Med. Biol. Eng. J. Med. Biol. Eng. **37**, 936–943 (2017)
37. Colorectal cancer statistics—World Cancer Research Fund International. http://www.wcrf.org/int/cancer-facts-figures/data-specific-cancers/colorectal-cancer-statistics
38. Zhan, T., Hielscher, T., Hahn, F., et al.: Risk factors for local recurrence of large, flat colorectal polyps after endoscopic mucosal resection. Digestion **93**, 311–317 (2016)
39. Dragicevic, A., Matija, L., Krivokapic, Z., et al.: Classification of healthy and cancer states of colon epithelial tissues using opto-magnetic imaging spectroscopy. J. Med. Biol. Eng. J. Med. Biol. Eng. **39**, 367–380 (2019)
40. Dragicevic, A., Krivokapic, Z., Dimitrijevic, I., et al.: 711 Ex vivo preclinical study of colon cancer using opto-magnetic imaging spectroscopy and dual speed spinner magnetometer. Eur. J. Cancer **51**, S130–S131 (2015)

41. Koruga, Đ., Miljkovic, S., Ribar, S., et al.: Water hydrogen bonds study by opto-magnetic fingerprint technique. Acta. Phys. Pol. A Gen. Phys. **117**, 777–781 (2010)
42. Koruga, Đ, Bandic, J., Janjic, G., et al.: Epidermal layers characterisation by opto-magnetic spectroscopy based on digital image of skin. Acta Phys. Pol. A Acta. Phys. Pol. A **121**, 606–610 (2012)
43. Campbell, I.D., Dwek, R.A.: Biological Spectroscopy. Benjamin/Cummings Pub. Co., Menlo Park, Calif (1984)
44. Koruga, Đ.: Apparatus for harmonizing light. US Patent, Pub. No.: US 2008/0286453 A1 (2008)
45. Lepeta, K., Lourenco, M.V., Schweitzer, B.C., et al.: Synaptopathies: synaptic dysfunction in neurological disorders—A review from students to students. J Neurochem **138**, 785–805 (2016). https://doi.org/10.1111/jnc.13713
46. Goadsby, P.J., Holland, P.R., Martins-Oliveira, M., et al.: Pathophysiology of migraine: a disorder of sensory processing. Physiol. Rev. **97**, 553–622 (2017). https://doi.org/10.1152/physrev.00034.2015
47. Kato, M.: Electromagnetics in Biology. Springer, Tokyo, New York (2006)
48. Tononi, G., Books, P.: Phi : a Voyage from the Brain to the Soul. Pantheon Books, New York (2012)
49. Weiss, H., Weiss, V.: The golden mean as clock cycle of brain waves. CHAOS</cja:jid> Chaos. Solitons and Fractals **18**, 643–652 (2003)
50. Basar, E., Bullock, T.H.: Chaos in Brain Function. Springer-Verlag, Berlin Heidelberg (1990)

Brownian Motion Fractal Nature Frontiers Within the Matter

Vojislav Mitić, Goran Lazović, Dušan Milošević, Jelena Manojlović, Elizabeta Ristanović, Dragan Simeunović, Shwu-Chen Tsay, Mimica Milošević, Marina Soković, and Branislav Vlahović

Abstract One of the main motivations for our research was to find a connection between the Brownian motion of microorganisms within fractal nature, with the

V. Mitić (Deceased)
Institute of Technical Sciences of the Serbian Academy of Science and Arts, Kneza Mihaila 35, 11000 Belgrade, Serbia

G. Lazović (✉)
Faculty of Mechanical Engineering, University of Belgrade, Kraljice Marije 16, 11000 Belgrade, Serbia
e-mail: glazovic@mas.bg.ac.rs

V. Mitić (Deceased) · D. Milošević
Faculty of Electronic Engineering, University of Niš, Aleksandra Medvedeva 14, 18106 Niš, Serbia
e-mail: dusan.milosevic@elfak.ni.ac.rs

J. Manojlović
Faculty of Mechanical Engineering, University of Niš, Aleksandra Medvedeva 14, 18106 Niš, Serbia

E. Ristanović
Faculty of Medicine of the Military Medical Academy, University of Defence, 11000 Belgrade, Serbia
e-mail: elizabet@eunet.rs

D. Simeunović
Faculty of Political Science, University of Belgrade, 11000 Belgrade, Serbia

S.-C. Tsay
Department of Chemistry, National Tsing Hua University, Hsinchu, Taiwan

M. Milošević
Faculty of Business Economics and Entrepreneurship, University of Belgrade, Mitropolita Petra 8, 11000 Belgrade, Serbia

M. Soković
Ministry of Education, Science and Technological Development, Nemanjina 22-26, 11000 Belgrade, Serbia
e-mail: marina.sokovic@mpn.gov.rs

S. Najman et al. (eds.), *Bioceramics, Biomimetic and Other Compatible Materials Features for Medical Applications*, Engineering Materials,
https://doi.org/10.1007/978-3-031-17269-4_16

idea of developing an appropriate procedure and method to control the microorganism's motion direction and predict the position of the microorganism in time. In this paper, we have followed the results of the very rear microorganism's motion sub-microstructures in the experimental microstructure analysis already observed and published. All of these data have been good basis to describe the motion trajectory by time interval method and fractals. We successfully defined the diagrams in two and three-dimensions and we were able to establish the control of Brownian chaotic motion as a bridge between chaotic disorders to control disorder. This significant study opens a new possibility for future investigation and the new potential of total control of the microorganism motion. These perspectives and findings provide significant data for getting more information from these bio systems. They can also be applied, based on self-similarities and biomimetics, to particle physical systems and matter, generally.

Keywords Coronavirus · Brownian motion · Fractals · Time interval method

1 Introduction

A fractal is a geometric figure that can be decomposed into smaller parts so that each of them is, at least approximately, reduced a copy of the whole. The term fractal was introduced by French mathematician Mandelbrot in the eighties of the past century. The word itself comes from the Latin word fractus, meaning fragmented, irregular. Mathematically, a fractal can be defined as the complete metric space invariant subset concerning the union of contractive mappings W. Thus, the equation holds for fractals. Applications show that fractals are more suitable for modeling many phenomena in nature and physics than the tools of Euclidean geometry. In this paper, we will use fractals to model the movement of microorganisms. Fractal Interpolation Curve (FIC) that simulates the trajectory of the microorganism has been constructed based on the localization of the microorganism position in discrete moments.

$$W(F) = F \tag{1}$$

To get the FIC curve, the Iterated Function System (IFS) has been applied [1–3]. In mathematics, an iterated function system, or IFS, is a fractal construction procedure in which the resulting constructions are always self-similar. The fractal

Institute for Biological Research "Siniša Stankovic", University of Belgrade, Belgrade, Serbia

B. Vlahović
North Carolina Central University, Durham, NC, USA
e-mail: vlahovic@nccu.edu

D. Simeunović
National Security Academy, 11000, Belgrade, Serbia

has been created with the union of several copies, transformed by an IFS. Formally, an Iterated Function System is a finite set of contraction mappings $\{w_1, w_2, \ldots, w_N\}$ of the complete metric space $(\mathbb{R}^m, d)$ into itself. Over IFS, Hutchinson operator can be defined as in [4]. For bounded set X from $\mathbb{R}^m$, Hutchinson operator over $\mathbb{R}^m\mathbb{R}^m$

$$W(X) = \bigcup_{i=1}^{N} w_i(X) \tag{2}$$

is a contraction in metric space $(H(\mathbb{R}^m), h)$, with the Hausdorff distance h. The corresponding fixed point

$$W(A) = A \tag{3}$$

is called the IFS attractor. The IFS always have at least one attractor [1].

1.1 Two Dimensional Case

Let us first consider two-dimensional case, metric space $\left(\mathbb{R}^2, d\right)$. For that purpose we have determine the set of points $\left\{(x_i, y_i) \in \mathbb{R}^2, \quad i = 0, 1, \ldots, N\right\}$ in plane and abscissas arranged in ascending order,

$$x_0 < x_1 < \cdots < x_N. \tag{4}$$

Over these points, there is a need to define IFS $\left\{\mathbb{R}^2; w_1, w_2, \ldots, w_N\right\}$ with affine transformation [5, 6]

$$w_i\begin{bmatrix} x \\ y \end{bmatrix} = \begin{bmatrix} a_i & 0 \\ c_i & d_i \end{bmatrix}\begin{bmatrix} x \\ y \end{bmatrix} + \begin{bmatrix} e_i \\ f_i \end{bmatrix}, \quad i = 1, \ldots, N \tag{5}$$

and constraints

$$w_i\begin{bmatrix} x_0 \\ y_0 \end{bmatrix} = \begin{bmatrix} x_{i-1} \\ y_{i-1} \end{bmatrix} \text{and } w_i\begin{bmatrix} x_N \\ y_N \end{bmatrix} = \begin{bmatrix} x_i \\ y_i \end{bmatrix}, i = 1, \ldots, N \tag{6}$$

From (5), we observe that every transformation $w_i, \quad i = 1, \ldots, N$ has five parameters a_i, c_i, d_i, e_i and f_i. Further, from Eq. (6), we see that for each transformation, two conditions, each with two equations, are given. Thus, four parameters are determined and one parameter is free. We selected the parameter d_i as free one because of his geometric interpretation [7, 8]. The transformation w_i. maps the straight line of length l parallel to the y-axis, to the straight line of length $w_i(l)$, also parallel to the y-axis. The absolute value of the quotient of the line lengths is equal $|d_i|$.

To ensure that the affine transformation w_i is a contraction, it is sufficient for the absolute value of the parameter d_i to be less than one. If all affine transformations $w_i, \quad i = 1, \ldots, N$ are contraction the attractor G of IFS

$$W(G) = \bigcup_{i=1}^{N} w_i(G) \tag{7}$$

is a graph of a continuous function passing through interpolation points $\{(x_i, y_i) \in \mathbb{R}^2, \quad i = 0, 1, \ldots, N\}$. This continuous function is the Fractal Interpolation Function (FIF). The Fractal Interpolation Function is self-affine for the reason that each of affine transformation w_i maps the whole function to the part between the interpolation points (x_{i-1}, y_{i-1}) and (x_i, y_i) for each $i = 1, 2, \ldots, N$.

When the ordinates x_i of the interpolation points $\{(x_i, y_i) \in \mathbb{R}^2, \quad i = 0, 1, \ldots, N\}$ are not in strictly ascending order, the case when conditions (4) are not fulfilled, direct application of IFS $\{\mathbb{R}^2; w_1, w_2, \ldots, w_N\}$, defined by (5) and (6), does not give interpolation curve that pass through the interpolation points.

In order to ensure that the condition (4) is satisfied, one can introduce additional coordinates in place of the ordinate x_i, for example, $x_i = i$ for each $i = 0, 1, \ldots, N$. Instead of increasing the dimension of the problem, by introducing an additional coordinate, the fulfillment of a condition (4) can be achieved by introducing a reversible transformation

$$T(x_i, y_i) = (u_i, v_i), \quad i = 0, 1, \ldots, N, \tag{8}$$

where

$$u_i = x_0 + \sum_{j=1}^{i} \left(|x_j - x_{j-1}| + p\right) = u_{i-1} + (|x_i - x_{i-1}| + c)$$

$$v_i = y_i. \tag{9}$$

With the expression (9) it is ensures that the ordinates u_i are in a strictly ascending order. The constant $c > 0$ is necessary only in the case when all interpolation points have the same ordinates x_i. In all other cases, it can be taken in (9) that $c = 0$.

In this way, it is ensures that the application of IFS $\{\mathbb{R}^2; w_1, w_2, \ldots, w_N\}$, defined by (5) and (6), gives the attractor which represent a graph of a continuous function that interpolates points $(u_i, v_i), \quad i = 0, 1, \ldots, N$.

In the last step, it is necessary to map the obtained attractor in (u, v)-plane by inverse transformation

$$T'(u', v') = (x', y'), \tag{10}$$

where

$$x' = x_{i-1} + (x_i - x_{i-1})\frac{u' - u_{i-1}}{u_i - u_{i-1}}, \quad u' \in [u_{i-1}, u_i]$$

$$y' = v', \tag{11}$$

back into the (*x*, *y*)-plane.

1.2 Three Dimensional Case

Let us now consider the case when $m = 3$. Suppose that a set of points $\{(x_i, y_i, z_i) \in \mathbb{R}^3, \quad i = 0, 1, \ldots, N\}$ are given, and abscissas of these points are arranged in ascending order, which means that the inequalities (4) are fulfilled.

Over these points, we will define IFS $\{\mathbb{R}^3; w_1, w_2, \ldots, w_N\}$ with affine transformations [3]

$$w_n \begin{bmatrix} x \\ y \\ z \end{bmatrix} = \begin{bmatrix} a_n & 0 & 0 \\ c_n^1 & s_n^{1,1} & s_n^{1,2} \\ c_n^2 & s_n^{2,1} & s_n^{2,2} \end{bmatrix} \begin{bmatrix} x \\ y \\ z \end{bmatrix} + \begin{bmatrix} d_n^1 \\ d_n^2 \\ d_n^3 \end{bmatrix} \tag{12}$$

and constraints

$$w_n \begin{bmatrix} x_0 \\ y_0 \\ z_0 \end{bmatrix} = \begin{bmatrix} x_{n-1} \\ y_{n-1} \\ z_{n-1} \end{bmatrix} \text{and } w_n \begin{bmatrix} x_N \\ y_N \\ z_N \end{bmatrix} = \begin{bmatrix} x_n \\ y_n \\ z_n \end{bmatrix} \tag{13}$$

In each affine transformation, $w_1, w_2, \ldots, w_N$, we can observe from (12), that there are ten parameters $a_n, c_n^1, c_n^2, d_n^1, d_n^2, d_n^3, s_n^{1,1}, s_n^{1,2}, s_n^{2,1}$ and $s_n^{2,2}$. As there are two conditions with three equations for each (see (13)), we conclude that six parameters are definite, so four parameters are free.

For free parameters, we will select parameters $s_n^{1,1}, s_n^{1,2}, s_n^{2,1}$ and $s_n^{2,2}$. These four parameters make up the matrix.

$$A = \begin{bmatrix} s_n^{1,1} & s_n^{1,2} \\ s_n^{2,1} & s_n^{2,2} \end{bmatrix} \tag{14}$$

For the affine transformation to be a contraction, it is sufficient for the norm of this matrix A to be less than one. As in the two-dimensional case, if all affine transformations $w_1, w_2, \ldots, w_N$ are contractions, the attractor of the IFS $\{\mathbb{R}^3; w_1, w_2, \ldots, w_N\}$ is a graph of a continuous function passing through interpolation points $\{(x_i, y_i, z_i) \in \mathbb{R}^3, i = 0, 1, \ldots, N\}$. The obtained FIF is self-affine, because each of affine transformation w_i maps the whole function to the part between the interpolation points $(x_{i-1}, y_{i-1}, z_{i-1})$ and (x_i, y_i, z_i), for each $i = 1, 2, \ldots, N$.

In the case when interpolation points $\{(x_i, y_i, z_i) \in \mathbb{R}^3, \quad i = 0, 1, 2, \ldots, N\}$, do not satisfy the condition (4), when their ordinates are not in a strictly ascending order, interpolation curve that pass through all the interpolation points $\{(x_i, y_i, z_i) \in \mathbb{R}^3, \quad i = 0, 1, 2, \ldots, N\}$ cannot be obtained by direct application of IFS $\{\mathbb{R}^3; w_1, w_2, \ldots, w_N\}$ defined by (12) and (13).

Similar to the two-dimensional case we will define reversible transformation

$$T(x_i, y_i, z_i) = (u_i, v_i, w_i), \quad i = 0, 1, \ldots, N, \tag{15}$$

where

$$u_i = x_0 + \sum_{j=1}^{i} \left(\left|x_j - x_{j-1}\right| + p\right) = u_{i-1} + (|x_i - x_{i-1}| + p)$$

$$v_i = y_i$$

$$w_i = z_i, \tag{16}$$

which achieves that the ordinates u_i have arranged in ascending order.

Obtained points $\{(u_i, v_i, w_i), \quad i = 0, 1, \ldots, N\}$ satisfy condition (4), that is, for them hold inequalities $u_0 < u_1 < u_2 < \ldots < u_N$.

Finally, it is necessary to apply the inverse transformation to each point of the obtained attractor (u', v', w').

$$T'(u', v', w') = (x', y', z'), \tag{17}$$

where

$$x' = x_{i-1} + (x_i - x_{i-1}) \frac{u' - u_{i-1}}{u_i - u_{i-1}}, \quad u' \in [u_{i-1}, u_i]$$

$$y' = v',$$

$$z' = w'. \tag{18}$$

Experimental Procedure

In our experimental work we have analyzed different samples of bacteria and certain data regarding Covid-19 virus. The main idea in the research was to study and make some generalizations within experimental results what could be useful for some other applications and analysis.

For that purpose, we have created a general experiment, related to bacteria and Covid-19 virus within the liquid in one chamber, described in Fig. 1.

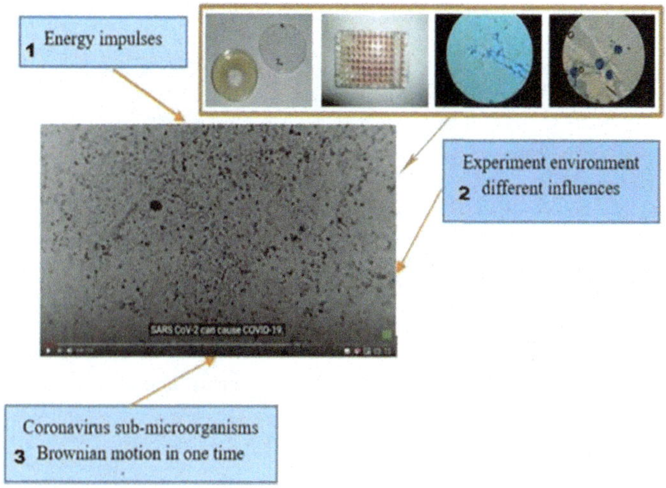

Fig. 1 The initial diagram of bacteria and coronavirus motion experiment. This experimental procedure demonstrates Brownian motions of living organisms in the liquid

Experimental parameters reflect the influence of the real experiment conditions of the observed experiment. There are 3 boxes in Fig. 1. The first box, marked with number 1, describes the precise influence of certain external energy. On the other hand, due to the interactions of Coronavirus in aerosol and liquid motion medium, there are significant energy impulses from the environment (box 2 in Fig. 1), that could not be neglected. Coronavirus is an extremely powerful super-microorganism. In order to analyze their very fine interactions even at the quantum-mechanical level, there is a need to record images of virus trajectories. For that purpose, we considered and discussed the influences of the environment which have micro-vibration character in the frame of energy impulses influences. The Brownian motion as a matter characteristic is represented by the third blue box (box 3, Fig. 1). This analysis is important because it has a significant impact on the formation of virus trajectories.

In order to follow the kinetics of sub-microorganisms, we have formed complex trajectories by selecting four groups of data. In the next step, we have applied the fractal interval nature analysis on the Brownian motion diagrams. We collected a large number of data points in a 0.1 s interval, and we began with six figures of the Covid-19 virus moving, as shown in Fig. 2.

Very similar results we have obtained and described in our previous experiments, are already published in our paper [6].

We have followed the trajectory of randomly selected Coronavirus in four time intervals and the changes in their positions have been presented by pictures in Fig. 2. The observation of the virus behavior and related conclusions can be applied to different modifications of this virus. In the pictures given in Fig. 2, we have selected a few parts of Covid-19 virus trajectories and detected their x and y coordinates, which are shown in Table 1.

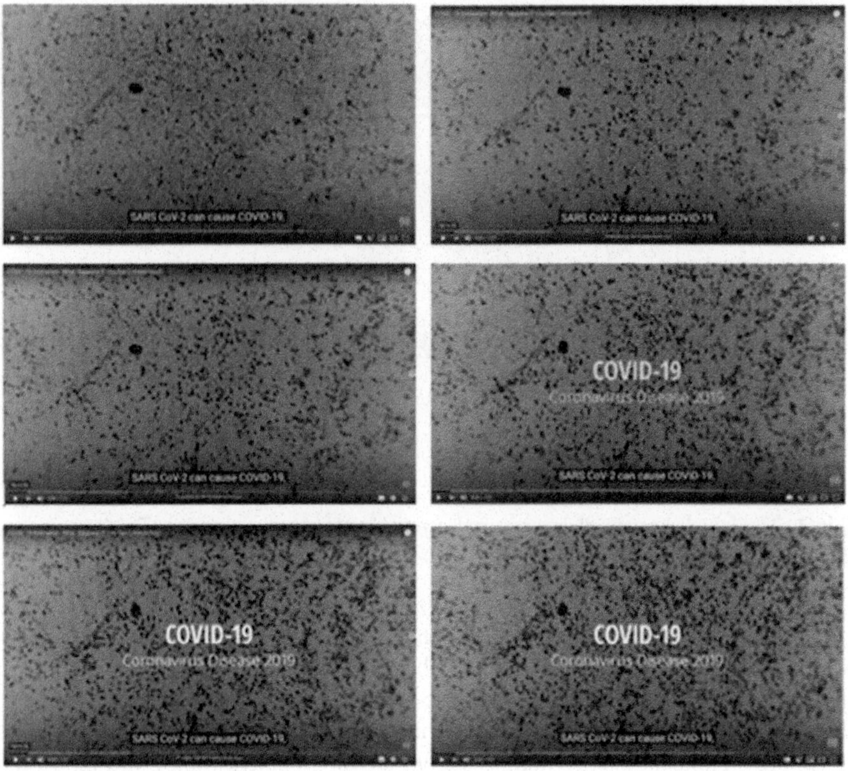

Fig. 2 Picture of Covid-19 virus moving recorded in successive time moments

Table 1 Coordinates of the COVID-19 virus position

x_1	0	0.560	0.9156	1.6157	0.6509	0.7868
y_1	0	−0.0705	0.2018	−0.1645	−0.0893	−0.1336
x_2	0	−0.2549	−0.5679	−1.171	−0.0706	−0.1155
y_2	0	−0.3407	0.6103	−0.176	0.365	−0.661
x_3	0	−0.0888	−0.90794	−1.93617	−1.2926	−1.7911
y_3	0	−0.1462	0.0513	−0.5102	0.197	−0.0833
x_4	0	−0.56757	−0.84831	−1.58725	−1.2254	−1.6697
y_4	0	0.9122	0.9588	0.7453	1.5856	1.2978

The numerical data is from the microscopy generated images, based on the scaled dimension. The values in Table 1 depend on the results of the microscope and can be applied on any scale.

Beside the experiments with Covid virus, we have organized certain number of experiments with bacteria. In order to monitor the influence of different energy signals on bacteria behavior (for example, music), we have selected two bacteria and three different music sounds. The data of bacteria's trajectories without and with sounds influence are described in the following tables.

2 Results and Discussion

As an illustration for two-dimensional case, we have organized an experiment related to Coronavirus behavior within the liquid phase of matter in one chamber. The goal of this experiment was to describe and illustrate the Brownian motions of Coronavirus in the liquid. In order to explore virus dynamics, we selected four parts of trajectories of one virus and examined their complexity. Additionally, we have given results regarding the analysis of the nature of the fractal interval applied to Brownian motion diagrams.

The aim of the experiment was to detect a trajectory of the Coronavirus motion. The positions of the specific viruses, their x and y coordinates, were obtained from six images of the virus obtained in a consecutive time interval of 0.1 s. The observation for this virus and related conclusions can be applied on different modifications of the virus.

The x and y coordinates of four selected Coronavirus trajectories parts are given in Table 1. It is important to emphasize that these numerical values can be defined for any microscopy characterization. Another important fact we have taken into account is that the size of bacteria is ten times bigger than the size of a virus. For the described experimental results, it is important to underline that those results are not the product of a simulation and they are obtained from actual experimental measurements, without simulation and prediction of the virus moving.

As we have already described in our previous work [8, 9] we have applied the interval method (explained in the section on the beginning of this paper) for the interpolation data given in Table 1. It is possible to construct the fractal interpolation function for each part of virus trajectory. The obtained trajectories of virus motion are presented on the Fig. 3 to the Fig. 7 [6]. These results can be good starting point to consider our next step in the virus and bacteria motion analysis.

For the data analysis it is important to describe that the sub-microorganisms Brownian motion we have analyzed in very short intervals and have extracted six figures. They are representing phase cross-section in this dynamic motion process. According to the results from the experiments with bacteria as a microorganism, we have recognized the fractal nature in Brownian motion of such a case. We can consider this conclusion as a general characteristic of the motions in the world of sub-microorganisms. Based on extracted coordinates, by using the algorithm presented in the previous section, we obtained motion trajectories given in the Fig. 3. Applying the interval fractal analysis, we can get information from the results that the virus forms a chaotic loop in very short time interval—0.5 s.

The second part of the virus trajectory is shown in Fig. 4. From this diagram we can observe that Brownian motion indicates its disordered circular motion. Another

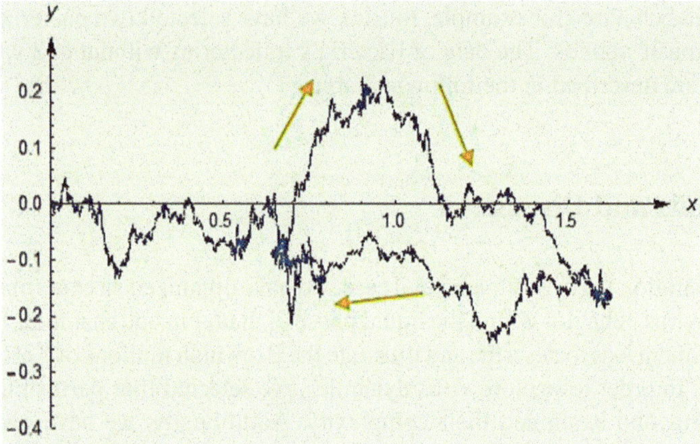

Fig. 3 The trajectory of the first coronavirus with scaling factors $d_i = 0.3, \quad i = 1, 2, \ldots, 6$

observation is that the virus after a very short period of time (around 0.4 s) returned to a point which is close to the starting point.

Following the third part of virus trajectory (Fig. 5), after the interval fractal analysis application, we can conclude that there is no return to the starting position in the interval of 0.5 s. Due to that, it is possible to conclude that the motion of the virus is evidently progressive.

The forth part of the virus trajectory, shown in Fig. 6, indicates its chaotic motion, there is no returning to the starting point in a certain time interval (0.5 s) and there is the progressive motion of the virus.

The purpose of demonstration the three-dimensional case we have analyzed the motion of bacterium in silence and in a situation when music is playing. From the research and experiments it is known that sounds could affect the structure of water

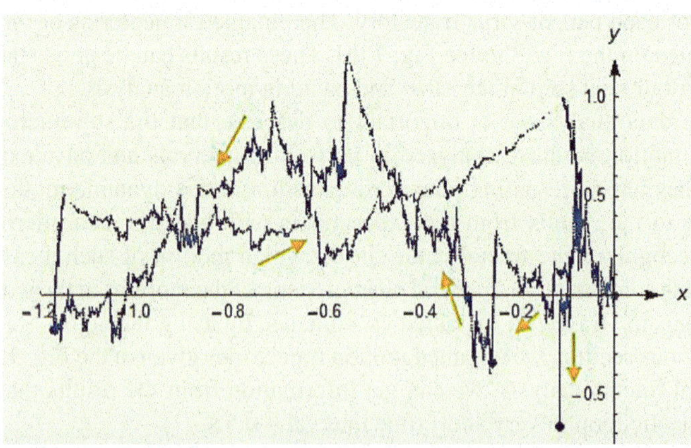

Fig. 4 The trajectory of the second coronavirus with scaling factors $d_i = 0.3, \quad i = 1, 2, \ldots, 6$

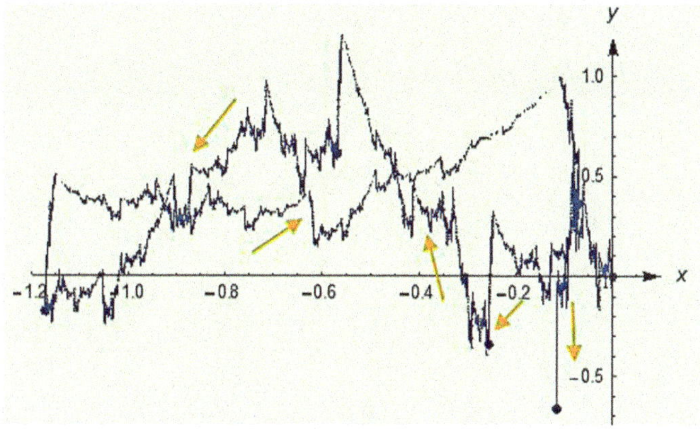

Fig. 5 The trajectory of the third coronavirus with scaling factors $d_i = 0.3, \quad i = 1, 2, \ldots, 6$

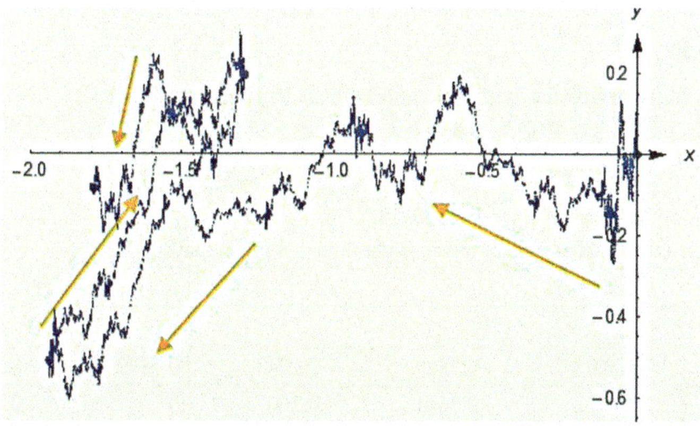

Fig. 6 The fourth part of coronavirus trajectory scaling factors $d_i = 0.4, \quad i = 1, 2, \ldots, 6$

molecules [9]. In particular, we have analyzed how bacterium behaves in the presence of three types of music. The goal of this experiment was to develop and illustrate the Brownian motions of bacterium, and find connection between biological and physical systems.

Tables 2 and 3 give the x, y and z coordinates of the first bacteria without music and with music played (Fig. 7).

From the obtained trajectory of the first bacteria from Fig. 7 and its Brownian chaotic motions, we can see that the bacteria were moving approximately in one direction. Also, we notice the length of its movement due to a later comparison.

The trajectory of bacteria motion with the first type of music played we can find in Fig. 8.

From the picture in Fig. 8, according to Brownian chaotic motions of these bacterium, we notice that the direction of the motion of the bacteria has changed

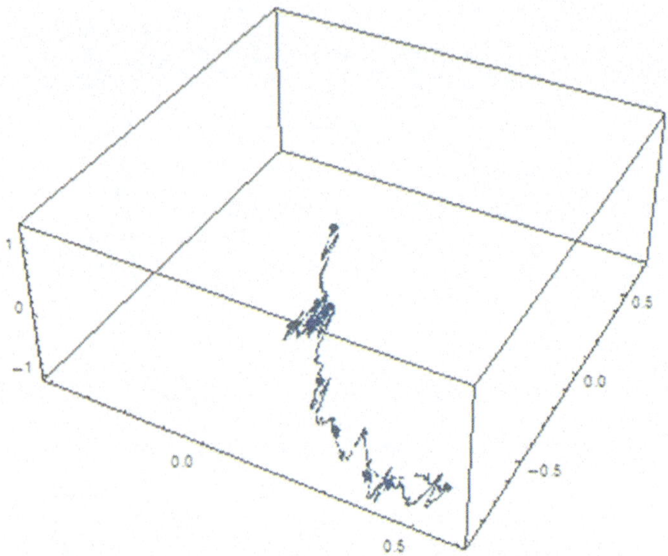

Fig. 7 The trajectory of the first bacterium without the music played on $s_i^{1,1} = 0.3,\ s_i^{1,2} = -0.1,\ s_i^{2,1} = 0.3,\ s_i^{2,2} = -0.1, \quad i = 1, \ldots, 10$

Table 2 Coordinates of the trajectory of motion of the first bacteria, without music on (left three columns) and with the first type of music (right three columns) played

x_i	y_i	z_i	x_i	y_i	z_i
0	0	0	0	0	0
0.1043	−0.3698	−0.2869	−0.1043	0.1849	−0.1882
0.0521	−0.4622	−0.3641	−0.2607	0	−0.1127
0.0521	−0.2773	−0.4809	−0.3649	0.3698	−0.0791
0.0521	−0.2773	−0.7842	−0.3128	0.4623	−0.1107
0.0521	−0.1849	−0.7605	−0.2607	0.2774	−0.0054
0.1564	−0.5547	−0.7709	−0.3128	0.1849	−0.1336
0.2607	−0.7396	−0.7757	−0.2607	0.1849	−0.1031
0.5213	−0.7396	−1.0163	−0.2607	0.1849	−0.0806
0.4170	−0.8320	−0.9330	−0.2607	0.0092	−0.0581
0.3649	−0.8320	−0.9349	−0.3649	0.3698	−0.1685

[5]. Also, we see that the trajectory has shortened, which means that the bacterium has calmed down after some time.

The bacterium motion with the second type of music played is shown in Fig. 9.

From the results given in Fig. 9 we can notice that the bacterium has a more restless movement with a distance of approximately the same as when there was no music on.

Table 3 Coordinates of the trajectory of motion of the first bacteria with the second (left three columns) and third (right three columns) music played on

x_i	y_i	z_i	x_i	y_i	z_i
0	0	0	0	0	0
−0.2085	0.0925	0.1239	0.1042	0.1849	0.0661
0.0521	0	0.0047	0.0521	−0.1849	−0.2426
0	0.0924	0.2852	0.1042	−0.1849	0.1681
0.1042	0.0925	0.4829	0.0521	−0.1849	−0.1278
0.1564	0.3698	0.4766	0.0521	−0.1849	0.0964
0.1564	0.5547	0.2986	0.0521	0.0925	0.2626
0.2606	0.2774	0.6912	0.0521	0.2774	0.4655
0.2085	0.2773	1.1927	0.0521	0.1849	0.4059
0.1564	0.3698	1.3380	0.1042	0.1849	0.3189
0.2606	0.2774	1.2783	0	0.6472	0.1834

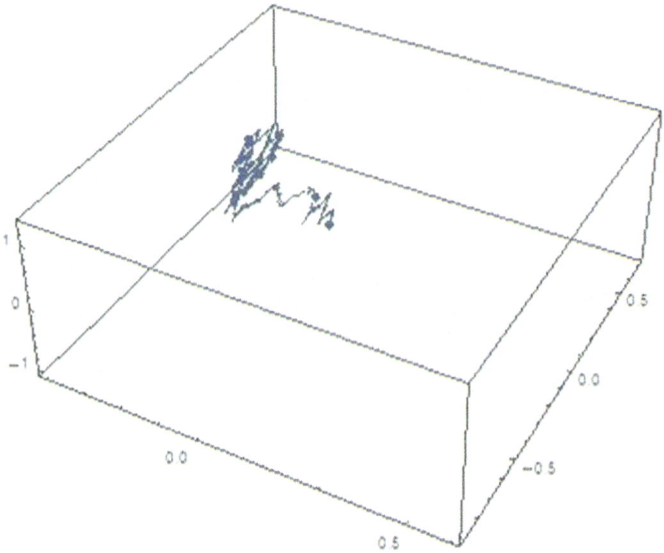

Fig. 8 The trajectory of the first bacterium with the first type of music played on $s_i^{1,1} = 0.3,\ s_i^{1,2} = -0.1,\ s_i^{2,1} = 0.3,\ s_i^{2,2} = -0.1, \quad i = 1, \ldots, 10$

Figure 10 shows the trajectory of the bacterium motion with the third type of music played on.

We notice the bacterium's calmer motion with a slightly shorter distance than without music played.

Finally, we can talk about the influence of the type of music on the motion of this bacterium. The first type of music has a calming effect on this bacterium, while

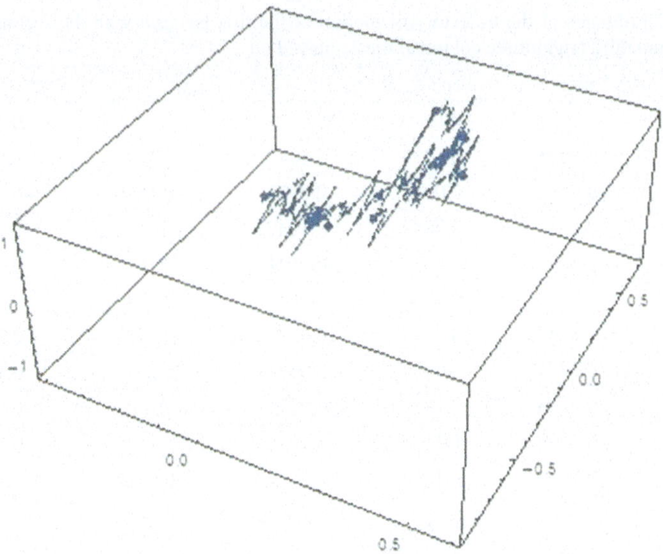

Fig. 9 The trajectory of the first bacterium with the second type of music played on $s_i^{1,1} = 0.3,\ s_i^{1,2} = -0.1,\ s_i^{2,1} = 0.3,\ s_i^{2,2} = -0.1, \quad i = 1, \ldots, 10$

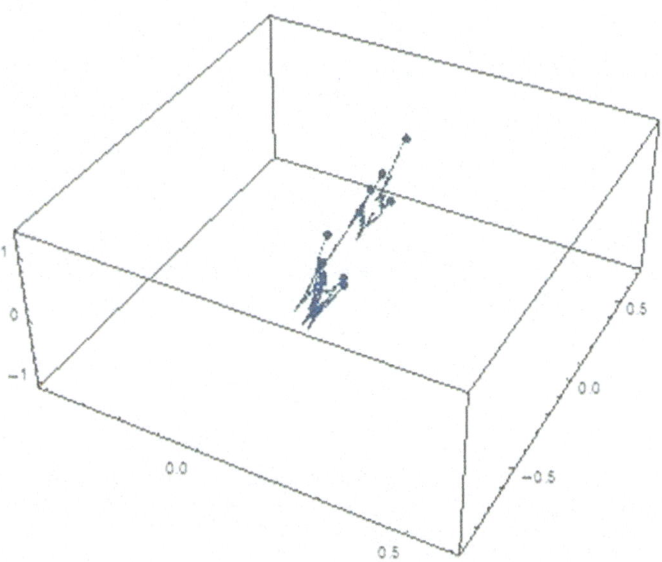

Fig. 10 The trajectory of the first bacterium with the third type of music played $s_i^{1,1} = 0.3,\ s_i^{1,2} = -0.1,\ s_i^{2,1} = 0.3,\ s_i^{2,2} = -0.1, \quad i = 1, \ldots, 10$

the second type disturbs it. The third type of music leads to a similar motion of bacterium, as when there is no music played.

Tables 4 and 5 give the coordinates of the trajectory of the second bacterium without music and with music played. Figure 11 shows the trajectory motion of the second bacterium without music played.

Compared to the motion of the first bacterium, we notice that this bacterium is more mobile and has traveled approximately five times the distance than the first bacterium.

Figure 12 shows the trajectory of the second (faster) bacterium motion with the first type of music played.

Table 4 Coordinates of the trajectory of motion of the second bacteria, without music on (left three columns) and with the first music (right three columns) played

x_i	y_i	z_i	x_i	y_i	z_i
0	0	0	0	0	0
−0.3127	0.4622	0.8545	−0.0521	0.1849	0.5398
−0.6776	−0.4622	1.7845	0.2607	0.7396	0.811
−1.1989	0.5547	2.1152	0.2085	0.5547	0.9604
−0.9383	−0.2773	2.6437	0.2085	0.9245	1.012
−0.9904	0.1849	2.9061	0.1564	0.6471	1.7786
1.0425	0.0092	3.662	0.1043	0.4623	1.9442
0.8862	0.2773	3.4277	0.4171	.4623	2.3245
1.1989	0.4622	3.8249	0.5213	.4623	2.3744
1.0947	0.2773	3.8952	0.5213	1.0169	2.7151
0.8862	0.3698	4.4158	0.5213	1.5716	2.1193

Table 5 Coordinates of the trajectory of motion of the second bacteria with the second type (left three columns) and third type (right three columns) of music played

x_i	y_i	z_i	x_i	y_i	z_i
0	0	0	0	0	0
−0.4692	−0.1849	0.9754	0.3649	0.9245	1.6788
−0.3649	0.5547	1.0555	−0.1042	1.5716	5.1865
−0.3649	0.8320	1.1972	0.3128	2.4037	7.0485
−0.7298	1.1094	2.0168	0.7298	3.3282	7.7127
−0.2085	0.6472	1.7007	0.4171	2.8660	9.6618
−0.2085	1.2018	1.0988	0.4171	2.5886	10.0423
−0.1564	0.8320	1.6857	0.0521	3.3282	10.1865
0.1564	1.0710	2.2625	−0.2606	3.4206	12.0405
0.5734	1.2943	2.6866	0	3.2358	12.7007
0.6255	2.1264	3.3115	−1.0947	3.7904	14.2342

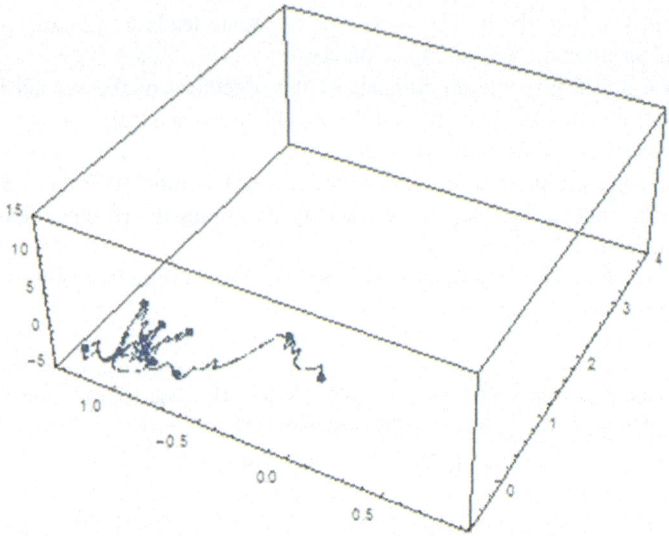

Fig. 11 The trajectory of the second bacterium without the music played $s_i^{1,1} = 0.2$, $s_i^{1,2} = -0.1$, $s_i^{2,1} = 0.1$, $s_i^{2,2} = -0.2$, $i = 1, \ldots, 10$

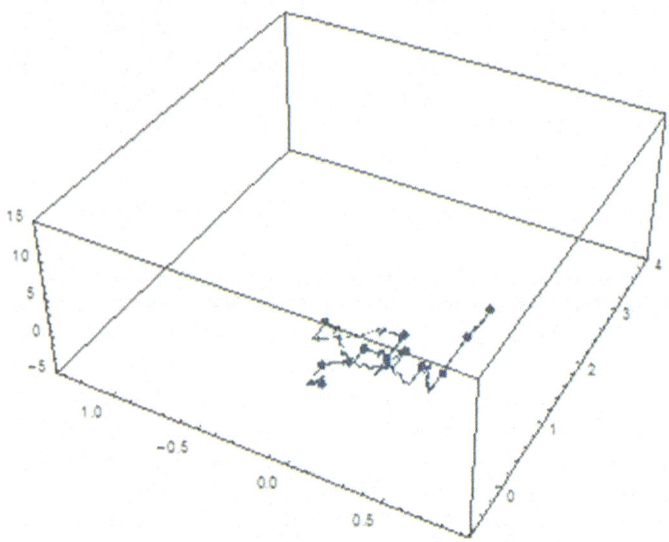

Fig. 12 The trajectory of the second bacterium with the first type of music played $s_i^{1,1} = 0.2$, $s_i^{1,2} = -0.1$, $s_i^{2,1} = 0.1$, $s_i^{2,2} = -0.2$, $i = 1, \ldots, 10$

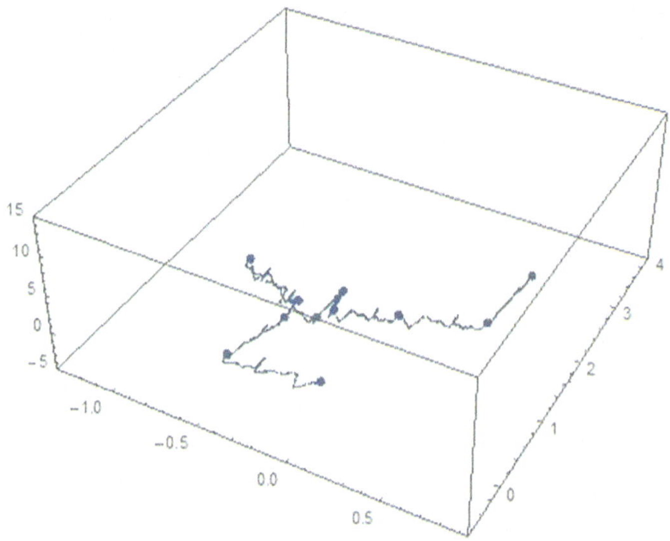

Fig. 13 The trajectory of the second bacterium with the second type of music played $s_i^{1,1} = 0.2$, $s_i^{1,2} = -0.1$, $s_i^{2,1} = 0.1$, $s_i^{2,2} = -0.2$, $i = 1, \ldots, 10$

We notice that the first type of music calms the motion of this fast bacterium. Figure 13 shows the trajectory of motion of second bacterium with the second type of music played.

From Fig. 13, we can notice that the second type of music does not significantly affect the movement of this bacterium.

Figure 14 shows the trajectory of motion of second bacteria with third type music played.

We notice that the third type of music disturbed this bacterium and caused it to move significantly faster with a distance of over ten times longer than when there was no music played.

According to our experiments and results analysis, we developed the original approach to get additional information about bacteria and coronavirus motion. Brownian motion as a creation in nature is recognized as the most similar one. All these results from the field of bacteria and coronavirus are very important tool for different applications in microbiology and clinical analysis in the process to get more information about the trajectories and microorganisms actions.

Future experimental and theoretical work would be in the direction of additional physics analysis, especially Heisenberg principle of indeterminism. This is very important if we asymptotically analyze the similarities between the motion of the living microorganisms and particles in condense matter. All of these penetrate through the biomimetic similarities in nature and generally matter, because many phenomena from the nature could be useful for some dynamic motions explanations

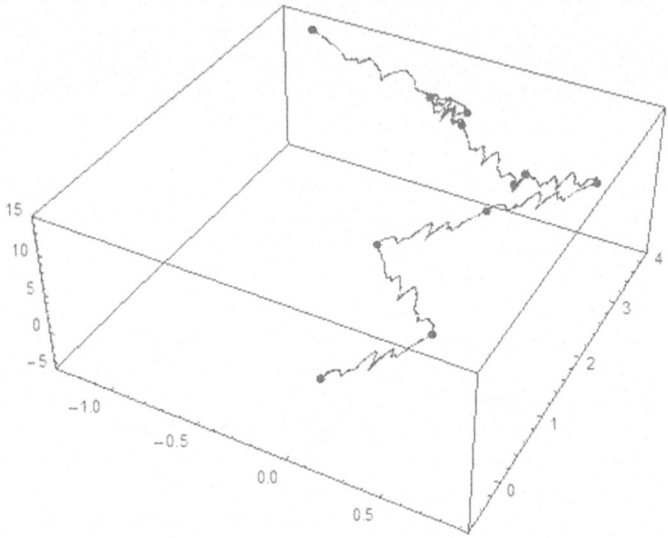

Fig. 14 The trajectory of the second bacterium with the third type of music played $s_i^{1,1} = 0.2,\ s_i^{1,2} = -0.1,\ s_i^{2,1} = 0.1,\ s_i^{2,2} = -0.2,\quad i = 1, \ldots, 10$

within the particles in condensed matter. It is evident that some sources of information and knowledge are biunivocally correspondence to the artificial mathematical points, recognized from the real nature as a fractal nature.

3 Conclusion

With the described research, we have opened a new approach to similar processes between particle motion in matter and microorganism's motion characterized by fractal nature, as just motions in matter like only one exists. Here, we have presented some methods and experimental results to simulate the motion of living microorganisms. According to the experimental results with viruses and bacteria, we were able to recognize their trajectories in two- and three-dimensions and opened a new frontier for understanding and predicting microorganisms in the real Brownian motion nature case. The results of our research can be applied in many scientific fields, such as medicine, microbiology, epidemiology and many others. Nowadays, we must strongly express new needs and intentions to research deeply into the relations between physical systems, generally, matter and biosystems. This is also very important from the biomimetic point of view, for it is a renewed source of inspiration from nature. On the other hand, there is a very important research analysis regarding the eventual existing life of different space bodies. For all of these reasons, the significance of the presented results, which illuminate very interesting directions for application in space research and biophysics in general, cannot be overstated. There is an additional, very significant field where we can use these results in the creation and prevention of potential bioweapon war. All of these results and methods are also very important from the aspect of antiterrorist actions against microbiological terrorism.

Acknowledgements The author gratefully acknowledges the financial support of Ministry for Education, Science and Technological Development of Serbia, and to NSF (The National Science Foundation) North Carolina, USA, for this work.

References

1. Barnsley, M.F.: Fractal functions and interpolation. Constr. Approx. **2**, 303–329 (1986)
2. Barnsley, M.F.: Fractals Everywhere, 2nd edn. Academic, San Diego (1993)
3. Secelean, N.A.: Countable iterated function systems. Far East J. Dyn. Syst. **3**(2), 149–167 (2001)
4. Hutchinson, J.: Fractal and self-similarity. Indiana Univ. J. Math. **30**, 713–747 (1981)
5. Mitic, V., Lazovic, G., Milosevic, D., Lu, C.A., Manojlovic, J., Tsay, S.C., Kruchinin, S., Vlahovic, B.: Brownian motion and fractal structure. Mod. Phys. Lett. B **34**(19&20), 2040061 (2020)
6. Mitic, V., Lazovic, G., Milosevic, D., Ristanovic, E., Tsay, S.C., Milosevic, M., Vlahovic, B.: Brownian fractal nature coronavirus motion. Mod. Phys. Lett. **35**(4), 2150076 (2021)
7. Marvasti, M., Strahle, W.: Fractal geometry analysis of turbulent data. Signal Process. **41**, 191–201 (1995)
8. Mazel, D.S., Hayes, M.H.: Using iterated function systems to model discrete sequences. IEEE Trans. Signal Process. **40**, 1724–1734 (1992)
9. Emoto, M.: The Hidden Messages in Water. Beyond Mind & Pseudoscience (2004)

Graph Theory Approach in Synthetized Diamonds Electrophysical Parameters Defining

Branislav Randjelović, Vojislav V. Mitić, Srdjan Ribar, Maria Čebela, Markus Mohr, Hans-Jörg Fecht, and Branislav Vlahović

Abstract There is an important novelty in biomaterials by innovative potential based on (ultra)nanocrystalline diamonds, what is almost the new result in scientific world, from the Institute of Functional Nanosystems, from Ulm University. The nanosynthetized diamonds are very new frontier application from the area biomedicine. From the other side, there is evident biocompatibility of the diamond layers, selectively improved by biomimetic 3D patterns structuring. From this point of view, graph theory approach is very inspirable new idea, already applied in some other systems, within material sciences, and electronic ceramics. By graphs, we already confirmed, also the first time in material sciences, that we can easily define the parameters values on the microstructure level between the structure constituencies grains and pores. So, now we originally apply all of this on the synthetized diamond structures. This novelty, graph applications, has the great importance in getting the additional ideas and directions for phenomena analysis of electrical and thermal conductivity grow, while electroconductivity goes down and opposite, better understanding. We

B. Randjelović (✉) · V. V. Mitić (Deceased)
Faculty of Electronic Engineering, University of Niš, Niš, Serbia
e-mail: branislav.randjelovic@elfak.ni.ac.rs

B. Randjelović
Faculty of Teachers Education, University of Priština in Kosovska Mitrovica, 38218 Leposavić, Serbia

V. V. Mitić (Deceased)
Institute of Technical Sciences of the Serbian Academy of Science and Arts, Belgrade, Serbia

S. Ribar
Faculty of Mechanical Engineering, University of Belgrade, Belgrade, Serbia

M. Čebela
Institute of Nuclear Science "Vinča", University of Belgrade, Belgrade, Serbia

M. Mohr · H.-J. Fecht
Institute of Functional Nanosystems, Ulm University, Ulm, Germany

B. Vlahović
North Carolina Central University (NCCU), Durham, NC, USA

S. Najman et al. (eds.), *Bioceramics, Biomimetic and Other Compatible Materials Features for Medical Applications*, Engineering Materials,
https://doi.org/10.1007/978-3-031-17269-4_17

already have done some analysis in this field by fractal nature approach, but here we add new methods based on very original graph theory.

Keywords Nanocrystallinity · Synthetized diamonds · Biomaterials · Biomimetics graph theory · Electrophysical parameters

1 Introduction

Materials science is spreading into all areas of fundamental and applied science. One such development, that will probably have the biggest impact on daily life is biomaterials—the development of new substrates for engineering and medicine. The most prominent bio-relevant properties of a biomaterial are chemical inertness and bio-durability, so nanocrystalline diamond is naturally coming into the focus of our attention. Nanocrystalline diamond is an incomparable biomaterial with unusual biocompatible properties, which are not explicable solely on the basis of its chemical and biological inertness. Physical and chemical determinants of biocompatibility, including information of the nanoscopic interfacial water layers can be defined on diamond substrates. Natural diamonds are produced by nature. But variations of synthetic diamond, for instance, nanocrystalline diamond, is biomimetic material. Fabrication of those biomimetic surface layers becomes viable, due to the unique properties of diamond and the possibility to synthesize and deposit homogenous films of nanocrystalline diamond.

1.1 Short Intro with Graph Theory New Frontiers

Many problems in mathematics, computer science, engineering and technics, as well as in nature, easily can be described and modeled using graph theory [1–4]. Graph theory, as one of the simplest and most applied field of mathematics, has special advantage among others—mathematical approach, visualization and visual connection to the problems, easy application of graph algorithms to some new problems, even if they are not closely related to graphs.

If we map some problems and processes from material science field onto graphs, then it would lead to more efficient simulation of those processes. Graph algorithms and graph operations, as well as parallel algorithms for fast calculations on a large data set, that is typical for multigrain models with a huge number of grains, opens a wide range of new possibilities. Matrices are god and very efficient tool for graph operations and for describing graph properties. In [5] we introduced "graph way of thinking" in research of intergranular impedances, using some simple examples and adjacency matrix and incidence matrix. Each grain is mapped into graph vertices. Relation between two grains is represented by edge (line) between two vertices in graph and number of grains in model is equal to the number of vertices in the graph. If there is some relation oer property, there is an edge in graph between corresponding vertices. Relation between pair of grains can be described with some numerical value, and then each edge has its own numerical value.

Having in mind that each interconnection or interaction between elements, will be mapped onto edge in graph, and that each of them can have some numerical value, it would be useful to use so called "weighted" graphs. Weighted graph is graph where each edge has its own numerical characteristic, some "weight". Weight matrix W, of dimensions $n \times n$ too, with elements defined as

$$w_{ij} = \begin{cases} value, & for\, i \neq j\, and\, there\, is\, relation\, between\, vertices \\ 0, & for\, i = j\, or\, for\, i \neq j\, and\, there\, is\, no\, relation\, between\, vertices \end{cases}$$

In [2, 2] we were focused on 1D and 2D planar graphs and in [5] we introduced novel approach, aiming to "granulate", distribute-disperse the grains, by associating graph vertices at the top of the grain and at the bottom of the grain. Vertices were located even in some imaginary points in the middle of a grain, or in the space between grains. v is some electrophysial or electrothermical property.

In previous papers we presented mapping of some simple $2 \times 2 \times 1$ sample, onto 1D graph with 2 vertices, onto 2D graph with four vertices, or onto 3D graph with 8 vertices, and also using some other geometrical shapes or vertices displacement, inside graph, especially in 3D case, we have various shapes (shown in [5]). Some examples of graph shapes are shown in Fig. 1.

Now, we can review that very important results based on 3D graph theory application within the measurements and calculation the values of some thermophysical parameters on microstructural level. Anyhow, this direction and road came over our previous results by implementation graph theory on 1D and 2D cases, which are considering, for example, capacity as the parameter. So, we are coming up to the top of the pyramidal hierarchy structure, with the essence of graph theory applied in electronic, ceramics, materials area.

According to results [3–5], this method of development, we disposed completely new approach for getting much more precise values calculations which are concretely connected with experimental sources. Based on this graph theory and previous research we can dispose one unique reviewed feature, which explains what have we done and what can we do in next steps.

2 Experimental Part

2.1 HFCVD for NCD and C-UNCD Films

Nanocrystalline diamond films (NCD, average grain size 10–100 nm) and conductive ultra-nanocrystalline diamond films (C-UNCD, average grain size about 5 nm) were deposited onto 4″ Si wafers, using hot filament chemical vapor deposition (HFCVD)

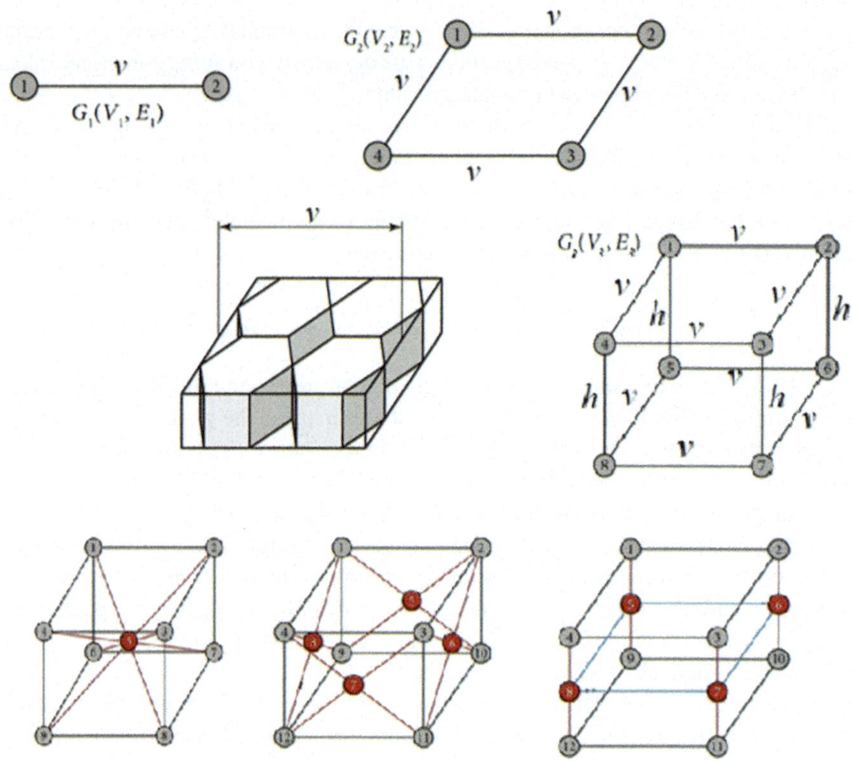

Fig. 1 Varieties of graph representations of 1D, 2D and 3D

process, before that, the Si-wafers were seeded inside a nanocrystalline diamond solution, with a seeding density of 10^{11} cm^{-2} and average seed size of 3–5 nm.

Tungsten was used as filament material, electrically heated up to around 2000 °C. The process gas was a mixture of methane (CH_4) and hydrogen (H_2). The process pressure and filament-current were not varied, while the gas flow ratio between methane and hydrogen was varied from 3 to 6% (sample to I–IV). In general, a higher methane to hydrogen ratio is leading to an increasing electrical conductivity.

Before the seeding and deposition process, the surface of Si wafers was oxidized in a heated oven, in order to build up an insulating thin SiO_2 layer, preventing the influence of wafer's electrical conductivity during the measurement of the diamond films conductivity.

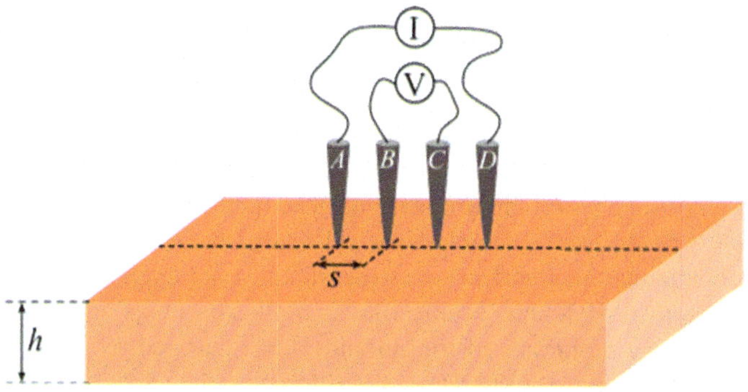

Fig. 2 Principle of four-points resistivity measurement [21]

2.2 Measurement of Film Surface Morphology, Roughness, Average Grain Size and Electrical Conductivity

The surface morphology and roughness of diamond films were captured and measured respectively by SEM (scanning electron microscopy) and AFM (atomic force microscopy). X-ray diffraction (XRD) was used, on the one sides for proofing the existence of diamond crystalline grains in the film, on the other side for evaluating the diamond film's average grain size, considering the FWHM (full width at half maximum) of the diamond (111)-peak by $2\theta = 43.9°$, in Scherrer's equation, using a standard Bragg–Brentano geometry and a Cu $K\alpha$ X-ray source.

The four-point method was applied for the measurement of the diamond films specific electrical conductivity (σ, in S/cm). For this, four sharp probes with identical distance "s" were placed onto the flat surface of the sample, and a current was passed through the two outer electrodes (A and D in Fig. 2), then the floating potential was measured across the inner pair (B and C in Fig. 2). And for an infinitely thin film, which means a small value of "h/s", the film's electrical specific resistivity "ρ" can be approached with following equation, as "h" is the thickness of film [20].

$$\rho = \frac{\pi}{\ln 2} * \frac{U}{I} * h$$

2.3 Samples Grown with Different Ammonia Conditions

The conductive UNCD films serials, were grown using the HFCVD technique by adding NH_3 to the gas mixture of H_2 and CH_4 under controlled deposition parameters. Ammonia was added as a nitrogen containing source to the process gas during the whole 10-h long deposition to enhance the electrical conductivity [26, 27]. The thin films were grown on silicon (100) substrates which were seeded ultrasonically in a nanodiamond solution. The synthetises of n-type conductive UNCD film details were given in [26]. To investigate the influence of NH_3 addition on the electrical conductivity of the UNCD film, samples were grown by introducing different NH_3 fractions ($NH_3/CH_4 + H_2$), ranging from zero up to 5%. More than 5% NH_3 addition completely suppressed the film growth. Scanning electron microscopy (SEM) of the surface of the grown samples was performed using a Zeiss Leo 1540. The roughness of the diamond surfaces was measured in the tapping mode by Atomic Force Microscopy (AFM, Dimension 3100, Digital Instruments) using $10 \times 10\ \mu m^2$ scans. The average grain size of the samples was measured by X-ray diffraction (XRD), using a Siemens D5005 X-ray diffractometer, the (111) diamond peak and the Debye–Scherrer equation.

For precise electrical measurements, conductive diamond thin films (1–2 μm) were grown on insulating substrates (silicon wafers with a thick thermal oxide layer on top). The diamond layer was then structured into rectangular van der Pauw [27] geometries (500 μm × 500 μm), with ohmic metal contacts at each corner. The contact system consists of a multilayer stack of electron beam evaporated Ti (50 nm)/Pt (50 nm)/Au (100 nm) with ohmic behaviour over a large voltage range as well as long term temperature stability.

Regarding measuring the temperature influence on the electrical conductivity and determination different conductive samples activation energies, a special vacuum chamber with an integrated electrical measurement setup was used. This setup allows temperature controlled measurements from room temperature up to 1200 K. High vacuum conditions of about 10^{-6} mbar were used to avoid reactions of the diamond film with oxygen at higher temperatures. Electronic structures of the as-deposited UNCD films were analysed by conducting near edge X-ray absorption fine structure (NEXAFS) experiments at beamline 8–2 of the Stanford Synchrotron Radiation Lightsource (SSRL), SLAC National Accelerator Laboratory. The linearly polarized and focused X-ray beam cross-section was approximately 500 μm in diameter. NEXAFS spectra at the carbon (C) and nitrogen (N) K-edges were recorded at normal incidence via the total electron yield (TEY) mode and normalized to incident X-ray beam intensity (using the I0 current signal generated by a gold grid located upstream in the beamline). The X-ray photon energy was calibrated by the position of the π^* resonance in the carbon K-edge NEXAFS spectrum on freshly cleaved highly oriented pyrolytic graphite (HOPG).

The graphitic carbon fraction (sp^2 hybridization) relative to the total number of carbon atoms in the UNCD samples was estimated by taking the intensity ratio of the π^* resonances to the step-edge at 315 eV with reference to the same ratio of HOPG, recorded close to a magic angle of 55, as a measure of 100% contribution of the graphitic carbon.

3 Experimental Data

For the purpose of our further analysis and implementing the theoretical experiment based on graph theory, we will use some of data from the experiment, presented in [22], with various fractions of NH_3 to the HFCVD process gas. Particulary, we will use values for electrical conductivity, for each of the samples, shown in Table 1.

3.1 Theoretical Experiment Based on Graph Theory Application

If we, theoreticaly, split diamond surface into small particles, we can implement similar approach like with grains in [19]. Let's discuss a infinitely small part of diamond surface, of "dimension" $2 \times 2 \times 1$, shown on Fig. 1. We can detect and assign graph vertices in upper surface of diamond, shown on Fig. 3, then vertices on lower surface of diamond. Additionally, we can assign some vertices in the middle of diamond sample.

Graph is shown on Fig. 4. Using that graph model we can calculate appropriate weight matrix. We can assume some property (any electrical, dielectrically

Table 1 Electrical conductivities for different samples of NH_3 fractions

Sample	1	2	3	4	5	6	7	8	9
% $NH_3/(CH_4 + H_2)$	0	0.1	0.3	0.7	1	1.3	1.6	3.2	5
Electrical conductivity (S/cm)	10^{-6}	1	1	10	1	1	10^{-1}	10^{-3}	10^{-4}

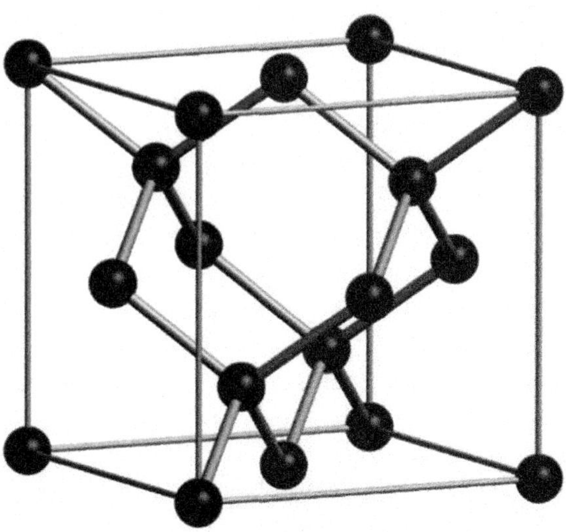

Fig. 3 Diamond internal structure

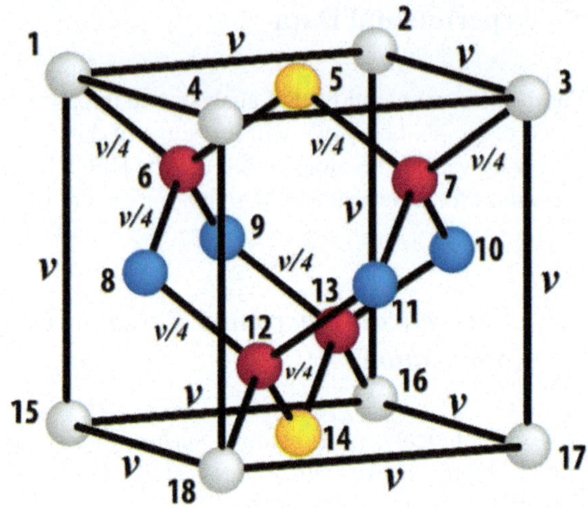

Fig. 4 3D graph model

or magnetic property), noted with v, and we can assign values on those graph edges, so we can represent this graph with weight matrix W.

Graph $G = (V, E)$, has a set of vertices $V = \{1, 2, 3, \ldots, 18\}$ and a set of edges $E = \{\{1, 2\}, \{1, 4\}, \{1, 6\}, \{1, 15\}, \{2, 3\}, \{2, 16\}, \{3, 4\}, \{3, 7\}, \{3, 17\}, \{4, 18\}, \{5, 6\}, \{5, 7\}, \{6, 8\}, \{6, 9\}, \{7, 10\}, \{7, 11\}, \{8, 12\}, \{9, 13\}, \{10, 13\}, \{11, 12\}, \{12, 14\}, \{12, 18\}, \{13, 14\}, \{13, 16\}, \{15, 16\}, \{15, 18\}, \{16, 17\}, \{17, 18\}\}$. Corresponding weight matrix of this graph is:

$$W = \begin{bmatrix}
0 & v & 0 & v & 0 & v/4 & 0 & 0 & 0 & 0 & 0 & 0 & 0 & 0 & v & 0 & 0 & 0 \\
v & 0 & v & 0 & 0 & 0 & 0 & 0 & 0 & 0 & 0 & 0 & 0 & 0 & 0 & v & 0 & 0 \\
0 & v & 0 & v & 0 & 0 & v/4 & 0 & 0 & 0 & 0 & 0 & 0 & 0 & 0 & 0 & v & 0 \\
v & 0 & v & 0 & 0 & 0 & 0 & 0 & 0 & 0 & 0 & 0 & 0 & 0 & 0 & 0 & 0 & v \\
0 & 0 & 0 & 0 & 0 & v/4 & v/4 & 0 & 0 & 0 & 0 & 0 & 0 & 0 & 0 & 0 & 0 & 0 \\
v/4 & 0 & 0 & 0 & v/4 & 0 & 0 & v/4 & v/4 & 0 & 0 & 0 & 0 & 0 & 0 & 0 & 0 & 0 \\
0 & 0 & v/4 & 0 & v/4 & 0 & 0 & 0 & 0 & v/4 & v/4 & 0 & 0 & 0 & 0 & 0 & 0 & 0 \\
0 & 0 & 0 & 0 & 0 & v/4 & 0 & 0 & 0 & 0 & 0 & v/4 & 0 & 0 & 0 & 0 & 0 & 0 \\
0 & 0 & 0 & 0 & 0 & v/4 & 0 & 0 & 0 & 0 & 0 & 0 & v/4 & 0 & 0 & 0 & 0 & 0 \\
0 & 0 & 0 & 0 & 0 & 0 & v/4 & 0 & 0 & 0 & 0 & 0 & v/4 & 0 & 0 & 0 & 0 & 0 \\
0 & 0 & 0 & 0 & 0 & 0 & v/4 & 0 & 0 & 0 & 0 & v/4 & 0 & 0 & 0 & 0 & 0 & 0 \\
0 & 0 & 0 & 0 & 0 & 0 & 0 & v/4 & 0 & 0 & v/4 & 0 & 0 & v/4 & 0 & 0 & 0 & v/4 \\
0 & 0 & 0 & 0 & 0 & 0 & 0 & 0 & v/4 & v/4 & 0 & 0 & 0 & v/4 & 0 & v/4 & 0 & 0 \\
0 & 0 & 0 & 0 & 0 & 0 & 0 & 0 & 0 & 0 & 0 & v/4 & v/4 & 0 & 0 & 0 & 0 & 0 \\
v & 0 & 0 & 0 & 0 & 0 & 0 & 0 & 0 & 0 & 0 & 0 & 0 & 0 & 0 & v & 0 & v \\
0 & v & 0 & 0 & 0 & 0 & 0 & 0 & 0 & 0 & 0 & 0 & v/4 & 0 & v & 0 & v & 0 \\
0 & 0 & v & 0 & 0 & 0 & 0 & 0 & 0 & 0 & 0 & 0 & 0 & 0 & 0 & v & 0 & v \\
0 & 0 & 0 & v & 0 & 0 & 0 & 0 & 0 & 0 & 0 & v/4 & 0 & 0 & v & 0 & v & 0
\end{bmatrix}$$

Each "horizontal" edge of this graph has weight v, direct "vertical" edge also has weight v, and "skew" edges, through structure has weight $v/4$. Why divided with 4? Because in this model every algebraic path through this graph, starting from upper surface down to lower surface, consist of 4 edges, length of algebraic path is 4.

4 Results and Discussion

If we take some particular case of electrical conductivity from Table 1, for example Sample A and appropriate electrical conductivity $1 * 10^{-6}$ S/cm, our graph, modelled and shaped like in Fig. 4, has set of 18 vertices and 28 edges. Corresponding weight matrix of this graph is:

$$W_A = \begin{bmatrix}
0 & 1 & 0 & 1 & 0 & 0.25 & 0 & 0 & 0 & 0 & 0 & 0 & 0 & 0 & 1 & 0 & 0 & 0 \\
1 & 0 & 1 & 0 & 0 & 0 & 0 & 0 & 0 & 0 & 0 & 0 & 0 & 0 & 0 & 1 & 0 & 0 \\
0 & 1 & 0 & 1 & 0 & 0 & 0.25 & 0 & 0 & 0 & 0 & 0 & 0 & 0 & 0 & 0 & 1 & 0 \\
1 & 0 & 1 & 0 & 0 & 0 & 0 & 0 & 0 & 0 & 0 & 0 & 0 & 0 & 0 & 0 & 0 & 1 \\
0 & 0 & 0 & 0 & 0 & 0.25 & 0.25 & 0 & 0 & 0 & 0 & 0 & 0 & 0 & 0 & 0 & 0 & 0 \\
0.25 & 0 & 0 & 0 & 0.25 & 0 & 0 & 0.25 & 0.25 & 0 & 0 & 0 & 0 & 0 & 0 & 0 & 0 & 0 \\
0 & 0 & 0.25 & 0 & 0.25 & 0 & 0 & 0 & 0 & 0.25 & 0.25 & 0 & 0 & 0 & 0 & 0 & 0 & 0 \\
0 & 0 & 0 & 0 & 0 & 0.25 & 0 & 0 & 0 & 0 & 0 & 0.25 & 0 & 0 & 0 & 0 & 0 & 0 \\
0 & 0 & 0 & 0 & 0 & 0.25 & 0 & 0 & 0 & 0 & 0 & 0 & 0.25 & 0 & 0 & 0 & 0 & 0 \\
0 & 0 & 0 & 0 & 0 & 0 & 0.25 & 0 & 0 & 0 & 0 & 0 & 0.25 & 0 & 0 & 0 & 0 & 0 \\
0 & 0 & 0 & 0 & 0 & 0 & 0.25 & 0 & 0 & 0 & 0 & 0.25 & 0 & 0 & 0 & 0 & 0 & 0 \\
0 & 0 & 0 & 0 & 0 & 0 & 0 & 0.25 & 0 & 0 & 0.25 & 0 & 0 & 0.25 & 0 & 0 & 0 & 0.25 \\
0 & 0 & 0 & 0 & 0 & 0 & 0 & 0 & 0.25 & 0.25 & 0 & 0 & 0 & 0.25 & 0 & 0.25 & 0 & 0 \\
0 & 0 & 0 & 0 & 0 & 0 & 0 & 0 & 0 & 0 & 0 & 0.25 & 0.25 & 0 & 0 & 0 & 0 & 0 \\
1 & 0 & 0 & 0 & 0 & 0 & 0 & 0 & 0 & 0 & 0 & 0 & 0 & 0 & 0 & 1 & 0 & 1 \\
0 & 1 & 0 & 0 & 0 & 0 & 0 & 0 & 0 & 0 & 0 & 0 & 0.25 & 0 & 1 & 0 & 1 & 0 \\
0 & 0 & 1 & 0 & 0 & 0 & 0 & 0 & 0 & 0 & 0 & 0 & 0 & 0 & 0 & 1 & 0 & 1 \\
0 & 0 & 0 & 1 & 0 & 0 & 0 & 0 & 0 & 0 & 0 & 0.25 & 0 & 0 & 1 & 0 & 1 & 0
\end{bmatrix} \cdot 10^{-6}$$

Similar calculation and appropriate graph model we can obtain and calculate for each particular set of data from Table 1, even with other experimental data.

If we take sample B or C or E or F, with electrical conductivity 1.00 S/cm, our graph, modelled and shaped like in Fig. 4, with 18 vertices and 28 edges have corresponding weight matrix:

$$W_B = \begin{bmatrix} 0 & 1.0 & 0 & 1.0 & 0 & 0.25 & 0 & 0 & 0 & 0 & 0 & 0 & 0 & 0 & 1.0 & 0 & 0 & 0 \\ 1.0 & 0 & 1.0 & 0 & 0 & 0 & 0 & 0 & 0 & 0 & 0 & 0 & 0 & 0 & 0 & 1.0 & 0 & 0 \\ 0 & 1.0 & 0 & 1.0 & 0 & 0 & 0.25 & 0 & 0 & 0 & 0 & 0 & 0 & 0 & 0 & 0 & 1.0 & 0 \\ 1.0 & 0 & 1.0 & 0 & 0 & 0 & 0 & 0 & 0 & 0 & 0 & 0 & 0 & 0 & 0 & 0 & 0 & 1.0 \\ 0 & 0 & 0 & 0 & 0 & 0.25 & 0.25 & 0 & 0 & 0 & 0 & 0 & 0 & 0 & 0 & 0 & 0 & 0 \\ 0.25 & 0 & 0 & 0 & 0.25 & 0 & 0 & 0.25 & 0.25 & 0 & 0 & 0 & 0 & 0 & 0 & 0 & 0 & 0 \\ 0 & 0 & 0.25 & 0 & 0.25 & 0 & 0 & 0 & 0 & 0.25 & 0.25 & 0 & 0 & 0 & 0 & 0 & 0 & 0 \\ 0 & 0 & 0 & 0 & 0 & 0.25 & 0 & 0 & 0 & 0 & 0 & 0.25 & 0 & 0 & 0 & 0 & 0 & 0 \\ 0 & 0 & 0 & 0 & 0 & 0.25 & 0 & 0 & 0 & 0 & 0 & 0 & 0.25 & 0 & 0 & 0 & 0 & 0 \\ 0 & 0 & 0 & 0 & 0 & 0 & 0.25 & 0 & 0 & 0 & 0 & 0 & 0.25 & 0 & 0 & 0 & 0 & 0 \\ 0 & 0 & 0 & 0 & 0 & 0 & 0.25 & 0 & 0 & 0 & 0 & 0.25 & 0 & 0 & 0 & 0 & 0 & 0 \\ 0 & 0 & 0 & 0 & 0 & 0 & 0 & 0.25 & 0 & 0 & 0.25 & 0 & 0 & 0.25 & 0 & 0 & 0 & 0.25 \\ 0 & 0 & 0 & 0 & 0 & 0 & 0 & 0 & 0.25 & 0.25 & 0 & 0 & 0 & 0.25 & 0 & 0.25 & 0 & 0 \\ 0 & 0 & 0 & 0 & 0 & 0 & 0 & 0 & 0 & 0 & 0 & 0.25 & 0.25 & 0 & 0 & 0 & 0 & 0 \\ 1.0 & 0 & 0 & 0 & 0 & 0 & 0 & 0 & 0 & 0 & 0 & 0 & 0 & 0 & 0 & 1.0 & 0 & 1.0 \\ 0 & 1.0 & 0 & 0 & 0 & 0 & 0 & 0 & 0 & 0 & 0 & 0 & 0.25 & 0 & 1.0 & 0 & 1.0 & 0 \\ 0 & 0 & 1.0 & 0 & 0 & 0 & 0 & 0 & 0 & 0 & 0 & 0 & 0 & 0 & 0 & 1.0 & 0 & 1.0 \\ 0 & 0 & 0 & 1.0 & 0 & 0 & 0 & 0 & 0 & 0 & 0 & 0.25 & 0 & 0 & 1.0 & 0 & 1.0 & 0 \end{bmatrix}$$

If we take case of Sample D and appropriate electrical conductivity $1 * 10^1$ S/cm, our graph, modelled and shaped like in Fig. 4, has set of 18 vertices and 28 edges. Corresponding weight matrix of this graph is:

$$W_D = \begin{bmatrix} 0 & 10 & 0 & 10 & 0 & 2.5 & 0 & 0 & 0 & 0 & 0 & 0 & 0 & 0 & 10 & 0 & 0 & 0 \\ 10 & 0 & 10 & 0 & 0 & 0 & 0 & 0 & 0 & 0 & 0 & 0 & 0 & 0 & 0 & 10 & 0 & 0 \\ 0 & 10 & 0 & 10 & 0 & 0 & 2.5 & 0 & 0 & 0 & 0 & 0 & 0 & 0 & 0 & 0 & 10 & 0 \\ 10 & 0 & 10 & 0 & 0 & 0 & 0 & 0 & 0 & 0 & 0 & 0 & 0 & 0 & 0 & 0 & 0 & 10 \\ 0 & 0 & 0 & 0 & 0 & 2.5 & 2.5 & 0 & 0 & 0 & 0 & 0 & 0 & 0 & 0 & 0 & 0 & 0 \\ 2.5 & 0 & 0 & 0 & 2.5 & 0 & 0 & 2.5 & 2.5 & 0 & 0 & 0 & 0 & 0 & 0 & 0 & 0 & 0 \\ 0 & 0 & 2.5 & 0 & 2.5 & 0 & 0 & 0 & 0 & 2.5 & 2.5 & 0 & 0 & 0 & 0 & 0 & 0 & 0 \\ 0 & 0 & 0 & 0 & 0 & 2.5 & 0 & 0 & 0 & 0 & 0 & 2.5 & 0 & 0 & 0 & 0 & 0 & 0 \\ 0 & 0 & 0 & 0 & 0 & 2.5 & 0 & 0 & 0 & 0 & 0 & 0 & 2.5 & 0 & 0 & 0 & 0 & 0 \\ 0 & 0 & 0 & 0 & 0 & 0 & 2.5 & 0 & 0 & 0 & 0 & 0 & 2.5 & 0 & 0 & 0 & 0 & 0 \\ 0 & 0 & 0 & 0 & 0 & 0 & 2.5 & 0 & 0 & 0 & 0 & 2.5 & 0 & 0 & 0 & 0 & 0 & 0 \\ 0 & 0 & 0 & 0 & 0 & 0 & 0 & 2.5 & 0 & 0 & 2.5 & 0 & 0 & 2.5 & 0 & 0 & 0 & 2.5 \\ 0 & 0 & 0 & 0 & 0 & 0 & 0 & 0 & 2.5 & 2.5 & 0 & 0 & 0 & 2.5 & 0 & 2.5 & 0 & 0 \\ 0 & 0 & 0 & 0 & 0 & 0 & 0 & 0 & 0 & 0 & 0 & 2.5 & 2.5 & 0 & 0 & 0 & 0 & 0 \\ 10 & 0 & 0 & 0 & 0 & 0 & 0 & 0 & 0 & 0 & 0 & 0 & 0 & 0 & 0 & 10 & 0 & 10 \\ 0 & 10 & 0 & 0 & 0 & 0 & 0 & 0 & 0 & 0 & 0 & 0 & 2.5 & 0 & 10 & 0 & 10 & 0 \\ 0 & 0 & 10 & 0 & 0 & 0 & 0 & 0 & 0 & 0 & 0 & 0 & 0 & 0 & 0 & 10 & 0 & 10 \\ 0 & 0 & 0 & 10 & 0 & 0 & 0 & 0 & 0 & 0 & 0 & 2.5 & 0 & 0 & 10 & 0 & 10 & 0 \end{bmatrix}$$

If we take sample G and appropriate electrical conductivity $1 * 10^{-1}$ S/cm, our graph, modelled and shaped like in Fig. 4, has set of 18 vertices and 28 edges. Corresponding weight matrix of this graph is:

$$W_G = \begin{bmatrix}
0 & 0.1 & 0 & 0.1 & 0 & 0.025 & 0 & 0 & 0 & 0 & 0 & 0 & 0 & 0 & 0.1 & 0 & 0 & 0 \\
0.1 & 0 & 0.1 & 0 & 0 & 0 & 0 & 0 & 0 & 0 & 0 & 0 & 0 & 0 & 0 & 0.1 & 0 & 0 \\
0 & 0.1 & 0 & 0.1 & 0 & 0 & 0.025 & 0 & 0 & 0 & 0 & 0 & 0 & 0 & 0 & 0 & 0.1 & 0 \\
0.1 & 0 & 0.1 & 0 & 0 & 0 & 0 & 0 & 0 & 0 & 0 & 0 & 0 & 0 & 0 & 0 & 0 & 0.1 \\
0 & 0 & 0 & 0 & 0 & 0.025 & 0.025 & 0 & 0 & 0 & 0 & 0 & 0 & 0 & 0 & 0 & 0 & 0 \\
0.025 & 0 & 0 & 0 & 0.025 & 0 & 0 & 0.025 & 0.025 & 0 & 0 & 0 & 0 & 0 & 0 & 0 & 0 & 0 \\
0 & 0 & 0.025 & 0 & 0.025 & 0 & 0 & 0 & 0 & 0.025 & 0.025 & 0 & 0 & 0 & 0 & 0 & 0 & 0 \\
0 & 0 & 0 & 0 & 0 & 0.025 & 0 & 0 & 0 & 0 & 0 & 0.025 & 0 & 0 & 0 & 0 & 0 & 0 \\
0 & 0 & 0 & 0 & 0 & 0.025 & 0 & 0 & 0 & 0 & 0 & 0 & 0.025 & 0 & 0 & 0 & 0 & 0 \\
0 & 0 & 0 & 0 & 0 & 0 & 0.025 & 0 & 0 & 0 & 0 & 0 & 0.025 & 0 & 0 & 0 & 0 & 0 \\
0 & 0 & 0 & 0 & 0 & 0 & 0.025 & 0 & 0 & 0 & 0 & 0.025 & 0 & 0 & 0 & 0 & 0 & 0 \\
0 & 0 & 0 & 0 & 0 & 0 & 0 & 0.025 & 0 & 0 & 0.025 & 0 & 0 & 0.025 & 0 & 0 & 0 & 0.025 \\
0 & 0 & 0 & 0 & 0 & 0 & 0 & 0 & 0.025 & 0.025 & 0 & 0 & 0 & 0.025 & 0 & 0.025 & 0 & 0 \\
0 & 0 & 0 & 0 & 0 & 0 & 0 & 0 & 0 & 0 & 0 & 0.025 & 0.025 & 0 & 0 & 0 & 0 & 0 \\
0.1 & 0 & 0 & 0 & 0 & 0 & 0 & 0 & 0 & 0 & 0 & 0 & 0 & 0 & 0 & 0.1 & 0 & 0.1 \\
0 & 0.1 & 0 & 0 & 0 & 0 & 0 & 0 & 0 & 0 & 0 & 0 & 0.025 & 0 & 0.1 & 0 & 0.1 & 0 \\
0 & 0 & 0.1 & 0 & 0 & 0 & 0 & 0 & 0 & 0 & 0 & 0 & 0 & 0 & 0 & 0.1 & 0 & 0.1 \\
0 & 0 & 0 & 0.1 & 0 & 0 & 0 & 0 & 0 & 0 & 0 & 0.025 & 0 & 0 & 0.1 & 0 & 0.1 & 0
\end{bmatrix}$$

If we take sample H, with electrical conductivity from Table 1 1 * 10^{-3} S/cm, our graph, modelled and shaped like in Fig. 4, has set of 18 vertices and 28 edges. Corresponding weight matrix of this graph is:

$$W_H = \begin{bmatrix}
0 & 1.0 & 0 & 1.0 & 0 & 0.25 & 0 & 0 & 0 & 0 & 0 & 0 & 0 & 0 & 1.0 & 0 & 0 & 0 \\
1.0 & 0 & 1.0 & 0 & 0 & 0 & 0 & 0 & 0 & 0 & 0 & 0 & 0 & 0 & 0 & 1.0 & 0 & 0 \\
0 & 1.0 & 0 & 1.0 & 0 & 0 & 0.25 & 0 & 0 & 0 & 0 & 0 & 0 & 0 & 0 & 0 & 1.0 & 0 \\
1.0 & 0 & 1.0 & 0 & 0 & 0 & 0 & 0 & 0 & 0 & 0 & 0 & 0 & 0 & 0 & 0 & 0 & 1.0 \\
0 & 0 & 0 & 0 & 0 & 0.25 & 0.25 & 0 & 0 & 0 & 0 & 0 & 0 & 0 & 0 & 0 & 0 & 0 \\
0.25 & 0 & 0 & 0 & 0.25 & 0 & 0 & 0.25 & 0.25 & 0 & 0 & 0 & 0 & 0 & 0 & 0 & 0 & 0 \\
0 & 0 & 0.25 & 0 & 0.25 & 0 & 0 & 0 & 0 & 0.25 & 0.25 & 0 & 0 & 0 & 0 & 0 & 0 & 0 \\
0 & 0 & 0 & 0 & 0 & 0.25 & 0 & 0 & 0 & 0 & 0 & 0.25 & 0 & 0 & 0 & 0 & 0 & 0 \\
0 & 0 & 0 & 0 & 0 & 0.25 & 0 & 0 & 0 & 0 & 0 & 0 & 0.25 & 0 & 0 & 0 & 0 & 0 \\
0 & 0 & 0 & 0 & 0 & 0 & 0.25 & 0 & 0 & 0 & 0 & 0 & 0.25 & 0 & 0 & 0 & 0 & 0 \\
0 & 0 & 0 & 0 & 0 & 0 & 0.25 & 0 & 0 & 0 & 0 & 0.25 & 0 & 0 & 0 & 0 & 0 & 0 \\
0 & 0 & 0 & 0 & 0 & 0 & 0 & 0.25 & 0 & 0 & 0.25 & 0 & 0 & 0.25 & 0 & 0 & 0 & 0.25 \\
0 & 0 & 0 & 0 & 0 & 0 & 0 & 0 & 0.25 & 0.25 & 0 & 0 & 0 & 0.25 & 0 & 0.25 & 0 & 0 \\
0 & 0 & 0 & 0 & 0 & 0 & 0 & 0 & 0 & 0 & 0 & 0.25 & 0.25 & 0 & 0 & 0 & 0 & 0 \\
1.0 & 0 & 0 & 0 & 0 & 0 & 0 & 0 & 0 & 0 & 0 & 0 & 0 & 0 & 0 & 1.0 & 0 & 1.0 \\
0 & 1.0 & 0 & 0 & 0 & 0 & 0 & 0 & 0 & 0 & 0 & 0 & 0.25 & 0 & 1.0 & 0 & 1.0 & 0 \\
0 & 0 & 1.0 & 0 & 0 & 0 & 0 & 0 & 0 & 0 & 0 & 0 & 0 & 0 & 0 & 1.0 & 0 & 1.0 \\
0 & 0 & 0 & 1.0 & 0 & 0 & 0 & 0 & 0 & 0 & 0 & 0.25 & 0 & 0 & 1.0 & 0 & 1.0 & 0
\end{bmatrix} \cdot 10^{-3}$$

If we take sample I, with electrical conductivity from Table 1 1 * 10^{-4} S/cm, our graph, modelled and shaped like in Fig. 4, has set of 18 vertices and 28 edges. Corresponding weight matrix of this graph is:

$$
W_I = \begin{bmatrix}
0 & 1.0 & 0 & 1.0 & 0 & 0.25 & 0 & 0 & 0 & 0 & 0 & 0 & 0 & 0 & 1.0 & 0 & 0 & 0 \\
1.0 & 0 & 1.0 & 0 & 0 & 0 & 0 & 0 & 0 & 0 & 0 & 0 & 0 & 0 & 0 & 1.0 & 0 & 0 \\
0 & 1.0 & 0 & 1.0 & 0 & 0 & 0.25 & 0 & 0 & 0 & 0 & 0 & 0 & 0 & 0 & 0 & 1.0 & 0 \\
1.0 & 0 & 1.0 & 0 & 0 & 0 & 0 & 0 & 0 & 0 & 0 & 0 & 0 & 0 & 0 & 0 & 0 & 1.0 \\
0 & 0 & 0 & 0 & 0 & 0.25 & 0.25 & 0 & 0 & 0 & 0 & 0 & 0 & 0 & 0 & 0 & 0 & 0 \\
0.25 & 0 & 0 & 0 & 0.25 & 0 & 0 & 0.25 & 0.25 & 0 & 0 & 0 & 0 & 0 & 0 & 0 & 0 & 0 \\
0 & 0 & 0.25 & 0 & 0.25 & 0 & 0 & 0 & 0 & 0.25 & 0.25 & 0 & 0 & 0 & 0 & 0 & 0 & 0 \\
0 & 0 & 0 & 0 & 0 & 0.25 & 0 & 0 & 0 & 0 & 0 & 0.25 & 0 & 0 & 0 & 0 & 0 & 0 \\
0 & 0 & 0 & 0 & 0 & 0.25 & 0 & 0 & 0 & 0 & 0 & 0 & 0.25 & 0 & 0 & 0 & 0 & 0 \\
0 & 0 & 0 & 0 & 0 & 0 & 0.25 & 0 & 0 & 0 & 0 & 0 & 0.25 & 0 & 0 & 0 & 0 & 0 \\
0 & 0 & 0 & 0 & 0 & 0 & 0.25 & 0 & 0 & 0 & 0 & 0.25 & 0 & 0 & 0 & 0 & 0 & 0 \\
0 & 0 & 0 & 0 & 0 & 0 & 0 & 0.25 & 0 & 0 & 0.25 & 0 & 0 & 0.25 & 0 & 0 & 0 & 0.25 \\
0 & 0 & 0 & 0 & 0 & 0 & 0 & 0 & 0.25 & 0.25 & 0 & 0 & 0 & 0.25 & 0 & 0.25 & 0 & 0 \\
0 & 0 & 0 & 0 & 0 & 0 & 0 & 0 & 0 & 0 & 0 & 0.25 & 0.25 & 0 & 0 & 0 & 0 & 0 \\
1.0 & 0 & 0 & 0 & 0 & 0 & 0 & 0 & 0 & 0 & 0 & 0 & 0 & 0 & 0 & 1.0 & 0 & 1.0 \\
0 & 1.0 & 0 & 0 & 0 & 0 & 0 & 0 & 0 & 0 & 0 & 0 & 0.25 & 0 & 1.0 & 0 & 1.0 & 0 \\
0 & 0 & 1.0 & 0 & 0 & 0 & 0 & 0 & 0 & 0 & 0 & 0 & 0 & 0 & 0 & 1.0 & 0 & 1.0 \\
0 & 0 & 0 & 1.0 & 0 & 0 & 0 & 0 & 0 & 0 & 0 & 0.25 & 0 & 0 & 1.0 & 0 & 1.0 & 0
\end{bmatrix} \cdot 10^{-4}
$$

5 Outlook

In future research we plan to continue with graph theory with thermal conductivity and connect the whole overview with electroconductivity in synthetized diamonds. Also, we will develop the concept of graph approach on fractal relation of fractalised the grains as vertices in direction of graph fractal electronics.

6 Conclusion

The ultra-nanocrystalline synthetized diamonds are very advanced materials for biomedical and other applications. In this chapter we present an overview of complex relation between graph theory and electrophysical parameters of the consolidated nano-diamonds. We performed and explained related experimental procedure with results data. The micrographs, based on the samples forming process are important for open doors in implementation of graphs. This novelty, graph applications, has the great importance in getting the additional ideas and directions for phenomena analysis of thermal conductivity grow, while electroconductivity goes down and opposite, better understanding.

By this method we provided way for defining the electrophysical parameters on micro and nano level of grains and pores, what is important for further designing microelectronic structures and advance miniaturization.

Acknowledgements This study was funded by Serbian Ministry of Education, Science, and Technological Development, under grants TR-32012, III-43007.

References

1. Mitić, V.V., Lazović, G., Randjelović, B., Paunović, V., Wu, J.M., Mancić, D.. Hwu, J.R.: Fractal microeletronic frontiers and graph theory applications. In: International Conference on MS&T 2019, Portland, USA, September 29–October 03 (2019)
2. Mitić, V.V., Lazović, G., Randjelović, B., Paunović, V., Radovic, I., Stajcic, A., Vlahovic, B.: Graph theory applied to microelectronic intergranular relations. Ferroelectrics **570** (2021)
3. Randjelovic, B., Mitic, V.V., Ribar, S., Radovic, I., Stajcic, A., Novakovic, I., Vlahovic, B.: Ceramics, materials, microelectronics and graph theory new frontiers. Modern Phys. Lett. B **34**(34), 2150159 (2020)
4. Randjelovic, B., Mitic, V.V., Ilic, I., Ribar, S., Stajcic, A., Fecht, H., Vlahovic, B.: 3D-graph approach for breakdown voltage calculation on $BaTiO_3$-ceramics. Int. J. of Modern Phys. B **35**(6), 2150103 (2021)
5. Randjelović, B., Nikolić, Z.: Graph theory applied to modeling and simulation of microstructure evolution in sintering. In: Mitić, V., Mančić, L., Obradović, N. (eds.) Advanced Ceramics and Applications VIII: New Frontiers in Multifunctional Material Science and Processing, Invited Lecture, Book of Abstracts, Belgrade, Serbian Ceramic Society, 23–25 September 2019, p 38 (2019)
6. Mitic, V.V., Lazovic, G., Paunovic, V., Cvetkovic, N., Veljkovic, S., Randjelovic, B., Vlahovic, B.: Fractal frontiers in microelectronic ceramic materials. Ceram. Int. **45**(7), Part B, 9679–9685 (2019)
7. Mitic, V.V., Lazovic, G., Paunovic, V., Veljkovic, S., Randjelovic, B., Vlahovic, B., Fecht, H.: Electronic ceramics fractal microstructure analysis—Minkowski Hull and grain boundaries. Ferroelectrics **545**(1), 184–194 (2019)
8. Mitic, V.V., Ribar, S., Randjelovic, B., Lu, C.-A., Radovic, I., Stajcic, A., Novakovic, I., Vlahovic, B.: Neural networks and microelectronic parameters distribution measurements depending on sinthering temperature and applied voltage. Modern Phys. Lett. B **34**(35), 2150172 (2020)
9. Mitic, V.V., Kocic, Lj.M., Tidrow, S., Fecht, H.J.: Structures, fractals and energy. In: Raj, B., Van de Vorde, M., Mahajan, Y. (eds.) Nanotechnology for Energy Sustainability, vol. 2. Wiley-VCH Verlag GmbH & Co. KGaA, Germany (2017)
10. Al-Allak, M., et al.: Effect of donor-dopant concentration on the room temperature resistivity of $BaTiO_3$ ceramics with positive temperature coefficients of resistance. J. Phys. D Appl. Phys. **21**(7), 1226 (1988)
11. Daniels, J., Hardtl, K.H., Wernicke, R.: The PTC effect of barium titanate. Philips Tech. Rev. **38**(3), 73 (1978/79)
12. Hari, N.S., Padmini, P., Kutty, T.R.N.: Complex impedance analyses of n-$BaTiO_3$ ceramics showing positive temperature coefficient of resistance. J. Mater. Sci. Mater. Electron. **8**, 15–22 (1997)
13. Heywang, W.: Bariumtitanat als Sperrschich-thalbleiter. Solid State Electr. **3**(1), 51 (1961)
14. Heywang, W.: Semiconducting barium titanate. J. Mater. Sci. **6**(9), 1214 (1971)
15. Singh, M., Yadav, B.C., Ranjan, A., Kaur, M., Gupta, S.K.: Synthesis and characterization of perovskite barium titanate thin film and its application as LPG sensor. Sens. Actuators BL Chem. **241**, 1170–1178 (2017)
16. Vosika, Z.B., Mitić, V.V., Lazović, G.M., Kocić, Lj.: Discrete temperature values in the sintering process as a $BaTiO_3$-ceramics properties parameter. Sci. Sintering **49**, 469–477 (2017)
17. Clark, A.E., Restorff, J.B., Wun-Fogle, M., Lograsso, T.A., Schlagel, D.L.: Magnetostrictive properties of body-centered cubic Fe-Ga and Fe-Ga-Al alloys. IEEE Trans. Magn. **36**(5), 3238–3240 (2000)
18. Amos, R., Rarity, J., Tapster, P., Shepherd, T., Kitson, S.: Fabrication of large-area face-centered-cubic hard-sphere colloidal crystals by shear alignment. Phys. Rev. E **61**(3), 2929–2935 (2000)

19. Randjelovic, B., Nikolic, Z.: A mathematical model for simulation of intergranular μ-capacitance as a function of neck growth in ceramic sintering. In: Daras, N., Rassias, T. (eds.) Computational Mathematics and Variational Analysis, Springer Optimization and Its Applications, vol. 159, pp. 403–420. Springer (2020)
20. Valdes, L.: Resistivity measurements on germanium for transistors. Proc. IRE **42**, 420–427 (1954)
21. Mohr, M.: Neuartige nanostrukturierte Diamantschichten mit optimierten mechanischen, elektrischen und thermischen Eigenschaften. Diss. Universität Ulm (2017)
22. Wiora, N., Mertens, M., Brühne, K., Fecht, H.-J., Tran, I. C., Willey, T., van Buuren, A., Biener, J., Lee, J.-S.: Grain boundary dominated electrical conductivity in ultrananocrystalline diamond. J. Appl. Phys. **122**, 145102 (2017)
23. Mitic, V.V., Fecht, H.-J., Mohr, M., Lazovic, G., Kocic, Lj.: Exploring fractality of microcrystalline diamond films. AIP Adv. **8**, 075024 (2018). https://doi.org/10.1063/1.5034469
24. Ilić, I.: Weak convergence of product of sums of independent variables with missing values. FILOMAT **24**(3), 73/81 (2010)
25. Ilić, I., Veličković, V.M.: Simple tail index estimation for dependent and heterogeneous data with missing values. Braz. J. Prob. Stat. **33**(1), 192–203 (2019)
26. Mertens, M., Mohr, M., Wiora, N., Bruehne, K. and Fecht, H.-J.: N-type conductive ultrananocrystaline diamond films grown by hot filament CVD. J. Nanomater. 527025 (2015)
27. Wiora, M., Bruehne, K., Floter, A., Gluche, P., Willey, T.M., Kucheyev, S.O., Van Buuren, A.W., Hamza, A.V., Biener, J., Fecht, H.-J.: Grain size dependent mechanical properties of nanocrystalline diamond films grown by hot-filament CVD. Diam. Relat. Mater. **18**, 927–930 (2009)

Neural Networks from Biophysical Applications in Microelectronics Parameters Measurements

Srdjan Ribar, Vojislav V. Mitić, Chun-An Lu, Goran Lazović, Jih Ru Hwu, Branislav Randjelović, Hans-Jörg Fecht, and Branislav Vlahović

Abstract Apply of artificial neural networks (ANN) in technology has started at the second half of the twentieth century. This arose as a consequence of extensive research in the field of biophysics carried out in the middle of the twentieth century. These biophysical researches have led to knowledge how a neuron as a basic element of a living being nervous system receives and processes signals. Living organisms use no mathematical model, the neurons processes signals by a simple algorithm, signals are massively parallel processed, the output is the superposition of all parallel processed signals. Artificial neural networks which are formed on these principles are used solving various problems such as pattern classification, clustering, function approximation and optimization. They can replace theoretical models that are hard to be presented analytically with data obtained using these models. In this paper we analyzed electrophysical parameters based on Murata powders and processing

S. Ribar (✉) · G. Lazović
Faculty of Mechanical Engineering, University of Belgrade, Kraljice Marije 16, 11120 Belgrade, Serbia
e-mail: sribar@mas.bg.ac.rs

V. V. Mitić (Deceased) · B. Randjelović
Faculty of Electronic Engineering, University of Niš, Aleksandra Medvedeva 14, Niš, Serbia

V. V. Mitić (Deceased)
Institute of Technical Sciences of Serbian Academy of Sciences and Arts, Kneza Mihaila 35, 11000 Belgrade, Serbia

C.-A. Lu
Material and Chemical Research Laboratories, Industrial Technology Research Institute, Hsinchu, Taiwan

J. R. Hwu
Department of Chemistry, National Tsing Hua University, Hsinchu, Taiwan

H.-J. Fecht
Institute of Functional Nanosystems, Ulm University, Ulm, Germany

B. Vlahović
North Carolina Central University (NCCU), Durham, NC, USA

S. Najman et al. (eds.), *Bioceramics, Biomimetic and Other Compatible Materials Features for Medical Applications*, Engineering Materials,
https://doi.org/10.1007/978-3-031-17269-4_18

consolidated samples technology. Between different electric, dielectric and ferroelectric characteristics we applied our neuro network approach on tgδ (loss factor) and for predicting the grain sizes in the function of T and time (τ) as distribution function between, the experimentally applied sintering temperatures (for example from 1190 to 1370 °C). Here, we continue to use neural networks to predict microelectronic parameters on the thin films around the grains based on the bulk surface measurements. All these extended applications are the quite new tool and method for getting the distributed parameters values at the real microstructure level what is opening new perspectives in microelectronics miniaturization designing.

Keywords Neural networks · Microelectronic parameters · Error back propagation

1 Back Propagation Method Basis

Back propagation algorithm presents generalization of least square algorithm which modifies network weight coefficients to minimize error between desired and actual network output [1]. Supervised learning is applied on set of input—desired output data [2]. Trained network have further on all constant weight coefficients and it is prepared to perform mapping of a new input data. Feedforward process implies introducing network inputs to an input layer and dispersing weighted values to a next layer. In the first phase each hidden layer node calculates its weighted input sum which is dispersed further on neurons of next layer. Second phase is characterized by spreading network error backwards including weight values correction. Weight coefficients are changed according error gradient. This method implies multiple iterations.

Algorithm calculates error function minimum in the state of weights. Weights combination that minimizes error function is adopted as a network learning solution. Since this method implies gradient function calculating in the each iteration step, error function has to be continuous and differentiable. Activation function [3] most often used in back propagation neural networks is sigmoid function, defined as:

$$f(v) = \frac{1}{1 + e^{-\lambda v}} \tag{1}$$

Two phases in error back propagation algorithm [4] are noticed. First phase implies input signal propagation starting in input layer through hidden layers finishing in output layer. As a result of this process network produces a signal at a network output. Further on, error signal which is difference between desired $d^{(k)}$ and calculated output $y^{(k)}$ is spread backwards starting from the output layer through hidden layers used to adapt weight coefficients.

Further example of three layered neural network is presented on Fig. 1.

Detailed structure of a neuron $(1, i)$ in hidden layer and a neuron $(2, j)$ in the output layer is presented on Fig. 2.

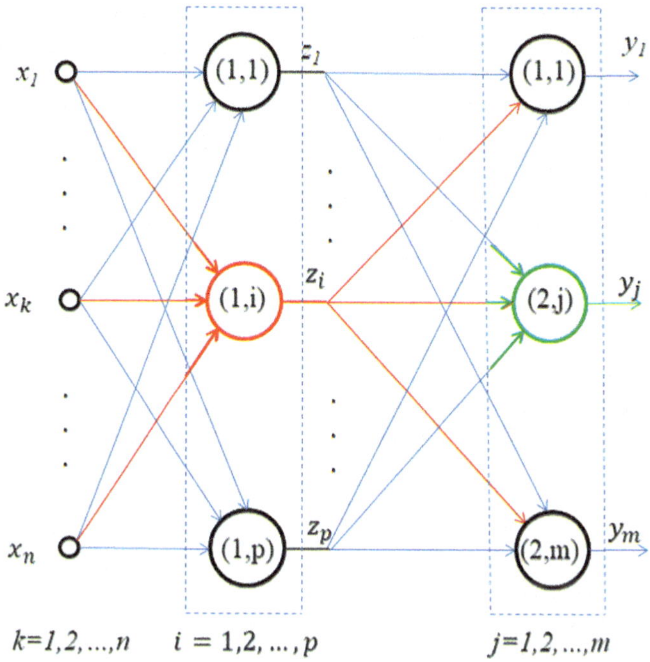

Fig. 1 Neural network structure with one hidden layer

For observed neurons extended input vectors and weights can be defined. Extended input vector and extended weight vector of neuron $(1, i)$ are:

$$\mathbf{x}_a = [x_0\ x_1\ x_2 \ldots x_n]^T \in R^{(n+1)}, \quad x_0 = 1 \tag{2}$$

$$\mathbf{w}_{ai}^{(1)} = \left[\mathrm{w}_{i0}^{(1)}\ \mathrm{w}_{i1}^{(1)}\ \mathrm{w}_{i2}^{(1)} \ldots \mathrm{w}_{in}^{(1)}\right]^T \in R^{(n+1)}, \quad i = 1, 2, \ldots, p \tag{3}$$

And for output layer neuron are:

$$\mathbf{z}_a = \left[z_0\ z_1\ z_2 \ldots z_p\right]^T \in R^{(p+1)}, \quad z_0 = 1, \tag{4}$$

$$\mathbf{W}_{aj}^{(2)} = \left[\mathbf{w}_{j0}^{(2)}\ \mathbf{w}_{j1}^{(2)}\ \mathbf{w}_{j2}^{(2)} \ldots \mathbf{w}_{jp}^{(2)}\right]^T \in R^{(p+1)}, \quad p = 1, 2, \ldots, m, \tag{5}$$

Asigning as an activation function input of neuron $(1, i)$ and neuron (2, j) as: $v_i^{(1)}$ and $v_j^{(2)}$ consequently, input–output equations of neurons $(1, i)$ and $(2, j)$ become:

$$neuron(1, i)(hidden\ layer) : \begin{cases} v_i^{(1)} = \sum_{k=0}^{n} \mathrm{w}_{ik}^{(1)} x_k = \left(\mathrm{w}_{ai}^{(1)}\right)^T \mathbf{x}_a \\ z_i = f\left(v_i^{(1)}\right), \quad i = 1, 2, \ldots, p \end{cases} \tag{6}$$

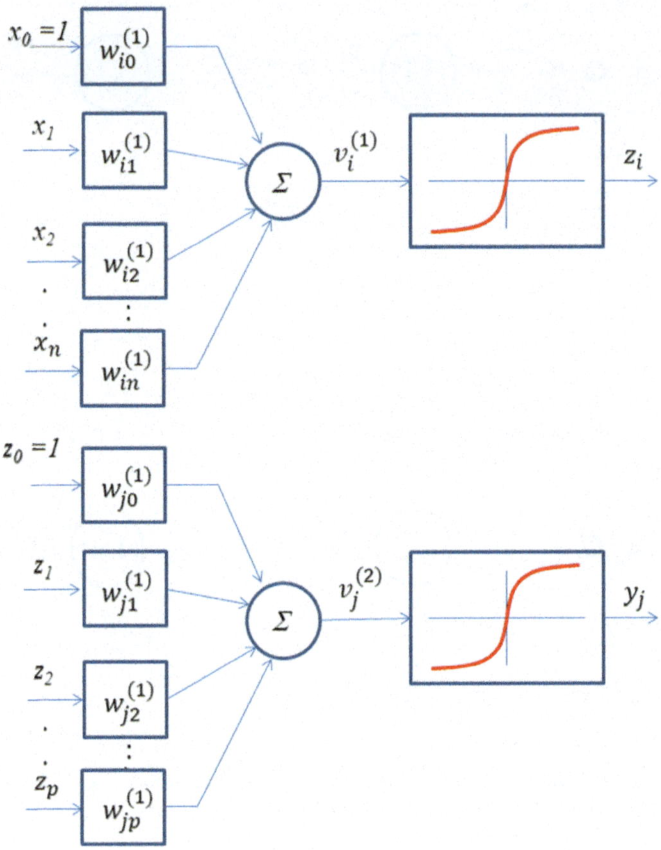

Fig. 2 Neuron with sigmoid activation function

$$neuron(2, j)(output\,layer) : \begin{cases} v_j^{(2)} = \sum_{q=0}^{p} \mathrm{w}_{jq}^{(2)} z_q = \left(\mathrm{w}_{aj}^{(2)}\right)^T \mathbf{z}_a \\ y_j = f\left(v_j^{(2)}\right), \quad j = 1, 2, \ldots, m \end{cases} \tag{7}$$

Extended weight matrices are:

$$\mathbf{W}_a^{(1)} = \left[\mathbf{w}_{a1}^{(1)}\ \mathbf{w}_{a2}^{(1)} \ldots \mathbf{w}_{ap}^{(1)}\right]^T = \begin{bmatrix} \mathrm{w}_{10}^{(1)} & \mathrm{w}_{11}^{(1)} & \cdots & \mathrm{w}_{1n}^{(1)} \\ \mathrm{w}_{20}^{(1)} & \mathrm{w}_{21}^{(1)} & \cdots & \mathrm{w}_{2n}^{(1)} \\ \vdots & \vdots & \ddots & \vdots \\ \mathrm{w}_{p0}^{(1)} & \mathrm{w}_{p1}^{(1)} & \cdots & \mathrm{w}_{pn}^{(1)} \end{bmatrix} \in R^{p\times(n+1)} \tag{8}$$

$$\mathbf{W}_a^{(2)} = \left[\mathbf{w}_{a1}^{(2)}\ \mathbf{w}_{a2}^{(2)} \ldots \mathbf{w}_{am}^{(2)}\right]^T = \begin{bmatrix} w_{10}^{(2)} & w_{11}^{(2)} & \cdots & w_{1p}^{(2)} \\ w_{20}^{(2)} & w_{21}^{(2)} & \cdots & w_{2p}^{(2)} \\ \vdots & \vdots & \ddots & \vdots \\ w_{m0}^{(2)} & w_{m1}^{(2)} & \cdots & w_{mp}^{(2)} \end{bmatrix} \in R^{m\times(p+1)} \tag{9}$$

Assigning vectors:

$$\mathbf{v}^{(1)} = \begin{pmatrix} v_1^{(1)} \\ v_2^{(1)} \\ \vdots \\ v_p^{(1)} \end{pmatrix}, \quad \mathbf{v}^{(2)} = \begin{pmatrix} v_1^{(2)} \\ v_2^{(2)} \\ \vdots \\ v_p^{(2)} \end{pmatrix} \tag{10}$$

Input–output equations in vectors form become:

$$hidden\,layer: \begin{cases} \mathbf{v}^{(1)} = \mathbf{W}_a^{(1)}\mathbf{x}_a \\ \mathbf{z}_a = \boldsymbol{f}_a\left(\mathbf{v}^{(1)}\right) \end{cases} \tag{11}$$

$$output\,layer: \begin{cases} \mathbf{v}^{(2)} = \mathbf{W}_a^{(2)}\mathbf{z}_a \\ \mathbf{y}_a = f\left(\mathbf{v}^{2)}\right) \end{cases} \tag{12}$$

Nonlinear mapping which perform three layered neural network can be presented as (Fig. 3):

$$\mathbf{y} = \boldsymbol{f}\left(\mathbf{W}_a^{(2)}\boldsymbol{f}_a\left(\mathbf{W}_a^{(1)}\mathbf{x}_a\right)\right) \tag{13}$$

Multilayered neural networks can process continuous as well as discrete signals using nonlinear mapping function. For discrete input–output signals mapping error is:

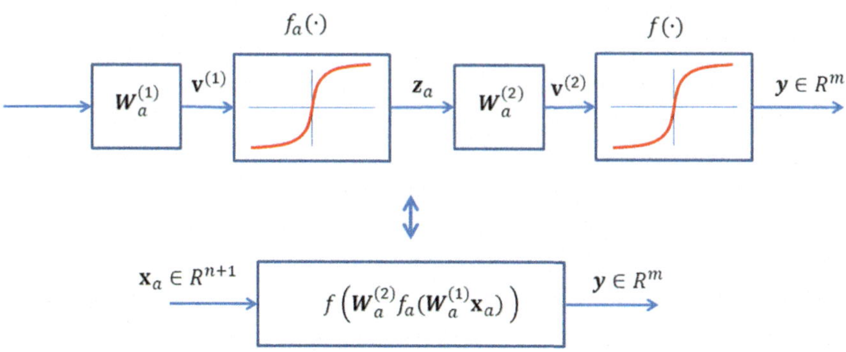

Fig. 3 Three layered neural network nonlinear input–output mapping

$$E = \frac{1}{2}\sum_{j=1}^{m}\left(d_j(k) - y_j(k)\right)^2 = \frac{1}{2}\sum_{j=1}^{m} e_j^2(k) \tag{14}$$

where e_j presents difference between desired and actual output of neuron (2, j):

$$e_j = d_j - y_j \tag{15}$$

Error function E value depends on all synaptic weights values and present performance index.

Weight values correction is proportional to error function negative gradient:

$$\triangle\, \mathbf{w}_{ai}^{(2)} = -\eta \nabla_{\mathbf{w}_{ai}^{(1)}} E = -\eta \frac{\partial E}{\partial \mathbf{w}_{ai}^{(1)}}, \quad i = 1, 2, \ldots, p \tag{16}$$

$$\triangle\, \mathbf{w}_{aj}^{(2)} = -\eta \nabla_{\mathbf{w}_{aj}^{(1)}} E = -\eta \frac{\partial E}{\partial \mathbf{w}_{aj}^{(2)}}, \quad j = 1, 2, \ldots, m \tag{17}$$

Value η is so called learning constant and it effects on convergence speed during weight coefficients adjustment.

Error signals on each neuron of output and hidden layer respectively are:

$$\delta_i^{(1)} = -\frac{\partial E}{\partial \mathrm{v}_i^{(1)}}, \quad i = 1, 2, \ldots, p \tag{18}$$

$$\delta_j^{(2)} = -\frac{\partial E}{\partial \mathrm{v}_j^{(2)}}, \quad j = 1, 2, \ldots, m \tag{19}$$

$\delta_i^{(1)}$ is a partial derivative of neuron $(1, i)$, $\delta_j^{(2)}$ is a partial derivative of neuron $(2, j)$.

In order to define partial derivatives in output layer Eqs. (19) and (14) it yields:

$$\delta_j^{(2)} = -\frac{1}{2}\frac{\partial \sum_{l=1}^{m}(d_l - y_l)^2}{\partial v_j^{(2)}} = -\frac{1}{2}\frac{\partial \sum_{l=1}^{m}\left(d_l - f\left(v_l^{(2)}\right)\right)^2}{\partial v_j^{(2)}}$$
$$= -\frac{1}{2}\sum_{l=1}^{m}\frac{\partial\left(d_l - f\left(v_l^{(2)}\right)\right)^2}{\partial v_j^{(2)}} \tag{20}$$

Since d_l, $v_j^{(2)}$ and $v_l^{(2)}$ are mutually independent it yields:

$$\delta_j^{(2)} = \left(d_j - f\left(v_j^{(2)}\right)\right)\frac{\partial f(v_j^{(2)})}{\partial v_j^{(2)}} = e_j^{(2)} f'\left(v_j^{(2)}\right) \tag{21}$$

In order to obtain weight coefficients correction expression gradient error function E has to be calculated relative to weight vector $\mathbf{w}_{aj}^{(2)}$

$$\nabla_{\mathbf{w}_{aj}^{(2)}} E = \frac{\partial E}{\partial \mathbf{w}_{aj}^{(2)}} = \sum_{l=1}^{m} \frac{\partial E}{\partial \mathrm{v}_l^{(2)}} \frac{\partial \mathrm{v}_l^{(2)}}{\partial \mathbf{w}_{aj}^{(2)}} \tag{22}$$

Since $\mathrm{v}_l^{(2)}(l \neq j)$ it does not depends on $\mathbf{w}_{aj}^{(2)}$ it yields:

$$\nabla_{\mathbf{w}_{aj}^{(2)}} E = \frac{\partial E}{\partial \mathrm{v}_j^{(2)}} \frac{\partial \mathrm{v}_j^{(2)}}{\partial \mathrm{w}_{aj}^{(2)}} \tag{23}$$

From:

$$\upsilon_j^{(2)} = \left(\mathrm{w}_{aj}^{(2)}\right)^T \mathbf{z}_a \tag{24}$$

It follows:

$$\frac{\partial \mathrm{v}_j^{(2)}}{\partial \mathrm{w}_{aj}^{(2)}} = \mathbf{z}_a \tag{25}$$

It becomes:

$$\nabla_{\mathbf{w}_{aj}^{(2)}} E = -\delta_j^{(2)} f'\left(\upsilon_j^{(2)}\right)\mathbf{z}_a \tag{26}$$

Adaptation weight vectors law finally becomes:

$$\begin{aligned} \nabla \mathrm{w}_{aj}^{(2)}(k+1) &= \mathrm{w}_{aj}^{(2)}(k) - \eta \nabla_{\mathrm{w}_{aj}^{(2)}} E(k) = \mathrm{w}_{aj}^{(2)}(k) + \eta \delta_j^{(2)}(k)\mathbf{z}_a(k) \\ &= \mathrm{w}_{aj}^{(2)}(k) + \eta e_j^{(2)}(k) f'\left(\upsilon_j^{(2)}\right)\mathbf{z}_a(k) \end{aligned} \tag{27}$$

Hidden layer error δ is:

$$\delta_i^{(1)} = -\sum_{l=1}^{m} \frac{\partial E}{\partial \mathrm{v}_l^{(2)}} \frac{\partial \mathrm{v}_l^{(2)}}{\partial \mathrm{v}_i^{(1)}} = \sum_{l=1}^{m} \delta_l(2) \frac{\partial \mathrm{v}_l^{(2)}}{\partial \mathrm{v}_i^{(1)}} \tag{28}$$

Using input–output Eqs. (6) and (7) it becomes:

$$\frac{\partial \mathrm{v}_l^{(2)}}{\partial \mathrm{v}_i^{(1)}} = \frac{\partial \sum_{q=0}^{p}\left(\mathrm{w}_{lq}^{(2)}\mathbf{z}_q\right)}{\partial \mathrm{v}_i^{(1)}} = \sum_{q=0}^{p} \frac{\partial\left(\mathrm{w}_{lq}^{(2)} f'(\upsilon_q^{(1)})\right)}{\partial \mathrm{v}_i^{(1)}} = \mathrm{w}_{li}^{(2)} f'\left(\upsilon_i^{(1)}\right) \tag{29}$$

It follows:

$$\delta_i^{(1)} = \sum_{l=1}^{m} \delta_l^{(2)} w_{li}^{(2)} f'\left(v_i^{(1)}\right) \tag{30}$$

Error $e_i^{(1)}$ is defined as:

$$e_i^{(1)} = \sum_{l=1}^{m} \delta_l^{(2)} w_{li}^{(2)} \tag{31}$$

This error presents error in the hidden layer which depends from errors of all output layer neurons. Replacing Eq. (31) into Eq. (30) it becomes:

$$\delta_i^{(1)} = e_i^{(1)} f'\left(v_i^{(1)}\right) \tag{32}$$

Gradient regarding hidden layer weights is calculated as:

$$\begin{aligned} \nabla_{\mathrm{w}_{ai}^{(1)}} E &= \frac{\partial E}{\partial \mathrm{w}_{ai}^{(1)}} = \sum_{j=1}^{m} \sum_{q=1}^{p} \frac{\partial E}{\partial \mathrm{v}_j^{(2)}} \frac{\partial \mathrm{v}_j^{(2)}}{\partial \mathrm{v}_q^{(1)}} \frac{\partial \mathrm{v}_q^{(1)}}{\partial \mathrm{w}_{ai}^{(1)}} = \sum_{q=1}^{p} \frac{\partial E}{\partial \mathrm{v}_q^{(1)}} \frac{\partial \mathrm{v}_q^{(1)}}{\partial \mathrm{w}_{ai}^{(1)}} \\ &= -\sum_{q=1}^{p} \delta_q^{(1)} \frac{\partial \mathrm{v}_q^{(1)}}{\partial \mathrm{w}_{ai}^{(1)}} \end{aligned} \tag{33}$$

Since $\mathrm{v}_q^{(1)} (q \neq i)$ is independent to $\mathrm{w}_i^{(1)}$:

$$\frac{\partial \mathrm{v}_q^{(1)}}{\partial \mathrm{w}_{ai}^{(1)}} = -\begin{cases} 0, & q \neq i, \\ \mathbf{x}_a, & q = i, \end{cases} \tag{34}$$

It follows:

$$\nabla_{\mathrm{w}_{ai}^{(1)}} E = -\delta_i^{(1)} \mathbf{x}_a \tag{35}$$

Replacing $\delta_i^{(1)}$ from Eq. (32) into previous Eq. (35)

$$\nabla_{\mathrm{w}_{ai}^{(1)}} E = -e_i^{(1)} f'\left(v_i^{(1)}\right) \mathbf{x}_a \tag{36}$$

So, hidden layer weights adaptation law is:

$$\begin{aligned} \mathrm{w}_{ai}^{(1)}(k+1) &= \mathrm{w}_{ai}^{(1)}(k) - \eta e_i^{(1)}(k) E(k) = \mathrm{w}_{ai}^{(1)}(k) + \eta \delta_i^{(1)}(k) \mathbf{x}_a(k) \\ &= \mathrm{w}_{ai}^{(1)}(k) + \eta e_i^{(1)}(k) f'\left(v_i^{(1)}\right)(k) \mathbf{x}_a(k) \end{aligned} \tag{37}$$

One can notice that weight vectors adaptation laws in output and hidden layer are similar. Equations (27) and (37) present generalized delta rule. Second element in both equations presents a part proportional to network error. Using these equations it is possible to calculate a new set of all weight values for all neural network neurons which should perform input–output mapping with minor error. In that way the contribution of the signal which is calculated on the network output (error) is distributed to the whole network. This procedure of spreading a signal through the whole network and calculating its components can be widened to any signal of interest. Electro-physical measurements imply various measurements on the sample surface.

Assuming sample structure as a granular, grains can be presented as neural network nodes—neurons. Transmission of measured electro physical quantities on sample surface through the structure can be presented by neurons interconnections. Introducing this analogy it is possible to spread any signal of interest through the neural network instead error signal.

Replacing electro physical measurements instead error signal it is possible to calculate its components through the whole structure.

2 Experimental Procedure

Special attention is paid to the preparation of ceramic powder, pressing and sintering, as parts of a complex process of $BaTiO_3$-ceramics consolidation samples Fig. 4 [5]. In this work, we presented the principle scientific-technological-research between different blocks schematic, as well as, laboratory process for consolidation.

As the starting material with high purity was used commercial $BaTiO_3$ Murata powder (99.9% purity, mean grain size <2 μm). For further investigations related to nanostructural and electrical characteristic interdependence optimization and for fractal application involvement, it was necessary to prepare sample series based on $BaTiO_3$-ceramics. We investigated the influence sintering conditions (temperature, sintering time) and additive content on the characteristics of the final $BaTiO_3$-ceramics.

It was measured $BaTiO_3$ with additive powders, and then the mixture was processed into a mill with balls and water. After that, organic binders were added and homogenization was performed for about 48 h. This mass was transported to the sprayer via the membrane pump and dried. On this we obtained and determined the powder granulation. Then material bulk density was measured every hour in a special vessel. It was used occasionally the vibrating sieve. The powder particles were roughly shaped (diameters ranging 10–130 μm).

We researched the influence of sintering temperatures, as well as different concentrations of CeO_2, $MnCO_3$, Bi_2O_3, Fe_2O_3, $CaZrO_3$, Nb_2O_5, Er_2O_3, Yb_2O_3, Ho_2O_3. In $BaTiO_3$-x-ceramics, different dielectric, ferroelectric effects were observed. Sintering times where 2 h, 3 h at a temperature (1190–1370 °C) and at a pressing pressures (86–150 MPa). In this paper we used the additives: CeO_2, $MnCO_3$, Bi_2O_3,

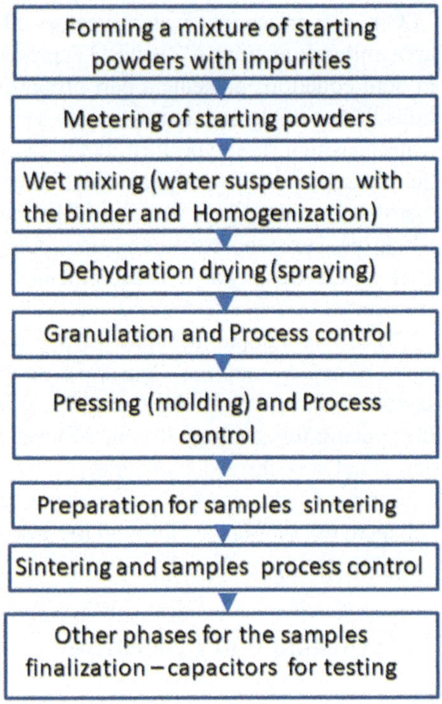

Fig. 4 Scheme of the process of consolidation of $BaTiO_3$-ceramics

Fe_2O_3. Within samples testing we measured different electric, dielectric and ferroelectric properties as tgδ (dielectric losses) (Table 1). A special interest was to analyze tgδ in our samples at which we applied our original neural network approach. Regarding the comparison, we applied our methods at the pure $BaTiO_3$ and as well as with additives.

Regarding the application of neural network method on experimental data we introduce, as theoretical experiment, the additional part where we practically develop the algorithm in novelties for parameters calculation.

2.1 *Theoretical Experiment by Neural Network Approach*

In this experiment dielectric losses tgδ measured on a bulk sample surface are used as a neural network input signal in a specific way. Back propagation neural network algorithm has a characteristic to spread calculated output error through the whole network determining contribution of all neurons to its value. Having in mind this network feature, arbitrary input–output data were used for neural network training. Since initial values of neural network parameters are set at random error absolute value is of interest and its sign in this analysis will be neglected. Set of various neural network

Table 1 Process and dielectric parameters: pressure (p), sintering temperature (T_{sint}), time (τ_{sint}) and dielectric losses (tgδ); pure $BaTio_3$ and with additives

Sample type	P (MPa)	T_{sint} (°C)	τ_{sint} (h)	tgδ
I-16 $BaTiO_3$-ceramics with no additives	86	1190	2	0.0032
	105	1190	2	0.0022
	130	1190	2	0.019
	150	1190	2	0.019
	86	1290	2	0.038
	105	1290	2	0.042
	130	1290	2	0.042
	150	1290	2	0.057
	86	1370	2	0.039
	105	1370	2	0.047
	130	1370	2	0.054
Basic mixture $BaTiO_3$-ceramics: composition: 0.1%CeO_2 + 0.14%$MnCO_3$		1190	2	0.009
		1190	2	0.01
		1190	2	0.007
		1190	2	0.0008
		1370	2	0.0074
		1370	2	0.007
		1370	2	0.0074
		1370	2	0.0074
Basic mixture $BaTiO_3$-ceramics: composition: 0.1%CeO_2 + 0.14%$MnCO_3$		1190	2	0.0014
		1240	2	0.0175
		1290	2	0.0076
		1370	2	0.0111
		1190	3	0.0296
		1240	3	0.0205
		1290	3	0.0087
		1370	3	0.0081
		1370	3	0.0061
		1370	3	0.0057
		1370	3	0.0085
		1370	3	0.0105
		1370	3	0.0065
		1370	3	0.0156

Table 2 Error for the neural network with two neurons in one hidden layer

Neuron	Hidden layer	Output neuron
1	0.730103	0.902102
2	−0.3426	

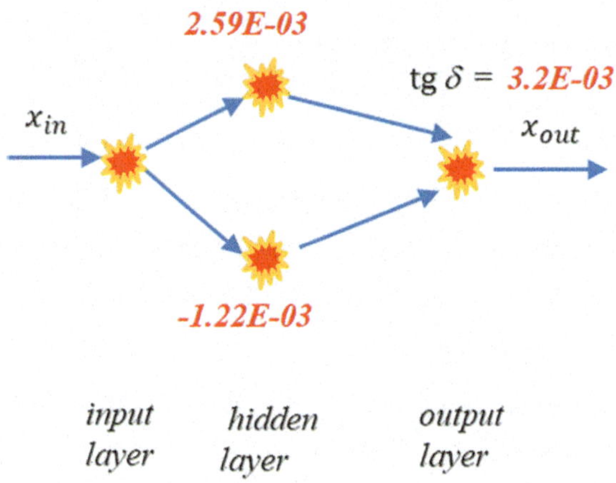

Fig. 5 The structure of the neural network with two neurons in one hidden layer

structures was applied to perform this input–output mapping. During training process neural network weights were changed to reduce input–output mapping error.

Assuming that measured dielectric losses tgδ on a grain surface present a total value of a whole sample grains losses they are spread through whole structure using back propagation of a error. Error signal is replaced with measured dielectric loss. In this example error is replaced by first value of tgδ in Table 1: 0.0032.

During training process for neural network with two neurons in a hidden layer error is presented in Table 2.

Calculated contribution to a measured dielectric loss $tg\delta = 0.0032$ in all hidden layer neurons are presented on Fig. 5.

Here, we developed experimental-theoretical model of neural networks application which later, we extended on several different neural network structures combinations. So, we continued all this analysis in 3. Results and discussion.

3 Results and Discussion

Further more we analyzed the neural network with three hidden layers with two neurons in each layer error is presented in Table 3.

Calculated contribution to a measured dielectric loss $tg\delta = 0.0032$ in all hidden layers neurons are presented on Fig. 6.

Neural network with four hidden layers with two neurons in each layer error is presented in Table 4.

Table 3 Error for the neural network with three hidden layers, two neurons per each layer

Neuron	First hidden layer	Second hidden layer	Third hidden layer	Output neuron
1	0.004886	0.012628	0.14495	0.855903
2	0.000836	0.05865	0.158095	

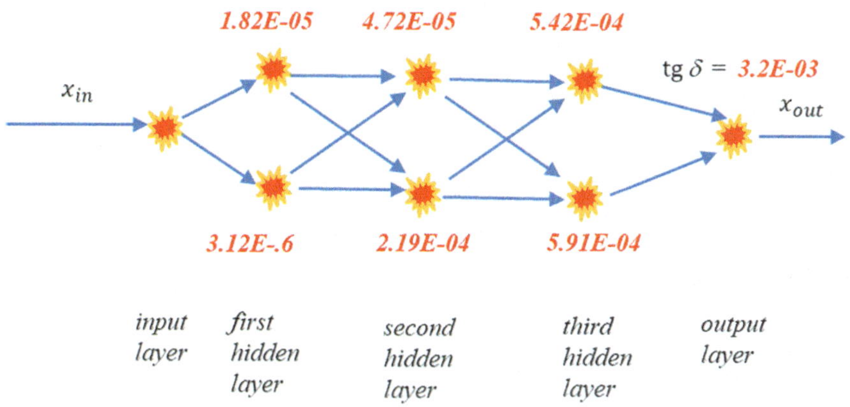

Fig. 6 The structure of the neural network with three hidden layers, two neurons per each layer

Table 4 Error for the neural network with four hidden layers, two neurons per each layer

Neuron	First hidden layer	Second hidden layer	Third hidden layer	Fourth hidden layer	Output neuron
1	0.002311	0.009875	0.043778	0.08036	0.796415
2	0.001608	0.005466	0.039936	0.146492	

Calculated contribution to a measured dielectric loss $tg\delta = 0.0032$ in all hidden layers neurons are presented on Fig. 7.

Neural network with two hidden layers with three neurons in first and one neuron in second hidden layer error is presented in Table 5.

Calculated contribution to a measured dielectric loss $tg\delta = 0.0032$ in all hidden layers neurons are presented on Fig. 8.

Neural network with three hidden layers with three neurons in each layer error is presented in Table 6.

Calculated contribution to a measured dielectric loss $tg\delta = 0.0032$ in all hidden layers neurons are presented on Fig. 9.

Neural network with three hidden layers with four neurons in each layer error is presented in Table 7.

Calculated contribution to a measured dielectric loss $tg\delta = 0.0032$ in all hidden layers neurons are presented on Fig. 10.

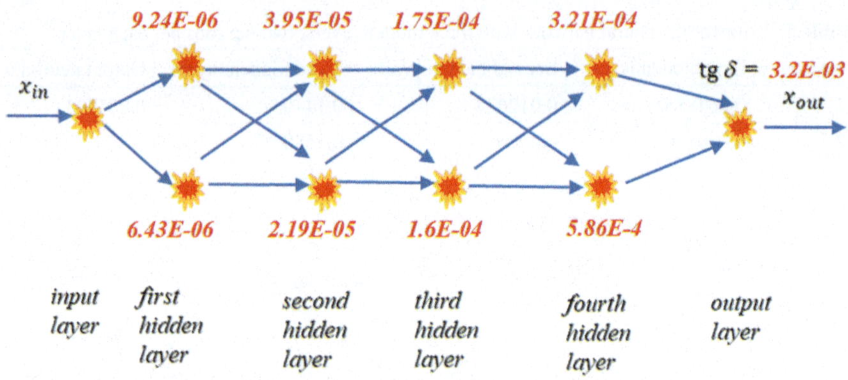

Fig. 7 The structure of the neural network with four hidden layers, two neurons per each layer

Table 5 Error for the neural network with two hidden layers, three neurons in first and one neuron in second hidden layer

Neuron	First hidden layer	Second hidden layer	Output neuron
1	−0.01393	−0.10363	1.096438
2	−0.00868	−0.11409	
3	−0.00158	/	

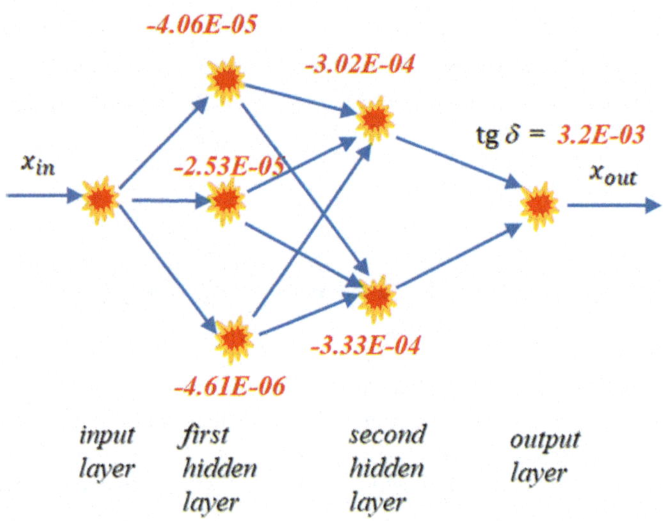

Fig. 8 The structure of the neural network with two hidden layers, three neurons in first and one neuron in second hidden layer

Table 6 Error for the neural network with three hidden layers, three neurons per each layer

Neuron	First hidden layer	Second hidden layer	Third hidden layer	Output neuron
1	0.004956	0.016444	0.044505	0.197486
2	0.004774	0.014836	0.047888	
3	0.008398	0.006215	0.046824	

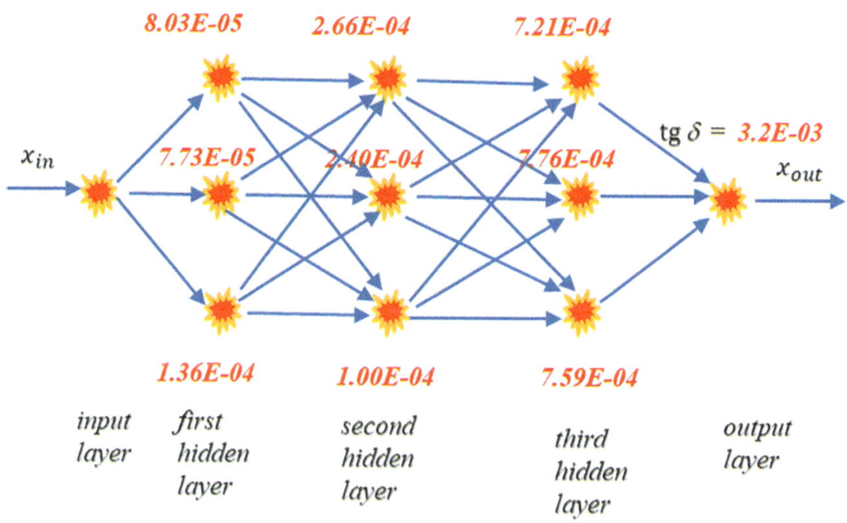

Fig. 9 The structure of the neural network with three hidden layers, three neurons per each layer

Table 7 Error for the neural network with three hidden layers, four neurons per each layer

Neuron	First hidden layer	Second hidden layer	Third hidden layer	Output neuron
1	0.008155	0.018785	0.007517	0.763601
2	0.006744	0.011126	0.087819	
3	0.00296	0.010913	0.112125	
4	0.009441	0.023366	0.032148	

From now on due to the simplicity of the network presentation lines between neurons are omitted. Neurons are fully interconnected namely all neurons from one layer are connected to all neurons of next layer.

Neural network with two hidden layers with five neurons in each layer error is presented in Table 8.

Calculated contribution to a measured dielectric loss $tg\delta = 0.0032$ in all hidden layers neurons are presented on Fig. 11.

Neural network with three hidden layers with five neurons in each layer error is presented in Table 9.

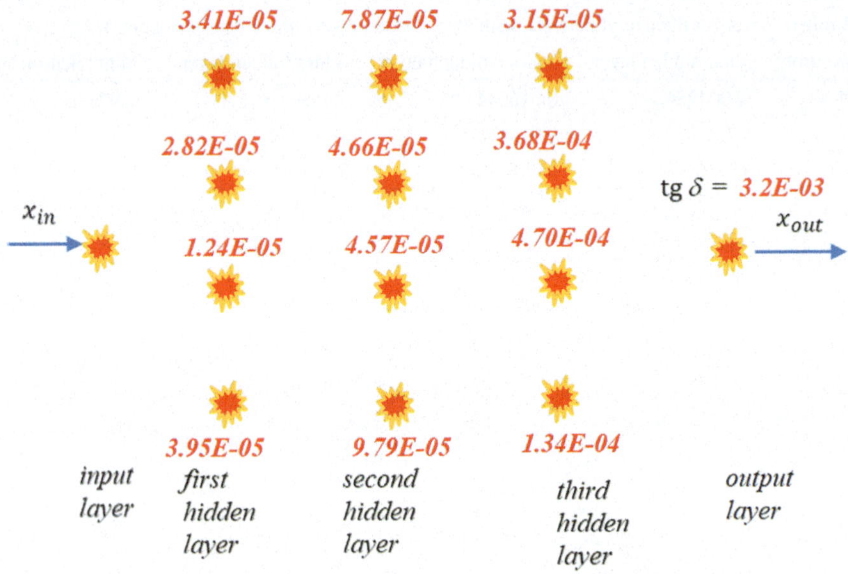

Fig. 10 The structure of the neural network with three hidden layers, four neurons per each layer

Table 8 Error for the neural network with two hidden layers, five neurons per each layer

Neuron	First hidden layer	Second hidden layer	Output neuron
1	0.023971	0.007538	0.883785
2	0.020625	0.05856	
3	0.018391	0.03675	
4	0.017613	0.054857	
5	0.018079	−0.00193	

Calculated contribution to a measured dielectric loss $tg\delta = 0.0032$ in all hidden layers neurons are presented on Fig. 12.

Neural network with two hidden layers with ten neurons in each layer error is presented in Table 10.

Calculated contribution to a measured dielectric loss $tg\delta = 0.0032$ in all hidden layers neurons are presented on Fig. 13.

Neural network with three hidden layers with ten neurons in each layer error is presented in Table 11.

Calculated contribution to a measured dielectric loss $tg\delta = 0.0032$ in all hidden layers neurons are presented on Fig. 14.

In this research a set of neural networks were used to propagate measured electrophysical parameter obtained in sintering process loss factor—tgδ. This signal is propagated through a network instead of network error which is calculated in network training process. On Fig. 5 are shown results of signal distribution through

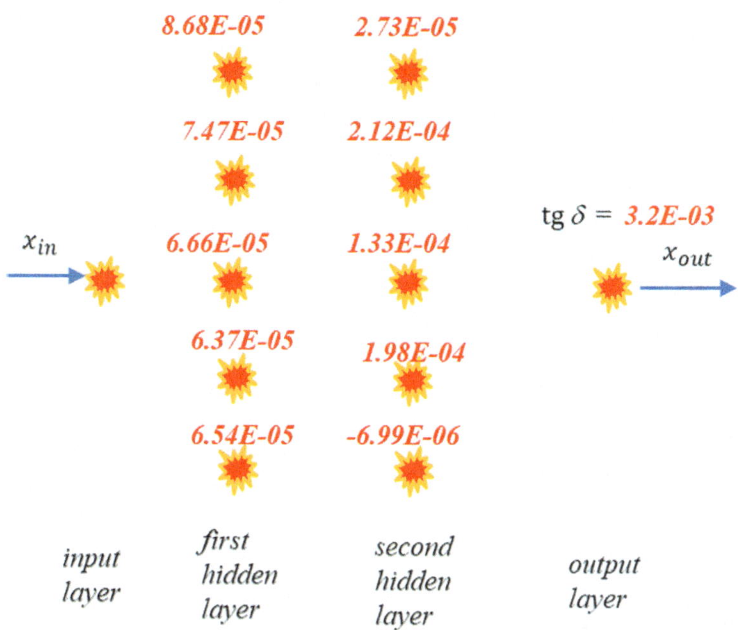

Fig. 11 The structure of the neural network with two hidden layers, five neurons per each layer

Table 9 Error for the neural network with three hidden layers, five neurons per each layer

Neuron	First hidden layer	Second hidden layer	Third hidden layer	Output neuron
1	−0.00134	−0.00181	0.025108	1.1256
2	−0.00112	−0.00791	−0.03733	
3	−0.00112	−0.0017	−0.01249	
4	−0.00163	−0.00333	−0.01635	
5	−0.00066	0.002042	0.000891	

the network. In this case for a network with one hidden layer it can be noticed that signals are the same order of magnitude as an input signal. All other network structures are with two or more hidden layers, Figs. 6, 7, 8, 9, 10, 11, 12, 13 and 14. In all these cases signals in all hidden layers neuron signals are lower order of magnitude than input signal. Further, increasing only number of hidden layers with the same number of neurons per layer Figs. 6 and 7, signal order of magnitude lowers from output to input layer regularly. We noticed that the order of values magnitude is lower or the same than input signal. This property could be also spotted in the network with different number of neurons per layer, Fig. 8. Neural network presented on Fig. 9 has a property that signals of all hidden layers neurons have the same order of magnitude: −4 except two upper neurons in the first hidden layer: −5.

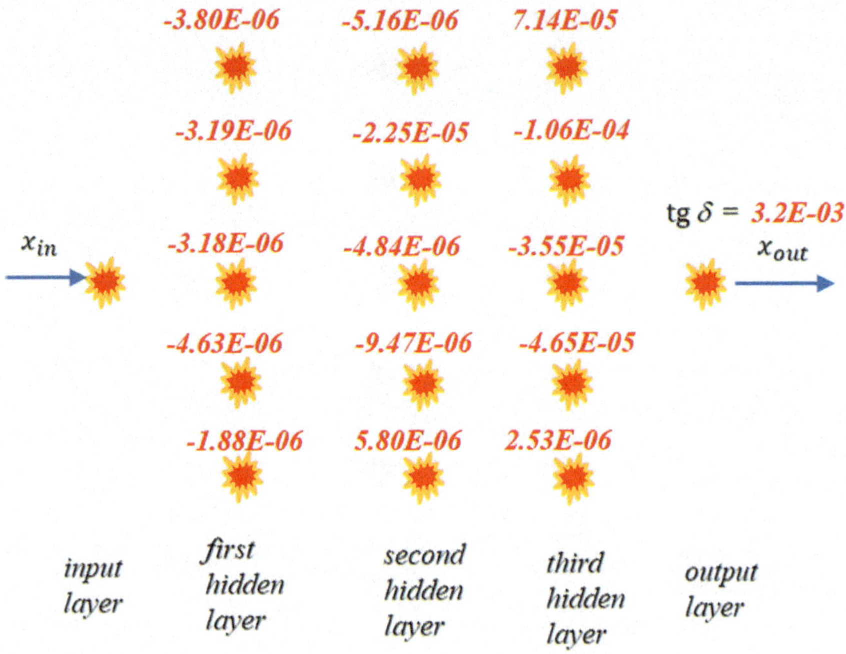

Fig. 12 The structure of the neural network with three hidden layers, five neurons per each layer

Table 10 Error for the neural network with two hidden layers, ten neurons per each layer

Neuron	First hidden layer	Second hidden layer	Output neuron
1	0.006696	0.006823	0.76158
2	0.008969	0.002514	
3	0.004025	0.016441	
4	0.00171	−0.00811	
5	0.002824	−0.00568	
6	0.006178	0.019705	
7	0.007034	0.000803	
8	0.005393	0.011224	
9	0.002613	−0.00247	
10	0.006653	−0.00357	

On Fig. 10 in this case we don't have the same network behavior like in previous sample. Here we noticed temporary change the signal values order of magnitude between −4 and −5.

On neural network presented on Fig. 10 property of lowering order of magnitude is violated because all neurons are the same order of magnitude: −5 except neurons: 2, 3 and 4 in the third hidden layer which have order of magnitude: −4. This is

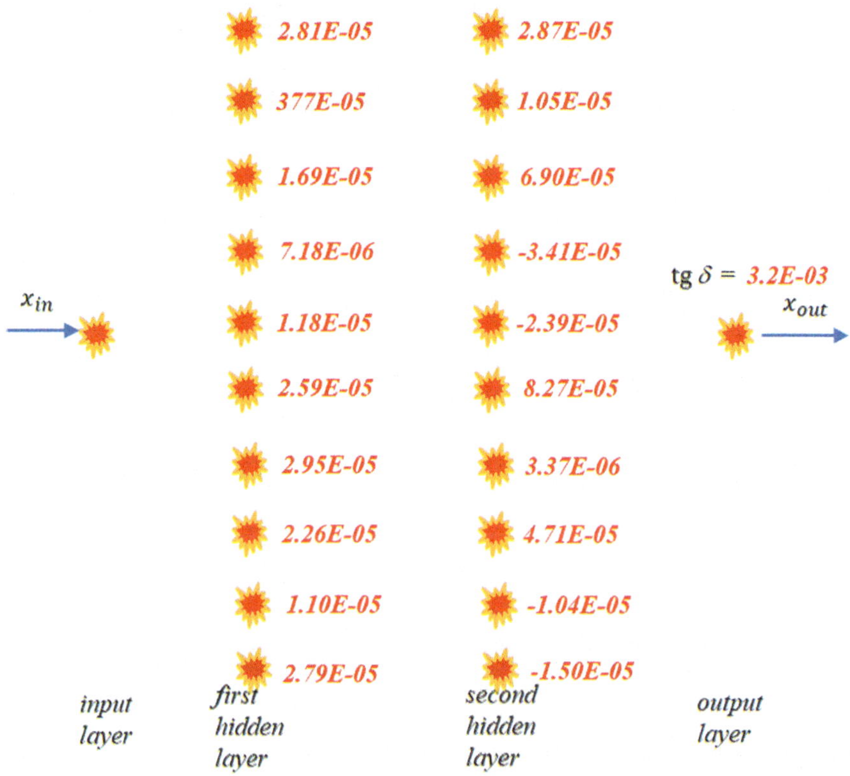

Fig. 13 Neural network structure with dielectric loss contribution marked red. The structure of the neural network with two hidden layers, ten neurons per each layer

Table 11 Error for the neural network with three hidden layers, ten neurons in each layer

Neuron	First hidden layer	Second hidden layer	Third hidden layer	Output neuron
1	−5.1E−06	−0.00052	−0.0051	1.127981
2	6.28E−05	−0.00038	−0.00449	
3	−9.2E−05	−0.00018	−0.00205	
4	−0.00022	0.000492	−0.01186	
5	−2.9E−05	0.000385	0.019647	
6	2.16E−05	−0.0001	0.007739	
7	−6.21E−05	−0.00033	−0.01686	
8	−7.55E−05	−9.4E−05	0.003588	
9	7.36E−06	0.000258	−0.00015	
10	−6.83E−05	0.000153	0.005105	

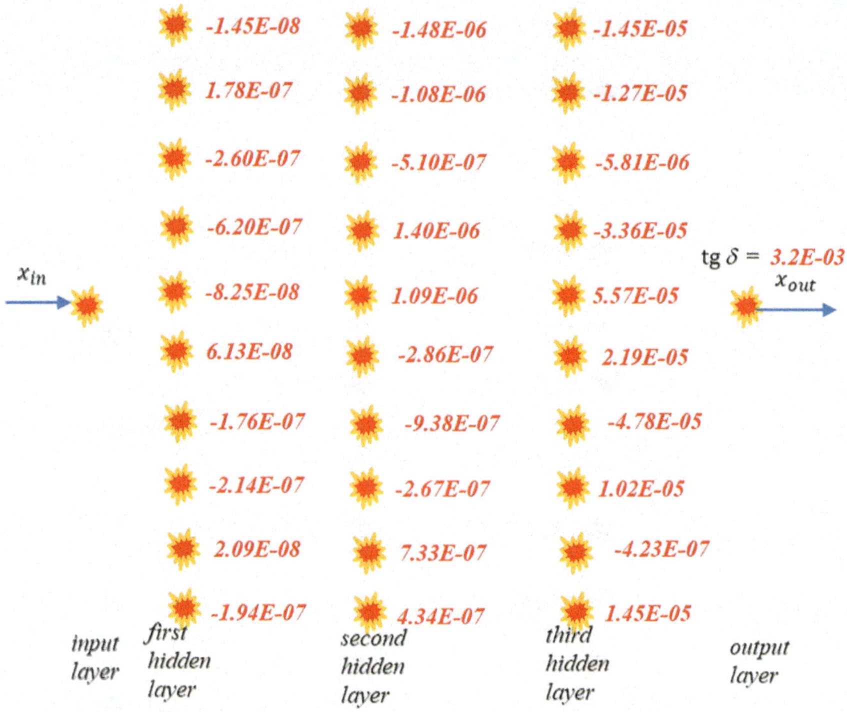

Fig. 14 The structure of the neural network with three hidden layers, ten neurons per each layer

repeated on Fig. 11 in the case of second hidden layer last neuron. Inserting just one more hidden layer to that structure, Fig. 12, regularity of diminishing order of magnitude through the layers remains valid. For two layered network with ten neurons per layer signals are the same lower magnitude then input signal, Fig. 13, except fourth neuron in first hidden layer which has a signal lower magnitude then all other neurons. Inserting one more hidden layer to that neural network, Fig. 14, signals are lower order except for seventh neuron in first and second hidden layer, eighth neuron in first and second hidden layer and tenth in first and second hidden layer which have same order of magnitude.

All these neural networks are trained on arbitrary input–output data and tested on the set with 30 elements. On Table 12 is presented neural networks back propagation average signal obtained on the whole test signals set for assumed output value: 0.0032.

Average signal propagation through the network layers for three layered network with three hidden layers is presented on Fig. 15.

We can evidently by Fig. 15 dispose how looks signal distribution from the input point deeper into different structures.

Table 12 Average signal

Network structure neurons per layer	First hidden layer	Second hidden layer	Third hidden layer	Fourth hidden layer	Output layer
2	1.00E−03	/	/	/	0.0032
2 2 2	1.07E−05	1.33E−04	5.67E−04	/	0.0032
2 2 2 2	7.75E−06	3.08E−05	1.68E−04	4.56E−04	0.0032
3 2	−2.32E−05	−3.17E−04	/	/	0.0032
3 3 3	1.01E−04	2.07E−04	7.55E−04	/	0.0032
4 4 4	2.81E−05	6.65E−05	2.50E−04	/	0.0032
5 5	6.86E−05	1.10E−04	/	/	0.0032
5 5 5	−3.63E−06	−7.60E−06	−2.31E−05	/	0.0032
10 10	2.20E−05	1.60E−05	/	/	0.0032
10 10 10	−2.05E−07	−1.48E−07	−1.30E−06	/	0.0032

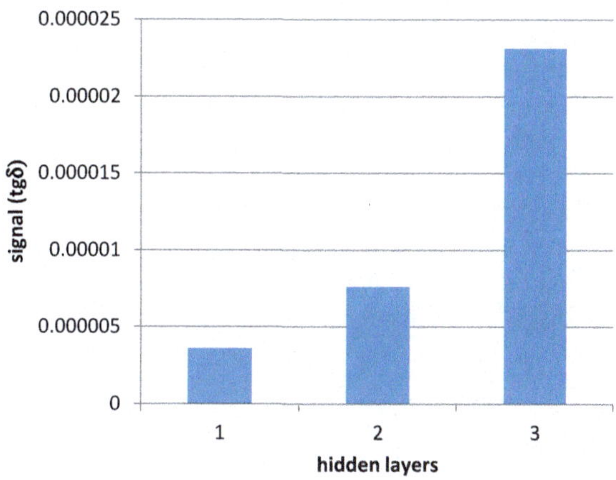

Fig. 15 Neural network backward average signal propagation

4 Conclusion

Definitely, this is one of the first papers that analyze and discuss the neural networks application on defining the electrophysical, dielectric and other parameters in material sciences especially electronic ceramics. Nowadays, in basic sciences, there is a trend in new perspectives for research and further application in matter research, different phenomena from biosystems [6, 7]. One of the best most interesting cases is neural network [8]. These biosystem structures are very successfully applied in the research on the signal processes in artificial electronic systems. The ideas of further miniaturization and higher level electronic parameters integrations demand the new ideas and solutions how to measure and define the electronic parameters on micro structure level, but to avoid the rough statistical approach and distribution from the global phenomenological measurements of the samples down to the level between grains and pores as microstructure elements.

In our recent fractals, graphs and neural networks research we develop new ideas and applications how to get the parameters values on this micro level [9, 10]. Definitely the subject of our paper is a quite original neural networks application in that direction. The novelty which is already present in few scientific plenary lectures and scientific papers, originally involve the error as a real positive signal which provide the parameters values at the micro structure level. We already published results as for an example neural networks application at brake down voltage [11].

Here in this chapter we completely analyzed the whole our innovation for the parameter like dielectric losses (tgδ). Definitely, if we plan to move forward and to improve the miniaturization, also by getting the results as electronic, dielectric, ferro electric parameters at the micro level there is a need for defining the tools for predicting the microelectronics structures and designing in directions, where the classic semiconductor technologies are not anymore applicable.

In our paper we discussed by several examples and structure combinations the neural networks approach behavior. These new extracted results provide very important new analysis which definitely establish the mechanisms of very fine procedure to get much more precise parameters results between grains and pores. We successfully explained some additional phenomena which contribute to get these results, especially in the sense of the parameters magnitude order changes deeper down to the materials structures levels. Significant number of analyzed samples is treated in results and discussion, so definitely we have very original important method in our research hands to provide the parameters defined values which could act in advance design, predicted electronics, ceramics structures with predicted properties for diversity applications.

References

1. Hecht-Nielsen: Theory of the backpropagation neural network. In: International Joint Conference on Neural Networks, vol. 1, pp. 593–605. IJCNN.1989.118638 (1989)
2. Erdogmus, D., Principe, J.C.: An error-entropy minimization algorithm for supervised training of nonlinear adaptive systems. IEEE Trans. Sig. Process. **50**(7), 1780–1786 (2002)
3. da Silva, I.N., Hernane Spatti, D., Andrade Flauzino, R., Liboni, L.H.B., dos Reis Alves, S.F.: Artificial neural network architectures and training processes. In: Artificial Neural Networks. Springer, Cham (2017)
4. Rumelhart, D., Hinton, G., Williams, R.: Learning representations by back-propagation errors. Nature **323**, 533–536 (1986)
5. Mitic, V.V.: Structure and electrical properties of $BaTiO_3$ ceramics. Andrejevic Foundation (2001)
6. Mitic, V.V., Randjelovic, B., Ribar, S., Lu, C., Radovic, I., Stajcic, A., Novakovic, I., Vlahovic, B.: Ceramics, materials, microelectronics and graph theory new frontiers. Mod. Phys. Lett. B **34**(34), 2150159 (2020)

7. Mitic, V.V., Lazovic, G., Randjelovic, B., Paunovic, V., Radovic, I., Stajcic, A., Vlahovic, B.: Graph theory applied to microelectronics intergranular relations. Ferroelectrics **570**(1), 145–152 (2021)
8. Ribar, S.: A hybrid software system for diagnosing the biophysical properties of the skin based on expert system, neural networks, fuzzy logic and genetic algorithms. PhD thesis, University of Belgrade (2011)
9. Mitic, V.V., Lazovic, G., Ribar, S., Lu, C., Radovic, I., Stajcic, A., Fecht, H., Vlahovic, B.: The artificial neural networks applied for microelectronics intergranular relations determination. Integr. Ferroelectr. **212**, 135–146 (2020)
10. Ribar, S., Mitic, V.V., Lazovic, G.: Neural networks application on human skin biophysical impedance characterisations. Biophys. Rev. Lett. (2020)
11. Mitic, V.V., Ribar, S., Randjelovic, B., Chun-An, L., Radovic, I., Stajcic, A., Novakovic, I., Vlahovic, B.: Neural networks and microelectronics parameters distribution measurements depending on sintering temperature and applied voltage. Mod. Phys. Lett. B **34**(35), 2150172 (2020)

Ceramics in Socio-political Fields

Bioceramics and Politics: (Un)likely Encounters

Ivana Damnjanović

Abstract The aim of this paper is to explore possible interactions and intersections between bioceramics research and applications and politics in its widest sense. It argues that ceramics was intimately tied to politics for much of human history, sometimes shaped by it and sometimes shaping it. This is illustrated by several examples: the role of ceramics in the Neolithic technological revolution and the formation of the first polities; the use of clay tablets for writing, thus demarcating barbarism from civilization; and the re-invention of porcelain in Europe and establishment of royal monopolies. In the recent decades, ceramics played, and will continue to play, an important role in technological races which are used as tools of politics. The paper then explores possible approaches to social study of bioceramics, with focus on political science paradigms such as biopolitics, especially the concept of cyborgs introduced by Haraway. Finally, some contemporary socio-political issues—changes in population structure and rise of inequality—are considered in relation to bioceramics.

Keywords Bioceramics · Politics · Biopolitics · Inequality

1 Introduction

However unlikely it may seem at the first glance, the development of different technologies has never been independent of nor divorced from politics. Since 1980s (a period that coincides with the acceleration of progress in the field of bioceramics), a body of literature, mainly from disciplines such as History of Technology, Anthropology and Science, Technology and Society Studies (see [1–3]) has convincingly demonstrated that technologies do not develop in vacuum. On the contrary, technologies are inevitably immersed in the society, therefore influenced by, but also exerting influence on, its political choices. This is the case for ceramics, being one of the oldest technologies, in general, but also for bioceramics as a more recent phenomenon.

I. Damnjanović (✉)
Faculty of Political Science, University of Belgrade, Belgrade, Serbia
e-mail: ivana.damnjanovic@fpn.bg.ac.rs

S. Najman et al. (eds.), *Bioceramics, Biomimetic and Other Compatible Materials Features for Medical Applications*, Engineering Materials,
https://doi.org/10.1007/978-3-031-17269-4_19

In this paper I shall endeavor to show the complicated relation between development and use of ceramics and politics trough history, and offer some questions, or research frameworks, that might be useful in further investigations of the socio-political side of bioceramics research and applications.

Practically speaking, inclusion of this type of research could potentially maximize social impacts of bioceramics innovations and applications, and bring them closer to making the full contribution to the human well-being.

First part of the paper describes points of intersection between ceramics and politics trough history. In the second part I shall try to investigate some possible lines of discussion of bioceramics through framework known as biopolitics. Finally, I intend to point out some of the wider political issues of our age and the possible place of bioceramics research and application in their development.

2 Ceramics and Politics: Tale as Old as Time

The invention of ceramics—the insight, probably coincidental—that fire irreversibly transforms clay into ceramic pottery [4, 5]—was among factors that had started far reaching changes in the way humans lived, and, subsequently, the ways in which their societies were organized: in other words, politics. Throughout history, ceramics drew attention of those in power, and was sometimes used as an instrument of political influence. But above everything else, invention of ceramics was instrumental in creation of the first polities and, later, civilizations and empires.

2.1 Neolithic Technological Revolution

Ceramic pottery was among technologies that transformed human societies from nomadic to sedentary, transforming economy from hunting and gathering to agriculture. Ceramic vessels, being fire resistant and waterproof, allowed for better storage and hitherto unimaginable methods of food processing [4]. They were important, albeit sometimes overlooked [6] part of the Neolithic technological revolution, which, while it "was an economic and technological milestone, it also was a dramatic social and symbolic transformation" [7].

Technological revolution, according to Bar-Yosef [8], occurs when "[t]he successful completion of the first phase of a crucial transition culminates in the reaching of 'a point of no return'". Neolithic revolution had started some 13,000 years ago,[1] and while agriculture and transformation of food production was the main generator of changes, many other important inventions can be traced back to this period—resulting in unprecedented flourishing of trade, architecture and art.

[1] There are certain disputes regarding precise definition and dating of the Neolithic period, some of them due to complexities of radiocarbon dating and interpretation of its results [7].

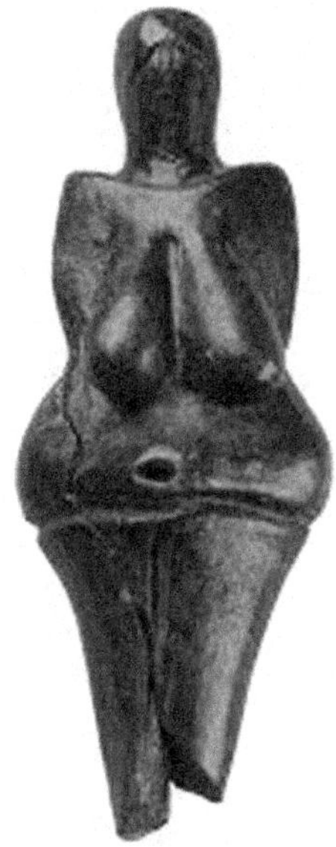

Fig. 1 The Venus of Dolní Věstonice, the oldest clay figurine. Moravské zemské muzeum [9]

Introduction of ceramic pottery into the material culture, occurring relatively late in the Neolithic period, has become a significant benchmark in itself. Not only that entire Late Neolithic period is usually referred to as the Pottery Neolithic (starting approximately 9000 years ago), but, at least in the Near East area, it meant increased diversification and rise of distinctly local cultures [7].[2] Even though most archeologists and other researchers of ancient ceramics used to "stress the physical, chemical and economic constraints within which the potter operates, and would see the choices he makes as primarily dictated by these constraints," [10] there is also literature suggesting that, especially in the early stages of this period, decorative features of the pottery were more important than their functionality. Thus, as shown in Simmons [7], those vessels were, in fact, "an elaboration of ideological expressions", communicating symbolic and social messages. Plasters, and later clay, were used throughout the period for sculptures and figurines, performing similar social functions.

While, as Mumford [6] convincingly demonstrates, the pottery itself—the production of vessels and similar household items—was, along with other technologies perceived as a "woman's domain"[3] frequently overlooked by researchers of technology, the *potter's wheel* was lauded as one of the first machines with moving parts.

[2] However, there are findings suggesting that ceramic pottery was invented in China much earlier, c. 16,000 BC, while the oldest clay figurine, the Venus of Dolni Vestonice [11, 12] was dated c. 26,000–24,000 BC. See Figs. 1 and 2.

[3] Interestingly, Foster [15] summarizes the dominant interpretation of the social consequences of the potter's wheel in a way very pertinent to this Mumford's [6] observation: "In pre-wheel times women made pots, primarily for their own domestic consumption. Pot-making techniques were laborious and time-consuming, so that absolute production was strictly limited. The wheel greatly shortened the time necessary to make a vessel, reduced the physical effort involved, and simultaneously improved the quality of the ware. Full-time male specialists essentially eliminated women from

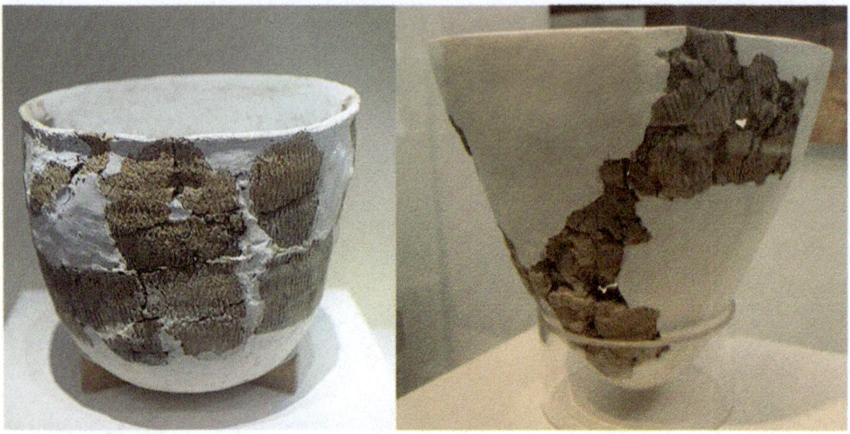

Fig. 2 Oldest Chinese pottery. Left: Xianrendong pot, National Museum of China. Right: Yuchanyan pot, Hunan Museum [13, 14]

Its origins are, however, in the somewhat later, Early Bronze period. Widespread throughout Eurasia, and improved on ever since, the potter's wheel has become one of the symbols of traditional, pre-industrial modes of production.

The potter's wheel and its operation can be easily and briefly described [15]: "[it] may be described in material terms as a pair of horizontal discs joined by an axle, supported in such fashion that it rotates easily and rapidly. Its mode of use may be described equally briefly: the potter places clay on the upper disc, sets the apparatus in motion by kicking the lower disc, and forms the vessel with his hands." However, as the same author rightfully notices, the essence and cultural consequences of this invention rest not in its form but in the idea—the recognition of possibilities of exploiting the centrifugal action of the flywheel. This same principle has yielded, as archeological and ethnological data suggest, at least four different forms or types of the potter's wheel: (1) the unpivoted turntable; (2) the pivoted turntable; (3) the simple wheel; and (4) the double or kick wheel [15]. Omnipresent in the ancient world, the potter's wheel also produced a set of distinct social practices and ideologies, exerting its own social and political influence [16].

After the Neolithic boom in the development of various technologies, the technological change was slowed down to almost nothing for the several centuries. This, along with the fact that Neolithic people, unlike the harbingers of the Industrial revolution had no notion of science as we understand it, has led anthropologist Levi-Strauss [16] to coin the term "Neolithic Paradox". Among the extraordinary achievements of this age he explicitly includes pottery: "[…] to make stout, water-tight pottery out of clay which is friable and unstable, liable to pulverize or crack (which, however, is possible only if from a large number of organic and inorganic materials, the one most suitable for refining is selected, and also the appropriate fuel,

pottery work, thus commercializing a home craft. Greatly increased production stimulated the development of trade and markets.

the temperature and duration of firing and the effective degree of oxidation) [...] there is no doubt that all these achievements required a genuinely scientific attitude, sustained and watchful interest and a desire for knowledge for its own sake."[4]

Within the wider context of Neolithic technological revolution, the invention and subsequent widespread use of pottery had led to the perhaps the vastest social transformation in human history. Establishment of permanent settlements and abandonment of the nomadic hunter-gatherer's way of life, resulted in the formation of the new social orders and stratifications, as well as of the first polities—societies in which politics was possible, necessary and, for the first time in history, tied to a certain territory. Even more important, pottery, with its novel qualities, allowed for more efficient storage of foodstuffs and liquids, making the societies more secure, and traveling as well as trade easier. It became commodity itself, traded throughout the ancient world. After millennia, it also became one of the most important ways to identify different ancient cultures and periods, as well as unique crumb trail for charting of the ancient trade routes [18].

This enormous technological revolution that took place in Neolithic perhaps had not directly lead to the birth of what we now call *a civilization*, but has certainly made its birth easier and earlier [6]. Ceramics, as we shall see in the following section, had an important part to play in this process as well.

2.2 Writing and the Rise of Civilization

Etymologically, civilization refers to an urban society, applying to "those who live in the cities". The true meaning of the concept was (and is), however, strongly disputed, even leaving aside its complicated colonizing connotations,[5] and the term was used as a synonym for culture, or human society as a whole. In his comprehensive analysis of different scholarly definitions of civilization, Targowski [21] lists a number of them which explicitly include writing, as one of the defining features. This includes definitions offered by Carroll Quigley (society becomes civilization only when it has writing and city life); Matthew Melko (sees civilization as a large society possessing, among other features, cities and writing or some other method of keeping long-term records); and Jaroslav Krejci (who claims that civilization starts with the process where people become urbanized and literate). According to McGaughe [22] civilization includes large-scale political organization and sophisticated expression in a medium such as writing. His classification of civilizations is based on two criteria, the communication technology being one of them—and other, incidentally, being the institution of power, which roughly translates to political authority (see Table 1).

Perhaps the strongest and far-reaching descriptions of writing as a condition sine qua non of civilization is found in Bosworth [23]: "Writing is the DNA of civilization. Writing permits for the organization of large populations, professional armies, and

[4] For additional discussion of the Neolithic Paradox, see also Fores [19].

[5] For the discussion on these issues see Duara [20].

Table 1 McGaughey's taxonomy of civilizations

Name of civilization	Communication technology	Institution of power
Civilization I	Ideographic writing	Imperial government
Civilization II	Alphabetic writing	World religion
Civilization III	Printing	Commerce and education
Civilization IV	Electronic recording and broadcasting	Media of news and entertainment
Civilization V	Computers	The internet

Adapted from Targowski [21]

the passing of complex information across generations. [...] The connection between writing and civilization could not be more intimate: writing and civilization share a mutual origin in the Sumerian city-states that emerged by 3000 BC. [...] In ordinary cultures, the passing of information and knowledge may depend upon imitation or oral communication; in civilizations, this cultural memory, etched into clay or drawn onto papyrus, takes on a life of its own."

Although sometimes it is hard to think about writing as a technology, it can be argued that it is, in fact, one of the most important technologies of all times. For Bosworth [23], writing systems are primarily "technologies of social organization", while Coulmas [24] sees them as "the single most consequential technology ever invented." Writing system was devised independently, it seems, only three times in history: in ancient Mesopotamia before 3000 BC, China no later than 1000 BC and Mesoamerica around 500 BC [24]. The writing system is usually defined as "a system of recording language by means of visible or tactile marks" [24] or "represented units of sound and meaning in systematic fashion" [25].

Various scholars convincingly argue that the emergence of writing was intrinsically related to the emergence and needs of the new type of political entity—an empire. Large territories, populated with people who sometimes did not necessarily share the same worldviews, religion, culture, or identity, demanded an efficient methods of record-keeping, as well as dissemination of decrees and orders. Some examples include Joyce Marcus, who sees complexity of writing as equivalent to complexity of state control; or Norman Yoffee, who suggests that complex polities use writing to achieve "the joint understanding, perception, and, ultimately, control of social arrangements" [25].

Diamond [26] continues this line of argumentation, claiming that the first writing systems emerged in highly stratified societies with centralized political institutions, and were, at first, used exclusively by professional scribes who were in the service of the temple or of the king. All of this scholarship, however, just echoes the memorable line of Levi-Strauss [27] that writing "seems to favor rather the exploitation than the enlightenment of mankind." He continues to hypothesize that "the primary function of writing, as a means of communication, is to facilitate the enslavement of other human beings" (Fig. 3).

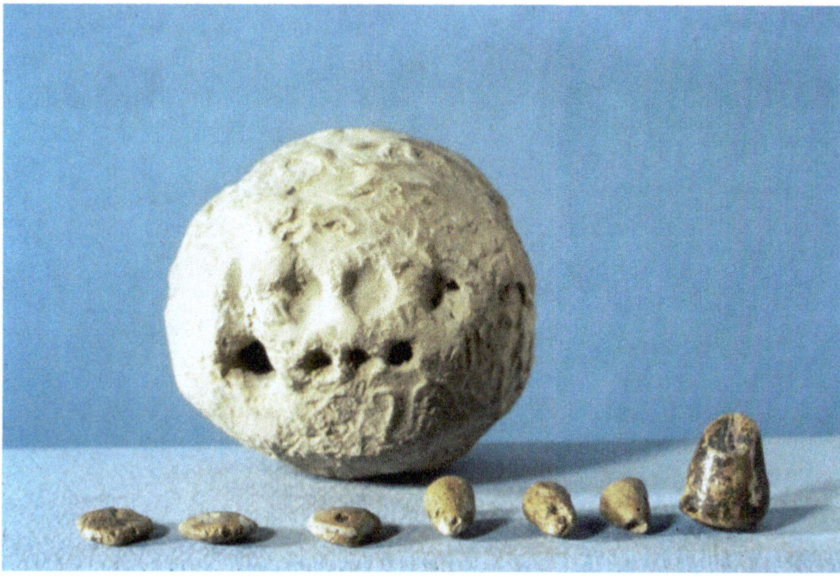

Fig. 3 Clay accounting tokens: envelope and contents from Susa, Iran, circa 3300 BC. Musée du Louvre [28]

If invention of writing was the demarcation line between barbarism and civilization [27], then ceramics was instrumental in the development of the oldest writing system—the Sumerian cuneiform. For centuries before the invention of writing as such, people of the Fertile Crescent had used clay tokens [26] or seals [29] for accounting purposes. These were usually in the shape of clay pebbles, or "hollow clay balls with the pebbles enclosed within" [27]. This has led some scholars to contend that "the use of clay to be at the basis of the invention of writing, the middle stages being made up by the use of geometric objects, clay pebbles (or tokens) and clay balls which are compared to clay envelopes." [26, 29]. Although this hypothesis is later disputed [29, 30], these archaeological findings shed some light on the features of ceramics that make it useful for writing—it is malleable, easily shaped, relatively light and easy to store and transport. They also seem to land support for the close relation between the complex society with centralized political power and the invention of writing as primarily record-keeping and accounting tool (Fig. 4).

The same can be said for some of the ancient Sumerian texts. The epic poem *Enmerkar and the Lord of Aratta* [33] depicts the origin of writing: "Because the messenger's mouth was heavy and he couldn't repeat (the message)/The lord of Kulaba patted some clay and put words on it, like a tablet/Until then, there had been no putting words on clay." This use of flat clay tablets as writing surface is seen by Diamond [26] as a key technological innovation, followed later by the development of the reed stylus.

Thus, clay tablets were instrumental in the birth of what we today colloquially call the Western Civilization. Their practicality made them widespread medium for

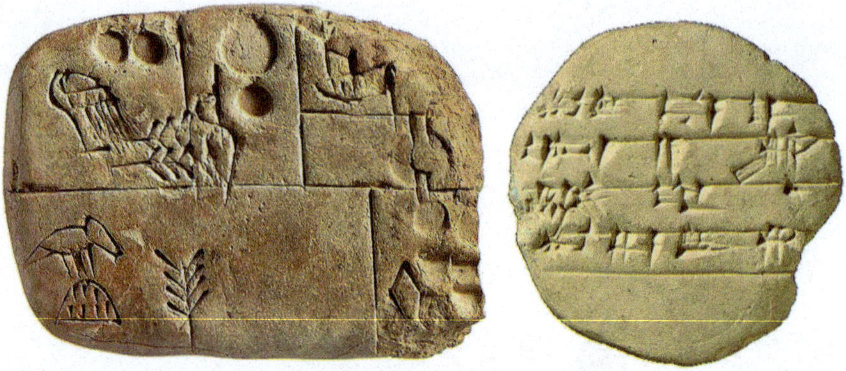

Fig. 4 Cuneiform tablets. Left: administrative account of the distribution of barley and grains, ca. 3100–2900 BC. The Metropolitan Museum of Art. Right: Practicing tablet with a proverb, Mesopotamia, ca.1700 BC. The British Museum [31, 32]

writing throughout the ancient world—from Mesopotamia to Greece, while their durability provides us with a glimpse into the daily lives of ancient civilizations, from accounting to schoolwork. Unique features of the clay tablets even allow us to distinguish the handwriting of different scribes—leading to insight that all of the Linear B tablets found in Knossos and Pylos palaces on Crete were written by only 75 and 40 different people, respectively [26]. Ever since the literal dawn of civilization, ceramics was the vehicle of human knowledge and political power.

2.3 *Glass, Porcelain and the Royal Power*

In Roman, Medieval and Early Modern times, ceramics and its production continued to intersect with politics and, to the various ends, attract attention of political rulers. Two instances of direct intervention of Roman emperors in the process of technological development were recorded—and one of them is about ceramics production.[6] After recounting processes of glass-making, Pliny [35] relates "a story that in the reign of Tiberius there was invented a method of blending glass so as to render it flexible. The artist's workshop was completely destroyed for fear that the value of metals such as copper, silver and gold would otherwise be lowered."

Luxury ceramic wares remained, on one hand, an insignia of royal wealth and power, and on the other a means to acquire said wealth and power. Perhaps the most illuminating example for this state of affairs is the story of establishment of the porcelain production in Europe.

[6] The other one, recorded by Suetonius [34], regards Vespasian's rejection of the column moving machine, with explanation that it will leave workers without bread.

The porcelain production was perfected in China at some point during the Han dynasty (25–220 AD). While the finesses of technological process itself are beyond the scope of this chapter, its features as well as socio-political functions bear some elaboration. As Marchand [36] puts it, "[i]t is the finest, whitest, and most difficult to make form of ceramics, and it enraptured Chinese emperors long before the first pieces made their way to Europe in the fourteenth century." Porcelain production was not only sponsored by the Chinese royalty, it added to their prestige—being one of the chief export articles. Since seventeenth century, European craftsmen are trying, and finally succeeding, to independently replicate the process. Interestingly, these workshops and factories were usually under royal or sometimes aristocratic patronage, in both France and (what is today) Germany, although not in England, where early attempts were made under the auspices of British Royal Society [37].

It seems that the first experimental recipes for porcelain in Europe were composed in Florence, at the Medici court, but it was unsuccessful. In France, the royal monopoly on porcelain production was enforced at first by the system of permits and charters, started by King Louis XIV at Rouen in 1673. However, fluctuation of the workforce throughout Europe had led to exchange of the trade secrets, thus endangering the royal income. In order to put a stop to such practices, King Louis XV legally forbade workers of the Royal Porcelain Manufactories to leave their employment without his express permission, under threat of criminal prosecution [37] (Fig. 5).

Nevertheless, Meissen is usually cited as the true "place of birth" of European porcelain. In this Saxon town, in 1708, the German alchemist Johann Friedrich

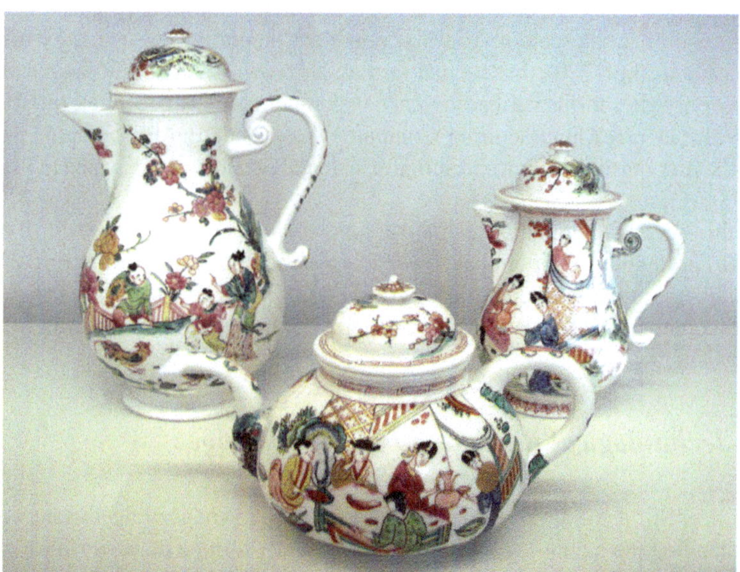

Fig. 5 Meissen teapots, ca. 1720. Musée des arts décoratifs [38]

Böttger, successfully replicated the white porcelain paste, necessary for production of so called hard-paste porcelain, while all the others at the time produced the soft-paste variant. The vessels from his workshop were promptly named "white gold" [35], and only two years later, Augustus II the Strong, Elector of Saxony, the King of Poland and the Grand Duke of Lithuania, has established, by decree, the first porcelain factory. Less than a decade after that, in 1718, a second factory was founded in Vienna, and its founder, Claudius Innocentius du Paquier, was for the next 25 years granted the imperial privilege of exclusive porcelain production [39]. Their example was promptly replicated elsewhere, and "[b]y the eighteenth century many heads of States were eager to sponsor a porcelain factory in their territory even if only as a status symbol" [40]. The porcelain plants soon were opened in Holy Roman Empire, Italy and England, and when Russia and Prussia rose in power and became important political players in Europe, the same plants were established in those countries as well. According to Reed [41], "[b]y 1785 important factories were scattered from Sweden to the Kingdom of Naples and from Russia to Portugal." While the key impetus for porcelain production (and for royal patronage as well as granting of patents and monopolies), in some instances they were directly in the function of royal prestige. For example, the factory of "Charles III of Spain at Buen Retiro, made during his lifetime only for the use of the royal family and persons it chose to honor with gift" [41]. Reed continues to recount the European rulers supporting the porcelain factories. Maria Theresa, Frederick the Great, Duke Charles I of Brunswick, Max Joseph III of Bavaria, John Frederick Charles, prince bishop of Mainz have been only the most notable. This royal support resulted in monopolies given to certain plants and adjustment of tariffs in order to maximize profits.

Interestingly, the eighteenth century saw the first, conditionally speaking, *bioceramical* use of the porcelain. The first porcelain dentures were made by a French apothecary in the 1770s, but its use in making crowns and single false teeth was possible only after further technological developments, in the late nineteenth century. S.S. White Dental Manufacturing Company was founded in Philadelphia in 1844, while the first European plant specializing in dental ceramics was opened in Germany in 1893 [36].

In this section, another facet of the long-standing close relationship between ceramics production and political power was highlighted. This relationship will once again change in the later centuries, but will not altogether disappear. The political uses of ceramics became less straightforward, but nevertheless important.

2.4 Technological Races and Political Prestige

The concept of technological race is quite recently introduced as a framework for understanding the technological change. It is usually limited to the forms of competition between companies for the position of technological leadership in a certain branch of industry—usually those deemed *high-tech*. Gottinger [42] defines the race as "an interactive pattern characterized by firms constantly trying to get ahead of their rivals, or trying not to fall too far behind." It is seen as behavior that recognizes the importance of strategic interactions between competing companies, which forces them to take into account their rivals' actions when making their own decisions [42]. Yet, these technological races have frequently been used for political purposes, taking place not only between companies, but also between countries, or even political blocs.

Politically speaking, technological races usually take the form of an *arms race*. It implies presence of at least two actors who perceive themselves to be in adversary relationship. They "are increasing or improving their armaments at a rapid rate and structuring their respective military postures with a general attention to the past, current, and anticipated military and political behavior of the other actors" [43]—thus displaying the behavior similar to companies engaged in technological race. Depending on their capacities and resources, political actors can opt not only to pursue quantitative advantage—in terms of increased numbers of troops and weapons available to them, but also qualitative one—trough research and development of technologically superior weapon systems. The most prominent arms race in the twentieth century was, of course, the one between United States of America and Soviet Union, and their respective political and military alliances. While the social and political aspects of production and use of military technology is probably the most widely researched topic within social sciences (see, for example, [44]), the inquiry into the role of the ceramics in this context is still underdeveloped. Ceramic materials, however, were and are used in military industry, especially in production of armors [45–47].

Another technological race with political significance, and predominantly political motives, was so called space race.[7] Ceramics had played a part in this endeavor as well. Ceramics composites were and are used in space propulsion, space power and space structures. They are crucial in production of combustion chambers and nozzles for liquid propellant rocket engines, thermal protection systems for space vehicles, leading edges of spacecraft, and the entire field was originally mostly driven by the demands of the space program [48] (Fig. 6).

The next potential technological race with political motives and implications is probably the race to achieve general artificial intelligence [50]. Given that, since the late nineteenth century, the technical and electrical uses of various ceramic compounds (including porcelain) were on the steady rise, being used in telegraph and railway construction [35], and that entire electronic industry, including computers and smartphones, relies heavily on various ceramic materials [51–55], inevitable conclusion is that ceramics will play its part in this technological race as well.[8]

[7] It is important to note that the term *space race* was in use almost exclusively in the USA, while the official Soviet paradigm of the time insisted on the label *space age*.

[8] On the other hand, the use of AI technologies in ceramics research has already yielded significant results [56–58].

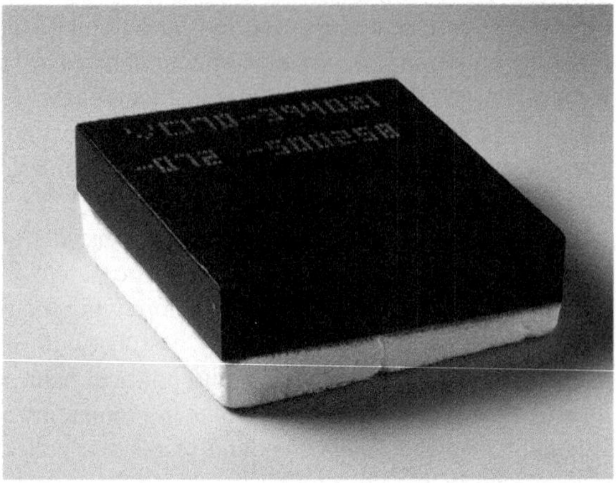

Fig. 6 Silica Space Shuttle thermal protection (TPS) tile, ca. 1980. Science Museum London [49]

3 Bioceramics and Biopolitics

Towards the end of the twentieth century, the new developments emerged in the fields of both ceramics and politics, changing their landscapes and providing opportunities for new encounter of a somewhat different kind. Significant breakthroughs in bioceramics were made in the 1970s and 1980s. At the same time, the concept of biopolitics achieved prominence in political science, opening new fields of inquiry and possible modes of explanation. In this section I will try to briefly highlight these new developments, and propose a way in which one version of biopolitics paradigm can be used in further research of political aspects of bioceramics.

3.1 Brief History of Bioceramics

In the early medical treatises of ancient Egypt and Greece, as well as Hindu civilizations, there are references to attempts of use of various implant materials, usually grafts, for healing purposes [59]. There is a body of literature, it should be noted, about ancient dental implants, although some of the presented evidence is highly disputed [60, 61].

As we have seen, the first use of porcelain in the production of dentures, inlays, and crowns dates back to nineteenth century [36]. About the same time, there are first attempts to use ceramic materials for healing various bone defects. The first published report about the use of Plaster of Paris for filling the defects in the bone dates around the same time—authored by Dreesman in 1892 [59]. Since that time, ever wider variety of materials was tested for use in the human body, marking the beginnings of bioceramics. Bioceramics is usually used to denote "ceramic materials designed to achieve a specific physiological behavior for use as a material of construction of prosthetic devices or artificial internal organs," [59] or, more briefly, "material within the class of medical implant" [62]. Bioceramical materials are ideal for this purpose, since they are "composed of ions commonly found in the physiological environment (calcium, potassium, magnesium, sodium etc.) and of ions showing limited toxicity to body tissue (aluminum and titanium)" [59]. Those materials are usually classified according to their reactive properties when interfaced with human tissues. Two main types are usually distinguished: *bioinert* and *bioactive* materials, while the bioactive ceramics can be resorbable or non-resorbable, the later sometimes referred to as surface-reactive.

The main clinical uses of bioceramics are in cranial repair, maxillofacial reconstruction, dental implants, alveolar ridge augmentation, periodontal pocket obliteration, percutaneous access devices, artificial heart valves, spinal surgery, iliac crest repair, bone space fillers, orthopedic load-bearing applications, orthopedic fixation devices, artificial tendons and ligaments [4]. There are also promising results of its use in cancer treatments [5, 63].

The last several decades have witnessed the accelerated developments in bioceramics, promising even more advanced and varied treatments and clinical applications.

3.2 *What is Biopolitics?*

The term biopolitics was coined at the beginning of twentieth century, to denote, primarily, an organicist concept of the state as a form of life [65]. It seemed to attract little attention until the publication of Michel Foucault's essay *Right of Death and Power over Life*, in 1976, and, perhaps even more, Giorgio Agamben's interpretation of this essay in his 1998 book *Homo Sacer: Sovereign Power and Bare Life*. This has produced "what might be called a 'biopolitical turn': a proliferation of studies, claiming Foucault as an inspiration, on the relations between 'life' and 'politics.'" [66]

The theoretical provenance and the meaning of biopolitics are still in a sort of flux—encompassing a number of theoretical perspectives, themes and definitions. Etymological definition is, not unusual occurrence in political science, only of limited use. While biopolitics, obviously, has something to do with the encounter of *life* and *politics*, the meanings of those very terms are highly contested [64–68].

Lemke [65] distinguishes two major conceptualizations of biopolitics, as shown on Fig. 7.

While the naturalist concept was present at least since the beginning of the twentieth century, and relies heavily on the nineteenth century "philosophy of life" [64, 69], the politicist concepts started to gain traction since the 1960s and 1970s. The ecological strand was fueled by the grim forecasts of the Club of Rome's report, predicting the breakdown of both natural and social environment, the technical concepts got their impetus from the rapid development of (primarily reproductive) medicine and other life sciences during these decades. These developments resulted in prenatal diagnoses of fetuses, in-vitro fertilization, as well as inter-species DNA

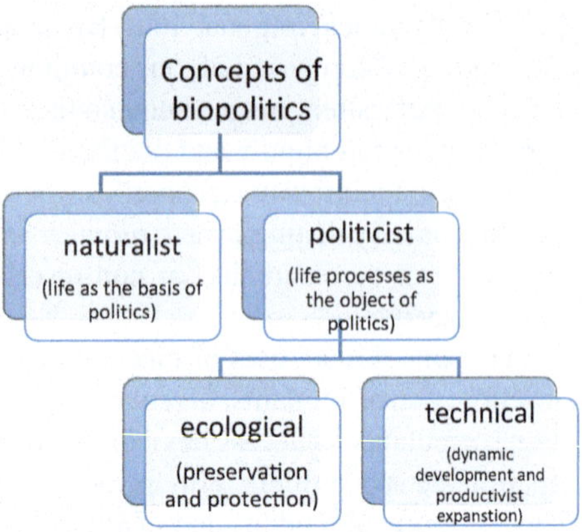

Fig. 7 Concepts of biopolitics according to Lemke [65]

transfer. Such innovations have raised new concerns about scientific and technological development, and prompted the need for new areas of collective decision making and new policies—now seen as the central field of biopolitics. Finally, this interpretation of biopolitics is the most pertinent for the possible study of bioceramics, since it implies "broadening of the political field—a field that encompasses sets of problems that were once understood as natural and self-evident facts but that are now open to technological or scientific intervention" [56]. Technologies brought about by life scientists inevitably produce serious challenges for public policy. As Somit [69] notes, "few of those issues [...] are purely scientific; few, purely political." There is, thus, a place for biopolitics as a connector between the two, providing for more comprehensive approach.

3.3 Bioceramical Cyborgs?

Within this strand of interpretation of biopolitics, one of the more influential frameworks was the one started by Donna Haraway [70] in her Manifesto for cyborgs, originally published in 1985. She posits a cyborg as a "hybrid of machine and organism, a creature of social reality as well as a creature of fiction." Originally standing as shorthand for *cybernetic organism*, the term was coined in 1964 [71], and cyborgs quickly became one of the staple features of modern science fiction. In Haraway's argument, they stand for beings who transgress the established borders and imposed dualities—dualities already challenged in the modern world, by the progress of science and technology. Borders between life and the machine, man and animal, etc. are increasingly blurred, making us "all chimeras, theorized and fabricated hybrids of machine and organism." Although that is not her main concern, she concedes that "machines can be prosthetic devices, intimate components, friendly selves."

Haraway's notion of cyborgs may be highly symbolic, a tool for understanding a modern condition of women (and men) in the contemporary, highly technological societies. It can, however, be taken much more literally—how many of us are, strictly speaking, unaltered human beings? Ever since the beginning of modern era, humans not only employ technologies as their "extensions" in the sense that McLuhan [72] famously claimed,[9] but integrate them *on*, or *in* their bodies. Eyeglasses; tooth fillings, implants, and dentures; contact lenses; pace-makers; artificial body parts and organs—they are more or less common feature of a modern human being. Even this very incomplete list of technologies incorporated into our bodies makes the presence of bioceramical materials obvious.

What are the consequences—psychological, social, and, most important for the argument of this paper, political consequences of such alterations? In the specific case of bioceramics, its very characteristics may make these issues less obvious. Because of its similarity, in composition, but sometimes also appearance, to human tissues—the very features that make its medical uses possible and desirable, as well as the fact that it is frequently hidden *inside* our bodies, it draws less attention than some other inorganic or technological enhancements. Another reason why bioceramics evades closer scrutiny from this point of view lays, probably, in the fact that it was not hitherto used in the most controversial fields of biotechnology and medicine—such as reproductive or neuro medicine. Not only that such uses are currently absent, but are also, at the time, hard to extrapolate.

Nevertheless, questions about self-identification, self-interest and so forth can, and probably will be asked. At which point does one cease to be fully human? How many bones, joints and teeth can we replace? This is the Plutarch's conundrum about the ship of Theseus[10] all over again, but with much graver potential consequences. Feminist political theory has demonstrated that bodies are political constructs, objects and subjects of politics. Haraway's concept of cyborg is going one step further, but can be useful as a point of view when discussing different types of relationships of human bodies with technologies, including bioceramics.

Illustrative as it may be, the utilization of biopolitical or cyborg framework to study bioceramics is only one possible, and not necessarily the most comprehensive, way of scrutinizing their relationship. In the next chapter, I shall try to put the research and application of bioceramics in wider political context, pointing out some issues of concern.

---

[9] McLuhan puts media in the title of his book, but it is clear that he uses the term not in everyday sense but as a synonym for technology.

[10] The famous question is, if every piece of the ship was replaced at one time or another, is it still the same ship?

4 Technological Versus Political Considerations: Equality and Distribution of the Future

What would be possible political aspects and considerations of the bioceramics research and applications? For one, probably the most obvious instance concerns research ethics. Ethical standards for research and, especially, testing, have evolved, and it is dubious that experimentation on sheep or mongrel dogs, described by Hulbert et al. [59] is defensible in the twenty-first century. It is the issue not related exclusively to bioceramics, of course, but it does illustrate how social—and political—values shape scientific research and technological development. With the shift of social values regarding animals, new policies and ethical research guidelines were developed to comply with them.

There are, however, at least two other questions that should be discussed—social and political drives behind the bioceramics research and access to its clinical applications.

4.1 Bioceramics and Its Applications: Why and for Whom?

As we have seen in the section describing the development of porcelain production in Europe, political power and political interests are sometimes the main driving forces behind the technological developments. At least since 1950s, the nation-states were an important actor and driver of technological change. Not only were most inventions in this period result of teamwork on state-sponsored projects, but state appears in at least three different roles in the process of technological production—as customer, as regulator and as underwriter [73]. In all these roles, it significantly influences and sometimes directs the development of specific technologies.

How can this be applied to bioceramics? This question can be broken down along the lines of Street's classification. Firstly, the state can be in the role of customer—through public health system, state owned hospitals, public health insurance. The state as a customer has much greater negotiating power than the other, corporate or private customers. It can, therefore, coerce lower prices for bioceramical materials and products used in healthcare. As regulator, the state not only proscribes patent law, key component of legislation concerning technology, but also clinical testing procedures and safety standards. Finally, as underwriter, state can support research or production by awarding grants or financial incentives.

The state priorities can be, and are, determined by the number of factors, extremely dependable on the wider context. Historically, research and clinical applications of bioceramics had very different social as well as political goals and motives. This is evident from the review of literature on the history of bioceramics. Given that main areas of clinical application of bioceramics have been dental implants and joint or bone reconstruction, the profile of patients, and the causes of their condition, changed dramatically.

In nineteenth and twentieth centuries, the main concern were injuries, frequently result of the warfare. The very invention and subsequent development of Bioglass® in 1967 was prompted by "the terrible cost of wounds sustained during the Vietnam War in terms of amputations" [62]. While injuries are still one of the main causes of conditions that can benefit from use of bioceramics in treatments, another, and increasingly important cause are "degenerative diseases which are often associated with ageing" [60]. For example, it is estimated that the 100,000–300,000 dental implants are placed per year, and the number of placed hip and knee joints is similar [74]—and the need for both procedures is closely related to increasingly ageing population.

While tooth decay was a condition known even in prehistoric times, its incidence increased dramatically with changes in diet, especially those which increased intake of fermentable carbohydrates. The highest increase rates coincided with the more widespread use of sugar cane and processed sugar. While preventive measures, primarily promotion of oral hygiene, have yielded remarkable results, the incidence of cavities is modern world is still higher than it was in antiquity [75]. While injuries were once the main cause of tooth loss, today its mostly result of tooth decay, gum disease, or a failed root canal. Statistics for the United States show that by age 74, 26% of adults have lost all of their permanent teeth [74].

Given that the population of the technologically advanced and rich countries in the global North is getting older—over 15% of the United States [76] and over 20% of the European [77] population is 65 or older—the need for treatments for age-related conditions, including implants and other bioceramic products will only increase. So will the burden for national health budgets, which will probably lead to pressure to decrease cost of both materials and procedures.

The point is, technological development does not occur in vacuum, independently of social needs and corresponding policy decisions. In the case of bioceramics, this means that development of new materials and products needs to take into account not only technical and medical characteristics, but also price and other socially determined factors. Of course, this is nothing new, although it does bear further attention: for example in 1991 Hench [5] noted that the situation in which the lifetime of bioceramical devices is shorter than the life of a patient is untenable—not only because of trauma of another surgery, but also because the expense to the health-care system.

4.2 *Price, Efficiency, Accessibility: Unequal Distribution of Future*

The aging population, however, is the problem generally limited to the global North. Even there, the accessibility of healthcare is sometimes unsatisfactory. In United States, a little over 9% of the population has no health insurance [76], while in the European Union 1.5% of population claims that their needs for health care were unmet due to high prices, geographic distance or waiting lists [77]. These inequalities are further exaggerated when it comes to dental care—it being with increasing frequency removed from the primary health care covered by insurance in a number of countries.

Disparities in availability of medical treatments are even greater when the global divide is taken into account. The problems are not limited to potentially prohibitive prices of the bioceramic materials, but also include the availability of trainings for medical professionals.

These issues stem from the wider problem—the global rise of inequality in wealth, both between and within the countries. World Inequality Report [78] shows that income inequality has increased worldwide during the past decades, with government growing poorer even as countries grow richer. However, the authors stress the importance of policy measures which they credit for the uneven tempo of this change.

The bioceramics has promised, and delivered, enviable results in healing, and, consequently, improvement of human condition, and even more remarkable achievements are yet to come. However, they may not be available to those who are in the greatest need for them. As the futurist William Gibson famously stated, "the future is already here, it's just not evenly distributed". It is the job of politics to make this distribution more equal.

5 Conclusions

Politics and bioceramics do seem, at the first glance, like completely separate fields, with little in common. They do, however, intersect, albeit not always directly. This is a continuation of the long history of encounters between ceramics and politics, dating back to the dawn of the humankind. Innovations in ceramics were driven by changing political conditions, and in turn shaped polities and policies. While one possibility for socio-political study of bioceramics is from the biopolitical paradigm, it can also be situated into the wider discussion about societal values and needs, and political means for fulfilling them.

Further research in this area could focus on particular technologies and applications of bioceramics, especially social factors in their construction, not forgetting that recent research in ceramics and fractals can help in dealing with other crises facing the modern world—such as energy and health crises [79–81]. But even more important, exploration of issues of availability and accessibility in wider social context should be a priority, if the bioceramics is to fully realize its potential for improving the human condition.

References

1. Hughes, T.: Networks of Power. Johns Hopkins University Press, Baltimore (1983)
2. Bijker, W., Law, J. (eds.): Shaping Technology/Building Society. MIT Press, Cambridge MA (1994)

3. Lemonnier, P. (ed.): Technological Choices: Transformation in Material Cultures since the Neolithic. Routledge, New York (2013)
4. Hench, L.L.: An Introduction to Bioceramics. World Scientific, Singapore (1999)
5. Hench, L.L.: Bioceramics: from concept to clinic. J. Am. Ceram. Soc. **74**(7), 1487–1510 (1991)
6. Mumford, L.: The Myth of the Machine 1: Technics and Human Development. Harcourt Brace Jovanovic, New York (1966)
7. Simmons, A.H.: The Neolithic Revolution in the Near East: Transforming the Human Landscape. University of Arizona Press, Tucson (2010)
8. Bar-Yosef, O.: On the nature of transitions: the middle to upper Palaeolithic and the Neolithic revolution. Camb. Archaeol. J. **8**(2), 141–163 (1998)
9. Novák, P.: Wikipedia, Wikimedia Commons. https://commons.wikimedia.org/wiki/File:Vestonicka_venuse_edit.jpg. Accessed 12 Mar 2021
10. van der Leeuw, S.: Giving potter a choice: conceptual aspects of pottery techniques. In: Lemonnier, P. (ed.) Technological Choices: Transformation in Material Cultures Since the Neolithic, pp. 238–288. Routledge, New York (2013)
11. Cohen, D.J., Bar-Yosef, O., Wu, X., Patania, I., Goldberg, P.: The emergence of pottery in China: recent dating of two early pottery cave sites in South China. Quatern. Int. **441**, 36–48 (2017)
12. Vandiver, P.B., Soffer, O., Klima, B., Svoboda, J.: The origins of ceramic technology at Dolni Věstonice Czechoslovakia. Science **246**(4933), 1002–1008 (1989)
13. Wikimedia Commons. https://commons.wikimedia.org/wiki/File:National_Museum_of_China_2014.02.01_14-43-38.jpg. Accessed 12 Mar 2021
14. Todd, G.L.: Wikimedia Commons. https://fr.wikipedia.org/wiki/Fichier:The_Pot_of_Yuchanyan._Hunan_Museum.jpg. Accessed 12 Mar 2021
15. Foster, G.M.: The potter's wheel: an analysis of idea and artifact in invention. Southwest. J. Anthropol. **15**(2), 99–119 (1959)
16. Choleva, M.: Travelling with the potter's wheel in the early bronze age Aegean. Ann. Brit. Sch. Athens **115**, 59–104 (2020)
17. Levi-Strauss, C.: The Savage Mind. University of Chicago, Chicago (1966)
18. Stanković, M.N., Krstić, N.S., Đorđević, D.M., Anastasijević, N., Mitić, V.V., Topličić-Ćurčić, G.A., Momčilović-Petronijević, A.J.: Chemical analysis of mortars of archaeological samples from Mediana locality Serbia. Sci. Sinter. **51**(2), 233–242 (2019)
19. Fores, M.: Science and the 'Neolithic Paradox.' Hist. Sci. **21**(2), 141–163 (1983)
20. Duara, P.: The discourse of civilization and decolonization. J. World Hist. **15**(1), 1–5 (2004)
21. Targowski, A.: Towards a composite definition and classification of civilization. Comp. Civilizations Rev. **60**(60), 79–98 (2009)
22. McGaughe, W.: Five Epochs of Civilization: World History as Emerging in Five Civilization. Thistlerose Publications, Minneapolis (2000)
23. Bosworth, A.: The genetics of civilization: an empirical classification of civilizations based on writing systems. Comp. Civilizations Rev. **49**(49), 9–27 (2003)
24. Coulmas, F.: Writing Systems: An Introduction to Their Linguistic Analysis. Cambridge University Press, Cambridge (2003)
25. Houston, S.D.: Overture to the first writing. In: Houston, S.D. (ed.) The First Writing: Script Invention as History and Process, pp. 3–15. Cambridge University Press, Cambridge (2004)
26. Diamond, J.: Germs, Guns, Germs and Steel: A Short History of Everybody for the Last 13,000 Years. Vintage, New York (1998)
27. Levi-Strauss, C.: Tristes Tropiques. Criterion Books, New York (1961)
28. University of Texas. https://sites.utexas.edu/dsb/tokens/tokens/. Accessed 21 Mar 2021
29. Shendge, M.J.: The use of seals and the invention of writing. J. Econ. Soc. Hist. Orient **26**(2), 113–136 (1983)
30. Lieberman, S.J.: Of clay pebbles, hollow clay balls, and writing: a Sumerian view. Am. J. Archaeol. **83**(3), 339–358 (1980)
31. Metropolitan Museum of Art. https://www.metmuseum.org/art/collection/search/327384. Accessed 21 Mar 2021

32. The British Museum. https://www.britishmuseum.org/collection/image/121754001. Accessed 21 Mar 2021
33. Cooper, J.S.: Babylonian beginnings: the origin of the cuneiform writing system in comparative perspective. In: Houston, S.D. (ed.) The First Writing: Script Invention as History and Process, pp. 71–99. Cambridge University Press, Cambridge (2004)
34. Suetonius, G.: The Lives of the Caesars. William Heinemann LTD/Harvard University Press, London (1959)
35. Pliny, G.S.: Natural History, Vol. 10, Books XXXVI–XXXVII. William Heinemann LTD/Harvard University Press, London (1971)
36. Marchand, S.L.: Porcelain: A History from the Heart of Europe. Princeton University Press, Princeton/Oxford (2020)
37. Edwards, H.G.M.: 18th and 19th Century Porcelain Analysis: A Forensic Provenancing Assessment. Springer, Cham (2020)
38. Wikimedia Commons. https://commons.wikimedia.org/wiki/File:Meissen_hard_porcelain_teapots_circa_1720_decorated_in_the_Netherlands_circa_1735.jpg. Accessed 21 Mar 2021
39. Lyakhovich, E.V.: Chinese porcelain interpretation in Europe: history of Chinese and European porcelain cultures relationships. In: Proceedings of the 3rd International Conference on Art Studies: Science, Experience, Education, pp. 49–54. Atlantis Press, Amsterdam (2019)
40. Gabay, E.: The politics and social implications of tableware for feasting. In: Walker, H. (ed.) Oxford Symposium on Food & Cookery, 1990: Feasting and Fasting: Proceedings, pp. 99–103. Prospect Books, London (1990)
41. Reed, I.H.: The European hard-paste porcelain manufacture of the eighteenth century. J. Mod. Hist. **8**(3), 273–296 (1936)
42. Gottinger, H.-W.: Global technological races. Jpn. World Econ. **18**(2), 181–193 (2006)
43. Gray, C.S.: The arms race phenomenon. World Polit. **24**(01), 39–79 (1971)
44. Smit, W.: Science, technology, and the military: relations in transition. In: Jasanoff, S., Markle, G.E., Peterson, J.C., Pinch, T. (eds.) Handbook of Science and Technology Studies, pp. 598–626. Sage, Los Angeles (1995)
45. Prokurat Franks, L. (ed.): Advances in Ceramic Armor IV. Wiley, Hoboken (2009)
46. Gong, W.L., Lutze, W., Ewing, R.C.: Zirconia ceramics for excess weapons plutonium waste. J. Nucl. Mater. **277**(2–3), 239–249 (2000)
47. Lee, W.E., Ojovan, M.I., Stennett, M.C., Hyatt, N.C.: Immobilisation of radioactive waste in glasses, glass composite materials and ceramics. Adv. Appl. Ceram. **105**(1), 3–12 (2006)
48. Bansal, N.P.: Handbook of Ceramic Composites. Kluwer Academic Publishers, Boston (2005)
49. Wikimedia Commons. https://commons.wikimedia.org/wiki/File:Silica_Space_Shuttle_thermal_protection_(TPS)_tile,_c_1980._(9663807484).jpg. Accessed 21 Mar 2021
50. Taddeo, M., Floridi, L.: Regulate artificial intelligence to avert cyber arms race. Nature **556**(7701), 296–298 (2018)
51. Swartz, S.L.: Topics in electronic ceramics. IEEE Trans. Electr. Insul. **25**(5), 935–987 (1990)
52. Mitic, V.V., Lazovic, G., Paunovic, V., Cvetkovic, N., Jovanovic, D., Veljkovic, S., Randjelovic, B., Vlahovic, B.: Fractal frontiers in microelectronic ceramic materials. Ceram. Int. **45**(7), 9679–9685 (2019)
53. Mitic, V.V., Paunovic, V., Jankovic, S., Pavlovic, V., Antolovic, I., Rancic, D.: Electronic ceramic structure within the Voronoi cells model and microstructure fractals contacts surfaces: new frontier applications. Sci. Sinter. **45**(2), 223–232 (2013)
54. Mitić, V.V., Paunović, V., Kocić, L.: Higher electronics circuit integrations within the fractal electronics frontiers. J. Ceram. Sci. Tech. **07**(04), 365–378 (2016)
55. Mitić, V.V., Lazović, G., Paunović, V., Veljković, S., Randjelović, B., Vlahović, B., Fecht, H.: Electronic ceramics fractal microstructure analysis—Minkowski Hull and grain boundaries. Ferroelectrics **545**(1), 184–194 (2019)
56. Mitic, V.V., Lazovic, G., Ribar, C., Chun-An, L., Radovic, I., Stajcic, A., Fecht, H., Vlahovic, B.: The artificial neural networks applied for microelectronics intergranular relations determination. Integr. Ferroelectr. **212**(1), 135–146 (2020)

57. Terzić, A., Pezo, L.L., Andrić, L.D., Pavlović, V.B., Mitić, V.V.: Optimization of bentonite clay mechano-chemical activation using artificial neural network modeling. Ceram. Int. **43**(2), 2549–2562 (2017)
58. Mitic, V.V., Ribar, S., Randjelovic, B., Lu, C.A., Radovic, I., Stajcic, A., Novakovic, I., Vlahovic, B.: Neural networks and microelectronics parameters distribution measurements depending on sintering temperature and applied voltage. Mod. Phys. Lett. B **34**(35), 2150172 (2020)
59. Hulbert, S.F., Hench, L.L., Forbers, D., Bowman, L.S.: History of bioceramics. Ceram. Int. **8**(4), 131–140 (1982)
60. Becker, M.J.: Ancient "dental implants": a recently proposed example from France evaluated with other spurious examples. Int. J. Oral Maxillofac. Implants **14**(1), 19–29 (1999)
61. Becker, M.J.: Spurious" Examples" of ancient dental implants or appliances: part two of a series. Dent. Anthropol. J. **9**(1), 5–10 (1994)
62. Best, S.M., Porter, A.E., Thian, E.S., Huang, J.: Bioceramics: past, present and for the future. J. Eur. Ceram. Soc. **28**, 1319–1327 (2008)
63. Vallet-Regí, M., Ruiz-Hernández, E.: Bioceramics: from bone regeneration to cancer nanomedicine. Adv. Mater. **23**(44), 5177–5218 (2011)
64. Ribar, S., Mitic, V.V., Lazovic, G.: Neural networks application on human skin biophysical impedance characterizations. Biophys. Rev. Lett., 1–11 (2021)
65. Lemke, T.: Biopolitics: An Advanced Introduction. New York University Press, New York/London (2011)
66. Campbell, T., Sitze, A.: Biopolitics: an encounter. In: Campbell, T., Sitze, A. (eds.) Biopolitics: A Reader, pp. 1–41. Duke University Press, Durham/London (2013)
67. Sartori, G.: What is "politics." Polit. Theory **1**(1), 5–26 (1973)
68. Heywood, A.: What is politics? Polit. Rev. **11**(2), 2–4 (2001)
69. Somit, A.: Biopolitics. Brit. J. Polit. Sci. **2**(2), 209–238 (1972)
70. Haraway, D.: Simians, Cyborgs, and Women: The Reinvention of Nature. Routledge, New York (1991)
71. Tomas, D.: Feedback and cybernetics: reimaging the body in the age of the cyborg. Body Soc. **1**(3–4), 21–43 (1995)
72. McLuhan, M.: Understanding Media: The Extensions of Man. MIT Press, Cambridge MA (1994)
73. Street, J.: Politics & Technology. The Guilford Press, New York (1992)
74. Gaviria, L., Salcido, J.P., Guda, T., Ong, J.L.: Current trends in dental implants. J. Korean Assoc. Oral Maxillofac. Surggeons **40**(2), 50–60 (2014)
75. Ettinger, R.L.: Epidemiology of dental caries: a broad review. Dent. Clin. North Am. **43**(4), 679–694 (1999)
76. United States Census Bureau. https://www.census.gov/data.html. Last accessed 28 Jan 2021
77. Eurostat. https://ec.europa.eu/eurostat/. Last accessed 28 Jan 2021
78. Alvaredo, F., Chancel, L., Piketty, T., Saez, E., Zucman, G. (eds.): World Inequality Report 2018. Belknap Press, Cambridge, MA/London (2018)
79. Mitić, V., Lazović, G., Paunović, V., Hwu, J.R., Tsay, S.C., Perng, T.P., Veljković, S., Vlahović, B.: Ceramic materials and energy—extended coble's model and fractal nature. J. Eur. Ceram. Soc. **39**, 3513–3525 (2019)
80. Mitić, V.V., Lazović, G., Manojlović, J.Ž, Huang, W.C., Stojiljković, M.M., Facht, H., Vlahović, B.: Entropy and fractal nature. Therm. Sci. **24**(3), 2203–2212 (2020)
81. Mitić, V.V., Lazović, G.M., Đorđević, D.M., Stanković, M.N., Paunović, V.V., Krstić, N.S., Manojlović, J.Ž: Butler-Volmer current equation and fractal nature correction in electrochemical energy. Therm. Sci. **25**(00), 232–232 (2020)

The manufacturer's authorised representative in the EU is Springer Nature Customer Service Centre GmbH, Europaplatz 3, 69115 Heidelberg, Germany. If you have any concerns regarding our products, please contact ProductSafety@springernature.com

Printed and bound by CPI Group (UK) Ltd, Croydon, CR0 4YY
28/09/2026
02224077-0013